WORKBOOK IN
# PRACTICAL
# NEONATOLOGY

# WORKBOOK IN
# PRACTICAL
# NEONATOLOGY

## SECOND EDITION

### Richard A. Polin, M.D.

Professor of Pediatrics, University of Pennsylvania School of
Medicine; Division of Neonatology, The Children's Hospital
of Philadelphia, Philadelphia, Pennsylvania

### Mervin C. Yoder, M.D.

Associate Professor of Pediatrics and of Biochemistry and
Molecular Biology, Indiana University School of Medicine;
Attending Neonatologist, James Whitcomb Riley Hospital for
Children, Indianapolis, Indiana

### Fredric D. Burg, M.D.

Vice Dean of Education, University of Pennsylvania School
of Medicine; Professor of Pediatrics, The Children's Hospital
of Philadelphia, Philadelphia, Pennsylvania

**W.B. Saunders Company**

*A Division of Harcourt Brace & Company*

Philadelphia  London  Toronto  Montreal  Sydney  Tokyo

**W.B. SAUNDERS COMPANY**

*A Division of*
*Harcourt Brace & Company*

The Curtis Center
Independence Square West
Philadelphia, PA 19106

**Library of Congress Cataloging-in-Publication Data**

Workbook in practical neonatology / [edited by] Richard A. Polin,
   Mervin C. Yoder, Fredric D. Burg.—2nd ed.
     p.  cm.
   Includes bibliographical references and index.
   ISBN 0–7216–4292–6
   1. Neonatology. I. Polin, Richard A. (Richard Alan).
  II. Yoder, Mervin C. III. Burg, Fredric D. (Fredric David)
   [DNLM:  1. Infant, Newborn, Diseases—programmed instruction. WS
18 W926 1993]
  RJ254.W66  1993
  618.92'01—dc20
  DNLM/DLC                                     92–48453

Workbook in Practical Neonatology           ISBN  0–7216–4292–6

Last digit is the print number:    9    8    7    6    5    4    3    2    1

*To our wives and children:*
*Helene, Allison, Mitchell, Jessica, and Gregory Polin*
*Deborah, Drew, and Caitlin Yoder*
*Barbara, Ben, Beth, David, Kate, Paul James, and Jennifer Burg*

# CONTRIBUTORS

WALTER C. ALLAN, M.D.
Clinical Associate Professor; Chief, Division of Pediatric Neurology, Maine Medical Center, Portland, Maine

STEPHEN BAUMGART, M.D.
Professor of Pediatrics, Thomas Jefferson University, Jefferson Medical College; Senior Staff Physician, Thomas Jefferson University Hospital, Philadelphia, Pennsylvania

JOANN BERGOFFEN, M.D.
Fellow, Human Genetics and Molecular Biology, The Children's Hospital of Philadelphia, Philadelphia, Pennsylvania

RONALD S. BLOOM, M.D.
Associate Professor, Department of Pediatrics, University of Utah School of Medicine; University Hospital, Primary Children's Medical Center, LDS Hospital, Salt Lake City, Utah

FREDRIC D. BURG, M.D.
Vice Dean of Education, University of Pennsylvania School of Medicine; Professor of Pediatrics, The Children's Hospital of Philadelphia, Philadelphia, Pennsylvania

ROBERT RYAN CLANCY, M.D.
Associate Professor of Neurology and Pediatrics, The University of Pennsylvania School of Medicine; Senior Neurologist, The Children's Hospital of Philadelphia, Philadelphia, Pennsylvania

ANDREW T. COSTARINO, Jr., M.D.
Assistant Professor of Anesthesiology and Pediatrics, The Children's Hospital of Philadelphia and The University of Pennsylvania, Philadelphia, Pennsylvania

CATHERINE CROPLEY, R.N., M.N.
Assistant Clinical Professor, School of Nursing, University of California, Los Angeles, California

SCOTT C. DENNE, M.D.
Associate Professor of Pediatrics, Indiana University School of Medicine; Department of Pediatrics, James Whitcomb Riley Hospital for Children, Indianapolis, Indiana

PHYLLIS A. DENNERY, M.D.
Assistant Professor of Pediatrics, Stanford University School of Medicine; Department of Pediatrics, Stanford University Medical Center, Stanford, California

DOUGLAS A. DRANSFIELD, M.D.
Clinical Assistant Professor, Department of Pediatrics, University of Vermont College of Medicine; Director, Division of Neonatology, Maine Medical Center, Portland, Maine

WILLIAM A. ENGLE, M.D.
Associate Professor of Pediatrics, Indiana University School of Medicine; James Whitcomb Riley Hospital for Children, Indianapolis, Indiana

JEFFREY S. GERDES, M.D.
Associate Professor of Pediatrics, University of Pennsylvania School of Medicine; Associate Pediatrician, Pennsylvania Hospital; Associate Physician, The Children's Hospital of Philadelphia, Philadelphia, Pennsylvania

MICHAEL H. GEWITZ, M.D.
Professor and Vice Chairman, Department of Pediatrics, Director, Pediatric Cardiology, New York Medical College; Director, Pediatrics and Pediatric Cardiology, Westchester Medical Center, Valhalla, New York

MARY CATHERINE HARRIS, M.D.
Associate Professor of Pediatrics, The University of Pennsylvania School of Medicine; Attending Neonatologist, The Children's Hospital of Philadelphia, Philadelphia, Pennsylvania

DAVID E. HERTZ, M.D.
Fellow in Neonatology, Indiana University School of Medicine, Indianapolis, Indiana

ROBERT M. KLIEGMAN, M.D.
Professor, Pediatrics, Case Western Reserve University School of Medicine; Associate Director and Vice Chairman, Rainbow Babies and Children's Hospital, Cleveland, Ohio

PATRICIA NEAL, M.D.
Clinical Assistant Professor, University of North Carolina, Chapel Hill; Neonatologist, Carolinas Medical Center, Charlotte, North Carolina

GEORGE J. PECKHAM, M.D.
Professor of Pediatrics, University of Pennsylvania School of Medicine; Senior Physician and Neonatologist, The Children's Hospital of Philadelphia, Philadelphia, Pennsylvania

GILBERTO R. PEREIRA, M.D.
Associate Professor of Pediatrics, University of Pennsylvania School of Medicine; Neonatologist, The Children's Hospital of Philadelphia, Philadelphia, Pennsylvania

RICHARD A. POLIN, M.D.
Professor of Pediatrics, University of Pennsylvania School of Medicine; Division of Neonatology, The Children's Hospital of Philadelphia, Philadelphia, Pennsylvania

FREDERICK J. RESCORLA, M.D.
Assistant Professor of Surgery, Section of Pediatric Surgery, Indiana University School of Medicine; J. W. Riley Hospital for Children; Wishard Memorial Hospital, Indianapolis, Indiana

JOSEPH R. SHERBOTIE, M.D.
Assistant Professor of Pediatrics, University of Pennsylvania School of Medicine; Attending Nephrologist, The Children's Hospital of Philadelphia, Philadelphia, Pennsylvania

ALAN R. SPITZER, M.D.
Professor of Pediatrics, Jefferson Medical College, Thomas Jefferson University; Director, Division of Neonatology, Director of Nurseries, Thomas Jefferson University Hospital, Philadelphia, Pennsylvania

JOHN STEFANO, M.D.
Assistant Professor, Jefferson Medical College, Philadelphia, Pennsylvania; Attending Neonatologist, Medical Center of Delaware, A.I. du Pont Institute, Newark, Delaware

DAVID K. STEVENSON, M.D.
Harold K. Faber Professor of Pediatrics, Stanford University School of Medicine; Chief, Division of Neonatal and Developmental Medicine; Director of Nurseries, Lucile Salter Packard Children's Hospital at Stanford, Stanford, California

JAMES A. STOCKMAN III, M.D.
President, American Board of Pediatrics, Chapel Hill, North Carolina; Clinical Professor of Pediatrics, University of North Carolina School of Medicine, Chapel Hill, North Carolina; Consultant Professor, Duke University School of Medicine, Durham, North Carolina

MERVIN C. YODER, M.D.
Associate Professor of Pediatrics and of Biochemistry and Molecular Biology, Indiana University School of Medicine; Attending Neonatologist, James Whitcomb Riley Hospital for Children, Indianapolis, Indiana

ELAINE H. ZACKAI, M.D.
Professor of Pediatrics, University of Pennsylvania; The Children's Hospital of Philadelphia, Philadelphia, Pennsylvania

# PREFACE

In the ten years since our workbook was first published, the practice of caring for critically ill infants has undergone a dramatic transformation. Natural and artificial surfactants are now routinely administered as treatment for respiratory distress syndrome in infants born prematurely. This single new therapy has lowered patient mortality and reduced many of the short- and long-term complications previously associated with this disorder. In a similar manner, the use of extracorporeal membrane oxygenation (ECMO) has significantly improved the outlook for term infants with respiratory failure. Further refinements in this technology may soon allow its application to selected preterm infants. Noninvasive pulse oximetry, Doppler echocardiography, and refinements in diagnostic ultrasound devices have altered the way that infants are monitored and have extended diagnostic capabilities into the prenatal period. In almost every other aspect of neonatal care, from gastroenterology and nutrition (where parenteral alimentation solutions *designed* for preterm infants are routinely used) to infectious disease (an area experiencing a rebirth in immunotherapeutic approaches to augment host defenses), the day to day practice of neonatology has significantly changed for the better.

Readers of this book will notice considerable differences from our first edition of the *Workbook in Practical Neonatology*. In the second edition, we have expanded our focus of common problems to include chapters dealing with pulmonary hypertension, anemia, renal failure, breathing disorders, intraventricular hemorrhage, the malformed infant, bronchopulmonary dysplasia, mineral metabolism, and surgical emergencies. Similarities to the first edition remain, however, as we have tried to make sure the book is still entertaining by preserving the interactive nature of the chapters. Patient case histories that ask the reader to make diagnostic or therapeutic decisions are presented in every chapter. We have also attempted to have the reader explain various scientific concepts as the concepts apply to each clinical problem. In addition to the nine new chapters, the ten original chapters have been extensively revised and updated. Furthermore, we have tried to make sure that each diagnostic or therapeutic recommendation represents "state of the art care" and is clearly grounded in a rationale provided by the authors.

As with any new book, there are several individuals to whom we owe our thanks. These include the outstanding group of contributors who have provided us with well written and informative chapters, Judith Fletcher and the staff at W. B. Saunders Company, and Carol Miller and Ellen Ramsay for their editorial and technical assistance. We are also indebted to the many medical students and housestaff who encouraged us to do a second edition.

R.A.P.
M.C.Y.
F.D.B.

# CONTENTS

# Chapter 1

# PRINCIPLES

# OF NEONATAL

# RESUSCITATION

*Ronald S. Bloom,* M.D.

*Catherine Cropley,* R.N., M.N.

*George J. Peckham,* M.D.

No age group is more susceptible to asphyxia or is as frequently in need of resuscitation than the neonate. The manner in which an asphyxiated infant is managed can have consequences that span an entire lifetime and that directly affect the quality of the infant's life. Facilities and individuals engaged in the care of newborn infants must recognize and meet the responsibility of being able to perform neonatal resuscitation using appropriate techniques in a timely manner. Regardless of the type or size of facility involved in the delivery and care of infants, each infant has the right to resuscitation that is performed at a high level of competency.

Effective resuscitation requires more than the availability of equipment and established protocols. It requires staff who have mastered resuscitation skills, are readily available, and are capable of working as a team. Each staff member should be aware of his or her role in neonatal resuscitation and must develop the specific skills related to that role. Furthermore, these individuals should be able to perform their resuscitation skills correctly and know when to use them. Each member must also be fully aware of the role of the other health professionals because resuscitation requires a team effort.

The individual techniques discussed, such as positive pressure ventilation (PPV) or cardiac massage, cannot be completely taught here, because the ability to execute them correctly requires not only knowledge, but also the acquisition of a great deal of skill. Just as you would not approach a freeway after reading a book on "how to drive a car," you would not be prepared to resuscitate infants merely by reading about how and when the procedures should be performed. Individual and team competency need to be developed through simulated situations and supervised application in a delivery room. Furthermore, these skills must be maintained with frequent practice. If the clinical load is not sufficient to maintain them, mock resuscitations should be practiced at regular intervals.

This chapter outlines an approach to resuscitation, emphasizing the major components of a neonatal resuscitation (Table 1-1). Although not all elements will be used in every resuscitation, you must be familiar with the entire resuscitative process.

The resuscitation of an infant, when per-

**Table 1-1** Elements of a Resuscitation

---

**Initial steps**
Thermal management
Clearing the airway
Tactile stimulation

**Establishment of ventilation**

**Chest compression**

**Medication**

---

formed effectively, consists of a highly disciplined series of well-ordered steps in response to the respiratory effort, heart rate, and skin color. Which steps are taken, however, depends on the responses of the infant. The resuscitation process involves evaluation, a decision based on the evaluation, and an action taken based on the decision. The process continues with another evaluation of the infant (Fig. 1-1).

## ANTICIPATION

There will always be some infants who unexpectedly require resuscitation at birth. In the majority of infants, however, the need for resuscitation can be anticipated if the prenatal and intrapartum histories are evaluated closely. We begin our discussion of resuscitation with a case study that emphasizes the need to anticipate the problem.

### CASE STUDY 1

Mrs. K is a 30-year-old gravida 2, para 1 woman, at 39 weeks' gestation. She was noted to be hypertensive during her previous pregnancy. Between pregnancies she was found to have essential hypertension for which she was treated with diuretics. During this pregnancy

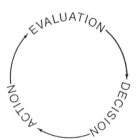

**Figure 1-1** Evaluation/decision/action cycle.

she has been maintained on diuretics but has developed a diastolic blood pressure of 90 to 95 mm Hg.

On arrival at the hospital, she is in active labor. Her cervix is 4 to 5 cm dilated and 70% effaced. Amniotic membranes are intact. The fetal heart rate is 140 beats per minute (BPM).

During the first 6 hours of labor, the contractions vary in frequency and intensity. Because of the poor progression of labor, an infusion of oxytocin is started. About 1.5 hours after starting the oxytocin, the fetal heart rate increases to 160 BPM with loss of beat-to-beat variability. At this point, the membranes are artificially ruptured and an internal monitor is attached. The amniotic fluid is clear and the cervix is fully effaced and 9 cm dilated. The fetal tracing continues to show a heart rate of 160 to 170 BPM, loss of beat-to-beat variability, and an occasional mild late deceleration. Within another 20 minutes, the cervix is fully effaced and dilated and the head is at +3 station. The mother is then moved to the delivery room where she delivers 20 minutes later.

### EXERCISE 1

---

**■ Question:**
Which elements might put the infant at risk for perinatal asphyxia?

**■ Answer:**
This mother has a history of hypertension for which she is receiving treatment, and currently has a diastolic blood pressure of greater than 90 mm Hg. Hypertension is frequently associated with a decrease in placental blood flow. There may be enough blood flow to supply the fetus adequately during baseline situations; however, with the stresses of labor some fetal compromise may result.

The rise in the fetal heart rate to 160 BPM and the loss of beat-to-beat variability are also indicators of potential asphyxia. Fetal tachycardia and loss of beat-to-beat variability may be the first signs seen when the utero-placental unit is compromised. It is not unusual for acceleration of the fetal heart rate and loss of variability to progress to late decelerations, which are considered more ominous and may be indicative of a compromised infant.

A concern in this case (as with many high-risk cases) is that the monitoring will end when the mother is taken to the delivery room. During the latter parts of the labor and the actual delivery, when the infant is subject to some of the greatest stresses of labor, there may be no way of telling whether or not the infant is undergoing further compromise.

Clearly, then, this is a situation where some risk for fetal asphyxia exists, and there may be a need to resuscitate the infant.

## PREPARATION OF DELIVERY ROOM

Not every resuscitation can be anticipated. Therefore, at every delivery trained staff and appropriate resuscitation equipment should be available and functioning properly if a resuscitation becomes necessary. With delivery of an infant in whom problems are anticipated, as with the infant in our initial case, someone must decide who should be available to manage the infant.

## EXERCISE 2

∎ **Question:**

Which of the following types of individuals are appropriate for the situation presented in Case Study 1?

1. a fully qualified individual "on call" to the delivery room, who can be called if the infant presents with a need for resuscitation

2. a fully qualified individual present at the delivery whose sole responsibility is the infant

3. an extra individual present at the delivery whose sole responsibility is the infant and who has been trained to assist with resuscitations

4. a delivery room nurse who is responsible to the mother and obstetrician and who can provide basic care to the infant until replaced by someone from the nursery

∎ **Answer:**

As we discuss next, 2 and 3 are the best choices and will ensure that the infant receives immediate and appropriate attention.

## Personnel

When neonatal resuscitation is likely, there should be an individual in the delivery room who has the infant as his or her *sole* responsibility. This person should not be the same individual who is taking care of the mother. In addition, a second individual should be in attendance to assist if the resuscitation becomes complicated. The second person need not be skilled in endotracheal intubation or administration of medications but should be able to assist with these procedures and should be competent in performing bag and mask ventilation and chest compression.

Even with an infant who is considered a routine delivery and not at risk, the person caring for the infant should, at a minimum, be competent in initiating a resuscitation and assisting if the resuscitation becomes more complex. There should also be someone close at hand who has all of the skills necessary to perform a complete resuscitation. Having people "on call" at home or in a remote area of the hospital prevents resuscitation from being carried out in a timely manner.

## Equipment

Having trained individuals at the delivery to manage the infant does not in itself ensure a smooth resuscitation. Care will be compromised if equipment is not readily available and functional. A decision must be made as to how much to prepare ahead of time, based on anticipated need. It is far cheaper to resterilize or discard an unused bag and mask, endotracheal tube, or vial of epinephrine than to deal with the financial, emotional, and social consequences of an infant damaged because of delay in initiating appropriate therapy.

To carry out a neonatal resuscitation, equipment is needed to establish thermal support, clear the airway, provide positive pressure ventilation, administer medications, and implement universal precautions. A minimal preparation of the delivery room should consist of the items listed in Table 1-2.

## INITIAL MANAGEMENT

The initial steps in managing any infant consist of preventing heat loss and establishing an open airway. These steps can take as little as 15 to 20 seconds and are appropriate for all

**Table 1-2**  Delivery Room Equipment Preparation

| PROCEDURE | EQUIPMENT | PREPARATION |
|---|---|---|
| Thermal protection | Radiant warmer<br>Towel/blanket | Preheat warmer<br>Warm towel/blanket |
| Clearing airway | Bulb syringe<br>Mechanical suction<br>Suction catheters:<br>  5 or 6, 8, and 10 Fr.<br>For meconium infants:<br>  Laryngoscope<br>   (#0 and 1 blade)<br>  ET tubes<br>   (2.5, 3.0, 3.5, 4.0 mm)<br>  Stylet<br>  ET tube suction adapter | Set pressure<br>  100 mm Hg<br><br>Attach appropriate size blade<br>and check light |
| Positive pressure<br>ventilation | Oxygen tubing/flowmeter<br>Resuscitation bag<br>Mask<br>Feeding tube, 8 Fr.<br>  20-cc syringe<br>ET tube<br>  (see Clearing airway) | Attach to bag<br>Check for function<br>Select appropriate size<br>On hand for gastric suction |
| Medications | Epinephrine 1 : 10,000<br>Sodium bicarbonate 0.5 mEq/mL<br>Naloxone<br>Volume expander<br>Syringes and needles | Prepare medications in syringe<br><br>Anticipate needing |
| Universal precautions | Gloves | |

infants. These initial steps are followed by a quick assessment to determine if further resuscitative measures are indicated.

### Thermal Management

Most delivery rooms are maintained at a temperature that provides comfort for the laboring mother and staff, but that is too cool for the infant. Neonates lose heat quickly in such an environment because they are born wet and have a very large body surface to mass ratio.

Infants who are excessively cooled increase their metabolic rate and consequently their requirements for oxygen and metabolic substrates. Cold stressed infants are therefore at risk for hypoglycemia and metabolic acidosis—serious problems for any infant and particularly those who are premature or otherwise compromised. Thermal protection is especially important for the infant who is sick or in need of resuscitation. Hypoxic infants are at risk for a greater than normal drop in temperature because hypoxia blunts the normal metabolic response to cold.

To prevent loss of heat, an infant should be placed in a suitable thermal environment on a preheated mattress under a radiant heater, dried thoroughly, and the wet towel removed. These simple measures will minimize considerably the drop in core temperature experienced at birth.

Refer to Exercise 3.

### Clearing the Airway

A clear airway is essential for ventilation and to prevent aspiration. It is attained at birth by suctioning and proper positioning. Most infants require some suctioning following delivery, even if the obstetrician suctioned the head when it presented on the perineum. With delivery of the body, secretions from the lungs and stomach are often forced into the upper airway.

Proper positioning helps to open the airway and facilitates early respiratory effort. With the infant supine, the neck should be *slightly extended* rather than hyperextended or flexed. If there are copious secretions, the head may

## EXERCISE 3

For each of the following situations, identify which methods of heat transfer are involved?

|  | Conduction | Convection | Evaporation | Radiation |
|---|---|---|---|---|
| Amniotic fluid on body |  |  |  |  |
| Cool room temperature |  |  |  |  |
| Overhead warmer |  |  |  |  |
| Cold mattress/blankets |  |  |  |  |

### ■ Discussion:

When the skin is moist with amniotic fluid, heat is lost through evaporation. Similarly, a cool air-conditioned room produces heat loss through convection. To counterbalance heat losses, almost all delivery rooms now use overhead radiant warmers. The overhead warmer provides heat through radiation. However, radiant warmer must be preheated. If the radiant warmer is not preheated (in addition to taking some time for the heater to produce heat), the mattress or blanket on which the infant is placed will be cool, and the infant will lose heat directly to these objects by conduction. In the delivery room, the newly born infant is at risk for heat loss from a number of sources. All can be minimized by thoroughly drying the infant and using a preheated radiant warmer. If the infant is stable, he or she can then be wrapped in a warm blanket.

---

be turned to the side, allowing the secretions to collect in the mouth where they can be easily reached.

Normally the airway can be cleared using either a bulb syringe or a suction catheter attached to mechanical suction. Suction pressures should not exceed 100 mm Hg. Suction devices that require oral suction should no longer be used because they are inconsistent with universal infection prevention precautions. Specific procedures for suctioning an infant born with meconium in the amniotic fluid are discussed later in this chapter, in the section entitled Prevention of Meconium Aspiration.

Refer to Exercise 4.

## ESTABLISHING VENTILATION

The actions of drying the infant and clearing the airway usually provide enough tactile stimulation to initiate respirations. If not, the soles of the feet may be slapped or the back rubbed in an effort to stimulate respirations. However, if the infant does not immediately respond with respiratory efforts sufficient to maintain a heart rate of 100 BPM or more, PPV should be initiated. Continued tactile stimulation of an infant who is not responding is not warranted and only delays establishing effective ventilation. Administering free-flow oxygen to an infant who is not breathing or one whose respirations are insufficient is of little value and, again, only delays appropriate management. The rationale for this lies in an understanding of the natural history of asphyxia.

### The Physiology of Asphyxia

*Primary and Secondary Apnea:* When infants become asphyxiated, they experience a well-defined sequence of events that consists of predictable changes in the heart rate and breathing patterns (Fig. 1-3). At the onset of an asphyxial episode, irregular gasping respirations replace regular breaths and the heart rate begins to fall. As the asphyxial process continues, the infant stops breathing and enters a period known as *primary apnea*. After primary apnea, irregular gasping-type respirations occur that are more erratic and not as strong or effective as during the previous period of irregular gasping (prior to primary apnea). If most

## EXERCISE 4

Choose the appropriate order for initially suctioning an infant at birth. Select the best way to position the head and neck from the diagrams shown in Figure 1-2.

Suctioning

1. Suction nose first, then mouth
2. Suction nose, then mouth and stomach
3. Suction mouth first, then nose

Positioning

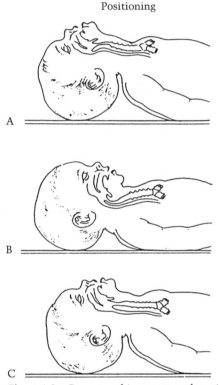

A

B

C

**Figure 1-2** Correct and incorrect neck positioning.
Reproduced with permission. *Textbook of Neonatal Resuscitation*, 1987, 1990. © Copyright American Heart Association.

### ■ Discussion:

After the infant is placed on a radiant warmer, the mouth should be suctioned, then the nose (answer #3). This removes secretions from the mouth, preventing aspiration if the infant gasps when the nose is suctioned. Care should be taken to suction the infant gently; vigorous suctioning and stimulation of the posterior pharynx in the first few minutes of life can induce a vagal response, resulting in bradycardia, apnea, or both. Because of the vagal response, gastric suctioning, which involves a catheter passed into the pharynx, should not be part of routine initial suctioning.

The proper position of the head is with the neck slightly extended, as illustrated in Figure 1-2C. This may be best achieved by placing a rolled towel, about 1-inch thick, under the shoulders. (Note that 1-2A is incorrect because the neck is hyperextended and 1-2B is incorrect because the neck is flexed.)

infants are exposed to oxygen prior to this point, the heart rate will rise and the respirations will even out. However, if the asphyxia continues, the infant enters a period called *secondary apnea.* The only way to reverse secondary apnea is with PPV with high concentrations of oxygen. The likelihood of brain damage occurring is significantly increased

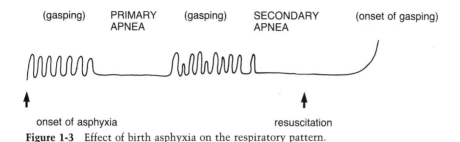

(gasping)   PRIMARY   (gasping)   SECONDARY   (onset of gasping)
            APNEA                  APNEA

onset of asphyxia                        resuscitation

**Figure 1-3**  Effect of birth asphyxia on the respiratory pattern.

when the infant reaches the stage of secondary apnea. This critical sequence usually occurs before the 1-minute Apgar score assessment is performed.

It is important to recognize that an infant may pass through any or all of the stages of asphyxia *in utero*. It is very difficult to judge whether the infant is in primary or secondary apnea. If you assume that an infant is in primary apnea and are wrong, the wasted time before establishing positive pressure ventilation increases the chances of brain injury. It will also extend the length of time that PPV will be required before spontaneous ventilation is established.

*Pulmonary Vasoconstriction:*  A further reason for rapid intervention is to prevent the accentuation of hypoxia and acidosis, which may result in pulmonary vasoconstriction and shunting of blood away from the lungs. During the asphyxial process, the infant's oxygen concentration in the blood ($PaO_2$) decreases, the carbon dioxide concentration ($PCO_2$) increases, and the pH falls because of the rise in $PCO_2$ (respiratory acidosis) and accumulation of organic acids (metabolic acidosis). The combination of a fall in pH and in $PaO_2$ results in pulmonary vasoconstriction, which diverts blood flow from the lungs through the foramen ovale and ductus arteriosus, thereby perfusing the systemic circuit, most importantly the head and heart.

A continuation of the asphyxial process results in a vicious cycle of pulmonary vasoconstriction, resulting in a marked decrease in pulmonary perfusion. Thus, when ventilation is begun late, although oxygen is entering the lungs, very little blood is flowing through the capillaries adjacent to the alveoli, and, consequently, the blood is inadequately oxygenated.

Three features of the asphyxial process should be emphasized. First, this entire sequence of events may begin *in utero* and continue after delivery. Second, the irregular gasps of an asphyxiated infant should not be interpreted as effective breathing and will not be sufficient to expand the lungs. Finally, to reverse the effects of intrauterine asphyxia, both ventilation and pulmonary perfusion must be present; either alone is insufficient.

### EXERCISE 5

Many pediatricians and obstetricians will tell you that they have taken care of infants who were not breathing at birth and that with continued stimulation and oxygen these infants eventually began to breath and did not need PPV.

■ **Questions:**

What stage of the asphyxial process do you suspect these infants were in?

Why should these infants have received positive pressure ventilation, rather than prolonged tactile stimulation?

■ **Answers:**

Infants in secondary apnea require PPV to recover. The infants referred to above eventually developed spontaneous respirations without PPV. Thus, we can be sure they were in primary apnea. We know this only in retrospect because of the later response of the infants. It is very difficult to distinguish primary apnea from secondary apnea simply by looking at an infant.

By continuing to provide tactile stimulation and free-flow oxygen, these physicians were gambling that the infants were in primary apnea. If their guess was wrong (and the infant was really in secondary apnea), the results would have been disastrous. The time consumed providing tactile stimulation would have increased the depth of the secondary apnea and the chances of brain injury. Furthermore, it would also have increased the amount of time that PPV would have to be given before the infant would begin to breath spontaneously.

**The Apgar Score**

As we have noted, the asphyxial process may begin *in utero* and continue into the neonatal period. Thus, resuscitation should begin as soon as there is evidence that the infant is not able to establish ventilations sufficient to sustain the heart rate at 100 BPM or more. This is usually determined well before 1 minute. Waiting until a 1-minute Apgar score is assigned before initiating resuscitation only delays the resuscitative efforts. Thus, the Apgar score should not be used as the primary indicator for resuscitation because it is not assigned until 1 minute of age.

## EXERCISE 6

In the following chart, check the appropriate action, given the condition of the child after drying and clearing the airway. Check as many boxes in each row as you believe are correct.

| | | Action | | |
|---|---|---|---|---|
| Condition | Heart Rate | Give Free-Flow O$_2$ | Initiate PPV with O$_2$ | Provide Tactile Stimulation |
| Crying | >100 | | | |
| Crying | 80–100 | | | |
| Crying | <80 | | | |
| Gasping | <100 | | | |
| Apnea | <100 | | | |
| Regular respiration | >100 | | | |
| Regular respiration | 80–100 | | | |
| Regular respiration | <80 | | | |

### ■ Discussion:

The fundamental principle to keep in mind is that if the infant is apneic or is gasping, or the respirations are regular but insufficient to sustain a heart rate at or more than 80 BPM, then PPV should be initiated immediately. If the infant is crying or has regular respirations, the heart rate should be checked to assure that the respirations are capable of sustaining the heart rate at 100 BPM or more. Free-flow oxygen and tactile stimulation can be used if the heart rate is between 80 and 100 BPM and the infant is ventilating well (crying or sustained regular respiration). If, however, the heart rate does not rise above 80 in 15 seconds, PPV should be used. Similarly, free-flow oxygen can be used in any infant who has a heart rate of more than 100 BPM (and is breathing) but who has not yet become pink.

## INITIAL EVALUATION

The process of drying the infant, clearing the airway, and providing initial tactile stimulation should take no more than 15 to 20 seconds. After these steps have been taken, respirations should be evaluated. If the infant is gasping or apneic, PPV *must* be initiated. If the infant has regular respirations, the heart rate should then be checked. If the respirations are insufficient to sustain the heart rate at 100 BPM or more, PPV with 100% oxygen should be started (Fig. 1-4).

Refer to Exercise 6.

## POSITIVE PRESSURE VENTILATION (PPV)

At delivery it is essential that ventilation be established quickly, either spontaneously or with PPV. PPV is indicated when, following tactile stimulation, the infant

- is apneic
- has gasping respirations
- is breathing with a heart rate less than 100 BPM

In the majority of infants requiring resuscitation at birth, a brief period of PPV is usually all that is needed to establish breathing.

In most circumstances, PPV can be adequately provided with a resuscitation bag and mask. Many individuals who possess the skill to intubate an infant rapidly prefer to use a bag and an endotracheal tube. However, unless you are skilled at intubation, a bag and mask should be used. Time spent at multiple attempts to intubate an infant is usually time

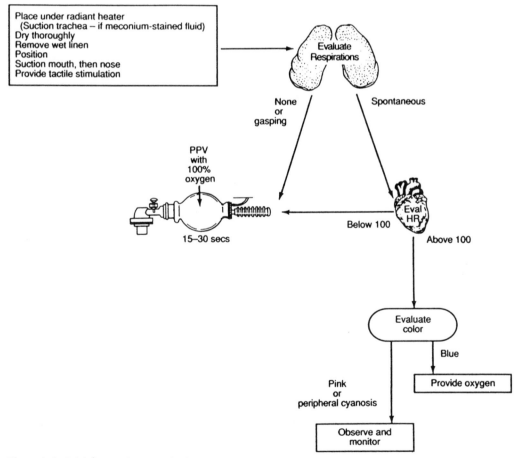

**Figure 1-4** Initial steps in resuscitation.
Reproduced and modified with permission. *Textbook of Neonatal Resuscitation*, 1987, 1990. © Copyright American Heart Association, p. 0-5.

better spent in providing adequate ventilation with a bag and mask. At a minimum, medical, nursing, and respiratory therapy staff involved clinically with the care of neonates in the delivery room, nursery, or elsewhere in the hospital should be skilled in using a resuscitation bag and mask.

The bag and mask procedure requires the following:

- selecting and assembling appropriate equipment
- providing 100% oxygen
- developing a seal between the mask and the face
- regulating the rate and pressure of the ventilations

### Bag and Mask Equipment

Various types of neonatal resuscitation bags are available. Each type has its limitations, capabilities, and idiosyncrasies. Knowledge of the specific bag being used is essential. The two basic types of bags are the anesthesia bag and the self-inflating bag (Fig. 1-5). The two types of bags differ mainly in their mechanism of inflation. The anesthesia bag, which resembles a balloon, requires a constant flow of gas to keep it inflated. The self-inflating bag reinflates spontaneously without being connected to a source of oxygen or compressed air. The type of bag chosen is mainly a matter of preference. Those who are experienced in the use of an anesthesia bag prefer it because they believe that it is more responsive and gives the individual greater control. However, an anesthesia bag takes more practice to use correctly than a self-inflating bag does. Unless the entire staff is trained and comfortable using an anesthesia bag, it is best to have self-inflating bags available.

Regardless of the type of bag selected, it should be equipped with either a pressure gauge or a pressure relief (pop-off) valve to minimize the chances of a pneumothorax, which can result from overinflation of the infant's lungs. Pressure relief valves are built into most self-inflating bags and are set to vent pressures greater than 30 to 40 cm water. Many pop-off valves can be temporarily occluded when higher pressures are desired. Any bag without a pop-off valve should have a pressure gauge to indicate to the operator pressures generated by the bag. Pressure gauges with adjustable pop-off valves are available and can be used with most bags.

Any bag used in a neonatal resuscitation should be capable of providing 90% to 100% oxygen. A self-inflating bag requires an oxygen reservoir to provide these high concentrations of oxygen. Without an oxygen reservoir, self-inflating bags cannot provide more than approximately 40% oxygen (Fig. 1-6). Oxygen reservoirs are not used with anesthesia bags because such bags are able to deliver 100% oxygen.

For delivery room resuscitation, the resuscitation bag should be connected to a 100% oxygen source and carefully checked for faults in the bag or mask before use. The bag can be checked by occluding the outlet with the palm of the hand and firmly squeezing the bag. Pressure should be generated on the pressure gauge, or the pop-off valve should open.

Face masks with cushioned rims are preferable to ones with noncushioned rims. The cushioned rim tends to conform to the contours of the face more easily and generally requires less pressure to obtain a seal. Masks should be available to accommodate infants ranging in weight from 500 to 4,500 g.

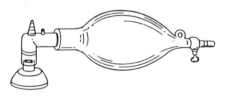

Anesthesia Bag

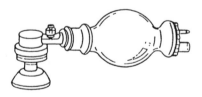

Self-Inflating Bag

**Figure 1-5** The two basic types of neonatal resuscitation bags.
Reproduced and modified with permission. *Textbook of Neonatal Resuscitation*, 1987, 1990. © Copyright American Heart Association, p. 3A-8.

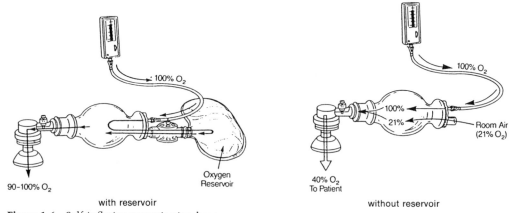

**Figure 1-6** Self-inflating resuscitation bags.
Reproduced and modified with permission. *Textbook of Neonatal Resuscitation*, 1987, 1990. © Copyright American Heart Association, p. 3A-23.

**Positive Pressure Ventilation Procedure**

Positioning prior to PPV is important in providing an open airway. The infant should be positioned with the neck slightly extended. The mask should be held on the face without excessive pressure. There should be no pressure over the eyes. The infant should be ventilated at a rate of 40 to 60 per minute, with just enough pressure to provide an *easy* rise and fall of the chest. The first breath may require significantly higher pressure than succeeding breaths (Table 1-3).

With the first several ventilations, particular attention should be paid to determining if the ventilation technique is adequate. One of the most useful guides is observing the adequacy of the rise and fall of the chest. If the chest does not rise, one of the following conditions is responsible:

1. There is an inadequate seal of the mask.
2. The airway is blocked.
3. The pressure is inadequate.

Any adjustment needed should be made quickly to prevent ongoing asphyxia. An as-

**Table 1-3** Pressures Required for Adequate Ventilation

| | |
|---|---|
| First breath | 30–40 cm $H_2O$ pressure |
| Succeeding breaths | 15–20 cm $H_2O$ pressure |
| If pulmonary disease exists | 20–40 cm $H_2O$ pressure |

sistant should auscultate breath sounds to assess ventilation if there is any doubt.

### EXERCISE 7

■ **Questions:**
What steps would you take to remedy

- an inadequate seal?

- a blocked airway?

- inadequate pressure?

■ **Answers:**
*Inadequate seal.* The most common problem is an inadequate seal. Repositioning the mask to the face and perhaps readjusting your hold on the mask usually helps correct an inadequate seal.

*Blocked airway.* Several things can contribute to a blocked airway. Reassess the position of the infant's head. In addition, try repositioning the head slightly, or suction secretions from the mouth, nose, and pharynx, if indicated. Ventilating through an open mouth can also relieve airway obstruction.

*Inadequate pressure.* When a bag with a pop-off valve is used, the valve may open before the needed pressure is reached. In such a circumstance, occlude the pop-off valve with your index finger as you squeeze the bag. Take care not to use excessive pressure. A pressure gauge is helpful in this situation.

If resuscitation with a bag and mask is needed for more than a couple of minutes, an orogastric tube should be inserted. This will prevent a buildup of air in the stomach and minimize the chance of aspiration or compromise of diaphragmatic excursion.

## ENDOTRACHEAL INTUBATION

As noted previously, under most circumstances PPV can be provided quickly and effectively with a bag and mask. However, many prefer to insert an endotracheal tube because it provides somewhat more control over ventilation, and because it eliminates the problems of gas entering the stomach during ventilation. In those infants born through thick meconium, insertion of the tube permits removal of secretions or meconium from the trachea as well as providing an effective route for ventilation if necessary.

Insertion of an endotracheal tube is best accomplished by two people. One person inserts the tube and ventilates the infant. The other assists with the procedure and, after placement of the tube, listens to the chest for the presence of bilateral breath sounds, which assures proper tube placement. Tube sizes ranging from 2.0 to 4.0 mm (inside diameter) should be available (Table 1-4).

The head of the infant should be slightly extended in preparation for intubation. Hy-perextending the neck, by hanging the head over the edge of a radiant warmer, moves the trachea anterior and makes the glottis harder to visualize. Flexion of the neck also impairs visualization of landmarks.

Much has been written about advancing the laryngoscope into the mouth and lifting the blade to visualize the glottis. In the last analysis, however, a skillful intubation relies on recognizing the position of the blade when it is first inserted and moving the blade to the proper position (Fig. 1-7). To maximize the view of the glottis, it is often helpful to apply gentle pressure over the larynx. This will lower the trachea and bring the glottis into view. After the glottis is visualized, the tip of the endotracheal tube should be inserted about 1 to 1.5 cm below the vocal cords. This should position the tip of the tube above the carina.

Two of the most common errors made in intubating an infant are not keeping the glottis in view during an intubation and inserting the tube through the center of the laryngoscope blade. Placing the tube alongside the blade preserves the line of sight.

A tip-to-lip distance for inserting the tube can be estimated by adding 6 to the weight (in kilograms) of the infant. This will approximate the centimeter marking that should appear at the lips of the infant when the tube is properly positioned.

Initial confirmation of the placement of the tube is done by listening for breath sounds while ventilating with a bag. If bilateral breath sounds are heard, the tube is correctly positioned in the trachea above the carina. Breath sounds heard over only one lung indicate that the tube is positioned in one of the mainstem bronchi. If this situation is suspected, the tube should be withdrawn approximately 0.5 cm and the infant ventilated again. If no breath sounds are heard, the tube is probably not positioned in the trachea. In this circumstance, the tube must be completely removed and re-inserted.

If an endotracheal tube is to be inserted, it must be done quickly. Prolonged attempts at inserting a tube will simply extend the asphyxial period and increase the chance of brain injury. If a tube has not been successfully inserted within 20 seconds and the infant is bradycardic, the attempt should cease and the infant should be ventilated with a bag and mask for about 30 seconds.

**Table 1-4** Endotracheal Tube Sizes

| TUBE SIZE (ID mm) | WEIGHT | GESTATION AGE |
|---|---|---|
| 2.0 | 500–750 g | <28 weeks |
| 2.5 | 751–1,000 g | <28 weeks |
| 3.0 | 1,001–2,000 g | 28–34 weeks |
| 3.5 | 2,001–3,000 g | 34–38 weeks |
| 3.5–4.0 | >3,000 g | >38 weeks |

| Position | Landmarks | Corrective action |
|---|---|---|
| Not inserted far enough | You see the tongue surrounding the blade | Advance the blade farther |

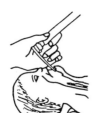 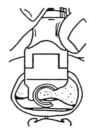 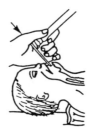

| Position | Landmarks | Corrective action |
|---|---|---|
| Inserted too far | You see the wall of the esophagus surrounding the blade | Withdraw the blade slowly until the epiglottis and glottis come into view |

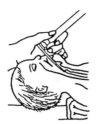 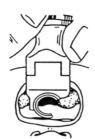 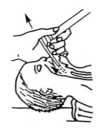

| Position | Landmarks | Corrective action |
|---|---|---|
| Inserted off to the side | In the posterior pharynx, you see part of the trachea to the side of the blade | Gently move the blade back to the midline, then advance or retreat according to the landmarks seen |

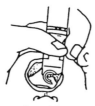 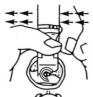

**Figure 1-7** Examples of incorrect positioning of the laryngoscope blade and how to take corrective action.
Reproduced and modified with permission. *Textbook of Neonatal Resuscitation*, 1987, 1990. © Copyright American Heart Association, p. 5-25.

Regardless of whether you choose to ventilate an infant with a bag and mask or a bag and an endotracheal tube, the procedure must be implemented at the appropriate time and in a skilled and efficient way. The use of either the bag and mask or bag and endotracheal tube requires practice. If adequate inflation of the lungs is not achieved with a properly positioned mask or if prolonged ventilation is anticipated, an endotracheal tube should be inserted for ventilating the infant.

## HEART RATE DECISIONS WITH POSITIVE PRESSURE VENTILATION

Regardless of whether a bag and mask or a bag and an endotracheal tube is used, after 15 to 30 seconds of PPV the heart rate should be checked. If the heart rate is at least 100 BPM, the infant should be checked for spontaneous respirations. If the infant is breathing, ventilation can be discontinued. As PPV is discontinued, free-flow oxygen should be given and withdrawn slowly if the infant remains pink.

If there are no spontaneous respirations, or the heart rate is less than 100 BPM, then PPV must be continued. The decision about whether to institute chest compressions and medications depends on the heart rate. If the heart rate is at or greater than 100 BPM, only PPV need be continued. If the heart rate is less than 60 BPM, chest compression and, if necessary, medications should be given. If the heart

rate is between 60 and 80 BPM and rising with PPV, then it is sufficient to continue to ventilate the infant and recheck the heart rate. However, if the heart rate is between 60 and 80 BPM, and not increasing, chest compressions should be started (Fig. 1-8).

## CASE STUDY 2

An infant is born after having severe late decelerations prior to birth. At birth the infant is apneic with a heart rate of 70 BPM, so PPV was immediately instituted and after 30 seconds of ventilation with 100% oxygen the heart rate is stable at 70 BPM.

## EXERCISE 8

### ■ Question:

What would be your next step, and why?

### ■ Answer:

This infant has a heart rate of 70 BPM, which is in the range in which the decision to initiate chest compressions will be determined by whether the heart rate is rising or not.

In this particular case, PPV with 100% oxygen was insufficient to cause enough of an increase in oxygen delivery to the myocardium to increase the heart rate. The infant heart rate is a very sensitive indicator of myocardial hy-

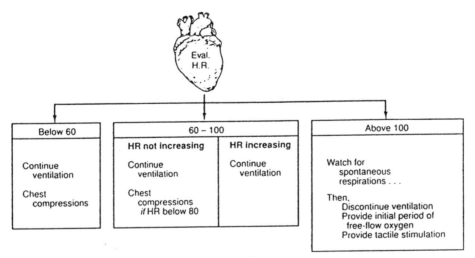

**Figure 1-8** Diagram summarizing the heart rate decisions.
Reproduced and modified with permission. *Textbook of Neonatal Resuscitation*, 1987, 1990. © Copyright American Heart Association, p. 3C-14.

poxia and ischemia. In addition to bradycardia, the infant will also exhibit poor myocardial contractility and decreased tissue perfusion. Because the heart rate (and probably myocardial contractility) is low enough to reduce cardiac output significantly and the heart rate is not increasing, chest compressions should be instituted and PPV with 100% oxygen continued.

## CHEST COMPRESSION

With continued hypoxia, the heart not only slows, but diminishes in function. The result is reduced cardiac output and systemic hypotension. This is manifested in the delivery room by a pale gray, mottled appearance with poor capillary filling and weak axillary and femoral pulses. To assist the heart in maintaining the circulation, chest compressions should be instituted. Resuscitation that has reached this point should be a coordinated process between two people: one ventilating the infant and the other providing chest compressions.

It must be stressed that chest compressions should be considered only after the establishment of PPV. Chest compression in the absence of ventilation is of little, if any, value.

Chest compression is performed by depressing the lower third of the infant's sternum one-half to three-quarters of an inch (which compresses the heart and forces blood into the systemic circulation). This can be accomplished in two ways (Fig. 1-9), and it is advantageous to know both methods.

***Thumb Technique:*** Both hands are used to encircle the chest, with thumbs compressing the sternum while the fingertips support the spine. The thumbs may be side by side or one placed over the other. The thumb technique is less tiresome to do for a prolonged period of time; however, it is difficult to use if the infant is large and the resuscitator's hands are small.

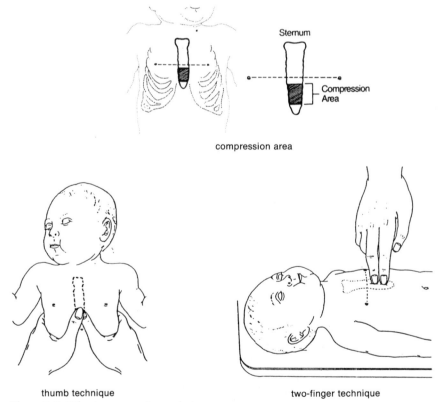

Sternum

Compression Area

compression area

thumb technique

two-finger technique

**Figure 1-9** Chest compression techniques.
Reproduced and modified with permission. *Textbook of Neonatal Resuscitation,* 1987, 1990.
© Copyright American Heart Association, p. 4-32.

***Two-Finger Technique:*** The index and middle finger of one hand are used to depress the sternum. The other hand may be placed under the infant to provide a firm surface. Care must be taken to maintain the fingers perpendicular to the chest and avoid a "stabbing" or "bounding" type of movement.

An area of considerable discussion is that of whether the ventilations should be interposed between the compressions. Although no consensus has been reached regarding this issue, we prefer to interpose a ventilation after every third compression. It is our belief that when ventilation and compression occur simultaneously, ventilation of the infant is compromised. The infant has a highly compliant chest, and compression of the chest makes it difficult to force air into the lungs at the same time—especially if ventilation occurs with a bag and mask, as opposed to a bag and an endotracheal tube.

Coordination between ventilation and compression can be enhanced if the compressor counts out each compression and release (e.g., "one–and–two–and–three–and–"). The number indicates the compression and the *and* indicates the release. A ventilation should occur following every third compression. Thus, when the count reaches ". . . three–and–," the ventilator will inflate the lungs simultaneously with the release indicated by the word *and*. The count then resumes and the new cycle begins. For example:

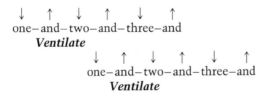

The American Academy of Pediatric's recommendation is to compress the chest at a rate of 120 times per minute, inserting a ventilation after every third chest compression.

The effectiveness of cardiac massage can be assessed by a third person who palpates the axillary or femoral pulses. Cardiac massage should be discontinued as soon as ventilation alone can sustain a heart rate of 80 BPM or greater.

Two essential points must be remembered when you are initiating chest compression. One is that the patient must be adequately ventilated with 100% oxygen while cardiac massage is performed. The second is that both individuals performing cardiac massage and ventilation must be skilled at their tasks. All persons taking part in the resuscitation must know exactly what they are to do and must have practiced coordinating their roles. The process represents the essence of a team approach. It is important to have resuscitation drills with mannequins. So-called *megacodes* are useful for this purpose. An actual resuscitation is not the time to practice or refine skills. The infant in need of PPV and cardiac massage requires staff who can perform competently and proceed without hesitation.

## MEDICATIONS

The most important step in any resuscitation is to establish adequate ventilation with enough oxygen to prevent cyanosis. In the majority of cases, ventilation and oxygenation are enough to resuscitate the infant. However, times will occur when medications will be necessary.

*Medications should be used if the infant has not responded to at least 30 seconds of PPV with 100% oxygen and chest compressions.* Many physicians believe that if there is no response to PPV, medications should be started simultaneously with chest compressions.

Depending on the medication, the umbilical venous, subcutaneous, intramuscular, or endotracheal route may be used. Table 1-5 displays the most commonly used drugs, their dosages and routes of administration, and how to prepare them for use in a neonatal resuscitation.

If a drug is administered through an umbilical venous catheter, extreme care must be taken to ensure that the tip is not wedged in the liver. The catheter can be inserted to a point where the tip is just beneath the skin level and blood returns easily upon aspiration. Alternatively, the tip can be placed into the inferior vena cava above the diaphragm. An estimate of the distance to the diaphragm from the umbilicus can be derived from Figure 1-10.

**Table 1-5**  Medications for Neonatal Resuscitation

| MEDICATION | CONCENTRATION TO ADMINISTER | PREPARATION | DOSAGE/ROUTE* | TOTAL DOSE/INFANT | | | RATE/PRECAUTIONS |
|---|---|---|---|---|---|---|---|
| | | | | **weight** | **total dose** | **total mLs** | |
| Epinephrine | 1 : 10,000 | 1 mL | 0.1–0.3 mL/kg IV or ET | 1 kg<br>2 kg<br>3 kg<br>4 kg | | 0.1–0.3 mL<br>0.2–0.6 mL<br>0.3–0.9 mL<br>0.4–1.2 mL | Give rapidly |
| Volume expanders | Whole blood<br>5% albumin<br>Normal saline<br>Ringer's lactate | 40 mL | 10 mL/kg IV | 1 kg<br>2 kg<br>3 kg<br>4 kg | | 10 mL<br>20 mL<br>30 mL<br>40 mL | Give during 5–10 minutes |
| Sodium bicarbonate | 0.5 mEq/mL (4.2% solution) | 20 mL or two 10-mL prefilled syringes | 2 mEq/kg IV | 1 kg<br>2 kg<br>3 kg<br>4 kg | 2 mEq<br>4 mEq<br>6 mEq<br>8 mEq | | Give *slowly*, during at least 2 minutes<br>Give only if infant is being effectively ventilated |
| Naloxone | 0.4 mg/mL | 1 mL | 0.1 mg/kg (0.25 mL/kg) IV, ET, IM, SQ | 1 kg<br>2 kg<br>3 kg<br>4 kg | 0.1 mg<br>0.2 mg<br>0.3 mg<br>0.4 mg | 0.25 mL<br>0.50 mL<br>0.75 mL<br>1.00 mL | Give rapidly IV, ET preferred IM, SQ acceptable |
| | 1.0 mg/mL | 1 mL | 0.1 mg/kg (0.1 mL/kg) IV, ET, IM, SQ | 1 kg<br>2 kg<br>3 kg<br>4 kg | 0.1 mg<br>0.2 mg<br>0.3 mg<br>0.4 mg | 0.1 mL<br>0.2 mL<br>0.3 mL<br>0.4 mL | |
| Dopamine | $6 \times \text{weight} \times \dfrac{\text{desired dose (mcg/kg/min)}}{\text{desired fluid (mL/hr)}}$ = mg of dopamine per 100 mL of solution | | Begin at 5 mcg/kg/min (may increase to 20 mcg/kg/min if necessary) IV | **weight** 1 kg<br>2 kg<br>3 kg<br>4 kg | **total mcg/min** 5–20 mcg/min<br>10–40 mcg/min<br>15–60 mcg/min<br>20–80 mcg/min | | Give as a continuous infusion, using an infusion pump<br>Monitor HR and BP closely<br>Seek consultation |

*Source:* Reproduced and modified with permission. *Textbook of Neonatal Resuscitation,* 1987, 1990. © Copyright American Heart Association, p. 6-55.

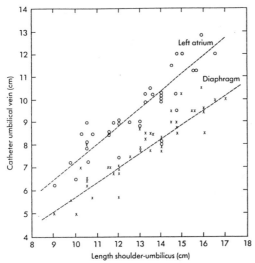

**Figure 1-10** The length of an umbilical venous catheter needed to reach the diaphragm (x) and the left atrium (o) in relation to the shoulder-umbilicus length.
From Dunn PM: Localization of umbilical catheters by post mortem measurement. *Arch Dis Child* 1966; 41:69. Reprinted with permission of the British Medical Association.

It is now well accepted that epinephrine should be the first drug used in a neonate requiring resuscitation. In addition to its ability to increase the heart rate and myocardial contractility, epinephrine also has a peripheral "alpha" effect: It increases peripheral vascular resistance, thus enhancing coronary blood flow and myocardial perfusion. Epinephrine can be given quickly through an endotracheal tube.

If the infant does not respond to epinephrine, consideration should be given to using sodium bicarbonate or a volume expander. You must recognize that the sodium bicarbonate will not stop the production of acid; only adequate ventilation, oxygenation, and circulation will do that. Sodium bicarbonate, however, will correct some of the metabolic acidosis, improving pulmonary blood flow and oxygen uptake. To prevent further $CO_2$ accumulation, you must establish ventilation *before* sodium bicarbonate is given because some of the bicarbonate is metabolized to $CO_2$, which diffuses readily into cells, thereby producing an intracellular acidosis.

In infants in whom there is evidence of hypovolemia or blood loss, a volume expander should be given. Finally, if the infant is still not responding, an isotropic agent such as dopamine can be used (see Table 1-5 for dosage).

## Drug-Depressed Infants

If an infant is suffering from respiratory depression as a result of a narcotic having been given to the mother, naloxone (0.1 mg/kg) should be given as soon as possible after ventilation is established. Because the half-life of the naloxone is shorter than almost all narcotics, naloxone may have to be repeated.

Naloxone should not be given to the infant of a mother who is a chronic narcotics user because it may result in acute withdrawal and seizures in the infant. It is important to understand that cocaine is not a narcotic and does not cause significant respiratory depression.

## CASE STUDY 3

An infant is born to a mother who experienced an abruptio placenta at 39 weeks' gestation. The mother is rushed to the local hospital where there are severe late decelerations with a baseline heart rate of 110 BPM. The infant is delivered by "crash" cesarean section. No meconium is found in the amniotic fluid. When the infant is placed on the radiant warmer, he is flaccid, pale, and apneic. The heart rate is 30 BPM. Ventilation is established.

## EXERCISE 9

■ **Question:**
What would be your next step(s), and why?

■ **Answer:**
This is obviously an infant who is profoundly depressed. There is no question about starting chest compression. In general, it is recommended that chest compressions be performed along with PPV. After 30 seconds, evaluate the heart rate. However, because of the profound compromise in cardiac output, many individuals in this case, would simultaneously administer epinephrine rather than wait to see if ventilation and chest compression alone raised the heart rate.

## CASE STUDY 4

A mother who is a known drug addict comes into the labor and delivery area. She admits to sniffing cocaine but claims she was clean for the past 2 weeks. About 45 minutes before delivery, she is given 125 mg meperidine for pain. At delivery the infant is apneic and PPV is started. The heart rate quickly rises to greater than 100 BPM, and the infant appears pink with good peripheral circulation, but has a poor respiratory effort.

## EXERCISE 10

### ■ Question:

Are further medications warranted in this case?

### ■ Answer:

This infant appears to be apneic, without other signs of significant compromise. If the child does not develop spontaneous ventilation in a short period of time, then naloxone is indicated because of the administration of meperidine. This mother was given a large dose of a narcotic 45 minutes prior to delivery. This is enough time for the drug to cross the placenta and cause respiratory depression in a newborn infant.

Naloxone is not contraindicated in infants born to cocaine-abusing women because cocaine does not have the same effects as a narcotic and does not compete for the same binding sites as naloxone. Thus, in these circumstances, it is probably safe to use naloxone. Any hesitation in using naloxone stems from the fact that many mothers who give a history of using one drug may frequently take others, so this mother may also have taken narcotics. Some feeling about the reliability of the mother and her story will dictate whether or not to use naloxone.

## PREVENTION OF MECONIUM ASPIRATION

Meconium passage *in utero* occurs in 10% to 15% of all infants born and is a major cause of morbidity and mortality in term and post-term infants. When meconium is present in the amniotic fluid, it could be taken into the mouth and subsequently into the lungs. Special steps are necessary to prevent the aspiration of meconium at birth.

A number of studies have been conducted that are related to delivery room management of the infant born of meconium-stained amniotic fluid. However, controversy still exists with regard to some aspects of care. One step in which there is consensus—and perhaps the most important step in preventing meconium aspiration—is for the obstetrician to suction the mouth, nose, and pharynx thoroughly when the head is delivered, before delivery of the shoulders. This applies to infants with either watery *or* particulate (thick) meconium in the amniotic fluid. Suctioning should be done with a 10 Fr. or larger suction catheter. If the meconium is thin or watery, an increasing body of opinion agrees that these infants need no further special management upon delivery.

A consensus also exists that, in the infant with thick or particulate meconium who is depressed at birth, the trachea should be suctioned as soon after delivery as possible to remove any meconium from the lower airway. Studies have demonstrated that meconium can be present below the cords even though there is no meconium visible in secretions suctioned from the upper airway.

The controversy exists over how to handle the vigorous crying infant born through thick or particulate meconium. The disagreement is about whether the difficulty of intubating an active infant can justify the advantages of the procedure.

The American Heart Association/American Academy of Pediatrics (AHA/AAP) program on neonatal resuscitation recommends that in any infant with thick or particulate meconium, the trachea should be intubated and suctioned as soon as possible after delivery to remove any meconium from the lower airway. The best way to accomplish this is to attach an adapter to the endotracheal tube so that suction can be directly applied as the tube is withdrawn (Fig. 1-11). The trachea can be reintubated and suctioned until the airway is clear. In a severely asphyxiated infant, careful attention to the heart rate should be given during this procedure. It may not be possible to clear the trachea of all meconium before the need to initiate PPV.

When tracheal suctioning is indicated, it should be done as quickly as possible after birth. This reinforces the need to have a trained individual capable of intubating an infant available for each delivery. Remember, in women with intact membranes, the status of

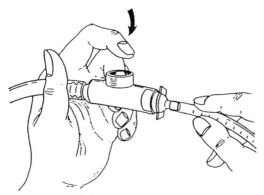

**Figure 1-11** Adapter for connecting an endotracheal tube to mechanical suction.
Reproduced and modified with permission. *Textbook of Neonatal Resuscitation*, 1987, 1990. © Copyright American Heart Association, p. 5-75.

the amniotic fluid will not be known prior to the actual delivery, too late to summon someone from afar.

To emphasize the various components of the resuscitation process, let us finish our discussion with a case study. As you read through the following clinical case presentation, consider the individual steps that are being taken and note the management so that you will be

able to respond to the various questions interspersed throughout the presentation.

Before you proceed to this final case study, look at Figure 1-12, which overviews the entire resuscitation procedure as outlined in the AHA/AAP *Textbook of Neonatal Resuscitation*. Keeping this outline in mind as you approach an infant will provide a foundation on which to make decisions as the status of the infant evolves.

### CASE STUDY 5

Mrs. W is a 26-year-old woman with diabetes who is in her third pregnancy. One pregnancy ended as a spontaneous abortion. The other produced a 9-lb term infant who had no difficulty after birth. Mrs. W is an insulin-dependent diabetic who is only moderately controlled. An ultrasound examination at 39.5 weeks estimated the fetal weight at 2,600 g.

A day or two past 40 weeks of gestation, Mrs. W goes into labor and enters the labor and delivery suite about 4 to 5 hours later with intact membranes and contractions that occur approximately every 4 minutes. When Mrs. W enters the hospital, the fetal heart rate is 165 BPM with some loss of beat-to-beat variability. Her cervix is 5 to 6 cm dilated and 80% effaced

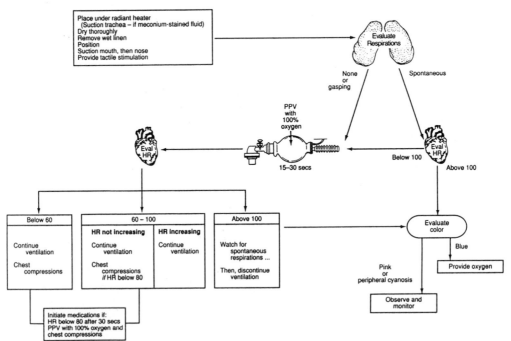

**Figure 1-12** Overview of resuscitation in the delivery room.
Reproduced and modified with permission. *Textbook of Neonatal Resuscitation*, 1987, 1990. © Copyright American Heart Association, p. 0-5.

and the infant is at +1 station. During the next 3 hours as labor progresses, the fetal heart rate ranges from 160 to 170 BPM with only an occasional mild late deceleration. Three hours after coming to the hospital, Mrs. W is fully dilated and at +3 to +4 station. Shortly afterward, however, a severe late deceleration is observed. Her membranes are ruptured and the amniotic fluid contains thick particulate meconium. Almost immediately after the membranes are ruptured, the infant develops a fixed bradycardia. The mother is rushed to the delivery room, where the infant is delivered with the aid of vacuum extraction. Upon delivery of the head, the obstetrician suctions the pharynx and nose and hands the baby to the nurse who places the infant on the bed of the radiant warmer. The infant appears to be about 2,500 g.

## EXERCISE 11

Identify the major points in this history that would lead you to believe that the infant might be in need of resuscitative support after delivery.

### ■ Discussion:

To begin with, this mother was a diabetic in only moderate control. This indicates that her blood sugar was out of control a reasonable portion of the time. Thus, one would expect a large-for-gestational-age (LGA) infant, as was true of her previous pregnancy. Yet, according to the ultrasound examination, the infant's weight was estimated to be only 2,600 g at 39.5 weeks. Although in absolute terms this does not represent a small-for-gestational-age (SGA) infant, in terms of an infant of a diabetic mother (in whom the mother is not in good control) this infant could be considered undergrown. The likely possibility is that there is some utero-placental insufficiency secondary to the diabetes that is compromising fetal growth. This is one reason to suspect an asphyxiated infant.

Further justification for anticipating a high-risk infant is the presence of thick meconium in the amniotic fluid. Another point of concern is the fetal heart rate. The tachycardia, the loss of beat-to-beat variability, and the occasional late decelerations are all associated with fetal asphyxia. The most ominous sign,

however, is the fixed bradycardia, which occurred immediately before delivery. A sudden fixed bradycardia is highly associated with a compromised infant.

Clearly, prior to the delivery there were enough indications to anticipate an infant who might be in need of resuscitation. The necessary steps should have been taken to ensure that appropriate personnel were in the delivery room and that the equipment was adequately prepared.

### CASE STUDY 5 continued

The nurse places the infant on the bed of the warmer and turns on the overhead radiant heater. The infant is noted to be limp and cyanotic and to have irregular gasping respirations. The nurse suctions the infant's nose and the mouth with a bulb syringe, connects oxygen tubing to the flowmeter, and provides free-flow oxygen to the infant. At the same time, she tactilely stimulates the infant by rubbing his back. At 1 minute of age, the infant remains motionless with only occasional gasping respirations and a heart rate of 70 BPM. An Apgar score of 2 is assigned and the obstetrician is notified. Because of the low Apgar score, the obstetrician asks that a pediatrician or anesthetist be called and orders bag and mask ventilation. The head nurse is also called into the delivery room. She unpacks and assembles the resuscitation bag and mask, connects it to oxygen, and begins to ventilate the infant.

### EXERCISE 12

Point out the errors in management and indicate how you would approach the first minute or so in the life of this infant.

### ■ Discussion:

A series of problems is associated with the way the initial stages of this resuscitation were approached.

**No Fully Trained Personnel Available:** It is obvious that there has been little preparation for a resuscitation that could have been easily anticipated. There are no trained personnel capable of performing a resuscitation available at the delivery, even though the history of the labor clearly indicates the potential for problems with the infant.

**Lack of Advance Preparation of the Equipment:** Precious time was lost setting up the equipment. For any infant, even for a normal delivery, basic resuscitation equipment should be set up prior to delivery and tested to ensure that it is functional.

**Inappropriate Management of Heat Loss:** The radiant warmer was not preheated. Preheating the warmer reduces conductive heat loss through the cold mattress pad. Because the heater takes some time to reach a maximum output, this is time during which the infant is exposed to excessive convective heat losses in the delivery room without any radiant heat input to compensate for such losses.

To compound the heat loss problem, the infant was not dried; this allowed evaporative heat loss as the amniotic fluid evaporated off the infant's skin.

**Management of Meconium:** Whenever an infant is delivered with thick meconium, especially if the baby is also depressed, it is necessary to perform laryngoscopy on the infant to remove any meconium that might be below the cords. This step was neglected, which left the infant at risk for meconium aspiration syndrome.

**Delayed Action:** The depth of the child's problem was not recognized until the 1-minute Apgar score was given. It was not until after the first Apgar score was given that any attempt at positive pressure resuscitation was made. The delay in providing PPV occurred despite the fact that the infant had only gasping respirations that were insufficient to sustain the heart rate at more than 100 BPM. This was an indication for immediate PPV after removing any residual meconium from the trachea through direct laryngoscopy.

**Inappropriate Actions:** Instead of immediately suctioning the trachea and initiating PPV, the nurse gave the infant tactile stimulation and free-flow oxygen for a prolonged time. PPV was instituted only late in the procedure, and the nurse did not ensure that the trachea was clear of meconium.

**What Should Have Happened:** As soon as the infant was born, he should have been placed on a preheated radiant warmer, a laryngoscope inserted, and any residual meconium removed from the trachea and the upper airway. The infant should have been dried and then evaluated for respiratory effort and heart rate. If the respirations were gasping or insufficient to sustain the heart rate at 100 PBM or more, the infant should have received PPV immediately. In the hands of a skilled team, all of this could have occurred well before 1 minute of life had passed.

---

**CASE STUDY 5 continued**

While waiting for the anesthetist or pediatrician to arrive, the head nurse continues to provide PPV, stopping periodically to assess the status of the infant. The infant continues to be hypotonic and cyanotic with only occasional gasping respirations. The heart rate falls to less than 60 BPM. By 3 minutes of age, the anesthetist arrives, intubates the infant, and provides PPV by means of a bag and an endotracheal tube. The infant appears slightly less cyanotic; however, peripheral perfusion remains poor and the heart rate remains less than 60 BPM. Ventilation continues until the arrival of the pediatrician at 6 minutes of age.

**EXERCISE 13**

---

■ **Question:**

What is the major problem presented in this last scenario and what should have been done?

■ **Answer:**

**Lack of Chest Compression:** Although the nurse and the anesthetist continued to provide PPV, no attempt was made to start chest compression or medications in an infant with a heart rate of less than 60 BPM.

---

**CASE STUDY 5 continued**

At 6 minutes of age, the pediatrician arrives and after assessing the situation inserts an umbilical catheter to just below the skin and injects 20 cc of 4.2% sodium bicarbonate (5 mEq/10 cc) during 1 minute. The infant remains mottled with poor perfusion and has a heart rate of less than 60 BPM. Following another minute of observation, the head nurse begins chest compression and the pediatrician injects 0.5 mL of

1:10,000 epinephrine by means of the umbilical vein.

The sodium bicarbonate and epinephrine are repeated again at about 8 minutes of age. At approximately 9 minutes of age, the heart rate begins to rise, although it is still only about 75 BPM, and there are no spontaneous respirations. By 12 minutes of age, the heart rate rises to 170 BPM and the infant's color begins to improve. By 20 minutes of age, the infant has spontaneous respirations. The endotracheal tube is removed at 23 minutes of age and the infant is transferred to the special care nursery.

## EXERCISE 14

Comment on the recent sequence of events, the appropriateness of the medications, their dosages, and the route of administration.

■ **Discussion:**

**Medications Without Chest Compression:** When the pediatrician arrived, it was appropriate to administer medications; however, he also should have insisted that chest compression be started simultaneously.

**Wrong Sequence of Medications:** The medications were administered in the wrong sequence. Epinephrine should have been the first drug used. Although it was eventually given in the appropriate dosage, time was wasted by inserting an umbilical vein catheter and giving sodium bicarbonate first. The epinephrine could have been given immediately by means of the endotracheal tube.

**Wrong Dose and Administration of Sodium Bicarbonate:** In addition to administering the sodium bicarbonate first, the doctor gave about twice the dose recommended. Furthermore, the rate of administration was very fast. The entire dose was given during 1 minute. It should have been given at a rate of 1 mEq/kg/minute, and it should have taken at least 2 minutes to administer the total dose.

**What Should Have Happened:** When the pediatrician arrived, he should have immediately instituted cardiac massage and given the epinephrine through the endotracheal tube. Then he could have inserted an umbilical vein catheter for administration of a correct dose (2 mEq/kg) of sodium bicarbonate over an appropriate time, about 2 minutes (1 mEq/kg/minute).

Unfortunately, scenarios similar to the one portrayed above occur all too often. However, in the presence of a skilled team of individuals who are available at the delivery, an infant can be resuscitated in a competent and efficient manner, hopefully reducing the chances of permanent brain damage.

# Chapter 2

# COMMONLY ENCOUNTERED FLUID AND ELECTROLYTE PROBLEMS IN THE PRETERM NEWBORN INFANT

*Stephen Baumgart,* M.D.

*Andrew T. Costarino, Jr.,* M.D.

The calculation of fluid and electrolyte requirements in newborn infants has traditionally been based on the concept of daily maintenance water, sodium, and potassium intakes. Historically, the stated goal of maintenance fluid therapy was to maintain an infant's body composition (including serum and urine chemistries) within an acceptable range of variation on a day-to-day basis. The clinical benchmarks of this strategy were the maintenance of body weight within a relatively narrow range each day (±2% to 5%) and the preservation of hydration. Hydration was determined clinically by assessing urine flow and by evaluating the appearance and perfusion of the peripheral capillary beds in the skin and mucous membranes.

To accomplish this objective, the principle of replacing daily urine water and salt losses, combined with accurate estimation and replacement of insensible water loss from the skin and upper respiratory passageways, was developed. However, as more premature babies began to survive, it became apparent that the traditional estimates for water and salt maintenance (i.e., replacement of daily fluid losses) had to be modified based on the degree of each patient's prematurity and the severity of his or her congenital or acquired disorders. Furthermore, numerous studies during the past two decades have suggested that the magnitude of insensible water evaporation from the skin of premature babies (particularly when subjected to phototherapy, nonhumidified incubator environments, and open radiant warmer beds) is truly immense, far exceeding the range of fluid volume prescriptions recommended for treating less ill and larger premature children. Estimating insensible losses has been further complicated by (1) the use of mechanical respirators with humidified gas systems (which may actually supplement water administration by condensation within the respiratory tubing) and (2) attempts to shield infants from excessive transcutaneous evaporation in dry environments by means of a variety of methods (plastic bubble-wrap, thin and transparent plastic sheets, body hoods, and double-walled incubators). Finally, the best estimation of parenteral maintenance or replacement fluid and electrolyte therapy has become even more uncertain with recognition of the *transitional phase in body fluid composition* that occurs on parturition. Recognition of these compositional changes in intracellular, extracellular, and circulating fluid compartments has become increasingly important in determining the correct fluid prescription for the critically ill infant.

In the following sections we present four fluid and electrolyte therapeutic conundrums encountered in the premature nursery. An approach to these problems based on the physiology (and pathology) of hydration is suggested, with the recognition that there may be no single way to solve them. Even though guidelines are presented, you must realize that no one recipe replaces the anticipation of problems and the thoughtful clinician's approach to the management of the premature neonate's fluid and electrolyte replacement needs.

### CASE STUDY 1 *The Premature Infant with Respiratory Distress Syndrome (RDS)*

An 18-year-old woman presents to the hospital emergency room in premature labor with fluid leaking from the vagina. Her previous care has been excellent, and her estimated fetal gestational age (by serial ultrasound determinations) is 29 weeks. She is afebrile, there is no uterine tenderness on examination, and her peripheral white blood cell count is within normal limits. As a precaution, she is hospitalized on strict bed rest and external fetal monitoring is begun. An attempt is made to stop labor with sympathomimetics. Nevertheless, contractions increase in frequency, and during the next 4 hours, labor is allowed to progress.

K.M., a 1,220-g, well-formed, premature male infant is delivered at 6 A.M. and is immediately placed on a radiant warmer bed. The nurse dries the infant and provides oxygen to the baby's face. The pediatrician, now present, assigns Apgar scores of 5 at 1 minute and 6 at 5 minutes with points off for tone, reflex irritability, respiratory effort, and color (which improves with supplemental oxygen). After transfer to the special care nursery, the infant's rectal temperature is noted to be 35.5°C, and he is placed in an incubator set on maximum to rewarm him.

Shortly thereafter, the baby's physical condition worsens. Air entry becomes poor, and he develops grunting, flaring, and chest retractions. Furthermore, the infant is cyanotic in 40% oxygen. A decision is made to transfer the baby to an open radiant warmer bed and to intubate the trachea for respiratory support. Artificial surfactant is administered.

Thereafter, the patient's respirations and color improve and a pulse oximeter indicates that the oxygen saturation is 90%. An umbilical arterial line is placed, and a blood gas sample is sent for analysis. While the nurse places a peripheral intravenous line for fluid administration, a bedside glucose test is taken and demonstrates a blood sugar level of 40 mg/dL.

### EXERCISE 1

#### ■ Questions:

1. What is your most immediate concern regarding the management of this infant's fluids? How should this problem be addressed?

2. What fluid and electrolyte solution would you select for your initial parenteral fluid therapy? At what rate would you administer it?

3. How would you modify your fluid plan during this infant's RDS?

4. What solution would you infuse through the umbilical arterial catheter? At what rate should the solution be infused?

#### ■ Answers:

1. Although the definition of *hypoglycemia* is somewhat controversial, these caretakers need to recognize that 40 mg/dL is a low

serum glucose value for this critically ill infant and that he needs immediate attention. We would recommend an initial infusion of 10% dextrose in water run at a rate of 4 mL/kg/hr (which provides 6.7 mg/kg/min of dextrose). Most newborn infants' blood glucose concentrations will stabilize between 45 and 90 mg/dL 1 to 3 hours postnatally. Although rates of glucose production in preterm infants normally range from 4 to 6 mg/kg/min, an infant who is thermally stressed and in respiratory distress may increase his or her rate of glucose consumption by as much as two to three times (necessitating an increase in the rate of glucose administration). The basal rate of glucose production may be somewhat higher in more mature infants, approaching 8 mg/kg/min near term gestation. The 4 mL/kg/hr infusion of 10% dextrose prescribed provides 6.7 mg/kg/min, which should be sufficient to correct the marginally depressed glucose value within 15 to 30 minutes. Blood sugar levels must be monitored at least every 30 minutes until stabilized, and the rate of dextrose infusion must be increased or decreased by 1 to 2 mL/kg/hr, as appropriate, to maintain a normal glucose concentration.

Bolus administration of dextrose solutions should be avoided in the absence of clinical signs compatible with hypoglycemia. Unfortunately, there is often a feeling of urgency among clinicians that they must acutely correct a low bedside sugar test by administering 200 to 500 mg/kg of dextrose (2 to 5 mL/kg of a 10% solution) as a bolus infusion, without consideration of potential adverse consequences. For example, the rapid administration of large amounts of dextrose in the presence of respiratory insufficiency (particularly hypoxemia) may actually increase the anaerobic production of lactic acid in the brain, and may further compromise the infant's cerebral metabolic status. Moreover, sudden infusions of hyperosmolar volumes directly into the infant's central venous or arterial circulation may potentiate intraventricular hemorrhage. In particular, 25% dextrose infusions should be avoided in this setting. Rather, we would increase the constant dextrose infusion rate by 1 to 2 mL/kg/hr, and repeat the bedside sugar testing every 15 minutes until a concentration of 45 to 90 mg/dL is

achieved in the serum. Thereafter, the concentration and rate of dextrose infusate may be adjusted accordingly.

2. Recommended volumes for parenteral water administration during the first day of life in premature infants range between 65 and 80 mL/kg/day. These recommendations originate from observations made in infants of 32 to 36 weeks' postconceptional age without respiratory distress or the need for mechanical ventilation, while being nurtured in incubators humidified to 50% relative humidity. Our case study infant, however, might be expected to have substantially greater fluid requirements because of a marked increase in insensible water loss, which results from his degree of prematurity and the environment in which he is nursed (under a radiant warmer bed surrounded by cool and dry ambient air).

An infant of this size and gestational age (nursed naked on a radiant warmer bed) would normally be expected to have an insensible water loss of 50 to 75 mL/kg/day (see Fig. 2-4 later in this chapter). Insensible water losses may not be as great for the infant in our case study because he is receiving nearly 100% humidified ventilatory gas through his endotracheal tube. The use of the endotracheal tube would reduce insensible water loss by about 30%. Moreover, we would recommend using a thin and pliable saran plastic blanket placed loosely over this baby (taking care not to obstruct the infant's airway) while he is nursed on an open bed platform and under a radiant heater. This plastic blanket would reduce transcutaneous water evaporation during the first week of life by an additional 30% to 50%, protecting the infant not only from cold air exposure, but also from excessive water evaporation from the immature skin.

Considering the infant's gestational maturity and the physical environment, we would begin fluid volume administration in the ranges prescribed in Figure 2-1 (i.e., between 60 and 80 mL/kg/day, depending on the degree of shielding). Concentrations of dextrose appropriate for the volume of fluid to be infused are shown at the left in Figure 2-1. An example is shown by the interrupted lines. A 1,000-g infant nursed in a conventional incubator should receive 65

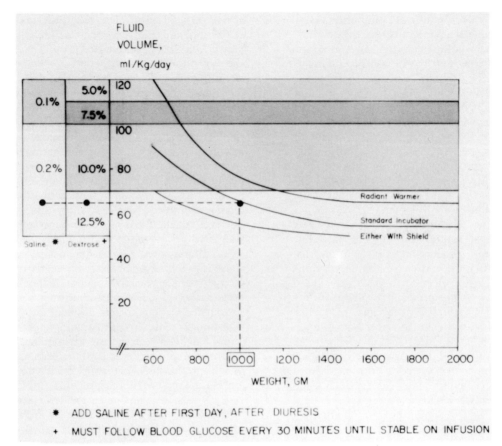

* ADD SALINE AFTER FIRST DAY, AFTER DIURESIS

+ MUST FOLLOW BLOOD GLUCOSE EVERY 30 MINUTES UNTIL STABLE ON INFUSION

**Figure 2-1** Recommendations for starting parenteral fluid therapy during the first day of life in preterm infants. Concentrations of dextrose appropriate for the volume of fluid to be infused are shown at the left. An example is shown by the interrupted lines. A 1,000-g infant nursed in a conventional incubator should receive 65 mL/kg/day of fluid volume. On the left side of this figure, this amount of fluid volume should contain 12.5% dextrose and 0.2% saline. Thereafter, during days 2, 3, and 4, and throughout the first week of life, the volume of this solution administered should be increased only sparingly to maintain clinical hydration. We do not recommend replacement of urine volume routinely or further fluid administration to cover increased but unmeasured insensible water losses (e.g., with phototherapy). Initiation of sodium chloride and potassium chloride may begin after the first day of life; however, in the very low birth weight subject of less than 700 to 800 g, addition of electrolytes should be delayed at least 48 to 72 hours, especially if serum electrolyte abnormalities are observed.

mL/kg/day of fluid volume. On the left side of this figure, this amount of fluid volume should contain 12.5% dextrose and 0.2% saline. Thereafter, during days 2, 3, and 4, and throughout the first week of life, the volume of this solution administered should be increased only sparingly to maintain clinical hydration. We do not recommend replacement of urine volume routinely or further fluid administration to cover increased but unmeasured insensible water losses (e.g., with phototherapy). Initi-

ation of sodium chloride and potassium chloride may begin after the first day of life; however, in the very low birth weight subject of less than 700 to 800 g, addition of electrolytes should be delayed at least 48 to 72 hours, especially if serum electrolyte abnormalities are observed.

3. By day 2 to 3 of life in infants with RDS, a *transitional* diuresis of an excess of extracellular fluid may occur. This diuresis precedes the improvement in lung compliance

and heralds the subsequent resolution of gas exchange abnormalities. (In infants that have received a surfactant preparation, the relationship between the onset of diuresis and the improvement in pulmonary function may not be clear). As Figure 2-2 demonstrates (top of graph), with the onset of diuresis, urine output increases to 80% to 100% of fluid intake. This diuresis is fol-

lowed by a reduction in the alveolar arterial oxygen difference (AaDO$_2$) within 12 to 36 hours. This increase in urine flow is due both to an increase in glomerular filtration and changes in renal tubular reabsorption of water, resulting in the formation of large volumes of urine ($\geq$4 to 6 mL/kg/hr). The composition of this urine is dilute and calculated free water clearances are high (middle of Fig. 2-2); nevertheless, an appreciable sodium diuresis occurs as well (especially late in the diuretic phase).

Concurrent with this diuresis, contraction of the extracellular fluid compartment occurs. Some investigators have advocated the use of furosemide to hasten pulmonary improvement by inducing this diuresis; however, beneficial changes in pulmonary function tests have proven to be both small and transient. We do not recommend routine furosemide therapy for the treatment of RDS.

We have adopted a modified approach toward providing fluid and electrolyte maintenance therapy as applied to premature babies with RDS (bottom of Fig. 2-2). Urine output is typically low during the first 1 to 2 days of this disease, and specific gravities vary widely. During this early *stabilization phase*, the goals of therapy are to establish vascular access, correct and prevent hypoglycemia, and to treat hypovolemic shock, if necessary, with transfusions of blood products or normal saline (10 to 20 mL/kg given during 30 minutes to 2 hours).

During the *restriction/maintenance* phase, which occurs next in the sequence (bottom of Fig. 2-2) and which is associated with the onset of diuresis, we do *not* replace all of the predicted fluid losses. Rather, we anticipate a 10% to 15% reduction in body weight reflecting the contraction of the extracellular fluid space, including the elimination of lung edema. *Fluid infusion rates are generally held constant during this phase.* We believe this conservative approach, which restricts parenteral fluid administration to the least volume required to maintain clinical hydration (i.e., adequate skin perfusion and normal serum and urine chemistries), simplifies fluid management and may prevent later development of pulmonary edema, patent ductus, arteriosus, heart failure, and bronchopulmonary dysplasia.

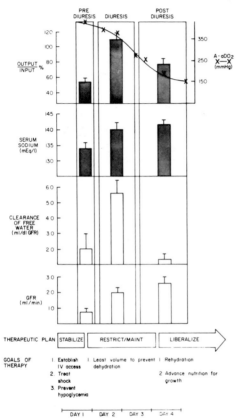

**Figure 2-2** Outline of the clinical course of respiratory distress syndrome (AaDO$_2$, X—X) in conjunction with a diuresis (percent urine output/input fluid volume). A rise in renal filtration (GFR) and serum sodium concentration are observed during the first week of life. Free water clearance appears to constitute the main physiological event during diuresis with improved lung function. Serum sodium concentration usually rises by 3 to 5 mEq/L, and a significant natriuresis occurs as well. At the bottom of this figure a therapeutic schema is presented in three phases: (1) initial stabilization, (2) maintenance with parenteral fluid volume restriction, and (3) careful liberalization of fluid volume administered only after a diuresis has been observed.

From Costarino AT, Baumgart S: Modern fluid and electrolyte management of the critically ill premature infant. *Pediatr Clin North Am* 1986; 33(1):162. Reprinted with permission of W.B. Saunders Company.

During the final phase of fluid management (*liberalization*, bottom of Fig. 2-2), the rate of parenteral fluid administration is increased cautiously as RDS resolves and the baby is weaned from mechanical ventilation. The goal now is to provide parenteral nutrition (70 to 100 kcal/kg/day) in amounts sufficient to induce anabolism and to achieve new tissue growth.

4. Management of the umbilical arterial catheter infusion varies with each nursery. We generally administer 5% dextrose and 0.2% normal saline at an infusion rate of 0.5 to 1 mL/hr in order to maintain catheter patency. We infuse dextrose and amino acids only by peripheral vein or central venous catheter. Most nurseries avoid infusing parenteral nutrition through the arterial site to avoid contamination associated with frequent line interruptions needed for blood gas or other blood sampling. Nevertheless, the volume of fluid infused through this catheter should be tabulated as part of the total parenteral fluid volume administered each day. Similarly, parenteral lipid infusions should be considered part of the total fluid volume administered. Blood removal and blood product administration, as well as medication volumes and line flushes, should also be recorded.

---

**CASE STUDY 1 continued** *Bronchopulmonary Dysplasia (BPD)*

Despite optimal nutritional, fluid, and ventilatory management, this infant develops a symptomatically significant patent ductus arteriosus at 12 days of age and ceases to wean from the mechanical ventilator. He receives three doses of indomethacin and the heart murmur and widened pulse pressures resolve by day 15. Despite the reintroduction of a relative fluid restriction (100 mL/kg/day) during this time to avoid congestive heart failure and pulmonary edema, chest roentgenograms Figure 2-3 demonstrate a hazy appearance of both lung fields consistent with edema accumulation. There is also streaky atelectasis in the upper poles and around the heart shadow. This film is consistent with the early signs of BPD now being observed in this patient.

The baby's oxygen requirement increases and, finally, ventilator settings are increased as well. The infant enters a static phase of his dis-

ease where, despite adequate nutritional support (110 kcal/kg/day), he is unable to wean from the respirator or achieve adequate weight gain (≥15 g/kg/day). Daily urine output volumes vary between 20 and 60 mL/kg/day, while fluid intakes range from 140 to 150 mL/kg/day when transfusions, medications, flushes, and intralipid volumes are totaled with the daily stock solution. Diuretics (usually furosemide) are administered intermittently in response to a diminishing urine output or periods of clinical deterioration manifested by wheezing, rales, and transient hypoxemia. At 21 days of age, the following serum chemistry values are obtained: sodium, 128 mEq/L; chloride, 89 mEq/L; potassium, 3.4 mEq/L; bicarbonate, 28 mEq/L; and serum albumin, 2.4 g/dL.

## EXERCISE 2

### ■ Questions:

1. What is the role of daily fluid administration in the pathogenesis of this infant's BPD?

2. Why is this infant hyponatremic and hypochloremic? Should the electrolyte disturbances be immediately corrected?

3. What is the role of chronic diuretic therapy in BPD?

### ■ Answers:

1. As a consequence of RDS, and often in association with a patent ductus arteriosus, premature babies all too frequently develop the syndrome of BPD. Depending on the severity of illness in a given newborn population, anywhere from 1 in 10 to as many as 1 in 3 infants develop chronic lung disease, the most often recognized complication of RDS. Current definitions of BPD vary. The American Academy of Pediatrics recognizes any premature infant receiving supplemental oxygen at 4 weeks of age as an infant with BPD. Most clinicians, however,

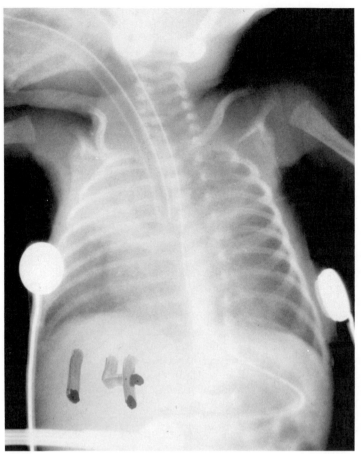

**Figure 2-3**  A chest roentenogram obtained during the second week of life.
Radiograph courtesy of The Children's Hospital of Philadelphia, Department of Radiology, Teaching File.

are satisfied that infants are developing BPD when, following 2 weeks of mechanical ventilation, more than 50% inspired oxygen is required to maintain a normal arterial oxygen concentration. Characteristic radiographic changes of BPD include hazy atelectasis (noted in Fig. 2-3) progressing to the development of cystic areas in both lower lobes and shifting areas of atelectasis in the upper lobes.

Regardless of definition, infants with chronic respiratory failure retain lung water as the result of high pulmonary capillary hydrostatic pressures (due to increased pulmonary vascular resistance) and low capillary oncotic pressures (attributable to low serum and lymphatic protein concentrations). Scarring and distortion of lung anatomy contribute to these physiological disturbances because of the high transpulmonary pressures that occur with both spontaneous and ventilator breaths. These high transpulmonary pressures favor movement of water and albumin out of the intravascular compartment and into the pulmonary interstitium. Administration of colloid-containing fluids may acutely promote the uptake of lung water back into the vascular compartment, but may also result in capillary leakage of albumin, which ultimately draws more crystalloid into the pulmonary interstitium, resulting in worsening lung edema and further decreasing pulmonary compliance. Edema also contributes to the increased airway resistance observed in infants with BPD and may contribute to the paroxysms of wheezing, hypoxemia, and rales commonly referred to as *BPD spells*.

The increased work of breathing and cardiac work associated with BPD, and treatment with theophylline or sympathomimetic bronchodilators, may increase the caloric requirement for growth in BPD patients. The clinician is thereby forced to increase the volume of fluid administration to meet caloric needs. Poor nutrition can lead to hypoalbuminemia and decreased capillary integrity, completing the picture of the edematous infant with chronic lung disease.

Controversy surrounds whether a high fluid volume intake, failure to generate a transitional diuresis during the early phase of RDS, a clinically symptomatic PDA, or all three promote the development of BPD. Similarly, the treatments of these conditions with fluid restriction (and therefore caloric restriction) and the use of diuretic therapy in the early phases of BPD as preventive measures are speculative. The incidence and duration of the disease seems unaltered by these therapeutic attempts, but its day-to-day severity and BPD spells may be ameliorated. We believe that short of massive fluid overload (150 to 200 mL/kg/day), exogenous water administration is probably *not* a primary factor in the early pathogenesis of BPD.

2. Analyzing daily or even weekly serum electrolytes in BPD patients is a frustrating exercise if daily sodium and water balances and appropriate renal function studies (e.g., fractional excretion of sodium) are not also routinely recorded. Clinicians are often left blindly responding to serum chemistry values that do not quite fit the laboratory's normal ranges. The role of aldosterone, arginine vasopressin, and atrial natriuretic factor in modulating water homeostasis in BPD varies among patients, and further research is required to define the role of these hormone modulators in the pathogenesis of electrolyte disturbances in BPD infants.

Chronic respiratory acidemia may contribute to bicarbonate retention and chloride wasting from the distal tubule of the kidney in these infants. This is particularly true in the underventilated patient with arterial $CO_2$ tensions greater than 50 to 55 mm Hg. Furthermore, it is not uncommon for BPD infants to be maintained chronically and mildly hypoxemic (50 to 55 mm Hg arterial oxygen tension) and hypercarbic (50 mm Hg arterial carbon dioxide tension) in order to minimize ventilatory requirements and decrease the risk of barotrauma. Hypochloremia and metabolic alkalemia, therefore, have become persistent components of this disease. Liberal use of systemic and inhalant bronchodilators in these patients may favorably alter the bicarbonate, chloride, and potassium exchange in the kidney by treating respiratory acidemia. However, these agents also permit weaning from high ventilator settings and theoretically minimize barotrauma. The clinician, therefore, chooses the optimal $PaCO_2$ for each patient and, in turn, "creates" the electrolyte disturbance.

Finally, the well-intentioned use of sodium restriction and the intermittent application of diuretics to minimize the complications of accumulated pulmonary edema may conspire to promote renal tubular wasting of sodium, potassium, and chloride. Hypotonic formulas used to ameliorate enteral feeding intolerances during periods of respiratory compromise may also inadvertently restrict salt intakes. As infants grow (even if slowly), new tissue formation requires that sodium and potassium occupy the newly formed extracellular and intracellular water volumes, respectively.

A sodium intake that is sufficient to compensate for salt losses and that meets the increment needed for growth should range between 3 and 4 mEq/kg/day (total enteral plus parenteral intake). The amounts of supplemental chloride and potassium needed to compensate for renal tubular wastage engendered by the use of intermittent diuretics is at best guesswork: 1 to 2 mEq/kg/day of potassium chloride (doubled if necessary) is where we generally begin. Serum chemistries are then monitored on a daily basis. We try to avoid administering sodium chloride (to replace chloride deficits) because diuretics are used first to eliminate excess sodium. We also avoid using ammonium chloride or hydrochloric acid because chronic acidemia is considered part of the pathophysiology of growth failure in this disease. A modest water restriction (120 to 130 mL/kg/day) seems warranted because at least some of the cause for the hyponatremia in infants with BPD is water overload in excess of the sodium overload and chloride depletion.

Our approach to BPD therapy is to establish priorities. The most important of these is the provision of adequate nutrition within a predetermined restricted fluid volume intake limit. Many of these infants will demonstrate an increased metabolic rate because of their underlying lung disease. Therefore, the use of calorically dense substrates to meet the increased metabolic needs in these infants (130 to 150 kcal/kg/day) is often necessary. Various calorically dense premature formulations are available and under intense investigation for the enteral management of the BPD patient. These formulas are augmented with glucose polymers, medium chain triglycerides, or long chain fats. The decision to use calorically dense parenteral mixtures of dextrose (20%), amino acids (3%), and lipid supplements (20%) may require the placement of a central venous line.

Normalization of serum electrolyte concentrations in severe BPD infants may be nearly impossible. Therefore, wider ranges of variation (serum sodium value ≥ 125 mEq/L) are frequently tolerated in the serum electrolyte profile. The consequences of chronic aberrations in electrolytes are largely unknown. In this case, the sodium concentration of 128 mEq/L would be acceptable.

3. The use of diuretic therapy to treat infants with BPD has become a standard part of the management plan. Unfortunately, chronic diuretic therapy results in myriad complications, including chloride, sodium, and potassium depletion; dehydration (with overdose); and urinary wasting of calcium and phosphate (resulting in bone demineralization and renal calculus formation). These complications have been most often associated with furosemide therapy. Furosemide is a widely used diuretic because it enhances free water clearance even more substantially in the neonate than in adult subjects. However, its pharmacokinetic half-life is significantly longer than in adults and its diuretic duration is similarly extended.

We advocate the use of chronic diuretic therapy with a combination of chlorothiazide and spironolactone in infants with chronic lung conditions. These two agents have proven as successful as furosemide therapy in improving lung mechanics acutely. We consider diuretic therapy with these drugs (supplemented with an occasional rescue dose of furosemide during BPD spells) as reasonable adjunctive therapy in BPD infants. Once or twice a week, scrutiny of serum electrolytes, bimonthly assessments of bone mineralization (by roentgenograms and alkaline phosphatase assays), and periodic renal ultrasound determinations to anticipate the formation of microcalcifications should become a routine part of the care of these patients. Furosemide is sometimes advocated every other day in the infant who cannot tolerate enteral medications, and it may avoid or delay the complications associated with its use.

## CASE STUDY 2 *The Very Low Birth Weight, Very Premature Infant*

A 25-year-old multiparous woman with a history of multiple, spontaneous, second-trimester abortions presents to the emergency ward in premature labor and precipitously delivers a 25-week-gestation female infant weighing 660 g. The infant, J.C., is vigorous at birth with spontaneous respirations and heartbeat. She is placed under a radiant heater and administered 100% oxygen by a cannula placed a few centimeters from the nares. The Apgar scores are 7 at 1 minute and 8 at 5 minutes. As the baby is warmed and gently dried, the oxygen is slowly withdrawn, revealing a pink and well-perfused infant.

The pediatrician, after arriving and talking briefly with both parents in the emergency ward, discovers that this is a much-wanted child, but given the previous loss of one such potentially viable infant, they are reluctant to consent to a prolonged course of mechanical ventilation. They request that parenteral fluids and warmth be provided and state that other life support measures (including mechanical ventilation for apnea) may be offered, but only after their consent is given.

Emergency transport to the intensive care nursery is accomplished using a prewarmed incubator with a saran blanket placed loosely over the infant's abdomen and lower extremities. The chest and head are left uncovered so that vital signs and spontaneous respirations can be evaluated. The infant remains in good condition and is placed under a radiant warmer on an open bed platform for further evaluation and therapy. The saran blanket is left in place. The infant's body temperature is 36°C (axillary) and other vital signs are considered normal. An umbilical arterial catheter is inserted and positioned below the fourth lumbar vertebra. A chest roentgenogram demonstrates clear lung fields and normal bony anatomy. Physical examination reveals that the skin is gelatinous and transparent; blood vessels and viscera are visible through the abdominal wall. A bedside glucose test is normal. The long hospital course begins as the baby becomes apneic for the first time and mechanical ventilation is begun. Initial blood gas values, serum chemistries, and hematology values are all normal.

### EXERCISE 3

#### ■ Questions:

1. What is the magnitude of this infant's expected insensible water loss?

2. What are the expected consequences of the large insensible water losses from this infant during the first 24 to 48 hours of life?

3. What quantities of fluid volume and electrolytes should this infant receive during the first 24 to 48 hours of life?

#### ■ Answers:

1. As shown in Table 2-1, the body surface area of this particular infant relative to body mass is nearly six times the adult's, and geometrically larger than the infant described in Case Study 1. Figure 2-4 demonstrates that insensible water loss for infants

**Table 2-1** Body Surface Area to Body Mass Ratio

| BODY MASS | BODY SURFACE AREA | SURFACE AREA‡ MASS RATIO |
|---|---|---|
| 70-kg adult | 1.73 m² | 250 cm²/kg |
| 1.5-kg premature | 0.13 m² | 870 cm²/kg |
| 0.5-kg micropremature | 0.07 m² | 1,400 cm²/kg |

‡ Body surface area to body mass ratio is represented for standard adult values and compared to premature babies weighing 1.5 to 0.5 kg at birth. Body surface area for premature infants was calculated from the weight and length formula of Haycock, Schwartz, and Wisotsky.[74] The higher relative proportion of neonatal body weight comprised of water is demonstrated in Figure 2-7 and the immaturity of the very premature infant's skin as a barrier to insensible water evaporation is described in the text. These comprise the three major factors contributing to the geometrically higher insensible water loss from very premature infants when compared to more mature babies.

in this weight range (during the first week of life) can be as much as 170 mL/kg/day when nursed on an open radiant warmer bed *without* a saran blanket. Figure 2-5 illustrates similar data from Scandinavia for infants nursed in conventional, convec-

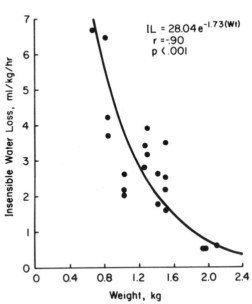

$$IL = 28.04 e^{-1.73(Wt)}$$
$$r = -.90$$
$$p < .001$$

**Figure 2-4** Insensible water loss increases with decreasing body weight in premature infants nursed under radiant warmers.
Reprinted with permission from Baumgart S, Langman CB, Sosulski R, et al: Fluid, electrolyte and glucose maintenance in the very low birthweight infant. *Clin Pediatr* 1982; 21:199.

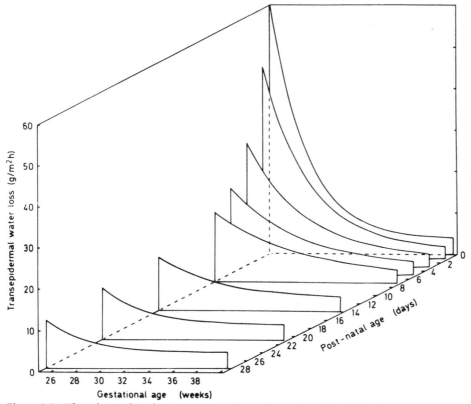

**Figure 2-5** The relationships between transepidermal water loss (g/m²/hr), the gestational age at birth, and increasing postnatal ages. Note the geometrically higher levels of insensible water loss in small premature infants, early in life.

From Hammerlund K, Sedin G, Stromberg B: Measurements of transepidermal water loss in newborn infants. *Acta Paediatr Scand* 1983; 72:723. Reprinted with permission of the Scandinavian University Press.

tively heated, modestly humidified incubators. Of note is that the magnitude of insensible water loss is similar under both sets of environmental conditions during the first day of life. These water losses occur free of sodium and chloride, and are derived from the interstitial fluid nearest the immature epidermal layer of the infant's skin, which is thin and poorly cornified.

2. Many of these very tiny infants demonstrate an acute dehydration syndrome during the first 24 to 48 hours of life. The syndrome is characterized by hypernatremia and hyperkalemia (and often by hypocalcemia and hyperglycemia). This syndrome occurs, however, without systemic blood pressure deterioration, oliguria, acidemia, or markedly abnormal renal function studies. Indeed, clinical perfusion of the skin of these infants usually is acceptable, blood pressure tracings on bedside monitors are

brisk, and urine flow rates are adequate (2 to 4 mL/kg/hr). Nevertheless, serum sodium concentrations commonly range between 150 and 160 mEq/L and serum potassium concentrations commonly exceed 6 mEq/L. Furthermore, hyperkalemia (≥7.0 mEq/L) even in the absence of acidemia may cause life-threatening dysrhythmias in these infants and should be treated aggressively. When hyperglycemia develops, it can usually be managed by decreasing the concentration of dextrose in parenteral fluid solutions.

3. Parenteral fluid and electrolyte management in these tiny babies is particularly critical during the first 24 to 48 hours of life to prevent the hyperosmolar, hypernatremic state described previously. As shown in Figure 2-6, the routine use of standard fluid and electrolyte solutions (10% dextrose and 0.2% normal saline),

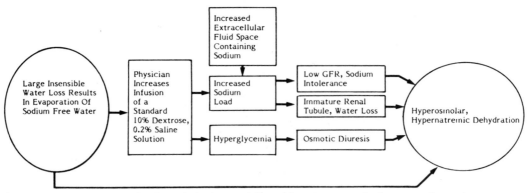

**Figure 2-6** Consequences of early underhydration followed by relative overhydration with a sodium overload in the very low birth weight preterm baby less than 800 g.

when infused at high rates, will increase the risk of hypernatremia and other fluid and salt overload-related complications. Water volume intakes in the range of 150 to 250 mL/kg/day are frequently needed to prevent dehydration and place these infants at increased risk to develop patent ductus arteriosus, congestive heart failure, and pulmonary edema (all of which may be important in the pathogenesis of BPD). If 0.2% normal saline is added routinely on the second day of life and infused at a rate approximating 200 mL/kg/day (providing 6.0 mEq/

kg/day to the infant in this case), salt overloading may occur—adding iatrogenic insult to this tenuous situation. Similarly, dextrose overloading and hyperglycemia (>180 mg/dL) may occur if 10% dextrose is routinely administered.

As shown in Figure 2-6 and dramatically indicated in Figure 2-7, the body fluid composition of these very low birth weight infants approximates that of fetal life (i.e., the body weight is comprised mainly of extracellular, salinated water). As the transition to extrauterine life occurs, this excess of

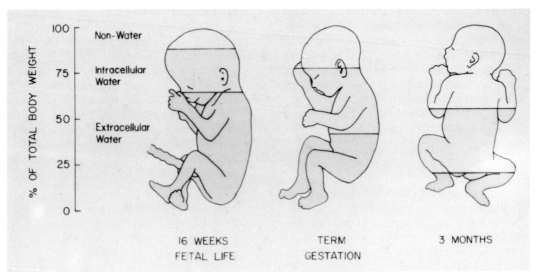

**Figure 2-7** Changes in the composition of body fluids occurring during normal fetal and neonatal development.
From Costarino AT, Baumgart S: Modern fluid and electrolyte management of the critically ill premature infant. *Pediatr Clin North Am* 1986; 33(1):156. Reprinted with permission of W.B. Saunders Company.

extracellular fluid is subject to the same transitional volume and salt diuresis observed in the more mature premature baby described in Case Study 1. This is probably why circulatory function is maintained despite the massive loss of water transcutaneously.

Our approach to fluid therapy in these infants is to first minimize the dehydration that occurs through the immature skin. Regular use of the saran blanket will decrease insensible water loss by 30% to 50%, simplifying the problem of intravascular replacement of large volumes of fluid. Many Europeans manage these infants in humidified incubators (50% to 80% relative humidity), which also reduces transcutaneous evaporation. This practice is usually limited only to the first week of life because bacterial infections in humidified environments may occur more frequently.

During the first 24 to 72 hours of life, we administer parenterally only the minimum volume of electrolyte free water (i.e., *no sodium, potassium, or chloride*) necessary to maintain serum sodium concentrations in a high-normal range (<150 mEq/L). We begin volume administration with 5% to 10% dextrose in water at the rates demonstrated in Fig. 2-2 (70 to 90 mL/kg/day). For tiny infants under radiant warmers, the saran shielding may be disturbed frequently during the infant's initial stabilization period and, therefore, may be less effective initially in reducing insensible water loss. Consequently, this volume may eventually prove too little. However, because serum electrolytes are assessed every 6 to 8 hours in these infants, the rate of water volume administration may be increased by 10 to 20 mL/kg/day as needed. Careful attention must be paid to umbilical line infusions because 1.0 mL/hr to maintain arterial line patency results in the delivery of 36 mL/kg/day in such low birth weight babies.

Only after the serum sodium concentration returns to a normal range (usually after 3 to 5 days) is salt supplementation considered appropriate for these babies. Notably, during this time, the fractional excretion of sodium is extraordinarily high and may exceed 10% of filtered sodium. Although it is relatively easy to restrict the amount of sodium provided by parenteral electrolyte solutions, it is important to remember that sodium (0.5 to 2.0 mEq/kg/day) is often given inadvertently during the early days of life as sodium bicarbonate, as sodium citrated blood product transfusions, as sodium ampicillin, or as sodium heparin. Therefore, carefully limiting *total* sodium administration to less than 3 mEq/kg/day is prudent, but may be very difficult during the first week of life in such patients.

Intravenous alimentation should begin with the first efforts to stabilize this infant's serum chemistries and body composition. As noted previously, however, many of these tiny infants will become hyperglycemic when they are administered sugar solutions containing standard amounts of dextrose (5% to 10%). Some preliminary investigations are now suggesting that the use of insulin infusions may augment glucose tolerance in these infants. Further research is clearly necessary before this strategy to promote early positive nutritional balance is routinely advocated.

---

**CASE STUDY 2 continued** *The Growing Premature Infant with Hyponatremia*

After several weeks in the intensive care nursery, mechanical ventilation is successfully discontinued. Enteral feedings have been advanced to meet the infant's nutritional requirements (weight gain of 15 to 20 g/kg/day), and she is transferred to a transitional care nursery where feeding, growing, and weaning from the incubator become the primary therapeutic goals. At age 5 weeks, a routine weekly set of serum chemistry studies unexpectedly reveals a mild to moderate hyponatremia (124 to 128 mEq/L).

### EXERCISE 4

---

#### ■ Questions:

1. Why is hyponatremia occurring at this postnatal age?

2. How should this electrolyte disturbance be managed?

## ■ Answers:

1. The pathogenesis of *late hyponatremia of prematurity* is incompletely understood. It may be in part attributable to our tendency to restrict the sodium intake and administer diuretics and theophylline to infants recovering from BPD. Late hyponatremia of prematurity does not necessarily result from a relative water excess. Therefore, this infant should not be water restricted. Rather, the infant's rapid growth at this stage of life, her need for expansion of the extracellular and intracellular compartments in association with developmental changes in renal tubular function, and a limited sodium intake (particularly in infants fed nonsupplemented human milk) all contribute to the development of this syndrome.

    Sodium balance studies have demonstrated that most of these infants exhibit a slightly positive sodium balance. Glomerular filtration and urinary flow are normal, and the fractional excretion of sodium is appropriate for the stage of renal development. Distal tubular solute delivery is high and free water excretion by the renal tubule is generally low. Renin and aldosterone levels are commonly high; however, distal tubular insensitivity to aldosterone may result in a relatively high and inappropriate sodium loss in the urine. Furthermore, diminished hematocrit values and a low oncotic pressure (due to a low serum albumin concentration) will tend to decrease proximal renal tubular resorption of sodium.

2. Infants with late hyponatremia of prematurity demonstrate a slightly positive sodium balance, which is insufficient to meet the demands of new tissue growth. Infants incorporate sodium into new tissue formation at a rate of 1.2 mEq/kg/day. The growing preterm infant's sodium balance (sodium intake minus urine and stool output) must include this amount of sodium in excess of basal requirements. Salt supplementation should be provided, therefore, when this entity has been identified and water overload is ruled out as a possible etiology. If the preterm infant is receiving human milk, it is appropriate to add a fortifier containing extra sodium. Formulas designed for preterm infants already contain supplemental amounts of sodium. After an evaluation of sodium balance has been undertaken, 1 to 2 mEq/kg/day of additional sodium chloride may then be added to the diet. Thereafter, careful titration of salt supplements upward by 1 mEq/kg/day increments may be considered.

## CLINICAL SUMMARY

Recommendations for fluid therapy in low birth weight neonates have been summarized in the figures within this chapter, particularly Figures 2-1 and 2-2. We believe the most important lesson in this chapter is the need for continuing reassessment of fluid and electrolyte balance accompanied by frequent adjustments of the rate of fluid administration and the concentrations of parenterally administered sodium and glucose.

During the acute phase of hospitalization, indices that should be carefully monitored each 6 to 8 hours include net fluid intake and urine volume output, body weight, urine specific gravity, urine tests for glucose, and serum glucose, sodium, and potassium concentrations. Fluids should be liberalized after the first few days of life by 1 to 2 mL/hr to maintain urine flow at ≥0.5 mL/kg/hr, and urine specific gravity between 1.012 and 1.016, and to maximize nutrition. We hasten to add that urine specific gravity and output may not be reliable indicators of the infant's hydration status during the first week of life. An increase in serum sodium of 10 mEq/L in a 24-hour period suggests fluid dehydration or sodium overload. Serial body weights do not usually reflect the degree of hydration during the short term, but may be useful in predicting trends during the first week of life: A 10% to 20% weight loss is commonly observed during this time. Additionally, we now assess serum and urine creatinine and sodium concentrations to calculate the fractional excretion of sodium and sodium balance in tiny premature infants.

As clinicians, we are faced with the dilemma of how much fluid and salt to provide to the premature infant with respiratory disease. To prevent pulmonary capillary interstitial leak and pulmonary edema, infants should be relatively fluid restricted. Conversely, to maintain cardiac output, to sustain caloric intake, and to provide adequate systemic perfusion, these patients require fluid volume.

Finding the proper balance between dehydration and fluid overload requires considerable clinical acumen and is the key to managing these infants successfully.

## BIBLIOGRAPHY

1. Winters RW: Maintenance fluid therapy. In Winters RW, ed: *The Body Fluids in Pediatrics.* Boston, Little, Brown and Co, 1973, pp. 113–133.
2. Holliday MA, Segar WE: Maintenance need for water in parenteral fluid therapy. *Pediatrics* 1957; 19:823.
3. Avery ME, Fletcher BD, Williams RG: *The Lung and Its Disorders in the Newborn Infant,* 4th ed. Philadelphia, WB Saunders Co, 1981, pp. 222–241.
4. Cornblath M, Forbes AE, Pildes RS, et al: A controlled study of early fluid administration on survival of low birthweight infants. *Pediatrics* 1966; 38:547.
5. Usher R: Treatment of respiratory distress syndrome. In Winters RW, ed: *The Body Fluids in Pediatrics.* Boston, Little, Brown and Co, 1973, pp. 303–337.
6. Bell EF, Warburton D, Stonestreet BS, et al: Effect of fluid administration on the development of symptomatic patent ductus arteriosus and congestive heart failure in premature infants. *N Engl J Med* 1980; 302:598.
7. Fanaroff AA, Wald M, Gruber HS, et al: Insensible water loss in low birthweight infants. *Pediatrics* 1972; 50:236.
8. Wu PYK, Hodgman JE: Insensible water loss in preterm infants: Changes with postnatal development and non-ionizing radiant energy. *Pediatrics* 1974; 54:704.
9. Williams PR, Oh W: Effects of radiant warmer on insensible water loss in newborn infants. *Am J Dis Child* 1971; 128:311.
10. Bell EF, Weinstein MR, Oh W: Heat balance in premature infants: Comparative effects of convectively heated incubator and radiant warmer with and without plastic heat shield. *J Pediatr* 1980; 96:460.
11. Baumgart S, Engle WD, Fox WW, et al: Radiant warmer power and body size as determinants of insensible water loss in the critically ill neonate. *Pediatr Res* 1981; 15:1495.
12. Sosulski R, Baumgart S: Respiratory water loss and heat balance in intubated premature infants receiving humidified air. *J Pediatr* 1983; 103:307.
13. Marks KH, Lee GA, Bolan CD Jr, et al: Oxygen consumption and temperature control of premature infants in a double-walled incubator. *Pediatrics* 1981; 68:93.
14. Baumgart S: Reduction of oxygen consumption, insensible water loss and radiant heat demand with use of a plastic blanket for low birthweight infants under radiant warmers. *Pediatrics* 1984; 74:1022.
15. Baumgart S, Fox WW, Polin RA: Physiologic implications of two different heat shields for infants under radiant warmers. *J Pediatr* 1982; 100:787.
16. Beard AG, Panos TC, Burroughs JC, et al: Perinatal stress and the premature neonate. I. Effect of fluid and calorie deprivation. *J Pediatr* 1963; 63:361.
17. Cassady G: Effect of caesarean section on neonatal body water spaces. *N Engl J Med* 1971; 285:887
18. Lorenz JM, Kleinman LI, Kotagal UR: Water balance in very low birthweight infants: Relationship to water and sodium intake and effect on outcome. *J Pediatr* 1982; 101:423.
19. MacLaurin JC: Changes in body water distribution during the first two weeks of life. *Arch Dis Child* 1966; 41:286.
20. Martin RJ, Fanaroff AA, Shalme MB: The respiratory distress syndrome and its management. Part 3 of the respiratory system. In Fanaroff AA, Martin RJ, eds: *Behrman's Neonatal-Perinatal Medicine.* St. Louis, CV Mosby Co, 1983, pp. 427–443.
21. Bland RD: Edema formation in the newborn lung. *Clin Perinatol* 1982; 9:593.
22. Jefferies AL, Coates G, O'Brodovich H: Pulmonary epithelial permeability in hyaline membrane disease. *N Engl J Med* 1984; 311:1075.
23. Lauweryns JM, Claessens S, Boussauw L: The pulmonary lymphatics in neonatal hyaline membrane disease. *Pediatrics* 1968; 41:917.
24. Moylan FMB, O'Connell KC, Todres TD, Shannon DC: Edema of the pulmonary interstitium in infants and children. *Pediatrics* 1975; 55:783.
25. Miranda LEV, Dweck HS: Perinatal glucose homeostasis: The unique character of hyperglycemia and hypoglycemia in infants of very low birthweight. *Clin Perinatol* 1977; 4:351.
26. Dweck HS, Cassady G: Glucose intolerance in infants of very low birthweight. *Pediatrics* 1974; 53:189.
27. Lilien LD, Rosenfeld RL, Baccaro MM, et al: Hyperglycemia in stressed small premature neonates. *J Pediatr* 1979; 94:454.
28. Stonestreet BS, Rubin L, Pollak A, et al: Renal functions of low birthweight infants with hyperglycemia and glucosuria produced by glucose infusions. *Pediatrics* 1980; 66:561.
29. Yang W, Segal S: 6,6-D,D-glucose labelled half-life determination in the human newborn. Personal communication. 1981
30. Vannucci RC, Yannucci KJ: Cerebral carbohydrate metabolism during hypoglycemia and anoxia in newborn rats. *Ann Neurol* 1978; 4:73.
31. Volpe JJ: *Neurology of the Newborn.* Philadelphia, WB Saunders Co, 1981.
32. Meyers RE, Yamaguchi S: Nervous system effects of cardiac arrest in monkeys. *Arch Neurol* 1977; 34:65.
33. Meyers RE: Anoxic brain pathology and blood glucose. *Neurology* 1976; 26:345.
34. Simmons MA, Adcock EW, Bard H, et al: Hypernatremia and intracranial hemorrhage in neonates. *N Engl J Med* 1974; 291:6.
35. Lauweryns JM, Claessens S, Boussauw L: The pulmonary lymphatics in neonatal hyaline membrane disease. *Pediatrics* 1968; 41:917.
36. Bhat R, Javed S, Malalis L, et al: Colloid osmotic

pressure in healthy and sick neonates. *Crit Care Med* 1981; 9:563.

37. Sola A, Gregory GA: Colloid osmotic pressure of normal newborns and premature infants. *Crit Care Med* 1981; 9:568.

38. Jefferies AL, Coates G, O'Brodovich H: Pulmonary epithelial permeability in hyaline membrane disease. *N Engl J Med* 1984; 31:1075.

39. Costarino AT, Baumgart S, Normal ME, et al: Renal adaptation to extrauterine life in patients with respiratory distress syndrome. *Am J Dis Child* 1985; 139:1060.

40. Rees L, Shaw JCL, Brook GD, et al: Hyponatremia in the first week of life in preterm infants. Part II: Sodium and water balance. *Arch Dis Child* 1984; 59:423.

41. Sinclair JC: Metabolic rate and temperature control. In Smith CA, Nelson NM, eds: *The Physiology of the Newborn Infant,* 4th ed. Springfield, IL, Charles C Thomas, 1976, pp. 354–415.

42. Northway WH, Rosan RC, Porter DY: Pulmonary disease following respiratory therapy of hyaline membrane disease. *N Engl J Med* 1967; 276:357.

43. Corbet A, Adams J: Current therapy in hyaline membrane disease. *Clin Perinatol* 1978; 5:299.

44. Kurzner S, Garg M, Bautista B, et al: Growth failure in bronchopulmonary dysplasia: Elevated metabolic rates and pulmonary mechanics. *J Pediatr* 1988; 112:73.

45. Wiriyathian S, Rosenfeld CR, Arant BS, et al: Urinary arginine vasopressin: Pattern of excretion in the neonatal period. *Pediatr Res* 1986; 20:103.

46. Rees L, Forsling ML, Brook CGD: Vasopressin concentrations in the neonatal period. *Clin Endocrinol* 1980; 12:357.

47. Leslie GI, Philips JB, Work J, et al: The effect of assisted ventilation on creatinine clearance and hormonal control of electrolyte balance in very low birthweight infants. *Pediatr Res* 1986; 20:447.

48. Tulassay T, Rascher W, Seyberth HW, et al: The role of atrial natriuretic peptide in sodium homeostasis in premature infants. *J Pediatr* 1986; 109:1023.

49. Findberg L: Furosemide—uses and abuses and unsolved puzzles. *Am J Dis Child* 1983; 137:1145.

50. Kao LC, Warburton D, Cheng MH, et al: Effect of oral diuretics on pulmonary mechanics in infants with chronic bronchopulmonary dysplasia. Results of a double-blind crossover sequential trial. *Pediatrics* 1984; 74:37.

51. Kao LC, Warburton D, Sargent CW, et al: Diuretics decrease airways resistance in chronic bronchopulmonary dysplasia. *J Pediatr* 1983; 103:624.

52. McCann EM, Lewis K, Deming DD, et al: Controlled trial of furosemide therapy in infants with chronic lung disease. *J Pediatr* 1985; 106:957.

53. Sniderman C, Clyman RI, Chang M, et al: Treatment of neonatal chronic lung disease with furosemide. *Pediatr Res* 1981; 15:682.

54. Surghol N, McMilan DD, Rademaker AW: Furo-semide improves lung compliance in infants with bronchopulmonary dysplasia. *Pediatr Res* 1983; 17:336A.

55. Tapia JL, Cerhardt T, Goldberg RN, et al: Furosemide and lung function in neonates with chronic lung disease. *Pediatr Res* 1983; 17: 338A.

56. Baumgart S, Langman CB, Sosulski R, et al: Fluid, electrolyte and glucose maintenance in the very low birthweight infant. *Clin Pediatr* 1982; 21:199.

57. Sedin G, Hammarlund K, Nilsson GE, et al: Measurements of transepidermal water loss in newborn infants. *Clin Perinatol* 1985; 12:79.

58. Gruskay J, Costarino AT, Polin RA, et al: Nonoliguric hyperkalemia in the premature infant weighing less than 1000 grams. *J Pediatr* 1988; 113:381.

59. Costarino AT, Gruskay JA, Corcoran L, et al: Sodium restriction vs. daily maintenance replacement in very low birthweight premature neonates, a randomized and blinded therapeutic trial. *J Pediatr* 1992; 120:99–106.

60. Costarino AT, Baumgart S: Modern fluid and electrolyte management of the critically ill premature infant. *Pediatr Clin North Am* 1986; 33:153.

61. Harpin A, Rutter N: Humidification of incubators. *Arch Dis Child* 1985; 60:219.

62. Day RL, Radde IC, Balfe JW, et al: Electrolyte abnormalities in very low birthweight infants. *Pediatr Res* 1976; 10:522.

63. Sulyok E: The relationship between electrolyte and acid base balance in premature infants during early postnatal life. *Biol Neonate* 1971; 95:227.

64. Honour JW, Shackleton CHL, Valman HB: Sodium homeostasis in preterm infants. *Lancet* 1974; 2:1147.

65. Gouyon JB, Guignard JP: Renal effects of theophylline and caffeine in newborn rabbits. *Pediatr Res* 1987; 21:615.

66. Sulyok E, Nemeth M, Teny IF, et al: Relationship between maturity, electrolyte balance, and the function of renin-angiotension-aldosterone system in newborn infants. *Biol Neonate* 1979; 35:60.

67. Kovacs L, Sulyok E, Lichardus B, et al: Renal responses to arginine vasopressin in premature infants with late hyponatremia. *Arch Dis Child* 1986; 61:1030.

68. Sulyok E, Kovacs L, Lichardus B, et al: Late hyponatremia in premature infants: Role of aldosterone and arginine vasopressin. *J Pediatr* 1985; 106:990.

69. Rees L, Brook GD, Shaw JCL, Forsling ML: Hyponatremia in the first week of life in preterm infants. Part I: Arginine vasopressin secretion. *Arch Dis Child* 1984; 59:414.

70. Leake RD, Trygstad CW: Glomerular filtration rate during the period of adaptation to extrauterine life. *Pediatr Res* 1977; 11:959.

71. Gruskin AB, Edelman CM Jr, Yuan S: Maturational changes in renal blood flow in piglets. *Pediatr Res* 1970; 4:7.

72. Strauss J: Fluid and electrolyte composition of

the fetus and newborn. *Pediatr Clin North Am* 1966; 13:1077.

73. Arant BS: Adaptation of the infant to an external milieu. In Gruskin AB, Norman ME, eds: *Pediatric Nephrology. Proceedings of the Fifth International Pediatric Nephrology Symposium 1980.* The Hague, Martinus Nijhoff, 1981, pp. 265–272.

74. Haycock GB, Schwartz GJ, Wisotsky DH: Geometric method for measuring body surface areas: A height-weight formula validated in infants, children and adults. *J Pediatr* 1978; 93:62.

# Chapter 3

# NORMAL AND ALTERED MINERAL BALANCE IN THE NEONATE

## *Patricia Neal,* M.D.

The purpose of this chapter is to review normal calcium, phosphorus, and magnesium physiology in term and low birth weight infants and to present several common problems that may be encountered involving the metabolism of these minerals. Disturbed calcium, phosphorus, and magnesium homeostasis may result from genetic or developmental disorders in the neonate or reflect an abnormal intrauterine environment. Patients may present with or without significant clinical symptoms. Abnormal serum mineral concentrations frequently alert the clinicians to problems in mineral balance. However, remember that serum levels reflect a single point in a complex homeostatic process involving serum proteins, several hormones, dietary intake, and other minerals. Furthermore, because serum concentrations represent only a small amount of the total mineral pool, significant variations in total body mineral concentrations and mineral balance may occur with little or no alterations in serum levels. Critical to optimizing mineral balance and defining the etiology of abnormalities in this patient population is a basic understanding of normal mineral physiology and nutritional requirements. In addition, an understanding of alterations in mineral balance in high risk neonates, for example, the neonate receiving diuretics or the low birth weight infant, allows dietary manipulations or closer surveillance to prevent or minimize problems days, weeks, or months later.

This chapter reviews the clinical presentation, course, and therapeutic interventions for neonates who present with common problems of altered calcium, phosphorus, and magnesium balance. Case presentations are provided, questions are asked, and the answers that follow are indicated in italics. A discussion of the material is included in the answer or may precede the case presentations in some instances.

## EARLY NEONATAL HYPOCALCEMIA

As you read these case histories, try to decide whether the serum calcium values listed are acceptable. What is the range of normal serum values at birth?

### CASE STUDY 1

Baby girl M (BGM) was born to a 37-year-old multiparous female at 32 to 33 weeks' gestation after a pregnancy that was unremarkable until the onset of preterm labor. Drugs to inhibit labor (tocolytics) and antibiotics were given to the mother; however, labor progressed and BGM was born vaginally. Apgar scores were 9 and 9 at 1 and 5 minutes, respectively. Her birth weight was 1,660 g. Because of her prematurity and small size, she was admitted to the neonatal intensive care unit (NICU). An infusion of a 10% dextrose solution was initiated intravenously at a rate providing 100 cc/kg daily. Serum for electrolytes was obtained at 20 hours of age. Her serum calcium concentration at that time was 8.1 mg/dL.

Laboratory results were reviewed by the pediatric resident and thought to be acceptable. Diluted and low-volume enteral feeds were initiated with a formulation appropriate for a preterm neonate. An intravenous infusion of 10% dextrose with supplemental calcium, sodium, and potassium was continued to maintain adequate total fluid intake. Calcium was administered enterally and parenterally at a rate providing 30 mg/kg/day of elemental calcium. A repeat serum sample for electrolytes was obtained at 31 hours of age. The serum calcium concentration was 7.7 mg/dL at that time.

The patient remained clinically stable with an unremarkable physical examination. She tolerated advancing feeds. The calcium concentration at 91 hours of age was 9.2 mg/dL. No further studies were obtained.

### CASE STUDY 2

Baby boy A (BBA) was born to a 42-year-old female at 27 weeks' gestation. The pregnancy had been unremarkable until Ms. A presented to the emergency room with premature rupture of membranes, preterm labor, and fever. The mother received tocolytic drugs, steroids, and antibiotics. Labor persisted and progressed. Thirty-six hours after the initial presentation, the child was delivered from a breech position by emergency cesarean section because of fetal distress. Apgar scores were 1, 4, and 7 at 1, 5, and 10 minutes, respectively. BBA was intubated for resuscitation and stabilization and transported to the NICU. His birth weight was 800 g. A catheter was placed in the umbilical artery and an infusion of 10% dextrose was initiated at a rate providing 120 cc/kg/day. When BBA was 7 hours of age, the first set of laboratory studies was obtained. His serum calcium concentration was 6.2 mg/dL.

Laboratory studies were reviewed by the resident and thought to be consistent with a diagnosis of early neonatal hypocalcemia. BBA's clinical condition precluded the initiation of feeds. Calcium supplementation was begun intravenously at a rate that provided 18 mg/kg of elemental calcium during the subsequent 24 hours.

Requirements for ventilatory support continued to increase. The patient remained active and responsive, calming with nursing measures. Arterial blood gases were within desired ranges and serum calcium concentrations are given in

**Table 3-1**  Serum Calcium Concentrations for BBA

| AGE (hrs) | SERUM CALCIUM CONCENTRATIONS (mg/dL) |
|---|---|
| 19 | 6.8 |
| 31 | 7.4 |
| 43 | 7.6 |
| 55 | 8.3 |
| 79 | 8.2 |
| 103 | 8.4 |
| 151 | 8.7 |

Table 3-1. Examination of the laboratory data of Table 3-1 demonstrates that calcium concentrations increased progressively after the initial low value.

### EXERCISE 1

■ **Questions:**

1. How would you interpret the serum calcium values in Case Study 1?

2. How would you interpret the serum calcium values in Case Study 2?

3. What is the definition of early neonatal hypocalcemia?

■ **Answers:**

*Normal serum calcium concentrations range between 8 and 11 mg/dL.*

Following delivery of the neonate, serum calcium concentrations decrease rapidly during the first 12 to 24 hours of life and reach a nadir by 24 to 72 hours of age. Levels increase starting at approximately 72 hours of age and return to normal by 5 to 10 days of age. *Early neonatal hypocalcemia appears to be an exaggeration of this normal fall in serum calcium concentrations and is defined as a serum cal-*

*cium concentration of less than 8 mg/dL in a term neonate and less than 7 mg/dL in a preterm neonate during the first 3 days of life.*

Approximately 3% of healthy term neonates have calcium levels of less than 8 mg/dL at 24 hours of age. The incidence in preterm neonates ranges between 30% and 50% and increases with decreasing gestational age. The incidence of early neonatal hypocalcemia is increased in asphyxiated neonates and in infants of diabetic mothers. Some investigators have also reported an increased incidence of early neonatal hypocalcemia in full-term growth retarded infants. Others deny any such association and attribute these calcium abnormalities to increased incidence of prematurity and birth depression in this population.

### ■ Question:

What is the pathophysiological basis for early neonatal hypocalcemia in preterm infants?

### ■ Answer:

This question is best answered by reviewing fetal calcium homeostasis and the physiological changes accompanying birth. During fetal growth, calcium ions are actively transported across the placenta and fetal serum calcium concentrations increase as gestation progresses. At midgestation, fetal calcium concentrations approximate 5.5 mg/dL. In preterm neonates, the serum concentrations of calcium average 8 to 9 mg/dL, while at term gestation, cord blood concentrations exceed maternal calcium levels by 1 to 2 mg/dL and may be as high as 13.8 mg/dL. Unlike calcium, the physiology of the calcitropic hormones is less well defined. Calcitonin and parathyroid hormone (PTH) do not cross the placenta. Placental production of these hormones may occur; however, the role of placentally produced calcitropic hormones in fetal calcium homeostasis is unclear.

Calcitonin is produced by the fetus early in gestation. Fetal and cord blood serum calcitonin concentrations equal or exceed maternal levels and the secretion of this hormone (at least in animal studies) occurs in response to appropriate stimuli. Because of the high serum fetal calcitonin levels, some researchers speculate that calcitonin is important in minimizing bone resorption in the fetus.

Fetal PTH homeostasis, on the other hand, is poorly defined. Widely varying fetal concentrations of PTH (and, therefore, ratios between fetal, or cord blood, and maternal concentrations of PTH) have been reported in the literature. Some of these discrepancies may be related to differences in the method of analysis (immunoassay versus bioassay) used in the various studies. Bioassays suggest that PTH activity is higher in the fetus compared to the mother. However, contrary results occur with immunoassays and many investigators have reported that fetal PTH activity is low. Because the fetus is developing in a hypercalcemic intrauterine environment, PTH activity would be expected to be minimal, as indicated by the immunoassay results.

The role of PTH in fetal growth and development is unclear, although its primary function may be to increase production of 1,25(OH)$_2$Vitamin D. Although placental passage and production of 1,25(OH)$_2$Vitamin D occurs in animals, the fetal kidney appears to be the primary source of this hormone. Studies in animals suggest that it plays a major role in placental calcium transport and is important in maintaining the maternal-fetal gradient of this ion.

At birth, the maternal supply of calcium is terminated and needs are met through absorption from dietary provisions. Serum calcium concentrations normally decline in the first 48 to 72 hours of life. In response to the fall in calcium, PTH concentrations rapidly and appropriately increase. However, calcitonin concentrations do not decrease but instead increase postnatally until approximately 12 to 72 hours of age, and then they progressively decline. The reasons for this postnatal surge in serum calcitonin concentrations and the consequences of this surge are unknown. However, some investigators suggest that calcitonin may contribute to the postnatal decline in serum calcium concentrations.

The pathophysiology of early neonatal hypocalcemia in preterm neonates, infants of diabetic mothers, and asphyxiated neonates is not completely understood, but likely to be different in each instance. *In preterm neonates, decreased end-organ responsiveness to PTH, hypercalcitonemia, the abrupt termination of calcium provision in the presence of significant demands for calcium, and calcium concentrations that are already low (relative to those found in the term newborn) may all* contribute to the increased incidence of early neonatal hypocalcemia. In infants of diabetic mothers, hypomagnesemia induced by the maternal diabetes can inhibit PTH secretion by altering the calcium-sensitive, magnesium-dependent adenylate cyclase involved in parathyroid secretion. In asphyxiated neonates, an increased phosphate load associated with catabolic responses to stress as well as medical measures to correct metabolic acidosis (e.g., sodium bicarbonate) may exacerbate normal postnatal changes in serum calcium concentrations.

### ■ Question:
What is the course of early neonatal hypocalcemia?

### ■ Answer:
*Earlier, we pointed out that calcium levels decrease rapidly during the first 12 to 24 hours of life and reach a nadir by approximately 72 hours of age. Calcium levels then correct spontaneously during the ensuing 5 to 10 days without intervention.* Although in general patients are asymptomatic, jitteriness and seizure activity have been noted in hypocalcemic neonates. However, because of the high-risk critically ill nature of the infants involved, these symptoms may result from other clinical problems.

### ■ Question:
What interventions are necessary in patients with early neonatal hypocalcemia?

### ■ Answer:
Because patients are generally asymptomatic and serum calcium concentrations frequently normalize without treatment, some investigators would argue that intervention is not necessary. Furthermore, ionized calcium concentration (the physiologically active form of calcium) frequently remains within an acceptable range despite depressed total calcium concentrations. However, *because of the many other medical problems frequently encountered in these high-risk neonates, as well as the central role calcium plays in normal physiology, most clinicians attempt to correct or minimize hypocalcemia.*

*Intravenous boluses of elemental calcium administered for a brief period of time will result in prompt increases in serum calcium concentrations; however, this effect may not persist.* This mode of calcium replacement is reserved for infants with low serum ionized calcium concentrations, infants with diminished cardiac function, or those with severe tremors or seizures. Generally, 10% calcium gluconate is administered at a rate of infusion that does not exceed 2 mL/kg/10 min. Continuous cardiac monitoring is necessary during bolus infusions of calcium.

*The continuous infusion of calcium as a constituent of maintenance fluids is safer and will ameliorate the postnatal fall in serum calcium levels.* If a continuous infusion of calcium is begun during the first few hours of life at a rate that provides 35 mg/kg/day of elemental calcium, serum calcium concentrations should remain >7 mg/dL in almost all low birth weight infants. If serum calcium levels do fall to <7 mg/dL, an infusion that provides 54 mg/kg/day of elemental calcium will result in a higher calcium level 24 hours later. Interestingly, however, when the neonate is 72 hours of age, the serum calcium concentration of the supplemented patient will equal that of neonates who were not given calcium supplementation. Some investigators have recommended that 75 mg/kg of elemental calcium be administered daily to high risk neonates to maintain normal serum calcium levels. Given the benign nature of early neonatal hypocalcemia in most infants we have not adopted that policy.

## LATE NEONATAL HYPOCALCEMIA AND HYPOMAGNESEMIA

### CASE STUDY 3
Baby boy W (BBW) was born to a 30-year-old female after a pregnancy complicated by prolonged and premature rupture of membranes and vaginal bleeding. The mother received betamethasone and ampicillin. BBW was born vaginally and had Apgar scores of 7 and 8 at 1 and 5 minutes, respectively. He required sup-

plemental oxygen. Because of prematurity, respiratory distress, and small size, he was admitted to the NICU for ongoing management. His physical examination was unremarkable except for an increased respiratory rate, nasal flaring, and grunting with respirations. On the initial chest radiograph, fluid was noted in the fissure, lung fields were minimally (diffusely) hazy and hyperinflated, and the cardiothymic shadow was within normal limits. Because of his history and problems with respiratory distress, infection was suspected. Therefore, blood and cerebrospinal fluid were obtained for culture and laboratory analyses. Antibiotics and intravenous fluids were initiated. His respiratory status improved and supplemental oxygen was discontinued at 24 hours of age. At this time, serum was obtained for an electrolyte panel (sodium, potassium, chloride, bicarbonate, calcium, and creatinine). These studies were unremarkable except for a serum calcium level of 6.5 mg/dL. Supplemental calcium was added to intravenous fluids and enteral feeds were initiated with dilute concentrations of a formulation developed for preterm neonates. Repeat serum calcium analyses at 36 and 48 hours of age were 6.8 and 7.1 mg/dL, respectively.

## EXERCISE 2

■ **Question:**

What two diagnoses of altered mineral balance should be considered in the patient at this time?

1.

2.

■ **Answer:**

*The first and most likely possibility is that this infant has early neonatal hypocalcemia.* As mentioned previously, calcium levels normally decrease in neonates after delivery. This pattern is exacerbated in select populations, including premature infants. Increases in serum calcium occur with or without intervention and, generally, there are no associated symptoms, per our earlier discussion.

*A second possibility is that this infant is magnesium deficient.* As in the case of calcium, magnesium is actively transported across the placenta and the bulk of neonatal magnesium stores is accrued during the latter part of gestation. Normal concentrations of magnesium in the serum range between 1.5 and 2.8 mg/dL; however, serum magnesium levels at birth are inversely related to gestational age. Thus, less mature neonates may have lower serum concentrations and tissues stores. Furthermore, with chronic maternal magnesium deficiency, magnesium stores in the fetus may be deficient as well.

Generally, the relationship between PTH and magnesium parallels, to a lesser degree, that between calcium and PTH. Thus, with decreasing magnesium levels, PTH secretion increases to normalize serum levels. However, with persistently diminished magnesium supplies, cellular levels are compromised and PTH secretion paradoxically decreases. Thus, in cases of hypocalcemia associated with hypomagnesemia, correction of hypomagnesemia is required before serum calcium levels will return to normal.

Historically, *late neonatal hypocalcemia* is a term that has been applied to hypocalcemia persisting or presenting beyond the first 2 to 4 days of life. In addition to magnesium deficiency, increased dietary phosphorus and diminished maternal vitamin D stores can result in hypocalcemia. Modification of mineral intake usually results in normalization of biochemical studies.

## CASE STUDY 3 continued

Repeat laboratory analyses of serum at 60 hours of age demonstrated a calcium concentration of 6.9 mg/dL and a serum magnesium level of 2.0 mg/dL. Feedings were rapidly advanced and BBW received 210 mg of elemental calcium/kg and 105 mg of phosphorus/kg daily. However, serum calcium levels remained low throughout the first 10 days of life and ranged from 6.5 to 6.8 mg/dL. No symptoms were noted. On day 10 of BBW's life, his phosphorus level was 10.2 mg/dL. Renal function studies and urine output were normal at that time. Serum was obtained to measure PTH levels on the patient as well as his mother. These samples were forwarded to an outside laboratory for analysis. In the interim, BBW was changed to a formula that provided a lower phosphorus intake and calcium salts were used to supplement his enteral mineral intake.

## EXERCISE 3

**■ Question:**

What diagnoses should be considered in this case?

**■ Answer:**

*Hypoparathyroidism* and *excess dietary phosphorous intake.*

## HYPOPARATHYROIDISM

Hypoparathyroidism is an infrequently diagnosed but important cause of persistent hypocalcemia. This problem may be primary, reflecting problems in the neonate, or secondary to maternal factors. Primary hypoparathyroidism may be inherited as an X-linked or autosomal dominant trait or may result from congenital abnormalities in the development of the third and fourth pharyngeal pouches, that is, DiGeorge syndrome. In this syndrome, thymic and parathyroid agenesis or hypoplasia as well as cardiac defects occur. Primary hypoparathyroidism may also occur sporadically and be transient in nature. In this case, generally, no other abnormalities are noted, although cardiac abnormalities have been reported. Laboratory analyses demonstrate increased serum phosphorus levels, decreased serum parathyroid hormone and calcium levels, and appropriate tissue responses to parathyroid hormone. With supportive care, biochemical abnormalities usually resolve during a period of days to weeks. Others suggest that short courses of supplemental vitamin D may be necessary. The pathogenesis of this problem is unknown. However, some authors suggest that it may represent true, although very mild, parathyroid hormone deficiency. Resolution of biochemical abnormalities reflects compensation by the newborn infant. However, hypocalcemia may recur with stresses in childhood and adolescence.

Secondary hypoparathyroidism may occur in neonates of mothers with hyperparathyroidism. In these instances, mothers are hypercalcemic and fetal calcium levels are elevated above the normal range. Intrauterine hypercalcemia results in further suppression of parathyroid gland secretion and hypocalcemia in the neonate.

### CASE STUDY 3 continued

Maternal serum PTH and calcium concentrations were within normal limits. BBW's PTH level was also within normal limits, although at the time his serum calcium level was 6.7 mg/dL. On day 18 of BBW's life, his serum calcium and phosphorus levels were 9.9 and 6.4 mg/dL, respectively. On day 28 of BBW's life, similar values were obtained. These findings were considered consistent with transient, neonatal hypoparathyroidism.

## EXERCISE 4

**■ Question:**

What should be done to treat this infant?

**■ Answer:**

*Supportive dietary therapy in the neonate suffices until normal parathyroid function returns.*

## HYPERMAGNESEMIA

The following cases describe two neonates exposed to high concentrations of magnesium. Included in the presentations are the risk factors, symptoms, and usual course associated with hypermagnesemia in the low birth weight infant. As you read these cases, try to decide why magnesium sulfate was administered to these mothers. Which mother is likely to exhibit higher serum magnesium levels?

### CASE STUDY 4

Ms. B is a 33-year-old female who presented at 34 weeks' gestation with preterm labor. Her past medical history was significant for the following reasons: (1) a previous episode of preterm labor associated with cervical effacement necessitating cerclage placement at 26 weeks' gestation and (2) gestational diabetes managed by dietary manipulations. On presentation, she received betamethasone, ampicillin, and continuous infusions of insulin. Magnesium sulfate ($MgSO_4$) was the agent used for tocolysis. She received a 4-g bolus of $MgSO_4$ followed by a continuous infusion of 2 to 4 g of $MgSO_4$ per hour. A maternal magnesium level obtained 10 hours after the initiation of therapy was 9.3 mg/dL.

## CASE STUDY 5

Ms. S is a 24-year-old female who presented at 28 to 32 weeks' gestation with findings consistent with preeclampsia. A bolus of $MgSO_4$ was given and followed by a continuous infusion that delivered 1 to 2 g of $MgSO_4$ per hour. Five days later the infusion was discontinued. Shortly afterward, however, the mother developed seizure activity and received a bolus of $MgSO_4$ and 100 mg of valium.

## EXERCISE 5

■ **Question:**

Why did these women receive $MgSO_4$?

■ **Answer:**

*A bolus of $MgSO_4$ followed by a continuous intravenous infusion may be administered to pregnant women with preeclampsia, eclampsia, or preterm labor. During preterm labor, $MgSO_4$ suppresses uterine activity by directly antagonizing cellular calcium metabolism and is, therefore, used as tocolytic therapy.* However, some investigators state that in the dosages used and with the serum levels achieved, no consistent or persistent evidence of suppression of myometrial contractions by $MgSO_4$ occurs. Infusions of $MgSO_4$ have also been noted to decrease blood pressure transiently. However, in women with preeclampsia and eclampsia, $MgSO_4$ is used to diminish neuromuscular irritability and prevent or eliminate seizures. Generally, serum magnesium levels between 5 and 8 mg/dL are rapidly achieved after the bolus. When a continuous infusion of magnesium is used, maternal serum magnesium levels rise and plateau 6 to 24 hours after initiation of therapy: The plateau reflects an equilibration between intake and output.

■ **Question:**

Which mother in these two cases is at increased risk for developing a markedly increased serum magnesium concentration and why?

■ **Answer:**

Magnesium homeostasis is a complex process involving interactions between gastrointestinal absorption, bone metabolism, and renal excretion. Gastrointestinal absorption is inefficient and occurs primarily in the ileum and jejunum. The role of calcitropic hormones (i.e., calcitonin, PTH, and vitamin D) in magnesium homeostasis appears to be minimal. Plasma magnesium levels are maintained by altering the reabsorption of magnesium in the thick ascending limb of the loop of Henle. Various factors, including increased serum magnesium levels, increase urinary magnesium losses. Thus, the size of the bolus and the rate of infusion of magnesium as well as the primary disorder necessitating this form of therapy in the mother will determine the maternal serum magnesium level. Decreased renal function, which may occur during eclampsia or preeclampsia, may result in a rapid elevation in the maternal magnesium level. *Therefore, the mother in Case Study 5 is at higher risk for developing an elevated serum magnesium concentration.*

■ **Question:**

What happens to magnesium balance in the fetus when the mother receives $MgSO_4$?

■ **Answer:**

Normally, magnesium crosses the placenta and concentrates in fetal tissues. At delivery, a maternal-fetal magnesium gradient exists with umbilical blood levels exceeding maternal levels. This gradient is reversed or eliminated with maternal hypermagnesemia. Investigators report a delay of only 2 hours in establishing an equilibrium between maternal and fetal plasma magnesium levels. Furthermore, after a single dose of magnesium in pregnant animals, magnesium gradually concentrates in fetal tissues, exceeding maternal concentrations at 24 hours. *Therefore, fetal magnesium levels, assessed with umbilical cord blood measurements, are increased above normal values when the mother is hypermagnesemic.*

### ■ Question:

What maternal or fetal conditions might alter magnesium homeostasis during the perinatal period?

### ■ Answer:

*Three conditions have been shown to alter magnesium homeostasis in the newborn infant. These include the presence of maternal diabetes, low neonatal birth weight, and birth asphyxia.* The first two instances have been associated with lowered cord magnesium levels, the latter with slightly increased magnesium levels. In the case of infants of diabetic mothers, Tsang et al. noted hypomagnesemia at birth in several of the neonates studied. These investigators described a significant correlation between maternal and cord magnesium levels in infants of diabetic mothers and also noted that the incidence of hypomagnesemia increased significantly with increasing severity of maternal diabetes. The etiology of hypomagnesemia in this case is unclear. Normally, maternal magnesium requirements increase during pregnancy because of fetal needs and increased protein synthesis. Interestingly, however, maternal magnesium serum levels during pregnancy actually decrease, possibly reflecting hemodilution. Furthermore, tissue magnesium levels may also be deficient in all pregnant women (and especially those with diabetes) as reflected by low red blood cell magnesium concentrations. All of this may be exacerbated by increased renal magnesium losses, which have been reported in insulin-dependent diabetics.

Lower magnesium levels have also been noted in the low birth weight infant, although there are conflicting reports regarding this finding. In the case of preterm neonates, abrupt termination of maternal-fetal magnesium transfer or an immature response of the parathyroid gland to a decreased serum magnesium concentration may be the etiology of the depressed levels observed during the perinatal period. Finally, hypermagnesemia has been documented in neonates who require resuscitative procedures, have delayed onset of

respiration, or have depressed Apgar scores, although the etiology of increased magnesium levels in these cases is unclear.

In Case Studies 4 and 5, both patients are premature (less than 37 weeks' gestation). In Case Study 4 the mother was receiving insulin for diabetes mellitus. In Case Study 5, a maternal seizure might have been associated with compromised fetal blood flow and asphyxia. Although these factors can alter magnesium levels, their significance in these two cases (where both mothers were markedly hypermagnesemic) is probably minimal. However, knowledge of these possible associations will assist the clinician in interpreting laboratory values and managing these kinds of high risk neonates.

As you read through the continuation of Case Studies 4 and 5 next, try to decide which of the patients' symptoms (if any) are due to hypermagnesemia.

### CASE STUDY 4 continued

Seventeen hours after the onset of labor and 7 hours after the spontaneous rupture of membranes, baby girl B (BGB) was delivered vaginally. One hour prior to delivery of BGB, her mother received Stadol (an intravenous narcotic). At delivery, BGB was floppy, had no spontaneous respirations, was poorly perfused, and had a heart rate of 80 beats per minute (BPM). Bag and mask ventilation was established and BGB's color and heart rate improved. However, respiratory effort remained inadequate and tone and activity were diminished. She received two doses of Narcan without improvement. BGB was intubated and taken to the intensive care unit for ongoing management. The initial physical examination demonstrated (1) a cephalohematoma at the occiput, (2) a grade I/VI systolic murmur, (3) slightly decreased pulse and perfusion, and (4) diminished muscle tone. During day 2 of life, the patient's physical examination improved and ventilatory support was discontinued.

### CASE STUDY 5 continued

Because of the mother's deteriorating status, baby boy S (BBS) was delivered by emergency cesarean section with general anesthesia. Rupture of membranes occurred at delivery. The patient required bag and mask ventilation initially for poor respiratory effort and bradycardia. He responded with clinical improvement. However, at about 3 minutes of age, his respiratory effort declined and he was intubated. Apgar scores were 5 and 8 at 1 and 5 minutes, respectively. His examination on admission was unremarkable except for prematurity. His ventilatory support was discontinued during day 2 of life because of clinical improvement.

## EXERCISE 6

### ■ Questions:
Were the initial presentations in these neonates a result of hypermagnesemia? If so, what symptoms of hypermagnesemia were exhibited?

### ■ Answers:
*Controversy continues regarding the effect, if any, of maternal MgSO₄ administration on the neonate.* When controlled studies are evaluated, it appears that maternal $MgSO_4$ administration can be associated with altered physical findings in the neonate. The majority of these symptoms appear to be mild when other factors that may compromise the intrauterine environment are eliminated. The signs and symptoms of hypermagnesemia result from the effects of magnesium ion on the neuromuscular junction. These include (1) a decrease in the amount of acetylcholine released from motor nerve terminals, (2) decreased depolarizing action of acetylcholine at the endplate, and (3) diminished excitability of the muscle fiber membrane. These actions result in muscle weakness and paralysis. Cardiovascular effects are attributed to decreased smooth muscle contraction. Symptoms attributed to hypermagnesemia include the following:

*Weak or absent cry*

*Decreased reflexes*

*Hypotonia*

*Muscle weakness*

*Lethargy/poor responses to stimuli*

*Poor respiratory effort/respiratory failure*

Poor suck

Poor swallowing/constipation

? Microcolon

*Vasodilation/hypotension/EKG changes*

Abnormal bone mineralization

### ■ Question:
What are normal neonatal serum magnesium concentrations?

### ■ Answer:
*Normal values in neonates are similar to those of adult subjects with 95% confidence intervals of 1.5 to 2.8 mg/dL.*

### ■ Question:
At what serum magnesium concentrations do clinical problems occur in the neonate?

### ■ Answer:
Randall et al., using normal adult subjects and adults with renal failure, demonstrated a relationship between serum magnesium concentrations and symptoms. Difficulty with micturation and defecation as well as altered sensorium (drowsiness, lethargy, slight slurring of speech, ataxic gait) were noted in some patients with magnesium concentrations as low as 5 mg/dL. With levels of 9 to 12 mg/dL, decreased reflexes or areflexia and respiratory depression were noted. EKG changes and cardiac arrest were also reported with increased magnesium levels; however, other electrolyte abnormalities (hypocalcemia, hyperkalemia) were also present.

Despite the relationship between serum magnesium concentrations and neurological symptoms in adults, no such relationship has been demonstrated in neonates. *Investigators have repeatedly failed to define a correlation between cord magnesium levels or magnesium levels in serial neonatal serum samples and the level of neurological or respiratory depression or Apgar scores in the neonate. Some investigators have suggested that with prolonged maternal MgSO₄ administration (more than 24 hours), neonatal symptoms are more likely to occur.*

■ **Question:**

What is the course of neonatal hypermagnesemia and what treatments are available?

■ **Answer:**

Renal excretion is the primary route of elimination of excess magnesium. Unfortunately, the newborn does not excrete a magnesium load as rapidly as adults. *Hence, symptoms associated with hypermagnesemia may persist longer in the neonate than in the mother. Some investigators have reported an improvement in sucking, crying, and neurological responses when hypermagnesemic neonates were 24 to 48 hours of age. Decreases in serum magnesium concentrations occurred during the same or slightly longer time frame (24 to 72 hours).*

Besides supportive therapy, other interventions are rarely required. In cases with significant symptoms, calcium administration may decrease the inhibitory effect of magnesium at the neuromuscular junction and improve the patient's clinical status. Diuretics, which increase magnesium excretion, such as furosemide, may also be useful.

## METABOLIC BONE DISEASE IN PREMATURE INFANTS

Because the bulk of calcium and phosphorus is stored in tissues, significant dietary deficiencies will not result in biochemical or clinical aberrations early in the postnatal period. However, with continued inadequate mineral intake, bone becomes dimineralized (osteopenic) and fractures and rickets may result. Osteopenia of prematurity is an exceedingly common problem among very low birth weight premature infants. Skeletal changes have been demonstrated in 17.5% to 30% of such infants (birth weights of less than 1,500 g) and, not surprisingly, the incidence of these radiographic abnormalities increases with decreasing birth weight and gestational age. While some investigators have questioned the adequacy of dietary vitamin D and its metabolism by the preterm neonate as the etiology of these problems, suboptimal substrate provision (i.e., calcium and phosphorous) is generally consid-

ered the cause. Thus, clinicians must be aware of the mineral requirements for high-risk preterm neonates as well as conditions modifying absorption and excretion of calcium and phosphorous.

The following three cases describe scenarios in which neonates are at nutritional risk of inadequate mineral intake. As you read through the cases, please try to identify those factors that place the infants at risk for altered calcium and phosphorous homeostasis.

## CASE STUDY 6

AY is a 1,060-g twin male born at 28 weeks' gestation to a 30-year-old female after a pregnancy complicated by preterm labor and premature and prolonged rupture of membranes. The mother received tocolytics, antibiotics, and narcotics. Unfortunately, labor progressed and the patient was delivered vaginally from the breech position with Apgar scores of 5 and 7 at 1 and 5 minutes, respectively. Ventilatory support was instituted at birth; however, the patient weaned rapidly and was extubated by 10 days of age. Enteral feeds were initiated on day 3 of life with a formulation designed for the preterm infant. Full enteral feeds were achieved by day 17 of life. At that time the patient was receiving 150 cc/kg/day.

## CASE STUDY 7

BZ is a 1,230-g female infant born at 30 weeks' gestation to a 30-year-old female. The pregnancy was unremarkable until the mother presented to the emergency room with a 6-hour history of labor pains. Apgar scores were 8 and 9 at 1 and 5 minutes, respectively. BZ had no respiratory problems, and enteral feeds were initiated with human milk on day 3 of life at low volume and advanced to full feeds by 10 days of age. BZ received 150 cc/kg/day of human milk and a multivitamin providing 400 IU/day of vitamin D.

## CASE STUDY 8

CN is a 750-g female newborn infant delivered at 27 weeks' gestation by emergency cesarean section to a 35-year-old female with eclampsia. The patient was intubated at birth and slowly weaned to moderate ventilatory support. Requirements for ventilatory support continued with radiographic changes consistent with bronchopulmonary dysplasia. Aminophylline and Lasix were added to optimize ventilatory function. At 21 days of age, Decadron was begun as well. Enteral feeds with diluted formula as well as peripheral intravenous hyperalimentation were initiated by day 5 of life. However, the enteral feedings were disrupted frequently because of fluid overload and feeding intolerance. In the interim, parenteral hyperalimentation through a centrally placed catheter was continued.

## EXERCISE 7

■ **Question:**

What are the calcium and phosphorus requirements in the preterm neonate?

■ **Answer:**

The foundation for daily calcium and phosphorus requirements for preterm neonates consists of data obtained by evaluating the mineral content of stillbirths, aborted fetuses, and neonates of varying gestational ages who have died shortly after delivery. Ideally such information should be obtained from analyses of a random population of patients with normal growth, from mothers who themselves are nutritionally replete, and from babies where the cause of death would not alter the nutritional status of the studied infant. In addition, the methods of analysis and reporting of data should be uniform. Unfortunately, a review of the reported information demonstrates that many of these standards were not achieved. In fact, gestational age is frequently poorly defined and anthropometric measurements, when compared to today's growth standards, suggest suboptimal intrauterine nutrient acquisition. Furthermore, in each report, only a small number of neonates were analyzed, and a wide variety of techniques were used to perform the analysis and report the information. Despite these shortcomings, vital information has been provided.

Researchers have reviewed the available data and combined all available information or selected those patients best described to define daily mineral accretion rates. At term gestation, neonates have accrued approximately 30 g of calcium and 16 g of phosphorus, the bulk of accretion occurring during the last trimester. During this period, *neonates receive approximately 90 to 150 mg of calcium/kg and 60 to 85 mg of phosphorus/kg daily. These values provide the basis for estimates of mineral requirements for the preterm neonate.*

■ **Question:**

How much calcium and phosphorus is provided by commonly used infant formulas or breast milk?

■ **Answer:**

*Figure 3-1* depicts the mineral content of human milk, standard milk formulas for term neonates, and milk formulas designed for the preterm neonate. By reviewing the information in the figure, clinicians can readily appreciate those feeding regimens that would not provide daily estimated mineral requirements for the low birth weight infant.

■ **Question:**

What endogenous factors influence mineral absorption?

■ **Answer:**

This question is of critical importance because nutrient provision does not guarantee nutrient accretion. When daily requirements are defined, mineral balance, that is, net and true absorption as well as net retention, must be considered. These terms are explained in Figure 3-2. Net mineral absorption and retention have been defined by measuring the amount of mineral excreted in stool and urine in an infant receiving a controlled mineral intake. From Figure 3-2, it is apparent that there are three sources of mineral loss:

Failure to absorb dietary provisions

Secretion of mineral into the intestines during normal digestive processes

Urinary losses

Calcium losses in urine are believed to be minimal under normal circumstances. However, calcium secretion into the intestinal tract as a constituent of digestive juices probably plays a key role in calcium metabolism in the neonate. Thus, even though true calcium absorption may be efficient, net calcium absorption may be diminished or vary over a

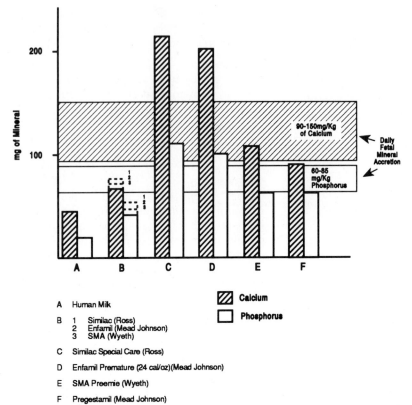

**Figure 3-1** Estimated daily *in utero* fetal calcium and phosphorus accretion and the concentration of these minerals in 150 cc of (A) human milk, (B) standard infant milk formulas, and (C–F) milk formulas for the preterm infant.

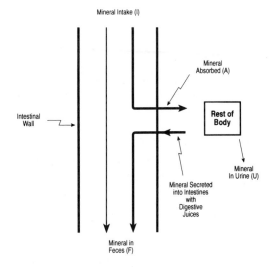

I - F = Net Mineral Absorption
I - (F + U) = Net Mineral Retention
A = True Mineral Absorption

**Figure 3-2** General factors that must be considered to understand why not all of the minerals provided in the diet are actually absorbed.

wide range because of calcium secretion into the intestinal tract. Factors influencing intestinal calcium secretion remain obscure. On the other hand, phosphorus secretion into the intestinal tract is thought to be minimal, since phosphorus retention generally approaches 90%, particularly with decreased dietary phosphorus provisions. Greer and Tsang have recently reviewed calcium and phosphorus absorption and retention in the low birth weight infant receiving a variety of enteral feeds. *With advancing gestational and postnatal age, or simply with increasing dietary calcium intake, calcium absorption is increased. Similarly, phosphorus absorption is increased by increasing phosphorus intake.*

■ **Question:**

How much dietary calcium and phosphorus should a preterm neonate receive?

■ **Answer:**

Two factors should be considered. First, the goal of phosphorous and calcium supplementation is to parallel intrauterine calcium and phosphorus accretion. Therefore, from Figure 3-1, it is apparent that there is insufficient calcium in human milk and in standard formulations designed for term neonates. Human milk is frequently supplemented to increase the preterm neonate's intake of calcium, phosphorus, and other nutrients.

Second, net mineral retention rates must also be considered. Even from those preterm formulations that contain sufficient amounts of calcium and phosphorous to parallel intrauterine accretion rates, only 60% to 70% of calcium and 70% to 80% of phosphorus provided is retained.

■ **Question:**

What are the risk factors for altered calcium and phosphorus homeostasis in Case Studies 6, 7, and 8?

■ **Answer:**

To define risk factors in our patients, the dietary provision and fetal accretion rates should be compared (Figures 3-1 and 3-3). Other risk factors for altered mineral balance can be derived from the patient's history. In

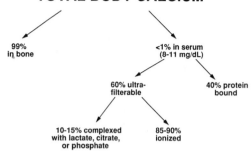

**TOTAL BODY CALCIUM**

**Figure 3-4**  Calcium distribution in total body and blood compartments.

summary, the risk factors for each patient follow:

| *Case Study 6* | *Case Study 7* | *Case Study 8* |
|---|---|---|
| *Prematurity* | *Prematurity* | *Prematurity* |
| *↓ Ca/Phos intake* | *↓ Ca/Phos intake* | *↓ Ca/Phos intake* |
| | | *Diuretic use* |

■ **Question:**

The clinicians, recognizing that the risk of altered calcium and phosphorus homeostasis was present, wanted to monitor their patients for altered skeletal metabolism. Which biochemical markers of bone metabolism should the clinicians monitor?

■ **Answer:**

Various chemical markers are available. They consist of enzymes involved in bone turnover as well as components of the bone matrix. *The biochemical indices most frequently followed in clinical settings are serum calcium, phosphorus, and total alkaline phosphatase levels.* Other markers less commonly used include the following:

Total and bone specific alkaline phosphatase

Osteocalcin

Procollagen I carboxy-terminal extension peptide

Plasma/urine hydroxyproline

From the distribution of calcium described in Figure 3-4, it is apparent that the bulk of the calcium pool is located within the skeleton.

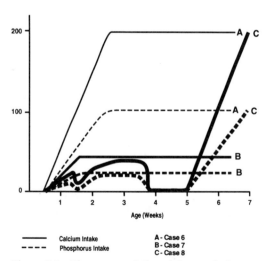

**Figure 3-3**  The average daily calcium and phosphorus (mg/kg) intake is indicated for each of the infants identified as (A) case 6, (B) case 7, and (C) case 8.

However, ionized calcium in serum is the metabolically active form of calcium and the major factor influencing hormonal systems important in calcium homeostasis. Calcium plays a central role in a variety of physiological functions such as neuronal conduction, blood coagulation, and muscle contraction and, thus, bone may become demineralized or mineralization of bone may be delayed to maintain normal serum calcium concentrations. Two hormones modulate gastrointestinal absorption of calcium and bone metabolism to maintain the desired serum calcium concentrations. These hormones are PTH and the biologically active component of vitamin D, 1,25-dihydroxycholecalciferol. PTH homeostasis is regulated directly by the serum ionized calcium concentration acting on the chief cells of the parathyroid glands. The major stimulus of PTH release is hypocalcemia. The actions of PTH to correct hypocalcemia are illustrated in Figure 3-5. Vitamin D (calciferol) is a lipid soluble vitamin serially hydroxylated in the liver and kidney to a metabolically active compound, 1,25-dihydroxy-cholecalciferol (Figure 3-6). Vitamin D and its metabolites [25OHD and 1,25(OH)$_2$D] increase calcium transport in the intestines and promote bone mobilization. PTH and deficiencies of serum calcium and phosphorus promote 1,25-dihydroxycholecalciferol production. While the effect of 1,25-dihydroxy-cholecalciferol on calcium is manifested anywhere from days to weeks, PTH minimizes alterations in serum calcium concentrations from moment to moment. Although, ionized calcium is the physiologically active form of calcium, the total serum calcium concentration is usually monitored when clinicians screen for metabolic bone disease.

Phosphorus, like calcium, is important to the structural integrity of bone and is also critical to a number of physiological functions including energy metabolism, muscle contractions, and nerve impulse propagation. As depicted in Figure 3-7, the bulk of the total body phosphorus pool is deposited in bone primarily as hydroxyapatite. Factors modulating phosphate homeostasis are not well understood. The effects of various factors on phos-

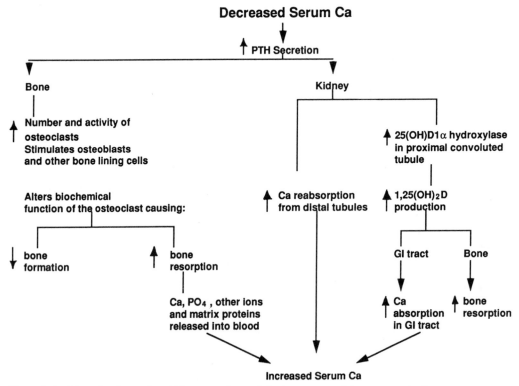

**Figure 3-5** The role of parathyroid hormone in modulating serum calcium concentrations.

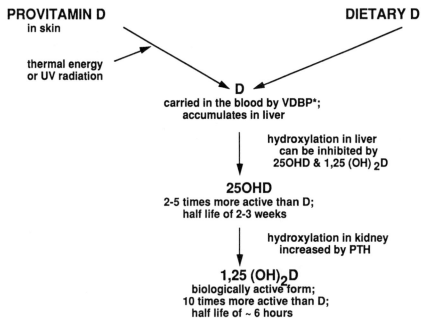

*VDBP: Vitamin D Binding Protein
**Figure 3-6** Vitamin D metabolism.

phate homeostasis are described in Table 3-2. Serum phosphate concentrations can vary over a broad range. Minimal dietary phosphate is lost in the stool, and although the skeleton is a major phosphate reservoir, the role of the skeletal system in daily phosphate homeostasis is overshadowed by that of the kidney.

Alkaline phosphatases are a group of isoenzymes that can be found in the placenta, intes-

tines, liver, kidney, and bone. These enzymes, which are membrane-bound glycoproteins, hydrolyze a variety of monophosphate esters at alkaline pH. The bone isoenzyme is secreted by osteoblasts and plays an as-yet poorly defined role in normal skeletal mineralization. This enzyme may increase local concentrations of inorganic phosphate or alter collagen secreted by osteoblasts to promote calcium salt deposition. At sites with active mineralization, marked increases in osteoblast alkaline phosphatase activity occur. Increased osteoblastic activity occurs with growth and, therefore, increased serum alkaline phosphatase concentrations are noted. Glass et al. surveyed serum alkaline phosphatase concentrations in 349 newborns 5 to 10 days of age with gestational ages ranging from 26 to 40 weeks to define normal values. This chronological age was selected to minimize the contribution of placental alkaline phosphatase to total values. If values exceeded 500 U/L, isoenzyme studies were performed. Alkaline phosphatase of bone origin was consis-

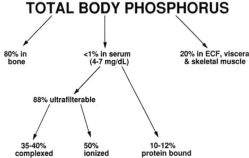

**Figure 3-7** Phosphorus distribution in total body and blood compartments.

**Table 3-2**  Factors Influencing Phosphate Metabolism

| | KIDNEY | INTESTINES | BONES |
|---|---|---|---|
| 1,25(OH)$_2$D | ? no direct effect {conflicting data due to difficulty controlling other metabolic responses to Vitamin D} | ↑ PO$_4$ absorption | In conjunction with PTH, ↑ bone resorption that releases phosphate {at higher concentrations may ↑ bone resorption without PTH} |
| Calcitonin | Normally, no major role | No important direct role | — |
| PTH | ↑ PO$_4$ excretion {tubular resorption inhibited; with ↓ PO$_4$ intake, no PTH effect} | No important direct role | ↑ bone resorption, which releases phosphate |
| Calcium | ↓ PO$_4$ excretion occurs with Ca infusion {? due to hormonal responses to ↑ serum Ca} | ↓ PO$_4$ absorption with large increases in dietary Ca | — |

1,25(OH)$_2$D = 1,25 dihydroxycholecalciferol, PO$_4$ = phosphate, Ca = calcium, PTH = parathyroid hormone.

tently the predominant fraction. Plasma values differed significantly between term and preterm neonates with values diminishing as gestational age increased. Mean values ranged between 164 (SD = 67) and 319 (SD = 142) U/L compared with values of 30 to 120 U/L in healthy adult subjects.

---

### CASE STUDY 6 continued

During the next 30 days, the infant experienced multiple episodes of feeding intolerance, which necessitated the administration of diluted formula for 24 to 48 hours. At 40 days of age his weight was 1,480 g. Serum was evaluated for calcium, phosphorus, and alkaline phosphatase concentrations. The results of these analyses are as follows:

| | |
|---|---|
| Calcium (mg/dL) | 10 |
| Phosphorus (mg/dL) | 6 |
| Alkaline phosphatase (U/L) | 300 |

### EXERCISE 8

---

■ **Question:**

Based on the preceding discussion, what would you do now?

■ **Answer:**

*These values are within acceptable limits and require no intervention.* Furthermore, after full enteral feeds were achieved, dietary calcium and phosphorus provisions exceeded fetal accretion rates for these minerals (Fig. 3-1). However, as noted previously, net calcium and phosphorus retention on formulations for preterm neonates can vary widely. Although the average retention for a large group of neonates may be adequate, examination of individual patient balance data demonstrates that some patients retain as little as 50 mg of calcium and 40 mg of phosphorus daily even though dietary provisions are much higher. Despite these variations, daily mineral requirements for normal bone mineralization and structure associated with growth, are never ending. Therefore, continued monitoring is indicated in all high-risk infants.

---

### CASE STUDY 7 continued

This patient tolerated human milk enteral feeds very well and his weight at 30 days of age was 1,330 g. Serum was obtained to assess calcium, phosphorus, and alkaline phosphatase levels. The values follow:

| | |
|---|---|
| Calcium (mg/dL) | 11 |
| Phosphorus (mg/dL) | 3 |
| Alkaline phosphatase (U/L) | 400 |

## EXERCISE 9

■ **Question:**

How would you manage this patient?

■ **Answer:**

In this case, calcium levels are slightly increased, phosphorus levels are depressed, and alkaline phosphatase levels are elevated. This pattern of laboratory findings as well as the patient's clinical history are consistent with the diagnosis of hypophosphatemia. Other laboratory findings that are commonly observed include the following:

Increased urinary calcium excretion

Enhanced tubular reabsorption of phosphorus

Normal 25(OH)Vitamin D and PTH levels

Increased 1,25(OH)$_2$Vitamin D levels

Normal or increased serum calcium

These findings were initially described by Rowe et al. in 1979 in a 595-g infant who received human milk as her primary source of nutrition starting at 12 days of age. When she was 5 months of age, overt rickets with fractures were noted. Subsequently, other investigators demonstrated these biochemical abnormalities in very low birth weight neonates receiving only human milk or formulations with a low phosphorus intake. The absorption and retention of phosphorus from human milk is very efficient—approaching 90% with and without vitamin D supplementation. Calcium retention is less efficient and ranges from 30% to 63%. However, as demonstrated in Figure 3-1, human milk provides inadequate amounts of calcium and phosphorus relative to that received in the intrauterine environment. The lowered phosphorus intake (and depressed serum phosphorous levels) stimulate 1,25-dihydroxycholecalciferol production. This active component of vitamin D promotes bone resorption, decreases bone formation, and increases calcium absorption from the gastrointestinal tract. As a result, hypercalcemia may occur in calcium-replete patients (e.g., low birth weight infants early in their postnatal course) even though calcium intake is inadequate. However, in the very low birth weight infant whose total calcium intake has been compromised for a prolonged period of time, normal or decreased serum calcium levels may occur. With phosphorus deficiency and the resulting altered hormonal milieu, excess calcium is not used for bone formation but instead is excreted in the urine.

In previous reports, the addition of phosphorus to human milk without calcium supplements did improve calcium retention. However, urinary phosphorus excretion increased, net phosphorus retention decreased, and in some cases, hypocalcemia resulted. *Therefore, it is recommended that patients who are hypophosphatemic, and who demonstrate a history of inadequate calcium and phosphorus intake, be supplemented with both calcium and phosphorus. Because of concerns regarding insoluble salt formation in the gastrointestinal tract with the addition of mineral solutions to human milk, the use of commercially prepared human milk fortifiers or formulations designed for preterm neonates is recommended.*

### CASE STUDY 8 continued

Dilute enteral feeds and intravenous peripheral hyperalimentation were begun on day 5 of life. Because of continued problems with feeding intolerance, enteral intake remained minimal. On day 15 of CN's life, a catheter was placed centrally to allow infusion of a hyperalimentation solution containing a higher glucose concentration. Calcium and phosphorus in the hyperalimentation were supplied in a 2:1 ratio. The daily parenteral calcium intake was approximately 40 mg/kg. The patient received full feeds for the first time on day 45 of life. At that time she weighed 1,180 g. Serum concentrations for calcium, phosphorus, and alkaline phosphatase were obtained. The results are as follows:

| | |
|---|---|
| Calcium (mg/dL) | 9 |
| Phosphorus (mg/dL) | 4.2 |
| Alkaline phosphatase (U/L) | 645 |

### EXERCISE 10

■ **Question:**

How would you manage this infant's case?

■ **Answer:**

These laboratory studies demonstrate a normal calcium level, a slightly decreased phosphorus serum concentration, and an elevated alkaline phosphatase activity. This pattern of laboratory studies and the nutritional history described previously suggests that this infant is also hypophosphatemic.

The alkaline phosphatase concentration exceeds values reported in the two previous cases. Since the activity of this enzyme increases with enhanced osteoblast activity, there should be concern about altered skeletal physiology. However, the alkaline phosphatase level at which pathological radiographic changes occur is unclear. Indeed, some investigators report normal alkaline phosphatase levels despite obvious radiographic abnormalities. Glass et al. monitored 51 low birth weight infants with weekly alkaline phosphatase levels during their hospitalization and then every 2 to 4 weeks after patients were discharged. Radiographic studies were available for review in 42 patients. Bone demineralization (arbitrarily graded 1 to 3), the presence or absence of metaphyseal changes (i.e., cupping, fraying, and expansion), and periosteal reactions were noted. These investigators concluded the following:

1. Maximal alkaline phosphatase concentrations occurred 2 to 4 weeks before the severest skeletal changes.

2. Radiographic abnormalities were significantly related to peak alkaline phosphatase concentrations.

3. No abnormalities in serum phosphate concentrations occurred and serum calcium concentrations were decreased only with severely affected preterm neonates.

Interestingly, one patient with normal radiographic findings had an alkaline phosphatase concentration exceeding 500 U/L. Kovar et al. also monitored calcium, phosphorus, and alkaline phosphatase levels serially (every 2 weeks starting at 2 weeks of age) in high-risk neonates, obtaining radiographs only to confirm rickets suspected because of clinical or biochemical criteria. No changes in plasma calcium or phosphorus values were noted in this patient population. From their data, these investigators concluded that alkaline phos-

phatase levels gradually increase and peak as bone growth outstrips substrate provision due to insufficient intake early in the patient's course. With adequate nutrition, mineral supply and demand reach equilibrium, and alkaline phosphatase levels diminish as bone mineralization normalizes. With continued inadequate intake, alkaline phosphatase levels continue to increase as active rickets develop. Thus, serial serum alkaline phosphatase activity may be useful in monitoring growing low birth weight infants. Because of varied nutrient intake, the timing of increases in this biochemical parameter are individualized. Therefore, at some institutions, serial determinations are begun 4 to 6 weeks after delivery and continued monthly. Values exceeding 400 to 500 U/L are considered abnormal. Some investigators, noting that alkaline phosphatase activity can vary with the method of analysis, have suggested that serum alkaline phosphatase levels 7.5-fold greater than the adult maximum normal value for that particular laboratory are of concern. When this biochemical abnormality occurs, the change from a fortified human milk or a preterm formulation to a standard formula should be delayed. *With increasing serum alkaline phosphatase values, radiographic studies should be obtained and the feeding volume increased to maximize calcium and phosphorus intake.*

A review of these patients' clinical courses demonstrates two important factors that contribute to the risk for altered calcium and phosphorus balance and, therefore, metabolic bone disease. First and foremost is that calcium and phosphorus intake had been inadequate. Note that, although hyperalimentation is an excellent method to provide calories as well as essential nutrients to neonates intolerant of enteral feeds, the pH of hyperalimentation solutions limits the solubility of calcium and phosphorus. Assuming that the desired calcium to phosphorus ratio is nearly 2 : 1, Fitzgerald et al. suggested that the maximal achievable calcium and phosphorus concentrations in intravenous fluids are 70 and 35 mg/dL, respectively. Other investigators have advocated a calcium to phosphorous ratio of 1.3 : 1 with concentrations as high as 80 mg/dL of calcium and 60 mg/dL of phosphorous. These concentrations, however, are exceedingly high and should be used with caution in tiny infants. Therefore, even with maximum parenteral supplementation, intrauterine calcium and phosphorus provisions are not achieved.

---

### CASE STUDY 8 continued

The patient continued on the preterm formulation receiving 150 to 175 cc/kg/day. Studies obtained are given in Table 3-3. Because of other clinical problems, the patient had several chest radiographs, which frequently included one or both humeri. The results of these studies and the patient's age follow:

Day 7:   Normal bones
Day 14:  Osteopenia
Day 41:  Osteopenia
Day 63:  Periosteal reactions involving the humerus, osteopenia
Day 70:  Periosteal reactions involving the humerus, osteopenia
Day 84:  Metaphyseal fraying in distal ulna; mild periosteal reactions surrounding distal radius and ulna; curvilinear deformity of diametaphyseal region of radius: findings consistent with rickets

### EXERCISE 11

---

■ **Question:**

What action is required in this case?

■ **Answer:**

These laboratory and radiographic results are consistent with continued mineral deficit in a growing neonate and are consistent with the diagnosis of metabolic bone disease or os-

teopenia of prematurity. This problem is frequently diagnosed as an incidental finding on radiographs obtained to monitor other clinical problems. Physical findings are usually absent but may include the following:

Prominent costochondral junctions (rachitic rosary)

Prominent wrists/ankles

Craniotabes

Enlarged anterior fontanelle

Bone formation begins with formation of an osteoid, which consists primarily of collagen secreted by osteoblasts. Following the formation of this matrix, the precipitation of calcium salts in the matrix occurs. Finally, these salts are reorganized into hydoxyapitite crystals. With insufficient calcium and phosphorus, osteoid formation continues; however, mineralization does not occur. The radiological features associated with metabolic bone disease in preterm neonates include the following:

Osteopenia

Submetaphyseal lucency

Periosteal reaction

Cortical thinning

Metaphyseal fraying, cupping, and splaying

Fractures

*In this patient, the mineral deficit gradually resolved during approximately 5 months. Note that the mineral deficit and, therefore, laboratory and radiographic studies cannot be corrected rapidly. Other than continued mineral provision no other intervention is required.*

---

**Table 3-3** Results of Serum Analyses

| Age (days) | 76 | 84 | 90 | 97 | 130 | 145 |
|---|---|---|---|---|---|---|
| Calcium (mg/dL) | 7.9 | 7.8 | 8.3 | 8.2 | 10.1 | 9.5 |
| Phosphorus (mg/dL) | 4.1 | 4.3 | 4.6 | 4.3 | 5.7 | 6.2 |
| Alkaline phosphatase (U/L) | 721 | 801 | 913 | 848 | 436 | 304 |
| Weight (g) | 1,770 | 1,920 | 2,240 | 2,270 | 3,480 | 3,660 |
| Height (cm) | 41 | 41 | 43 | 43 | 49.5 | 51 |

## NEPHROCALCINOSIS

As you read through this case history, try to identify the factors that increase the probability that this infant will develop nephrocalcinosis. You will be asked to list those factors later.

### CASE STUDY 9

AS was born at 26 weeks' gestation, weighing 930 g to a 15-year-old mother by cesarean section for maternal indications. He had severe hyaline membrane disease and required significant ventilatory support. Chest radiographic findings quickly became consistent with bronchopulmonary dysplasia. Therefore, parenteral furosemide and dexamethasone as well as inhaled albuterol were initiated by 14 days of age. Theophylline was added on day 25 of life. Ventilatory support was slowly weaned and AS was extubated and placed on supplemental oxygen per hood on day 60 of life. Dexamethasone was gradually weaned and discontinued; however, furosemide, theophylline, and albuterol were continued.

From a nutritional standpoint, parenteral hyperalimentation was begun when AS was 4 days of age and continued as enteral feeds were advanced. Attempts were made to maximize parenteral mineral intake. He received approximately 40 mg of calcium and 20 mg of phosphorus per kilogram daily. Although enteral feeds (minimal volume, dilute concentration) were initiated on day 6 of life, they were frequently interrupted because of deterioration in his clinical status. By day 45 of life, AS was tolerating full enteral feeds and parenteral fluids had been discontinued. An abdominal ultrasound study was obtained on day 61 of life.

### EXERCISE 12

#### ■ Question:
What renal complications can arise with long-term diuretic use in patients with chronic lung disease?

#### ■ Answer:
*Nephrocalcinosis (deposits of calcium in the renal tubules) and nephrolithiasis (presence of calculi in the kidney) may develop in some* *patients with chronic pulmonary disease who require diuretic administration.*

#### ■ Question:
List the clinical factors that increase the risk that this infant will develop nephrocalcinosis.

#### ■ Answer:
Urinary calcium reflects a balance between filtration and resorption with no calcium secretion occurring. Most of the filtered calcium is reabsorbed in the proximal tubule (approximately 60%) and the loop of Henle (approximately 25%). In these two sites, reabsorption appears to be primarily passive (voltage dependent) and independent of direct hormonal influences. A smaller percentage of calcium is reabsorbed in the distal tubule. At this site, the method is active, saturable, and responsive to hormonal influences, particularly parathyroid hormone, which acts directly to increase the tubular reabsorption of calcium. Although calcitonin transiently increases renal calcium losses, its role in renal calcium physiology appears to be minimal. Hypervitaminosis D increases renal calcium losses by increasing the filtered load (i.e., by increasing bone reabsorption or by increasing absorption of dietary calcium). Thus, the bulk of filtered calcium is reabsorbed.

Walter et al. reviewed data from older pediatric patients and defined factors associated with urolithiasis. The primary factors identified by these investigators included infection (with or without genitourinary tract abnormalities) and immobilization. Metabolic disorders (e.g., renal tubular acidosis), which increased urinary calcium losses, were rarely noted; however, urinary calcium excretion was not consistently evaluated. Other investigators cite hypercalciuria as the primary metabolic abnormality associated with nephrolithiasis in children. In many cases, the precipitating factor is never defined. Stones in pediatric patients may consist of calcium oxalate, calcium phosphate, or magnesium ammonium phosphate.

In neonates, factors increasing urinary calcium losses appear to be of primary importance in stone formation; however, other factors such as urinary flow rate, increased urine pH, and a lack of urinary stone inhibitors (e.g., magnesium, citrates, inorganic phosphates) also play an as-yet poorly defined role. Stones received from neonates and analyzed generally consist of calcium oxalate or calcium phosphate.

Normal urine calcium excretion in children is defined as an excretion of less than 4 mg/kg/day. Mean daily urinary calcium losses reported in preterm neonates can be minimal; however, a variety of nutritional factors and medications commonly encountered in this high-risk population can increase renal calcium losses. These include the following:

### Nutritional Factors
1. *hypophosphatemia/decreased phosphate intake*

2. *parenteral nutrient and calcium administration*

3. *hypervitaminosis D*

In studies completed in older children and adults, increased urinary calcium losses have been associated with increased protein intake and parenteral nutrient administration. It is unclear, however, how this effect is mediated. A similar problem has also been encountered in the low birth weight infant. Furthermore, some studies suggest that with increasing calcium intake, urinary calcium content also increases. However, it has been difficult to separate excessive calcium intakes from other factors, such as inadequate phosphorous intake, known to cause calciuria.

### Medications
1. *theophylline*

Ong et al. evaluated urinary calcium losses ($\mu$g/kg/min and urinary calcium/creatinine ratios) in preterm neonates before and after boluses of theophylline had been administered for the management of apnea of prematurity. Increased calcium losses exceeding those expected from the diuresis associated with theophylline were demonstrated. Studies in animals demonstrate a persistence of this effect.

2. *furosemide; ? other diuretics*

Furosemide is a potent diuretic that inhibits calcium reabsorption in Henle's loop. Urinary calcium losses increase two- to tenfold with furosemide administration. This effect does not decrease with time but may indeed increase. Conflicting information has been reported with other diuretics. The administration of spironolactone along with hydrochlorothiazide (but not spironolactone alone) to neonates has been associated with increased urinary calcium losses compared to preterm neonates receiving no diuretics. However, in children with calciuria induced by vitamin D administration, the addition of hydrochlorothiazide has been reported to reduce urinary calcium losses. Furthermore, decreased urinary calcium with resolution of renal calculi with the use of hydrochlorothiazide has been reported. This effect is noted even with continued use of furosemide, although calcium excretion continues to exceed that of patients on no diuretic.

3. *? dexamethasone*

In a single report, the development of nephrocalcinosis in a low birth weight infant was attributed to dexamethasone administration. Increased urinary calcium losses due to bone reabsorption have been reported with chronic steroid use. However, in this case the patient had also received furosemide, theophylline, increased daily vitamin D intake, and parenteral nutrition. These factors can all contribute to increased urinary calcium losses, hence, the role of dexamethasone in the etiology of nephrocalcinosis in this patient is unclear.

---

**CASE STUDY 9 continued**

The first abdominal ultrasound examination was normal. On day 80 of life, AS became increasingly irritable and his respiratory status deteriorated. He stabilized with increased levels of ambient oxygen. Studies to clarify the etiology of his deterioration were unremarkable and his decline was attributed to a viral illness. Although his respiratory status initially stabilized, AS required increasing respiratory support and continued to have intermittent episodes of irritability. As part of his ongoing care, his urine was screened for a variety of substances and hematuria was noted. Because of his irritability and hematuria, a renal ultrasound was obtained and demonstrated renal papillary calcifications.

## EXERCISE 13

### ■ Question:
How is nephrocalcinosis diagnosed radiographically?

### ■ Answer:
*Renal calculi may be diagnosed by abdominal radiograph or ultrasound. Confirmation of these findings requires an excretory urogram.*

### ■ Question:
How and when does nephrocalcinosis present?

### ■ Answer:
*Investigators performing serial studies on high-risk neonates report a broad range of ages at which nephrocalcinosis may be demonstrated. Jacinto et al. noted renal calcifications in preterm neonates with birth weights less than 1,500 g at the mean age of 39 days. Short et al. also monitored this high-risk population with serial ultrasounds of the urinary tract. The mean age at which these investigators demonstrated renal calculi was 47 days (SD = 14 days). Others, noting that hypercalciuria increases the risk of developing nephrocalcinosis, correlate the timing of stone appearance to initiation of furosemide. Gilsanz et al., retrospectively reviewing abdominal radiographs, identified renal calcifications 11 to 50 days after the initiation of this diuretic.*

*Although hematuria, pyuria, and crystals have been reported in some neonates with nephrocalcinosis, abnormalities in the urinalysis and clinical signs are conspicuously absent in most infants.*

*The incidence of nephrocalcinosis in preterm neonates has been evaluated by several investigators and appears to vary widely, but generally increases with decreasing gestational age and birth weight. Gilsanz reviewed the abdominal radiographs of 393 of 779 neonates admitted to the NICU. Renal calcifications were demonstrated in 10 neonates. Nine of these 10 neonates had birth weights of less than 1,250 g. Other investigators have reported an incidence ranging from 10% to 64%.*

## CASE STUDY 9 continued
AS's respiratory status continued to deteriorate. The frequency and severity of episodes of agitation increased. He was intubated and positive pressure ventilation was reinstituted. Furosemide was discontinued and Aldactone and Diuril started. Because of persistent requirements for ventilatory support, a tracheostomy was placed approximately 1.5 months after ventilator sup port was restarted. During this period AS had several episodes of severe agitation. These epi sodes were frequently associated with significant hematuria and were attributed to the passage of renal stones. No stones were recovered. Repeat renal ultrasounds 1 and 2 months after the initial study continued to demonstrate renal calcifications without hydronephrosis or hydroureter. Because of concerns that AS was in pain, as well as deteriorations in his respiratory status associated with these episodes, he received narcotics and sedatives. During the next 1.5 months, his respiratory status continued to improve and stabilize and ventilatory support was weaned. His episodes of agitation also diminished. Hematuria was no longer a problem. A renal ultrasound 5 months after the onset of hematuria continued to demonstrate nephrocalcinosis without hydronephrosis or hydroureters and normal-sized kidneys.

## EXERCISE 14

### ■ Question:
What is the usual course of nephrocalcinosis in affected infants?

### ■ Answer:
Most investigators report no evidence of obstruction in the urinary tract with demonstration of renal calculi. *Generally, resolution occurs during several months, usually without alterations in renal growth or diminished renal function.* However, an obstructive uropathy and decreased GFR may result and surgical intervention has been reported. It remains unclear whether altered renal function is due to the calculi themselves or reflects complications of other therapies instituted in this high-risk population.

With the discovery of calculi, elimination of factors promoting hypercalciuria are employed. Some investigators may also substitute hydrochlorothiazide for furosemide to decrease urinary calcium excretion.

# BIBLIOGRAPHY

## Early Neonatal Hypocalcemia

1. Itani O, Tsang RC: Calcium, phosphorus and magnesium in the newborn: Pathophysiology and management. In Hay WW, ed: *Neonatal Nutrition and Metabolism.* St. Louis, Mosby-Year Book, 1991, p. 171.
2. Salle BL, Delvin E, Gloriexs F, et al: Human neonatal hypocalcemia. *Biol Neonate* 1990; 58(suppl 1):22.
3. Tsang RC, Chen I, Friedman M, et al: Parathyroid function in infants of diabetic mothers. *J Pediatr* 1975; 86:399.
4. Loughead JL, Mimouni F, Tsang RC: Serum ionized calcium concentrations in normal neonates. *Am J Dis Child* 1988; 142:516.
5. Tsang RC, Kleinman LI, Sutherland JM, et al: Hypocalcemia in infants of diabetic mothers. Studies in calcium, phosphorus, and magnesium metabolism and parathormone responsiveness. *J Pediatr* 1972; 80:384.
6. Salle BL, David L, Chopard JP, et al: Prevention of early neonatal hypocalcemia in low birth weight infants with continuous calcium infusion. Effect on serum calcium, phosphorus, magnesium and circulating immunoreactive parathyroid hormone and calcitonin. *Pediatr Res* 1977; 11:1180.
7. Hillman LS, Rojanasathit S, Slatopolsky E, et al: Serial measurements of serum calcium, magnesium, parathyroid hormone, calcitonin and 25-hydroxy-vitamin D in premature and term infants during the first week of life. *Pediatr Res* 1977; 11:739.
8. Demarini S, Tsang RC: Disorders of calcium and magnesium metabolism. In Fanaroff AA, Martin RJ, eds: *Neonatal-Perinatal Medicine—Diseases of the Fetus and Infant.* St. Louis, Mosby-Year Book, 1992, p. 1181.
9. Scott SM, Ladenson JH, Aguanna JJ, et al: Effect of calcium therapy in the sick premature infant with early neonatal hypocalcemia. *J Pediatr* 1984; 104:747.
10. Mimouni F, Loughead JL, Tsang RC, et al: Postnatal surge in serum calcitonin concentrations. No contribution to neonatal hypocalcemia in infants of diabetic mothers. *Pediatr Res* 1990; 28:493.
11. Romagnoli C, Zecca E, Tortorolo G, et al: Plasma thyrocalcitonin and parathyroid hormone concentrations in early neonatal hypocalcemia. *Arch Dis Child* 1987; 62:580.
12. Tsang RC, Light IJ, Sutherland JM, et al: Possible pathogenic factors in neonatal hypocalcemia of prematurity. *J Pediatr* 1973; 82:423.
13. Venkataraman PS, Tsang RC, Chen I, et al: Pathogenesis of early neonatal hypocalcemia: Studies of serum calcitonin, gastrin and plasma glucagon. *J Pediatr* 1987; 110:599.
14. Pitkin RM: Calcium metabolism in pregnancy and the perinatal period: A review. *Am J Obstet Gynecol* 1985; 151:99.
15. Brunette MG: Calcium transport through the placenta. *Can J Physiol Pharmacol* 1985; 66:1261.
16. Pitkin RM: Calcium metabolism in pregnancy: A review. *Am J Obstet Gynecol* 1975; 121:724.
17. Kuoppala T, Tuimala R, Parviainem M, et al: Can the fetus regulate its calcium uptake? *Br J Obstet Gynaecol* 1984; 91:1192.
18. Paulson SK, DeLuca HF: Review article. Vitamin D metabolism during pregnancy. *Bone* 1986; 7:331.
19. Brommage R, DeLuca HF: Placental transport of calcium and phosphorus is not regulated by vitamin D. *Am J Physiol* 1984; 246:F526.
20. Venkataraman PS, Blick KE, Fry HD, et al: Postnatal changes in calcium-regulating hormones in very-low-birth weight infants. *Am J Dis Child* 1985; 139:913.
21. Mimouni F, Tsang RC, Hertzberg VS, et al: Polycythemia, hypomagnesemia, and hypocalcemia in infants of diabetic mothers. *Am J Dis Child* 1986; 140:798.
22. Tsang RC, Chen I, Hays W, et al: Neonatal hypocalcemia in infants with birth asphyxia. *J Pediatr* 1974; 84:428.
23. Brown DR, Steranka BH, Taylor FH: Treatment of early onset neonatal hypocalcemia. *Am J Dis Child* 1981; 135:24.
24. Roberton NRC, Smith MA: Early neonatal hypocalcemia. *Arch Dis Child* 1975; 50:604.
25. Brown DR, Salsburey DJ: Short-term biochemical effects of parenteral calcium treatment of early-onset neonatal hypocalcemia. *J Pediatr* 1982; 100:777.

## Late Neonatal Hypocalcemia and Hypomagnesemia; Hypoparathyroidism

26. Demarini S, Tsang RC: Disorders of calcium and magnesium metabolism. In Fanaroff AA, Martin RJ, eds: *Neonatal-Perinatal Medicine—Diseases of the Fetus and Infant.* St. Louis, Mosby-Year Book, 1992, p. 1181.
27. Koo WWW, Tsang RC: Calcium, magnesium, and phosphorus. In Tsang RC, Nichols BL, eds: *Nutrition During Infancy.* Philadelphia, Hanley and Belfus, 1988, p. 175.
28. Itani O, Tsang RC: Calcium, phosphorus and magnesium in the newborn: Pathophysiology and management. In Hay WW, ed: *Neonatal Nutrition and Metabolism.* St. Louis, Mosby-Year Book, 1991, p. 171.
29. Rosenblatt M, Kronenberg HM, Potts JT: Parathyroid hormone physiology, chemistry, biosynthesis, metabolism and mode of action. In DeGroot LJ, ed: *Endocrinology.* Philadelphia, WB Saunders Co, 1989, p. 848.
30. Tsang RC: Neonatal magnesium disturbances. *Am J Dis Child* 1972; 124:282.
31. McKusick V: *Mendelian Inheritance in Man.* Baltimore, Johns Hopkins University Press, 1990.
32. Mallette LE, Cooper JB, Kirkland JL: Transient congenital hypoparathyroidism: Possible association with anomalies of the pulmonary valve. *J Pediatr* 1982; 101:928.
33. Bainbridge R, Mughal Z, Mimouni F, et al: Transient congenital hypoparathyroidism: How transient is it? *J Pediatr* 1987; 111:866.
34. Kooh SW, Binet A: Partial hypoparathyroid-

ism. A variant of transient congenital hypoparathyroidism. *Am J Dis Child* 1991; 145:877.

35. Hanukoglu A, Chalew S, Kowarski A: Late-onset of hypocalcemic rickets and hypoparathyroidism in an infant of a mother with hyperparathyroidism. *J Pediatr* 1988; 112:751.

## Hypermagnesemia

36. Elliot JP: Magnesium sulfate as a tocolytic agent. *Am J Obstet Gynecol* 1983; 147:277.
37. Hutchinson HT, Nichols MM, Kuhn CR, et al: Effects of magnesium sulfate on uterine contractility, intrauterine fetus and infant. Am J Obstet Gynecol 1964; 88:747.
38. Pritchard JA, Cunningham G, Pritchard SA: The Parkland Memorial Hospital protocol for treatment of eclampsia: Evaluation of 245 cases. *Am J Obstet Gynecol* 1984; 148:951.
39. Pritchard JA, Pritchard SA: Standardized treatment of 154 consecutive cases of eclampsia. *Am J Obstet Gynecol* 1975; 23:543.
40. Cruikshank DP, Pitkin RM, Reynolds WA, et al: Effects of magnesium sulfate treatment on perinatal calcium metabolism. *Am J Obstet Gynecol* 1979; 134:243.
41. Worley RJ: Pregnancy-induced hypertension. In Danforth RN, Scott JR, eds: *Obstetrics and Gynecology.* Philadelphia, JB Lippincott Co, 1986, p. 446.
42. Shils ME: Magnesium. In Shils ME, Young VR, eds: *Modern Nutrition in Health and Disease.* Philadelphia, Lea and Febiger, 1988, p. 159.
43. McGuinness GA, Weinstein MW, Cruikshank DP, et al: Effects of magnesium sulfate treatment on perinatal calcium metabolism. II. Neonatal responses. *Obstet Gynecol* 1980; 56:595.
44. Lipsitz PJ: The clinical and biochemical effects of excess magnesium in the newborn. *Pediatrics* 1971; 47:501.
45. Donovan EF, Tsang RC, Steichen JJ, et al: Neonatal hypermagnesemia: Effect on parathyroid hormone and calcium homeostasis. *J Pediatr* 1980; 96:305.
46. Tsang RC, Strub R, Brown DR, et al: Hypomagnesemia in infants of diabetic mothers: Perinatal studies. *J Pediatr* 1976; 89:115.
47. Mimouni F, Tsang RC, Hertzberg VS, et al: Polycythemia, hypomagnesemia and hypocalcemia in infants of diabetic mothers. *Am J Dis Child* 1986; 140:798.
48. Engel RR, Elin RJ: Hypermagnesemia from birth asphxia. *J Pediatr* 1970; 77:631.
49. Mimouni F, Miodovnik M, Tsang RC, et al: Decreased maternal serum magnesium concentration and adverse fetal outcome in insulin-dependent diabetic women. *Obstet Gynecol* 1987; 70:85.
50. Tsang RC, Kleinman I, Sutherland JM, et al: Hypocalcemia in infants of diabetic mothers. Studies in calcium, phosphorus and. magnesium metabolism and parathormone responsiveness. *J Pediatr* 1972; 80:384.
51. Stone SR, Pritchard JA: Effect of maternally administered magnesium sulfate on the neonate. *Obstet Gynecol* 1970; 35:574.
52. Liptsitz PJ, English IC: Hypermagnesemia in the newborn infant. *Pediatrics* 1967; 40:856.
53. Brady JP, Williams HC: Magnesium intoxication in a premature infant. *Pediatrics* 1967; 40:100.
54. Rasch DK, Huber PA, Richardson CJ, et al: Neurobehavioral effects of neonatal hypermagnesemia. *J Pediatr* 1982; 100:272.
55. Ghoneium MM, Long JP: The interaction between magnesium and other neuromuscular blocking agents. Anesthesiology 1970; 32:23.
56. Itani O, Tsang RC: Calcium, phosphorus and magnesium in the newborn: Pathophysiology and management. In Hay WW, ed: *Neonatal Nutrition and Metabolism.* St. Louis, Mosby-Year Book, 1991, p. 171.
57. L'Hommedieu CS, Huber PA, Rasch DK: Potentiation of magnesium-induced neuromuscular weakness by gentamicin. *Crit Care Med* 1983; 11:55.
58. Amodio J, Berdon W, Abramson S, et al: Microcolon of prematurity: A form of functional obstruction. *Am J Roentgenol* 1986; 146:239.
59. Cumming WA, Thomas VJ: Hypermagnesium: A cause of abnormal metaphyses in the neonate. *Am J Roentgenol* 1989; 152:1071.
60. Lamm CI, Norton KI, Murphy RJC, et al: Congenital rickets associated with magnesium sulfate infusion for tocolysis. *J Pediatr* 1988; 113:1078.
61. Tsang RC: Neonatal magnesium disturbances. *Am J Dis Child* 1972; 124:282.
62. Randall RR, Cohen MD, Spray CC, et al: Hypermagnesemia in renal failure. Etiology and toxic manifestations. *Ann Intern Med* 1964; 61:73.

## Metabolic Bone Disease in Premature Infants

63. Koo WWK, Gupta JM, Nayanar VV, et al: Skeletal changes in preterm infants. *Arch Dis Child* 1982; 57:447.
64. Koo WWK, Oestreich A, Tsang RC, et al: Natural history of rickets and fractures in very low birth weight infants during infancy. *J Bone Miner Res* 1986; 1:123.
65. Koo WWK, Sherman R, Succop P, et al: Sequential bone mineral content in small preterm infants with and without fractures and rickets. *J Bone Miner Res* 1988; 3:193.
66. Iob V, Swanson WW: Mineral growth of the human fetus. *Am J Dis Child* 1934; 47:302.
67. Widdowson EM, Spray CM: Chemical development in utero. *Arch Dis Child* 1951; 26:205.
68. Fee BA, Weil WB: Body composition of infants of diabetic mothers by direct analysis. *Ann NY Acad Sci* 1963; 110:869.
69. Sparks JW: Human intrauterine growth and nutrient accretion. *Semin Perin* 1984; 8:74.
70. Kelly HJ, Sloan RE, Hoffman W, et al: Accumulation of nitrogen and six minerals in the human fetus during gestation. *Hum Biol* 1951; 23:61.
71. Ziegler EE, O'Donnell AM, Nelson SE, et al: Body composition of the reference fetus. *Growth* 1976; 40:329.
72. Shaw JCL: Parenteral nutrition in the manage-

ment of sick low birthweight infants. *Pediatr Clin North Am* 1973; 20:333.

73. Koo WWK, Tsang RC: Calcium, magnesium and phosphorus. In Tsang RC, Nichols BL, eds: *Nutrition During Infancy.* Philadelphia, Hanley and Belfus, 1988, p. 175.

74. Greer FR, Tsang RC: Calcium, phosphorus, magnesium and vitamin D requirements for the preterm infant. In Tsang RC, ed: *Vitamin and Mineral Requirements in Preterm Infants.* New York, Marcel Dekker, 1985, p. 99.

75. Lemons JA, Moya L, Hall D, et al: Differences in the composition of preterm and term human milk during early lactation. *Pediatr Res* 1982; 16:113.

76. Vaughan LA, Weber CW, Kemberling SR: Longitudinal changes in the mineral content of human milk. *Am J Clin Nutr* 1979; 32:2301.

77. Picciano MF: Mineral content of human milk during a single nursing. *Nutrition Reports Int* 1978; 18:5.

78. Fransson G, Lonnerdal B: Zinc, copper, calcium and magnesium in human milk. *J Pediatr* 1982; 101:504.

79. Greer FR, Tsang RC, Levin RS, et al: Increasing serum calcium and magnesium concentrations in breastfed infants. Longitudinal studies of minerals in human milk and in sera of nursing mothers and their infants. *J Pediatr* 1982; 100:59.

80. Senterre J: Endogenous faecal calcium, total digestive juice calcium, net and true calcium absorption. In Stembera Z, Polacek K, Sabata V, eds: *Perinatal Medicine Fourth European Congress of Perinatal Medicine.* Stuggart, Georg Thieme, 1975, p. 287.

81. Barltrop D, Mole RH, Sutton A: Absorption and endogenous faecal excretion of calcium by low birthweight infants on feeds with varying contents of calcium and phosphate. *Arch Dis Child* 1977; 52:41.

82. Ehrenkranz RA, Ackermann BA, Nelli CM, et al: Absorption of calcium in premature infants as measured with stable isotope $^{46}$Ca extrinsic tag. *Pediatr Res* 1985; 19:178.

83. Hillman LS, Tack E, Covell DG, et al: Measurement of true calcium absorption in premature infants using intravenous $^{46}$Ca and oral $^{44}$Ca. *Pediatr Res* 1988; 23:589.

84. Allen L: Calcium bioavailability and absorption: A review. *Am J Clin Nutr* 1982; 35:783.

85. Younoszai MK: Development of intestinal calcium transport. In Lebenthal E, ed: *Textbook of Gastroenterology and Nutrition in Infancy.* New York, Raven Press, 1981, p. 623.

86. Atkinson SA, Shah JK, McGee C, et al: Mineral excretion in premature infants receiving various diuretic therapies. *J Pediatr* 1988; 113:540.

87. Giles MM, Fenton MH, Shaw B, et al: Sequential calcium and phosphorus balance studies in preterm infants. *J Pediatr* 1987; 110:591.

88. DeVizia B, Fomon S, Nelson SE, et al: Effect of dietary calcium on metabolic balance of normal infants. *Pediatr Res* 1985; 19:800.

89. Delmas PD, Malaval L: New biochemical markers of bone turnover. In Cohen DV, Martin TJ, Meunier PJ, eds: *Calcium Regulation and Bone Metabolism: Basic and Clinical Aspects.* Amsterdam, Elsevier Science Publishers, 1987, p. 105.

90. Bringhurst FR: Calcium and phosphate distribution, turnover, and metabolic actions. In De-Groot LJ, ed: *Endocrinology.* Philadelphia, WB Saunders Co, 1989, p. 805.

91. Gertner JM: Disorders of calcium and phosphorus homeostasis. *Pediatr Clin North Am* 1990; 37:1441.

92. Rosenblatt M, Kronenberg HM, Potts JT: Parathyroid hormone: Physiology, chemistry, biosynthesis, secretion, metabolism, and mode of action. In DeGroot LJ, ed: *Endocrinology.* Philadelphia, WB Saunders Co, 1989, p. 848.

93. Holick MF: Vitamin D. In DeGroot LJ, ed: *Endocrinology.* Philadelphia, WB Saunders Co, 1989, p. 902.

94. Weiss MJ, Ray K, Henthorn PS, et al: Structure of the human liver/bone/kidney alkaline phosphatase gene. *J Biol Chem* 1988; 263:12002.

95. Koo WWK, Succop P, Hambidge KM: Serum alkaline phosphatase and serum zinc concentrations in preterm infants with rickets and fractures. *Am J Dis Child* 1989; 143:1342.

96. Register TC, Wuthier RE: Effect of pyrophosphate and two diphosphonates on $^{45}$Ca and $^{32}$Pi uptake and mineralization by matrix vesicle enriched fractions and by hydroxyapatite. *Bone* 1985; 6:307.

97. Guyton AC: Parathyroid hormone, calcitonin, calcium and phosphate metabolism, vitamin D, bone and teeth. In Guyton AC, ed: *Textbook of Medical Physiology.* Philadelphia, WB Saunders Co, 1991, p. 868.

98. Posen S: Do alkaline phosphatases have a physiological function? In *Vitamin D, Basic Research and Its Clinical Application.* New York, Walter de Gruyten and Co, 1979, p. 983.

99. Glass EJ, Hume R, Hendry GMA, et al: Plasma alkaline phosphatase activity in rickets of prematurity. *Arch Dis Child* 1982; 57:373.

100. Rock RC, Miller RE: Reference values for laboratory procedures. In Harvey A, Johns RJ, McKusick VA, eds: *The Principles and Practice of Medicine.* Connecticut, Appleton and Lange, 1988, p. 1215.

101. Cordano A, Bancalari E, Hansen JW, et al: Nutritional balance studies: Evaluation of a premature infant formula. *Arch Latinoam Nutr* 1985; 35:221.

102. Shenai JP, Reynolds E, Babson SG: Nutritional balance studies in very-low-birth-weight infants: Enhanced nutrient retention rates by an experimental formula. *Pediatrics* 1980; 66:233.

103. Rowe JC, Carey DE: Phosphorus deficiency syndrome in very low birth weight infants. *Pediatr Clin North Am* 1987; 34:997.

104. Rowe JC, Wood DH, Rowe DW, et al: Nutritional hypophosphatemic rickets in a premature infant fed breast milk. *N Engl J Med* 1979; 300:293.

105. Koo WWK, Antony G, Stevens LHS: Continuous nasogastric phosphorus infusion in hypophosphatemic rickets of prematurity. *Am J Dis Child* 1984; 138:172.

106. Sagy M, Birenbaum E, Balin A, et al: Phos-

phate-depletion syndrome in a premature infant fed human milk. *J Pediatr* 1980; 96:683.

107. Senterre J, Putet G, Salle B, et al: Effects of vitamin D and phosphorus supplementation on calcium retention in preterm infants fed banked human milk. *J Pediatr* 1983; 103:305.

108. Rowe J, Rowe D, Horak E, et al: Hypophosphatemia and hypercalciuria in small premature infants fed human milk: Evidence for inadequate dietary phosphorus. *J Pediatr* 1984; 104:112.

109. Senterre J, Salle B: Calcium and phosphorus economy of the preterm infant and its interaction with vitamin D and its metabolites. *Acta Paediatr Scand* 1982; 296(suppl): 85.

110. Miller RR, Menke JA, Mentser MI: Hypercalcemia associated with phosphate depletion in the neonate. *J Pediatr* 1984; 105:814.

111. Carey DE, Goetz CA, Horak E, et al: Phosphorus wasting during phosphorus supplementation of human milk feedings in preterm infants. *J Pediatr* 1985; 107:790.

112. Evans JR, Allen AC, Stinson DA, et al: Effect of high dose vitamin D supplementation on radiographically detectable bone disease of very low birth weight infants. *J Pediatr* 1989; 115:779.

113. Kovar I, Mayne P, Barltrop D: Plasma alkaline phosphatase activity: A screening test for rickets in preterm neonates. *Lancet* 1982; 1:308.

114. Fitzgerald KA, MacKay MW: Calcium and phosphate solubility in neonatal parenteral nutrient solutions containing Aminosyn PF. *Am J Hosp Pharm* 1987; 44:1396.

115. Fitzgerald KA, MacKay MW: Calcium and phosphate solubility in neonatal parenteral nutrient solutions containing TrophAmine. *Am J Hosp Pharm* 1986; 43:88.

116. Brooke OG, Lucas A: Metabolic bone disease in preterm infants. *Arch Dis Child* 1985; 60:682.

117. Itani O, Tsang RC: Calcium, phosphorus and magnesium in the newborn: Pathophysiology and management. In Hay WW, ed: *Neonatal Nutrition and Metabolism.* St. Louis, Mosby-Year Book, 1991, p. 171.

## Nephrocalcinosis

118. Bringhurst FR: Calcium and phosphate distribution, turnover, and metabolic actions. In DeGroot LJ, ed: *Endocrinology.* Philadelphia, WB Saunders Co, 1989, p. 805.

119. Walter PC, Lamm D, Kaplan GW: Pediatric urolithiasis: A ten-year review. *Pediatrics* 1980; 65:1068.

120. Garcia CD, Miller LA, Stapleton FB: Natural history of hematuria associated with hypercalciuria in children. *Am J Dis Child* 1991; 145:1204.

121. Ezzedeen F, Adelman RD, Ahlfors CE: Renal calcification in preterm infants. Pathophysiology and long-term sequelae. *J Pediatr* 1988; 113:532.

122. Noe HN, Bryant JF, Shane R, et al: Urolithiasis in pre-term neonates associated with furosemide therapy. *J Urol* 1984; 132:93.

123. Glasier CM, Stoddard RA, Ackerman NB, et al: Nephrolithiasis in infants: Association with chronic furosemide therapy. *AJR* 1983; 140: 107.

124. Hufnagle KG, Khan SN, Penn D, et al: Renal calcifications: A complication of long-term furosemide therapy in preterm infants. *Pediatrics* 1982; 70:360.

125. Langman CB, Moore ES: Hypercalciuria in clinical pediatrics. *Clin Pediatr* 1984; 23:135.

126. Lipkin EW, Ott SM, Chesnut CH, et al: Mineral loss in the parenteral nutrition patient. *Am J Clin Nutr* 1988; 47:515.

127. Bengoa JM, Sitrin MD, Wood RJ, et al: Amino acid–induced hypercalciuria in patients on total parenteral nutrition. *Am J Clin Nutr* 1983; 38:264.

128. Zennel MB: Calcium utilization: Effect of varying level and source of dietary protein. *Am J Clin Nutr* 1988; 48:880.

129. Chessex P, Pineault M, Zebiche H, et al: Calciuria in parenterally fed preterm infants: Role of phosphorus intake. *J Pediatr* 1985; 107:794.

130. Vileisis RA: Effect of phosphorus intake in total parenteral nutrition infusates in premature neonates. *J Pediatr* 1987; 110:586.

131. Pelegano JF, Rowe JC, Carey DE, et al: Simultaneous infusion of calcium and phosphorus in parenteral nutrition for premature infants: Use of physiologic calcium/phosphorus ratio. *J Pediatr* 1989; 114:115.

132. Ong MJ, Yeh JK, Yadoo M, et al: Theophylline induced hypercalciuria in the preterm infants: A pilot study. *Pediatr Res* 1988; 23:262A.

133. Whiting SJ, Whitney HL: Effect of dietary caffeine and theophylline on urinary calcium excretion in the adult rat. *J Nutr* 1987; 117:1224.

134. Jacinto JS, Houchang D, Modanlou HD, et al: Renal calcification incidence in very low birth weight infants. *Pediatrics* 1988; 81:31.

135. Savage MO, Wilkinson AR, Baum JD, et al: Frusemide in respiratory distress syndrome. *Arch Dis Child* 1975; 50:709.

136. Atkinson SA, Shah JK, McGee C, et al: Mineral excretion in premature infants receiving various diuretic therapies. *J Pediatr* 1988; 113:540.

137. Santos F, Smith MJV, Chan JCM: Hypercalciuria associated with long-term administration of calcitriol [1,25-dihydroxyvitamin D$_3$] action of hydrochlorothiazide. *Am J Dis Child* 1986; 140:139.

138. Kamitsuka MD, Peloquin D: Renal calcification after dexamethasone in infants with bronchopulmonary dysplasia. *Lancet* 1991; 337: 626.

139. Woolfield N, Haslam R, Quesne G, et al: Ultrasound diagnosis of nephrocalcinosis in preterm infants. *Arch Dis Child* 1988, 63:86.

140. Short A, Cooke RWI: The incidence of renal calcification in preterm infants. *Arch Dis Child* 1991; 66:412.

141. Gilsanz V, Fernal W, Reid BS, et al: Nephrolithiasis in premature infants. *Radiology* 1985; 154:107.

142. Ramey SL, Williams JL: Nephrolithiasis and cholelithiasis in a premature infant. *J Clin Ultrasound* 1986; 14:203.

# Chapter 4

# NEONATAL HYPOGLYCEMIA

*David E. Hertz,* M.D.

*Scott C. Denne,* M.D.

Glucose is the major energy source throughout fetal life. At the moment of birth, however, the constant maternal supply of glucose delivered to the fetus *in utero* is discontinued and the neonate must rely on his or her own homeostatic mechanisms to maintain a euglycemic state. This requires the orchestrated activation of various hormonal, neural, and enzymatic systems, which if disturbed may result in abnormal blood glucose levels.

This chapter begins with a review of neonatal glucose metabolism and concludes with six case studies. Each case exemplifies a clinical situation in which neonatal hypoglycemia may be encountered and is followed by several questions pertaining to that case. Each set of questions is answered in detail in the paragraphs that immediately follow. Answers to specific questions are shown in italicized print.

## GLUCOSE METABOLISM IN THE NEWBORN INFANT

During gestation, the fetus continuously receives almost 7 g/kg/day of glucose from the mother through the placenta. In contrast with older infants and children, fetal glucose metabolism is nearly independent of the traditional glucoregulatory hormones, insulin and glucagon. Although both of these hormones are present early in gestation, their regulation and activity differ from that seen in the newborn infant and the adult (i.e., under normal conditions the fetal liver is relatively insensi-

tive to the actions of insulin and glucagon). In contrast, the fetus does exhibit an ability to mobilize glucose and free fatty acids in response to certain catecholamines. Fetal glucose metabolism is also unique in that several key enzyme activities involved in glycolysis and gluconeogenesis are either present in low concentrations or absent prior to delivery.

At the time of delivery the neonate's glucose requirement continues to remain high (in the range of 4 to 6 mg/kg/min); however, clamping the umbilical cord removes the maternal source of glucose. Thus, in every infant the concentration of glucose falls postnatally, reaching a nadir at or between 1 and 3 hours of age (Fig. 4-1). During this time certain key glucoregulatory hormonal, neural, and enzymatic changes occur. For example, plasma glucagon and growth hormone values rapidly increase after birth, while the concentration of insulin falls. The rise in plasma glucagon levels is mediated in large part by adrenergic mechanisms, and probably does not represent a response to hypoglycemia. Similarly, the concentrations of the catecholamines, epinephrine, and norepinephrine also increase postnatally, though the increase in epinephrine is much greater than that of norepinephrine. The increased concentrations of epinephrine and glucagon stimulate lipolysis and increase the activity of phosphorylase, a key enzyme in glycolysis. The increased glucagon concentration also results in increased activity of phosphoenolpyruvate carboxykinase (PEPCK), a rate-limiting enzyme in gluconeogenesis. All these changes

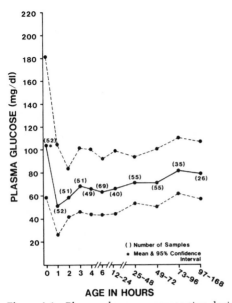

**Figure 4-1** Plasma glucose concentration during the first 168 hours of life in healthy, term, appropriate-for-gestational-age infants.
From Srinivasan G, Pildes RS, et al: Plasma glucose values in normal neonates: A new look. *J Pediatr* 1986; 118(5):115. Reprinted with permission of Mosby-Year Book, Inc.

act in concert to mobilize glucose in the newly born infant.

Numerous situations can occur that may lead to deviations in this normal transition and result in neonatal hypoglycemia. However, in most cases, the underlying etiology can be attributed to decreased production of glucose, increased utilization of glucose, or a combination of these (Table 4-1). In the following case studies, common causes of hypoglycemia are discussed in relation to how each results in aberrations in normal glucose homeostasis.

## CASE STUDY 1

Baby girl Brown is a 2-hour-old 3,200-g term infant who was precipitously delivered at home to a 30-year-old mother of five other children. Mother and baby were transported to a hospital immediately following the birth. On arrival, the infant's examination was within normal limits; however, the axillary temperature was only 35.9°C. The infant responded to routine warming measures and was transferred to the nursery. A whole blood glucose concentration obtained at the bedside was reported as 25 mg/dL. The infant appears vigorous and alert.

**Table 4-1** Risk Factors for Hypoglycemia

***Decreased glucose production/impaired mobilization***
Adrenocortical insufficiency
Congenital hypopituitarism
Fructose-1,6-diphosphatase deficiency
Fructose intolerance
Galactosemia
Glucagon deficiency
Glycogen storage disease, Type 1
Intrauterine growth retardation
PEPCK deficiency
Prematurity

***Increased glucose utilization***
Hypothermia
Hypoxia
Sepsis

***Hyperinsulinism***
Beckwith-Wiedemann syndrome
Islet cell adenoma/adenomatosis
Maternal beta-sympathomimetics
Maternal diabetes mellitus
Maternal thiazides
Nesidioblastosis
Rh incompatibility
Umbilical artery catheter placement

***Mixed***
Congenital heart disease
Exchange transfusion
Maternal propanolol

## EXERCISE 1

### ■ Questions:

1. Is this patient hypoglycemic?

2. Does this infant exhibit any symptoms that would suggest that she is hypoglycemic?

3. Does the history suggest any risk factors for the development of hypoglycemia?

4. How should this infant's hypoglycemia be managed?

## ■ Answers:

There is no universally accepted definition of neonatal hypoglycemia. *Many textbooks define hypoglycemia as a plasma glucose level <35 mg/dL in a term infant, <25 mg/dL in a preterm infant, and <45 mg/dL in any infant older than 72 hours of age.* Confounding this issue is the observation that some infants may be asymptomatic at plasma glucose concentrations less than these, while other infants may be symptomatic at values above those levels. Figure 4-1 displays the range of plasma glucose concentrations seen during the first 168 hours of life in healthy term infants who are appropriate for gestational age. Unfortunately, no similar data exist on preterm infants. Therefore, we and others believe that *the most prudent approach clinically may be to view any plasma glucose <40 mg/dL with suspicion and worthy of further investigation and probable intervention.* In any case, remember that corresponding whole blood glucose concentrations, such as those measured by standard bedside techniques, will be 10% to 15% lower than plasma glucose concentrations due to the dilutional effect of the red blood cell mass.

The diagnosis of hypoglycemia is first suggested by recording an abnormally low value on a bedside blood glucose screening test. Such screens must be confirmed by laboratory determinations because they may be abnormal if meticulous attention to detail is not observed when the sample is obtained. Delay in testing the sample can result in artificially low values due to red cell oxidation of glucose, whereas mixing the sample with isopropyl alcohol, which is commonly used to cleanse the sample site, will result in abnormally high values.

The signs and symptoms of hypoglycemia in the newborn range from subtle to profound and a high index of suspicion must be maintained (Table 4-2). Indeed, *a significant number of hypoglycemic infants have no recognizable signs or symptoms.* The symptomatic hypoglycemic infant may manifest lethargy, jitteriness, hypotonia, tachypnea, apnea, cyanosis, bradycardia, temperature instability, and seizures. Long-term follow-up of hypoglycemic infants has suggested that affected infants manifesting seizures are at greatest risk for neurodevelopmental abnormalities.

After the diagnosis is confirmed, immediate corrective measures must be undertaken, as are described in later paragraphs. However, a simultaneous effort must be made to uncover the underlying etiology of the hypoglycemia. In this regard the maternal and perinatal histories are invaluable. The maternal history should address the possible presence of diabetes mellitus (or any history of glucose intolerance), maternal use of medications, any history of preterm labor (especially requiring treatment with β sympathomimetics), preeclampsia, and the possibility of maternal-fetal blood group incompatibility. The perinatal history may suggest cold stress, asphyxia, or trauma. Physical examination of the newborn infant may reveal macrosomia or organomegaly, midline defects, or congenital anomalies, or may suggest abnormal prenatal growth. Initial laboratory testing should include measurement of plasma glucose, sodium, and potassium (to rule out adrenal insufficiency) and a complete blood count (as a screen for infection). Further studies that may be indicated—though not commonly necessary—include insulin, glucagon, and cortisol and growth hormone concentrations and thyroid function tests. More specialized tests are occasionally

**Table 4-2** Signs and Symptoms of Hypoglycemia

Apnea

Bradycardia

Cyanosis

Hypotonia

Jitteriness

Lethargy

Poor feeding

Seizures

Tachypnea

Temperature instability

needed when inborn errors of metabolism are suspected.

In the case just described, the perinatal history is important. *It suggests that hypothermia was a significant contributing factor to the development of hypoglycemia.* Stressed infants experiencing hypothermia or hypoxia may develop hypoglycemia, which is believed to result from an increase in anaerobic glycolysis. Furthermore, hypoglycemia may prolong the hypothermic event by affecting the central thermoregulatory center in the hypothalamus.

In Case Study 1 the infant is hypoglycemic but asymptomatic. In asymptomatic and otherwise healthy infants who appear vigorous and able to take a bottle, correction may be attempted with oral feedings. *The infant should be given 5% dextrose and water (D₅W) or formula, following which the blood glucose concentration should be checked every 30 minutes to monitor the response.* If the patient responds with rapid correction of blood glucose values, he or she should be allowed to feed ad lib. However, continued close monitoring of the blood glucose concentration (before and between feedings) should continue for at least 48 hours. If the blood glucose values continue to fall prior to feedings, the infant should be fasted (for as long as 8 hours), and blood glucose concentrations should be determined every 2 hours to make sure that the infant remains in a euglycemic state between feedings. The fasting study should be immediately terminated if hypoglycemia develops. Further evaluation is needed if the infant is unable to maintain a blood glucose concentration within acceptable limits. Recurrent or recalcitrant hypoglycemia may require continuous intravenous glucose infusions, steroid therapy to stimulate gluconeogenesis from noncarbohydrate sources, or diazoxide if the hypoglycemia is due to hyperinsulinism (Table 4-3).

---

**CASE STUDY 2**

Baby girl Smith is an 800-g infant born at 29 weeks' gestation to a 22-year-old primigravida woman. During the week prior to delivery, this woman was treated for 6 days with terbutaline in an attempt to stop preterm labor. Spontaneous rupture of membranes occurred 28 hours prior to delivery and the labor was allowed to progress. Delivery occurred without complication and Apgar scores of 7 and 8 were assigned. Her course was unremarkable until 6 hours of age when she appeared "jittery" and a bedside blood glucose screening test strip indicated a "low value." A corresponding laboratory determination of the plasma glucose concentration was 15 mg/dL.

**EXERCISE 2**

---

**■ Questions:**

1. What risk factors for hypoglycemia does this infant exhibit?

---

**Table 4-3**  Treatment of Hypoglycemia

| | |
|---|---|
| Asymptomatic | If infant is able to take oral feedings, allow him or her to bottle feed D₅W or formula and frequently check glucoses to monitor response. |
| Symptomatic | Give 200 mg/kg intravenous glucose (the equivalent of 2 cc/kg D₁₀W)* and simultaneously begin a constant glucose infusion to deliver 4 to 6 mg/kg/min. Increase the rate of the infusion as needed to maintain euglycemia. |
| Persistent | If greater than 15 to 20 mg/kg/min is required, hydrocortisone 5 mg/kg/day (IV or po) or prednisone 2 mg/kg/day po may be given to stimulate gluconeogenesis from noncarbohydrate sources. If the hypoglycemia remains recalcitrant and apparently due to hyperinsulinism, diazoxide at a dose of 10 to 15 mg/kg/day may be given to suppress pancreatic insulin secretion. |

* Glucagon 1 mg IM may be administered as a temporizing measure while establishing IV access is attempted.

2. How should this infant's hypoglycemia be managed?

■ **Answers:**

*This patient is premature* and *small for gestational age.* Both conditions are commonly associated with hypoglycemia. Premature infants have decreased glycogen stores and often have limited intakes. Their gluconeogenic and glycogenolytic systems also exhibit functional immaturity to varying degrees. Small for gestational age (SGA) infants are at particular risk for hypoglycemia. Almost one-third of growth-retarded infants demonstrate hypoglycemia in the immediate postnatal period. This incidence is almost doubled in infants who are both premature and SGA. The SGA infant is similar to the premature infant in that both have decreased glycogen stores and decreased levels or activities of certain key gluconeogenic enzymes. Serum levels of gluconeogenic substrates (alanine and lactate) and several gluconeogenic amino acids are increased in hypoglycemic SGA infants. Furthermore, compared to their nongrowth-retarded counterparts, SGA neonates exhibit a poor glycemic response to loading with alanine. Another important causative factor in the SGA infant may be the high ratio of cerebral glucose use to glucose production, which results from suboptimal hepatic glucose production and decreased glycogen stores.

*This infant was also born to a mother who had been receiving terbutaline for preterm labor.* Several maternal medications have been associated with neonatal hypoglycemia. The use of $\beta$ sympathomimetics such as terbutaline or ritodrine, which inhibit preterm labor, or benzothiadiazide diuretics may contribute to the development of hypoglycemia, by promoting fetal insulin production or release. Maternal use of propranolol has also been associated with hypoglycemia in the neonate. While the pathophysiological mechanism of propranolol-induced hypoglycemia is unclear, hypotheses include prevention of sympathetic stimulation of skeletal muscle glycogenolysis, inhibition of the increase in free fatty acids and lactate associated with epinephrine release, or increased secretion of growth hormone in the face of neonatal hypoglycemia.

Premature and prolonged rupture of membranes increase the likelihood of sepsis in this infant. *Sepsis, like hypoxia and hypothermia, places the neonate at risk for hypoglycemia, probably because of an increase in anaerobic glycolysis.* It has also been proposed that there may be an impairment in the mobilization of glucose in septic infants, which is suggested by the occurrence of hypoglycemia in septic infants with apparently adequate glycogen stores.

The infant in this case is significantly hypoglycemic and symptomatic, and immediate corrective measures should be taken. Given this patient's history and degree of hypoglycemia, an attempt at oral therapy would not be appropriate. *Intravenous administration of glucose would be the most efficacious therapy. The slow administration of glucose [200 mg/kg—the equivalent of 2 cc/kg of 10% dextrose and water ($D_{10}W$)] should restore the serum glucose concentration to a normal range. At the same time, a continuous infusion of glucose should be initiated to provide 4 to 6 mg/kg/min of glucose.* This constant infusion may then be increased as needed to maintain the patient's glucose concentration within the normal range.

---

**CASE STUDY 3**

Baby boy Jones is a 4,000-g infant who was born at term gestation to a poorly controlled insulin-dependent diabetic mother. Spontaneous vaginal delivery of this macrosomic infant was complicated by a right clavicular fracture. The infant was assigned Apgar scores of 7 and 8 at 1 and 5 minutes of life, respectively. Initially, the infant did well, but at 2 hours of age he was noted to be lethargic and a bedside glucometer reading revealed a value of 23 mg/dL. A laboratory plasma glucose sample sent at the same time confirmed the diagnosis of hypoglycemia with a glucose value of 20 mg/dL. The infant was given 8 cc of $D_{10}W$ intravenously and then allowed to take regular formula as tolerated. The blood glucose level obtained following the bolus dose of dextrose was 60 mg/dL. Two hours later a laboratory plasma glucose sample was sent and was again 20 mg/dL. A repeat intravenous bolus dose of 8 cc of $D_{10}W$

was repeated, following which the plasma glucose value was 65 mg/dL. Two hours following the last bolus dose of dextrose, the plasma glucose value was again low at 18 mg/dL.

## EXERCISE 3

### ■ Questions:

1. What is the mechanism responsible for this infant's recurrent hypoglycemia?

2. This infant is large for gestational age, which probably explains why his delivery was traumatic and complicated by a clavicular fracture. What other abnormalities or complications are commonly observed in infants of diabetic mothers?

3. How can the large "swings" in blood glucose levels be avoided?

### ■ Answers:

Infants of diabetic mothers (IDM) are another group of neonates who are at increased risk for experiencing hypoglycemia. Maternal diabetes mellitus, whether chronic or gestational, results in fetal blood glucose concentrations reflective of the mother's. However, maternal insulin does not cross the placenta. Therefore, *fetuses of poorly controlled diabetic mothers are exposed to chronic hyperglycemia, which ultimately increases fetal insulin production. This hyperinsulinism suppresses endogenous glucose release, increases peripheral glucose utilization, and, after birth, attenuates the normally seen rise in lipolysis. Therefore, following delivery the persistence of this hyperinsulinemic state in association with a sudden drop in glucose supply can result in a refractory hypoglycemia.* Typically hypoglycemia occurs shortly after birth, but in some cases it may not present until after 24 hours of age. The condition may persist for more than 48 hours.

Hypoglycemia is only one of a multitude of problems that may be experienced by these infants. Fetal insulin acts as an anabolic hormone and these infants commonly exhibit organomegaly (especially of the heart and liver) and overall macrosomia, which places them at increased risk for birth trauma or asphyxia. *Furthermore, a number of congenital anomalies have been observed in these infants, including congenital heart disease, caudal regression syndrome, small left colon syndrome, and musculoskeletal anomalies. Isolated cardiac septal hypertrophy may occur and present as a form of subaortic stenosis. Hypocalcemia and hypomagnesemia also commonly occur.*

*Polycythemia* is frequently observed in infants of diabetic mothers and it has been suggested that this may be due to chronic hypoxia or increased production of erythropoietin in response to chronic hyperinsulinism. *Hyperbilirubinemia*, another frequently observed problem, may be due to, or exacerbated by, increased bilirubin production secondary to the increased red cell mass. *Renal vein thrombosis*, a rare complication, may result from hyperviscosity secondary to the increased hematocrit. *Respiratory distress syndrome* may occur even in term infants of diabetic mothers and is believed to be secondary to an antagonistic effect of insulin on surfactant synthesis.

The most effective treatment for infants of diabetic mothers who are experiencing recurrent hypoglycemia is to provide an adequate continuous source of glucose as the hyperinsulinism resolves. *The repeated bolus doses of glucose that the infant in this case received induced a reactive hypoglycemia (i.e., each bolus was followed by an endogenous insulin surge, which rapidly ameliorated the transient improvement in the blood glucose concentration). A more effective treatment would have been to administer the initial intravenous bolus dose of glucose and to begin simultaneously a constant intravenous glucose infusion.* These infants may have high glucose requirements, and the need for rates of ≥12 mg/kg/min is not unusual. After the blood glucose concentration has stabilized, the infusion may be slowly weaned over a matter of days as the infant's oral intake increases. Data suggest that the maintenance of maternal euglycemia during gestation will result in a lower incidence of congenital anomalies and perinatal complications. Therefore, the best "treatment" for these infants is to control carefully maternal glucose values prior to delivery.

## CASE STUDY 4

Baby girl Gray is a 3,100-g female infant born at 39 weeks' gestation to a 31-year-old multiparous mother whose blood type is A⁻. The infant's early course was complicated by a rapidly rising unconjugated hyperbilirubinemia. During evaluation of this problem, the infant's blood type was found to be A⁺, and the direct Coombs test was strongly positive. On the second day of life, the infant's indirect bilirubin concentration rose to 26 mg/dL, necessitating a double volume exchange transfusion with whole blood collected in citrate-phosphate-dextrose. The patient tolerated the procedure well, but 2 hours following completion of the exchange transfusion a laboratory glucose concentration of 20 mg/dL was reported.

## EXERCISE 4

### ■ Questions:

1. What are possible etiologies for this infant's hypoglycemia?

2. How should this infant's hypoglycemia be managed?

### ■ Answers:

In this case, the hypoglycemia is probably secondary to hyperinsulinemia; however, there may also be an iatrogenic component. The hyperinsulinemic state can be seen in a number of conditions other than infants of diabetic mothers. *Infants with Rh incompatibility experience chronic red blood cell hemolysis. It is speculated that the release of reduced glutathione from the lysed red blood cells may act as a stimulus for pancreatic islet cell hyperplasia.* Hyperinsulinism also occurs in infants with nesidioblastosis, islet cell

adenomas, and adenomatosis. Similarly, hypoglycemia secondary to hyperinsulinism is commonly observed in infants with Beckwith-Wiedemann syndrome. This syndrome is characterized by omphalocele, muscular macroglossia, visceromegaly, and islet cell hyperplasia that results in hyperinsulinism.

Hypoglycemia in the newborn infant may also be iatrogenic in origin. *Exchange transfusion can result in decreased blood glucose concentrations for a variety of reasons.* Heparinized blood, which is frequently used for this procedure, contains no glucose and may result in hypoglycemia during or following completion of the procedure. In contrast, citrated blood contains a high sugar content and may result in a reactive hypoglycemia. In a similar fashion, the placement of an umbilical artery catheter in a "high" position has been associated with the occurrence of hypoglycemia, presumably from delivery of a high glucose load directly into the celiac axis.

*This infant's hypoglycemia can most effectively be treated by administering a 200 mg/kg bolus of intravenous glucose (the equivalent of 2 cc/kg of $D_{10}W$) followed by a constant glucose infusion to provide 4 to 6 mg/kg/min of glucose. This infusion rate can be increased as needed to maintain euglycemia.* If more than 15 mg/kg/min of glucose is required, it may be necessary to administer hydrocortisone (5 mg/kg/day intravenously or enterally) or prednisone (2 mg/kg/day enterally) in an attempt to mobilize glucose from noncarbohydrate sources. In this particular case, where hyperinsulinism may play an etiologic role, it may ultimately be necessary to administer diazoxide (10 to 15 mg/kg/day) to suppress pancreatic insulin secretion.

## CASE STUDY 5

Baby boy Gray was a 3,700-g, 40-week gestational age male born by repeat cesarean section following an uncomplicated pregnancy. The patient's immediate perinatal course was uneventful until 4 hours of age, at which time the infant was noted to be hypotonic and did not feed well. As part of an evaluation to assess this change in behavior, a blood glucose determination was ordered and a laboratory value of 15 mg/dL was obtained. The infant was given 7.4 cc of $D_{10}W$ intravenously, and a glucose infusion was begun to provide 6 mg/kg/min.

The maternal history was obtained and did not reveal any history of diabetes, preeclampsia, preterm labor, or use of medications. The mother was Rh positive. The delivery was a scheduled uncomplicated repeat cesarean section and the baby received Apgar scores of 9 and 9 at 1 and 5 minutes of life, respectively. The infant's physical examination was within normal limits, except for a body weight and length that were at the 90th percentile for the infant's gestational age. Electrolytes, calcium and magnesium concentrations, and a complete blood cell count were all within normal ranges.

One hour after the initiation of the glucose infusion, the infant was asymptomatic and a blood glucose concentration of 25 mg/dL was obtained. During the next 12 hours, the glucose infusion was gradually increased to a rate of 15 mg/kg/min in order to maintain marginally acceptable glucose values. The next blood glucose level obtained was 15 mg/dL. Intravenous hydrocortisone (5 mg/kg/day) was begun in an attempt to mobilize glucose from noncarbohydrate sources. This intervention had no effect on the blood glucose concentration. An insulin concentration drawn while the child was hypoglycemic was 160 μU/mL (normal is 5 to 40 μU/mL).

## EXERCISE 5

### ■ Questions:

1. What is the differential diagnosis of hyperinsulinemia in this infant?

2. What additional studies may be helpful in determining the etiology of this recalcitrant hypoglycemia?

3. How should this infant be managed at this point?

4. What other therapy remains if medical management fails?

### ■ Answers:

*As discussed in the preceding case, hyperinsulinism can be seen in infants of diabetic mothers; in those with Rh incompatibility; in infants with nesidioblastosis, pancreatic islet cell adenoma, and adenomatosis; and in infants with Beckwith-Wiedemann syndrome.* In this case, the history and physical examination argue against diabetes, Rh incompatibility, or Beckwith-Wiedemann syndrome, suggesting that pancreatic islet cell hyperplasia of some sort is responsible for the hypoglycemia. *An abdominal ultrasound or CT scan would be helpful in screening for abnormalities of pancreatic structure.*

If steroids fail to correct the hypoglycemia, *the next step would be to administer diazoxide in order to suppress pancreatic insulin secretion. This drug is usually administered in doses of 10 to 15 mg/kg/day.* Medical therapy may be ineffective in cases of nesidioblastosis where surgical intervention is usually necessary to correct the hyperinsulinemic state. *The surgical treatment of nesidioblastosis is 95% pancreatectomy.* Following this procedure, recurrence is rare and any postoperative hypoglycemia or hyperglycemia that may occur is usually transient and responsive to medical therapy. Long-term developmental follow-up in these infants appears to correlate with their preoperative condition.

## CASE STUDY 6

Baby boy Thomas is a 3,200-g male born following an uneventful term gestation to a 26-year-old mother. The vaginal delivery was spontaneous and uncomplicated, and Apgar scores of 9 at 1 minute and 9 at 5 minutes were assigned. The infant's initial course was unremarkable except for recurring asymptomatic preprandial hypoglycemia (laboratory glucose concentrations ranged from 25 to 30 mg/dL), which responded to oral feedings. At 3 days of age the infant developed a conjugated hyperbilirubinemia, which rose progressively during several days and peaked at a total serum bilirubin concentration of 17.2 mg/dL and a direct reacting fraction of 15.8 mg/dL. When the infant was 6 days of age, the recurrent hypoglycemia and hyperbilirubinemia persisted and he was transferred to a tertiary care center for further evaluation.

Physical examination at that time was remarkable for the presence of jaundice, undescended testes, and a penile corpora measuring 0.5 cm in length. Laboratory evaluation of serum electrolytes, calcium and magnesium concentrations, and a complete blood count were all within normal limits. A preprandial blood glucose concentration was 17 mg/dL and the direct bilirubin concentration was 15.1 mg/dL.

## EXERCISE 6

### ■ Questions:

1. What diagnosis is suggested by the triad of hypoglycemia, hyperbilirubinemia, and micropenis?

2. What other physcial findings though not present in this case would be supportive of the diagnosis?

3. What laboratory studies would you order at this point?

4. What is the treatment for this disorder?

### ■ Answers:

Certain endocrinologic and metabolic disorders may present during the newborn period with hypoglycemia. *Congenital hypopituitarism results in deficiencies of growth hormone and cortisol, which both normally stimulate gluconeogenesis. These infants may manifest associated midline defects and males commonly exhibit micropenis and undescended testes secondary to deficiency of gonadotro-*

*pins.* Cortisol deficiency can also be seen in adrenocortical insufficiency and will result in a ketotic hypoglycemia. Hypothyroidism is also associated with the occurrence of neonatal hypoglycemia, although the mechanism is currently unknown.

Congenital defects in gluconeogenesis or glycogenolysis can also result in hypoglycemia. Congenital deficiencies of glucagon and PEPCK, though rare, have been reported. Glycogen storage disease, Type 1, is an autosomal recessive disorder that results in hypoglycemia due to a deficiency of glucose-6-phosphatase, the enzyme catalyzing the final step in glycogenolysis. Galactosemia, hereditary fructose intolerance, and fructose-1,6-diphosphatase deficiency are other inborn errors of metabolism that may present with hypoglycemia.

In Case Study 6, the combination of recurrent hypoglycemia, hyperbilirubinemia, and micropenis is suggestive of congenital hypopituitarism. *Abnormally low growth hormone, cortisol, and thyroid hormone levels would all support the diagnosis, whereas a diagnosis of adrenocortical insufficiency would be supported by low cortisol concentrations in the face of elevated levels of ACTH.* Provocative testing and sophisticated radiographic testing such as MRI will permit a definitive diagnosis. *In cases of chronic hypoglycemia due to inborn errors of metabolism or endocrine disorders, therapy is directed at replacement of the deficient hormones or alterations in diet.*

## BIBLIOGRAPHY

1. DiGiacomo JE: Carbohydrates: Metabolism and disorders. In Hay WW, ed: *Neonatal Nutrition and Metabolism.* St. Louis, Mosby-Year Book, 1991, pp. 93–109.
2. Sann L: Neonatal hypoglycemia. *Biol Neonate* 1990; 58(suppl 1):16–21.
3. Menon RK, Sperling MA: Carbohydrate metabolism. *Semin Perin* 1988; 12(2):157–162.
4. Denne SC: Carbohydrate requirements. In Polin RA, Fox WW, eds: *Fetal and Neonatal Physiology.* Philadelphia, WB Saunders Co, 1992, pp. 234–236.
5. Kalhan SC: Metabolism of glucose and methods of investigation in the fetus and newborn. In Polin RA, Fox WW, eds: *Fetal and Neonatal Physiology.* Philadelphia, WB Saunders Co, 1992, p. 366.
6. Cornblath M, Schwartz R, Aynsley-Green A, et al, eds: Hypoglycemia in infancy, the need for a rational definition. *Pediatrics* 1990; 85(5):834–837.

7. Cowett RM: Hypoglycemia and hyperglycemia in the newborn. In Polin RA, Fox WW, eds: *Fetal and Neonatal Physiology.* Philadelphia, WB Saunders Co, 1992, p. 406.

8. Cowett RM: Pathophysiology, diagnosis and management of glucose homeostasis in the neonate. *Curr Probl Pediatr* 1985; 15(3):1–47.

9. Pildes RS, Lilien LD: Metabolic and endocrine disorders. In Fanaroff A, Martin RJ, eds: *Neonatal-Perinatal Medicine: Diseases of the Fetus and Infant.* St. Louis, Mosby Co, 1987, pp. 1049 and 1066.

10. Stiles AD, Cloherty JP: Hypoglycemia and hyperglycemia. In Cloherty JP, Stark AR, eds: *Manual of Neonatal Care.* Boston, Little, Brown, and Co, 1985, p. 339.

11. Koivisto M, Blanco-Sequeiros M, Krause U: Neonatal symptomatic and asymptomatic hypoglycaemia: A follow-up study of 151 children. *Develop Med Child Neurol* 1972; 14:603–614.

12. Lubchenco LO, Bard H: Incidence of hypoglycemia in newborn infants classified by birth weight and gestational age. *Pediatrics* 1971; 47(5):831–837.

13. Hay WW: Fetal and neonatal glucose homeostasis and their relation to the small for gestational age infant. *Semin Perin* 1984; 8(2):101–116.

14. Epstein MF, Nicholls E, Stubblefield PG: Neonatal hypoglycemia after beta-sympathomimetic tocolytic therapy. *J Pediatr* 1979; 94(3):449–553.

15. Procianoy RS, Pinheiro CEA: Neonatal hyperinsulinism after short-term maternal beta sympathomimetic therapy. *J Pediatr* 1982; 101(4): 612–614.

16. Senoir B, Slone D, Shapiro S, et al: Benzothiadiazides and neonatal hypoglycaemia. *Lancet* 1976; 2:377.

17. Cottrill CM, McAllister RG, Gettes L, et al: Propranolol therapy during pregnancy, labor, and delivery: Evidence for transplacental drug transfer and impaired neonatal drug disposition. *J Pediatr* 1977; 91(5):812–814.

18. Habib A, McCarthy JS: Effects on the neonate of propranolol administered during pregnancy. *J Pediatr* 1977; 91(5):808–811.

19. Yeung CY: Hypoglycemia in neonatal sepsis. *J Pediatr* 1970; 77(5):812–817.

20. Jovanovik L, Druzin M, Peterson CM: Effect of euglycemia on the outcome of pregnancy in insulin dependent women as compared with normal control subjects. *Am J Med* 1981; 71:921–927.

21. Nagel JW, Sims JS, Alpin CE II, et al: Refractory hypoglycemia associated with a malpositioned umbilical artery catheter. *Pediatrics* 1979; 64:315.

22. Willberg B, Muller E: Surgery for nesidioblastosis—indications, treatment, and results. *Prog Pediatr Surg* 1991; 26:76–83.

23. LaFranchi S: Hypoglycemia of infancy and childhood. *Pediatr Clin North Am* 1987; 34(4):961–982.

24. Vidnes J, Sovik O: Gluconeogenesis in infancy and childhood. *Acta Paediatr Scand* 1976; 65:307–312.

# Chapter 5

# NEONATAL

# HYPERBILIRUBINEMIA

*Phyllis A. Dennery, M.D.*

*David K. Stevenson, M.D.*

Jaundice or hyperbilirubinemia is a transient, yet ubiquitous, clinical condition in the neonate. Nonetheless, values exceeding 15 mg/dL are seen in only a small percentage of infants weighing more than 2,500 g. Given the high incidence of clinically apparent physiological hyperbilirubinemia, the clinician must be able to anticipate and assess situations that deviate from those normally observed and to formulate a differential diagnosis and institute appropriate therapy in a timely fashion. The goal of this chapter is to give the reader an organized approach to pathological jaundice in the neonate by presenting three clinical cases. By considering which steps of bilirubin metabolism are altered in each of the clinical scenarios, the participant will then be able to make the correct diagnosis and choose an appropriate management strategy.

## CASE STUDY 1

A 25-year-old Oriental primigravida, blood type O$^+$, presents to the hospital with ruptured membranes at 39 weeks' gestation. She is admitted and allowed to go into labor. Twelve hours after admission, a vaginal examination reveals that the cervix is 50% effaced and only 2 cm dilated. The patient is then given oxytocin to augment labor. Twenty-four hours after admission, she is noted to have a temperature of 101°F. At this point, a vaginal exam reveals a completely effaced cervix and dilation to 10 cm. A forceps-assisted vaginal delivery is attempted after an unsuccessful trial of pushing. A male infant is born with Apgar scores of 7 at 1 minute and 9 at 5 minutes. He has a fairly large collection of blood on the occiput and bruising about the face. The infant is admitted to the term newborn nursery. He does well on the first day of life, but at 36 hours of age he is feeding very poorly and appears somewhat lethargic and icteric. The nurses draw a complete blood count, a blood culture, a bilirubin level as well as a blood type, and a Coombs test. The results show a total serum bilirubin of 15 mg/dL, blood type A$^+$, and Coombs positive serology. You are asked to evaluate this infant.

### EXERCISE 1

1. List the factors that might be responsible for the elevated bilirubin level in this infant.

2. Describe the mechanisms by which each of these factors alters bilirubin metabolic pathways.

### ■ Discussion:

Heme or iron protoporphyrin is a component of hemoglobin that is released from red blood cells upon lysis. This molecule undergoes a two-step catabolic process that results in the formation of bilirubin (Fig. 5-1). The first step

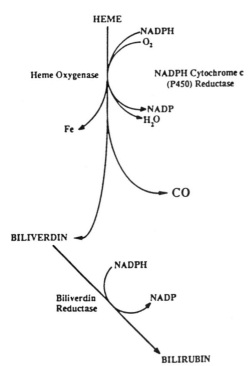

HEME

NADPH
O₂

Heme Oxygenase

NADPH Cytochrome c
(P450) Reductase

NADP
H₂O

Fe

CO

BILIVERDIN

NADPH

Biliverdin
Reductase

NADP

BILIRUBIN

**Figure 5-1** Heme degradation pathway. The microsomal enzymes heme oxygenase and cytochrome c(P450) reductase form a complex with cytosolic enzyme biliverdin reductase in the catabolism of heme to bilirubin.
From Rodgers PA, Stevenson DK: Developmental biology of heme oxygenase. *Clin Perinatol* 1990; 17:276. Reprinted with permission of W.B. Saunders Company and P.A. Rodgers.

is rate-limiting and involves the heme oxygenase enzyme. In this reaction, the protoporphyrin ring is opened, and there is release of free iron, biliverdin (a blue-green pigment), and carbon monoxide in equimolar amounts. The iron is recycled, carbon monoxide is excreted by the lungs, and biliverdin is readily excreted in the bile. In mammals, biliverdin is further metabolized by biliverdin reductase to form bilirubin, a toxic molecule that is not readily excreted and needs further metabolism. This molecule is transported to the liver, conjugated to glucuronic acid, and excreted in the bile. Physiological jaundice in newborn infants results from multiple abnormalities of the heme degradation and bilirubin excretion pathways. For example, neonates have a higher circulating red cell volume, a shortened red cell lifespan, and a diminished ability to conjugate bilirubin compared to adults. As a consequence, newborn infants have bilirubin production rates that are much higher than

adults and contribute to the development of physiological jaundice. Furthermore, other clinical circumstances that occur during the neonatal period can aggravate physiological hyperbilirubinemia by interrupting one or more of the steps along the bilirubin formation pathway (Table 5-1). These factors can be subdivided into five major categories: (1) disorders of bilirubin production, (2) disorders of bilirubin uptake into the liver, (3) disorders of conjugation, (4) disorders of excretion, and (5) alterations in enterohepatic circulation. The infant presented in Case Study 1 has several disorders of bilirubin production, which are discussed individually in the following discussion.

Forty percent of infants born to type O mothers have either type A or type B blood. The cord blood Coombs test is positive in 14% to 32% of these pregnancies. It is important to remember that although anti A and B antibodies are primarily 19 S globulins (IgM) and do not cross the placenta, there is some naturally occurring anti A activity in type O and type B individuals that can be demonstrated in the IgG fraction. These naturally occurring IgG antibodies can readily cross the placenta, interact to antigen on fetal red blood cells, and cause increased clearance from the circulation. Therefore, ABO hemolytic disease may occur following the first pregnancy in an unsensitized mother. Blood group A appears to be the most strongly antigenic. The potential for hemolysis is varied, and some infants have few to no symptoms, whereas others exhibit greater degrees of hemolysis. Release of hemoglobin leads to an increased production of bilirubin through the pathway described earlier.

Physiological jaundice differs greatly between races, with black Americans having the lowest values. Mean maximum serum unconjugated bilirubin concentrations in Chinese, Japanese, Korean, and American Indian newborns range between 10 and 14 mg/dL, which is approximately double those of non-Oriental populations. This occurs even if you correct for the presence of glucose-6-phosphate dehydrogenase (G6PD) deficiency, which is more common in Orientals. Bilirubin production, indexed by serum carboxyhemoglobin, is significantly higher in Japanese infants at 2 to 3 days of life than in Caucasian control subjects without any associated hemolysis. Other populations that are at risk for increased hyperbilirubinemia without associated hemolysis are

**Table 5-1** Pathological Causes of Neonatal Hyperbilirubinemia

| DISORDER | CLINICAL CONDITIONS |
| --- | --- |
| Production | *Isoimmunization:* Rh, ABO, minor blood groups |
| | *Erythrocyte biochemical defect:* G6PD, pyruvate kinase, hexokinase, porphyria |
| | *Structural abnormalities of red blood cells (RBCs):* hereditary spherocytosis, eliptocytosis |
| | *Infection:* bacterial, viral, protozoal* |
| | *Sequestered blood:* subdural hematoma, cephalohematoma, ecchymoses, hemangiomas |
| | *Polycythemia:* maternal-fetal or fetal transfusion, delayed cord clamping |
| | *Other:* infants of diabetic mothers, obstructive jaundice,† galactosemia,* hemolysis (DIC, vitamin K deficiency) |
| Uptake | Gilbert's syndrome |
| | Hypothyroidism* |
| | Galactosemia* |
| Conjugation | Crigler-Najjar syndromes (Types I and II) |
| | Transient familial neonatal hyperbilirubinemia |
| | Galactosemia, hypothyroidism |
| Excretion | Galactosemia |
| | Hypothyroidism |
| Enterohepatic circulation | Breast milk jaundice (early–late onset) |
| | Starvation |
| | Pyloric stenosis |
| | Intestinal obstruction |

* Mixed jaundice.
† Secondary to increased hemolysis due to RBC injury in the liver.

inhabitants of the Greek islands of Lesbos and Rhodes. It is believed that the increased incidence of hyperbilirubinemia, and also kernicterus in these populations, is due to environmental factors and genetic predisposition. It is interesting to note that Orientals living in the United States exhibit an increased incidence of hyperbilirubinemia similar to their counterparts in the Orient. Therefore, geographical factors alone cannot account for the differences between Caucasian and Oriental infants.

In this case study, the maternal fever of 101°F and the clinical presentation of the infant after the first 24 hours strongly suggest the likelihood of sepsis. Bacterial infections are known both to increase bilirubin production by promoting red cell hemolysis and to decrease bilirubin excretion by altering liver enzymes for conjugation. Bilirubin crystals have been observed in the granulocytes of septic infants with hyperbilirubinemia but not in their noninfected counterparts, suggesting an abnormal disposition of bilirubin in septic illness. Systemic infection with viruses, bacteria, and fungi can also lead to a toxic hepatitis by directly invading hepatocytes resulting in increases of the direct component of bilirubin. *E. coli*, in particular, can produce cholestasis in infants. Therefore, depending on the infectious agent and the age of onset of jaundice, you may see both an elevated indirect and direct component of bilirubin in a septic infant.

Subdural hematomas, cephalohematomas, ecchymoses, and hemangiomas can result in increased red blood cell breakdown and enhanced bilirubin production. This phenomenon can also be seen with any occult hemorrhage. Hyperbilirubinemia has also been observed in infants receiving fetal transfusions prior to birth because of delayed absorption of intraperitoneal blood. Removal of the red blood cells by peritoneal lavage is required to halt the production of bilirubin.

There have been several reports of an association between neonatal hyperbilirubinemia and the use of oxytocin to induce or augment labor. Davies et al. speculated that use of oxytocin may increase the incidence of hyperbilirubinemia by shortening the duration of pregnancy, resulting in the delivery of an infant who is unable to conjugate indirect bilirubin. Other investigators have suggested that neonatal hyperbilirubinemia associated with the use of oxytocin may be due to maternal and fetal hypoosmolarity with subsequent red cell swelling and deformation. Red cell swelling might occur because of the vasopressin-like effect of oxytocin along with sodium-free water administered to the patient. In fact, most of the reports demonstrating an association between oxytocin administration and neonatal hyperbilirubinemia were conducted in the United Kingdom, where it is common practice to administer large volumes of sodium-free water to mothers receiving oxytocin. Not all studies have demonstrated an association between oxytocin administration and neonatal hyperbilirubinemia. A study conducted by Johnson et al. reported no significant differences in bilirubin values, carbon monoxide excretion rates, serum sodium, and serum osmolarity between control infants without hemolytic disease and infants whose mothers received oxytocin. Although some correlation appears to exist between the amount of oxytocin used and neonatal hyperbilirubinemia, there also seems to be an association between the administration of relatively large volumes of electrolyte-free (or low-sodium) intravenous fluid and elevated bilirubin values.

### ■ Answers:

1. ABO, sepsis, race, oxytocin, and bruising.

2. *ABO:* Increased red blood cell (RBC) lysis.
   *Sepsis:* Increased RBC lysis, decreased liver function.
   *Race:* Orientals are more susceptible to hyperbilirubinemia than Caucasians or blacks; mechanism is unclear.
   *Oxytocin:* May or may not cause hemolysis and subsequent hyperbilirubinemia. Depends on vehicle of administration (large volumes of sodium-free fluid).

*Bruising:* Sequestration of blood, increased breakdown of RBC.

### EXERCISE 2

The infant is placed under phototherapy for a bilirubin value of 18 mg/dL at 48 hours of life.

1. Explain three mechanisms by which light photodegrades or modifies bilirubin.

2. List three ways to maximize the effectiveness of phototherapy.

### ■ Discussion:

Phototherapy has been used on millions of infants during the last 30 years with little to no significant toxicity. Cremer, Perryman, and Richards in 1958 first described the influence of sunlight and an artificial light on hyperbilirubinemia in newborn infants. Since then, phototherapy has been considered a treatment of choice for exaggerated physiological jaundice or pathological jaundice of the newborn throughout the world. Furthermore, in a national collaborative trial, phototherapy proved to be as safe and efficacious as exchange transfusion in preventing kernicterus and lowering serum bilirubin values.

Bilirubin (Fig. 5-2) is a tetrapyrrole molecule consisting of nearly identical (light-absorbing) halves joined by a saturated carbon. The outer two carbon bridges ($C_4–C_5$ and $C_{15}–C_{16}$) are doubly bonded to the outer two pyrrole rings. Therefore, on each side of the bilirubin molecule two different arrangements or configurations are possible. Newer nomenclature has adopted the chemical symbols Z and E to describe the two possible configurations around each of the double bonds. The abbreviations Z and E (derived from the German words for *together* and *opposite*) are analogous to the older chemical terms *cis* and *trans*. Native bilirubin is commonly referred to as 4Z,15Z-bilirubin to indicate that the bilirubin molecule is in the Z configuration at the $C_4–C_5$ and $C_{15}–C_{16}$ double bonds.

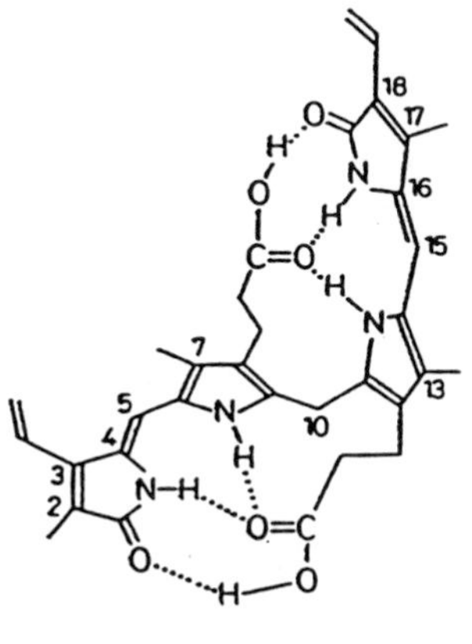

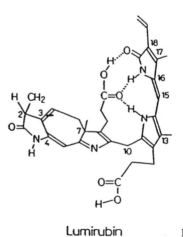

**4Z, 15Z-Bilirubin**

**Figure 5-2** Three-dimensional structure of 4Z,15Z-bilirubin demonstrating intramolecular hydrogen bonds.
From Ennever JF: Linear representation of 4Z,15E bilirubin and lumirubin. *Clin Perinatol* 1990; 17:467–483. Reprinted with permission of W.B. Saunders Company.

Three chemical reactions occur when bilirubin is exposed to light: photo-oxidation, structural isomerization, and configurational isomerization. Until relatively recently, photo-oxidation was thought to be the primary mechanism of action of phototherapy. In fact, photo-oxidation accounts for the decrease in the intensity of the yellow color of serum containing bilirubin when exposed to light *in vitro*. However, it now appears that this pathway is minor in its contribution to the overall photodegradation of bilirubin.

Configurational isomerization (the fastest photoisomerization reaction) is a process in which the atoms in the bilirubin molecule are rearranged (Fig. 5-3A). In this process the molecule absorbs a photon of light and rotates around either the $C_4$–$C_5$ double bond (producing 4E,15Z-bilirubin), the $C_{15}$–$C_{16}$ double bond (producing 4Z,15E-bilirubin), or around both double bonds if two photons of light are absorbed (yielding 4E,15E-bilirubin). In humans and other primates, configurational isomerization is regioselective (i.e., only the 4Z,15E isomer of Fig. 5-3A is produced in appreciable quantities). The E isomers are more water soluble than native bilirubin because internal hydrogen bonding is prevented. However, they are not very stable and spontaneously revert to the native state in the dark. It is not believed that configurational isomerization contributes greatly to the excretion of bilirubin in humans.

Structural isomerization results in the rearrangement of atoms in bilirubin by formation of new bonds between vinyl groups on the pyrolle ring and other bonds, making a new seven-member ring referred to as *lumirubin* (Fig. 5-3B). There are many forms of this compound, but it has not been determined which of the four possible lumirubin isomers is preferentially formed *in vivo*. In contrast to 4Z,15E-bilirubin, lumirubin does not readily revert to native bilirubin and is easily excreted. Furthermore, lumirubin is the major photoproduct that is excreted in the bile of newborn infants receiving phototherapy.

Because lumirubin is formed irreversibly, it makes sense that the intensity (or dose) of the light source should be a major determinant of

**4Z, 15E-Bilirubin**          A

**Lumirubin**          B

**Figure 5-3** (A) Configurational isomer of bilirubin and (B) structural isomer of bilirubin (lumirubin).
From Ennever JF: Linear representation of 4Z,15E bilirubin and lumirubin. *Clin Perinatol* 1990; 17:467–483. Reprinted with permission of W.B. Saunders Company.

the quantity of lumirubin produced. Most standard neonatology textbooks have recommended irradiances ranging between 6 and 12 $\mu W/cm^2/nm$, and for the majority of jaundiced infants that recommendation is satisfactory. There have been very few studies in the pediatric literature evaluating the efficacy of higher light intensities. However, studies from Tan indicate that light intensities up to 40 $\mu W/cm^2/nm$ may be increasingly effective in lowering serum bilirubin concentrations. Therefore, it seems reasonable to use higher light intensities when the serum bilirubin continues to rise and exchange transfusion is imminent. The physician must be careful, however, not to bring light sources emitting heat too close to the infant's skin.

One of the most controversial issues regarding phototherapy deals with the choice of color of the light source. Various investigators have recommended green lights, blue lights, or combinations of several different-colored lights. Despite theoretical arguments by some investigators that longer wavelength light (green light) may be more efficacious, studies to date have not demonstrated an advantage of green light phototherapy over the current "gold standard" Super Blue lights. In fact, Super Blue lights may be superior. The disadvantage of these lights, however, is that they are very irritating to work around, and they make the assessment of changes in the patient's oxygenation status difficult. Halogen lamps have also proved efficacious; however, they are more likely to generate a significant amount of heat.

A new mode of therapy that has evolved in the last few years is the fiber optic blanket. Two types of "blankets" are currently being marketed. The Wallaby™ is a fiber optic pad that can be wrapped around the infant and provides an irradiance of approximately 7 $\mu W/cm^2/nm$. Several studies have demonstrated that this mode of therapy is as effective as conventional phototherapy. Recently, a new fiber optic pad that delivers high-intensity light (up to 50 $\mu W/cm^2/nm$ in the 425 to 475 nm) has been available on the market under the name of Biliblanket™. If lumirubin formation is truly the most important pathway in the elimination of bilirubin during phototherapy and if higher-intensity phototherapy results in more rapid formation of lumirubin, this aforementioned device could yield very favorable results. Thus far, no controlled trials compar-

ing the effectiveness of the Biliblanket™ to either conventional therapy or to the Wallaby™ have been performed. Fiber optic pads may have their greatest value in permitting early discharge from the hospital and home therapy. This approach, however, is not suitable for all infants. The American Academy of Pediatrics has set stringent guidelines for determining suitable populations. This mode of therapy should be reserved for term infants with non-hemolytic disease.

Some concerns have arisen regarding the potential genotoxic effect of phototherapy. Although these concerns have a strong laboratory basis, they do not appear to have any clinical importance. An additional concern is the potential for retinal damage with phototherapy; this toxicity also has not been definitely proven. It is, however, recommended that the infant's eyes be shielded from light to prevent any retinal injury. Acute side effects of phototherapy include increased insensible water losses, diarrhea, hypocalcemia, riboflavin deficiency, free tryptophan decrease, hyperpigmentation, bronzing, and overheating. Therefore, it is important to monitor the infant's hydration and temperature status during phototherapy. Because of the potential for adverse side effects, it is reassuring that follow-up studies have demonstrated no long-term ill effects in infants treated with this mode of therapy.

### ■ Answers:

1. Photo-oxidation, structural isomerization, and configurational isomerization.

2. Increased irradiance, maximize skin exposure, choose an optimal wavelength.

---

### CASE STUDY 2

A 20-year-old G2PO Ab1 white female presents to the emergency room at 34 weeks' gestation with complaints of abdominal pain and light vaginal bleeding. A vaginal examination reveals total cervical effacement and dilation to 9 cm. She precipitously delivers a female infant weighing 2,200 g with Apgar scores 3 at 1 minute and 8 at 5 minutes. The infant has acrocyanosis, nasal flaring, grunting, and tachypnea. She is given oxygen by mask and transferred to the intensive care nursery. Because of persistent acidosis and hypoxia despite 100% oxygen by mask, the infant is intubated and placed on a ventilator. She remains acidotic and hypoxemic, and is given three doses of surfactant. She improves during the next 2 days. At 72 hours of life, the infant has a total serum bilirubin value of 15 mg/dL. Phototherapy is begun. On day 4 of life, the infant has a total serum bilirubin value of 19 mg/dL.

## EXERCISE 3

### ■ Questions:

1. What are six factors in preterm infants that predispose them to bilirubin toxicity?

2. When should an exchange transfusion be considered in this infant?

### ■ Discussion:

Bilirubin is a polar compound with low solubility in aqueous solutions. It binds strongly to albumin at a primary site but may also bind at secondary lower affinity sites. While in plasma, bilirubin is usually transported bound to albumin. Data from laboratory animals suggest that the albumin binding capacity is very important in preventing bilirubin deposition in the brain. In the term infant, 1 mole of albumin has the capacity to tightly bind 0.2 to 1 mole of bilirubin. In the preterm infant, there is lower binding capacity of albumin for bilirubin, and there is usually a lower serum albumin concentration as well. Furthermore, data from laboratory animal experiments suggest that the albumin binding capacity is very important in preventing bilirubin deposition in the brain.

Several agents can displace bilirubin from albumin or reduce bilirubin binding (Fig. 5-4):

1. *Free fatty acids:* These compounds competitively inhibit bilirubin-albumin binding. Some debate exists as to whether bilirubin-albumin binding is affected by the molar ratio of free fatty acids to albumin commonly present in serum. Starvation,

hypothermia, hypoglycemia, infection, and anoxia can all increase free fatty acid concentrations in the serum and can, therefore, theoretically lead to increased displacement of bilirubin from albumin.

2. *pH: In vitro* studies have shown that there is a decreased binding of bilirubin to albumin with a pH less than 7.4. *In vivo* observations corroborate these findings. There is some controversy as to whether bilirubin deposition in the brain is affected only by respiratory acidosis or also by metabolic acidosis.

3. *Drugs:* Several drugs can displace bilirubin from albumin: Sulfa drugs, benzyl alcohol, salicylates, indomethacin, ampicillin (when injected rapidly), and even stabilizers of albumin have been shown to decrease bilirubin albumin binding.

Bilirubin can also enter the brain through disruption of the blood-brain barrier (Fig. 5-4). In the neonate the integrity of the blood-brain barrier can be compromised by anoxia, hypercarbia, and infusion of hypertonic solutions. In these conditions both free bilirubin and bilirubin bound to albumin are deposited in the brain. As the concentration of free bilirubin in the brain increases, there is increased likelihood that cellular binding will occur.

Bilirubin also has the capacity to enter the brain of the infant who is entirely healthy. Bilirubin at low concentrations has been shown to diffuse into the brain because of a high passive permeability of the blood-brain barrier in the fetus and neonate. In this situation, however, bilirubin is not likely to cause any toxicity because of the very low level of bilirubin in the brain and the normal bilirubin clearance mechanisms. In the damaged brain there may be a more ready accumulation of bilirubin. Furthermore, if an acid environment exists, bilirubin will become less soluble and may even crystallize.

When deciding whether to perform an exchange transfusion, you should not simply rely on formulas (such as birth weight in kilograms × 10 = serum bilirubin level at which an exchange transfusion should be performed). Although formulas such as these can provide general guidelines for exchange transfusion, it is obvious that multiple factors can affect the entry and ultimate deposition and toxicity of bilirubin in the brain of the neonate. Healthy

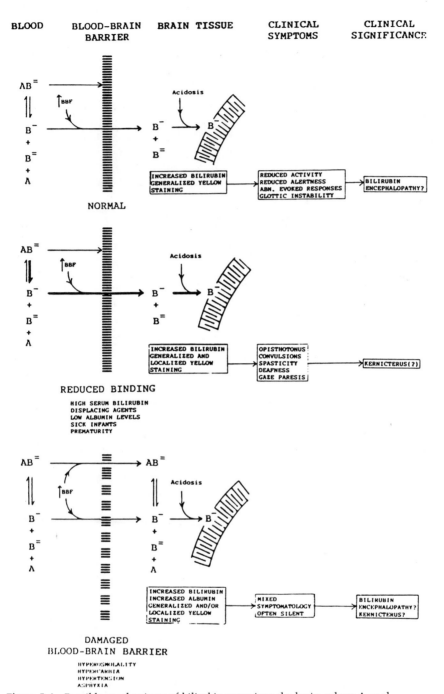

**Figure 5-4** Possible mechanisms of bilirubin entry into the brain, where A = albumin, AB$^=$ = albumin-bilirubin complex, B$^-$ = bilirubin-monoanion, B$^=$ = bilirubin dianion, BBF = brain blood flow.
From Bratlid D: How bilirubin gets into the brain. *Pediatr Clin North Am* 1990; 17:460. Reprinted with permission of W.B. Saunders Company.

preterm infants have a higher incidence of hyperbilirubinemia than healthy term infants. Furthermore, preterm infants are more likely to develop bilirubin encephalopathy at lower serum bilirubin values because they have lower serum albumin concentrations and are more likely to be subjected to poor nutrition, cyanosis, acidosis, hypoxia, hypothermia, hypoglycemia, and sepsis. Additionally, the blood-brain barrier of the premature infant is more vulnerable to disruption. Thus, it is logical to intervene at lower serum bilirubin values in preterm infants. Prior to instituting therapy, you should assess the patient's clinical status, nutritional status, albumin levels, and degree of maturity. Exchange transfusion is a procedure known to have serious complications, including necrotizing enterocolitis, cardiopulmonary arrest, electrolyte disturbances, and even a 0.5% to 1% mortality. Sicker preterm infants are more likely to experience a significant morbidity. It is extremely important to proceed with caution and to weigh the risks of exchange transfusion against the benefits.

## ■ Answers:

1. Premature infants are at high risk for bilirubin toxicity because (1) they exhibit a decreased ability to conjugate bilirubin, (2) they experience higher levels of serum bilirubin, (3) they have diminished serum albumin concentrations, (4) their blood-brain barrier is more prone to disruption, (5) the likelihood of hypothermia and hypoglycemia in preterm infants is greater, and (6) the likelihood of sepsis in preterm infants is greater.

2. Considering the infant's birth weight of 2,200 g, most clinicians would perform an exchange transfusion at a serum bilirubin concentration ranging from 15 to 20 mg/dL. A more precise answer would require knowledge of whether other risk factors for kernicterus exist (e.g., acid-base status, albumin level, degree of illness, etc.)

## EXERCISE 4

List the clinical features of kernicterus in term and preterm infants.

| TERM | PRETERM |
| --- | --- |
|  |  |

## ■ Discussion:

*Kernicterus* is a term first used by Schmorl in 1903 to describe the yellow staining of the basal ganglia of newborn infants dying with severe jaundice. This term is also used to describe the syndrome of bilirubin toxicity (primarily bilirubin encephalopathy) that is manifested by stupor, hypotonia, and fever, associated with an acute rise in bilirubin. Three phases of kernicterus have been described: Phase 1, stupor, hypotonia, poor sucking; phase 2, hypertonia, fever, opisthotonos; and phase 3, resolution of hypertonia. Poor feeding, high-pitched cry, gaze abnormalities, athetosis, and hearing defects are also observed in infants with chronic bilirubin encephalopathy. There is usually sparing of the intellect. In a term infant, this syndrome has been described at length, although the full-blown picture is rarely seen in today's everyday practice. Preterm infants exhibit different symptomatology. They may present with stupor and look otherwise ill; however, the classic phases of bilirubin encephalopathy are more difficult to establish. The condition is often fatal in preterm infants. Chronic signs of bilirubin encephalopathy in the preterm infant include delayed motor development, hearing loss, and static encephalopathy.

The histopathological findings of kernicterus at autopsy include staining of the basal ganglia and a yellow cast throughout the viscera, including liver, kidney, heart, and adrenal glands. Microscopic examination reveals bilirubin staining, necrobiosis (shrunken neurons), and swollen nuclei, which later become pyknotic. Late changes include gliosis and neuronal loss in the basal ganglia and subthalamic nuclei. In premature infants, staining of the basal ganglia with bilirubin at autopsy is of controversial clinical significance. Burgess et al. described a group of 750- to 1,500-g infants of 26 to 32 weeks who died of various causes and who were noted to have bilirubin staining in the basal ganglia despite low serum bilirubin concentrations, and no overt signs of kernicterus. Their basal ganglia appear to be more susceptible to diffusion of bilirubin because of their rich blood supply. Turkel also described bilirubin staining of the hyaline membranes and brains of infants dying with respiratory distress syndrome who had low serum bilirubin values. The frequency of low bilirubin kernicterus has decreased in the 1980s, perhaps due to improvement in neonatal care. Its significance still remains elusive.

■ **Answers:**

| TERM | PRETERM |
|---|---|
| Phase 1: Stupor hypotonia, poor suck | No specific phases are delineated |
| Phase 2: Hypertonia, fever, opisthotonos | Possible signs: Stupor, hypotonia, shock |
| Phase 3: Resolution of hypertonia | Nonspecific signs and symptoms |
| Other signs: Poor feeding, high-pitched cry, gaze disturbances, hearing loss | |

### CASE STUDY 3

You are asked to evaluate a 15-day-old infant born to an insulin-dependent diabetic. The infant was delivered by cesarean section for failure to progress. The initial hospital course was benign. The mother states that the infant has been nursing very well at home. At 2 days of life, the infant was noted to be icteric. A total serum bilirubin value was 13 mg/dL with a direct component of 1.0 mg/dL. The Coombs test was negative and the reticulocyte count was 2%. The infant was discharged on day 3 of life with a total serum bilirubin value of 14 mg/dL. At a follow-up visit at 2 weeks of age, the baby appears well other than intense icterus. He is referred to your hospital for a determination of serum bilirubin. The total serum bilirubin value is now 22 mg/dL with a direct component of 1.2 mg/dL.

### EXERCISE 5

■ **Questions:**

1. What are the possible causes of this infant's hyperbilirubinemia?

2. Of the following factors, which are associated with breast-milk jaundice or with exaggerated jaundice in infants of diabetic mothers?

| | INFANT OF DIABETIC MOTHER | BREAST-MILK JAUNDICE |
|---|---|---|
| (a) Birth weight: 4,500 g | | |
| (b) Jaundice at 48 hours | | |
| (c) Jaundice at 2 weeks | | |
| (d) Increased RBC breakdown | | |
| (e) Increased enterohepatic circulation | | |
| (f) Delayed hepatic conjugation | | |
| (g) Delayed transition to adult hemoglobin | | |
| (h) Increased bilirubin production | | |

3. How should this infant be managed?

■ **Discussion:**

Prior to assigning a diagnosis of breast-milk jaundice to the infant in the case presented, you should review the potential causes of pathological jaundice in the newborn and rule out any other possibilities that might explain the exaggerated jaundice (see Table 5-1). Usually, the likely etiologies of hyperbilirubinemia in the newborn fall under disorders of bilirubin production or disorders of enterohepatic circulation. The disorders of bilirubin production were discussed in Case Study 1. Breast-milk jaundice belongs in the category of disorders of enterohepatic circulation. In a study comparing bottle-fed with breast-fed infants, the mean bilirubin concentration was $5.7 \pm 3.3$ mg/dL in bottle-fed babies and $7.3 \pm 3.9$ mg/dL in breast-fed infants. Only 2.2% of formula-fed infants had a serum bilirubin concentration of greater than 12.9 mg/dL versus 9% of breast-fed infants. In the first few days of life, the infant who is exclusively breast fed is usually less well hydrated and relatively undernourished compared to his or her bottle-fed counterpart. Higher peak bilirubin values are thus encountered in breast-fed infants (Fig. 5-5). We do not yet understand how starvation induces unconjugated hyperbilirubinemia, but it is believed that in breast-fed infants there may be increased reabsorption of bilirubin from the intestine, a decreased bilirubin content in the stools, and delayed passage of meconium, leading to an increased enterohepatic circulation. Some studies have shown an inverse correlation between frequency of nursing and bilirubin concentration on the third day of life, but other investigators have not demonstrated any significant difference between a 3-hour feeding regimen and a 4-hour feeding regimen on the level of jaundice in breast-fed infants.

Early onset breast-milk jaundice, which follows the time course of physiological hyperbilirubinemia, must be differentiated from late onset breast-milk jaundice, a condition characterized by a relatively late onset of exaggerated unconjugated hyperbilirubinemia. Late onset breast-milk jaundice occurs in 1 in 50 to 1 in 200 breast-fed infants and is usually seen after the third day of life. Bilirubin values as high as 20 to 25 mg/dL may be observed by the end of the second week of the infant's life. These infants do not appear sick, and they have a gradual decline of bilirubin during the first 4 months of life. Interruption of nursing for 24 to 72 hours will usually result in a fall in the serum bilirubin concentration. Resumption of breast feeding will cause a cessation of the previous decline, but the rise in bilirubin should be minimal. This form of jaundice was originally believed to be due to an unusual hormone (pregnanediol) in breast milk that decreased or interfered with hepatic glucuronyl transferase. However, this is no longer thought to be the case. The pathophysiology of late onset breast-milk jaundice has still not been determined; however, possible mechanisms of action are thought to include (1) inhibition of hepatic conjugation by increased serum concentrations of free fatty acids (FFA) because of high lipoprotein lipase levels in some breast-milk samples and (2) an increased enterohepatic absorption of unconjugated bilirubin from the gut because of increased beta

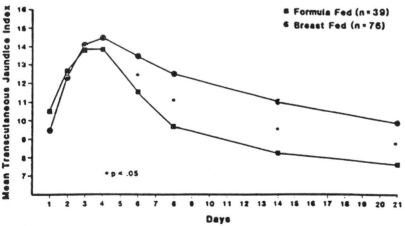

**Figure 5-5** Natural history of jaundice in white breast-fed and formula-fed infants. The transcutaneous jaundice index was measured with a Minolta jaundice meter. From Kivlahan C, James EJP: The natural history of neonatal jaundice. *Pediatrics* 1984; 74:364. Reproduced by permission of *Pediatrics*, vol. 74, page 364, copyright 1984.

glucuronidase activity in the breast milk of these mothers. Beta glucuronidase is known to deconjugate bilirubin glucuronides yielding unconjugated bilirubin. Recent observations suggest that infants with breast-milk jaundice syndrome may also have increased fasting serum bile acids and other abnormalities of liver function. However, there are no differences in the rate of bilirubin production between breast- and bottle-fed infants. Therefore, it appears that differences exist only in the bilirubin conjugating mechanism and enterohepatic circulation between breast-fed and bottle-fed babies. Some authors believe that treatment of this condition is not necessary because no cases of kernicterus have occurred in breast-fed babies and aggressive intervention leads only to maternal anxiety and disruption of bonding. Nonetheless, current recommendations are that nursing be interrupted for 24 to 72 hours and then resumed. These infants may be fed formula or a balanced electrolyte solution until breast feeding is reinstituted.

Infants of diabetic mothers (IDM) have bilirubin levels that are slightly, but significantly, higher than normal control subjects at similar gestation and weight. Factors contributing to the higher serum bilirubin concentrations include polycythemia, excessive weight loss, and prematurity. Peevy found that only large-for-gestational-age (LGA) infants of diabetics are at increased risk for hyperbilirubinemia. Additionally, Jahrig et al. observed that increased weight-to-length ratios were a more important predictor of jaundice in IDMs. It has been shown that carboxyhemoglobin concentrations and pulmonary excretion of carbon monoxide are higher in LGA infants compared to normal full-term infants. This implies that LGA infants of diabetics have increased bilirubin production rates. Furthermore, IDMs demonstrate a delayed transition from fetal to adult hemoglobin and exhibit a delayed clearance of bilirubin. As a consequence, hyperbilirubinemia is observed in about 20% to 40% of IDM infants.

■ Answers:

1. This infant appears well and has no laboratory evidence of hemolysis. Therefore, the most likely diagnosis is late onset of breast-milk jaundice syndrome. A urine specimen should be examined to rule out a urinary tract infection. More unusual causes of hyperbilirubinemia (e.g., metabolic disease)

should be considered if the bilirubin does not decline with interruption of breast feedings.

2.

| | INFANT OF DIABETIC MOTHER | BREAST-MILK JAUNDICE |
|---|:---:|:---:|
| (a) Birth weight: 4,500 g | X | |
| (b) Jaundice at 48 hours | X | X |
| (c) Jaundice at 2 weeks | | X |
| (d) Increased RBC breakdown | X | |
| (e) Increased enterohepatic circulation | | X |
| (f) Delayed hepatic conjugation | X | X |
| (g) Delayed transition to adult hemoglobin | X | |
| (h) Increased bilirubin production | X | |

3. Breast feedings should be interrupted for 24 to 72 hours and replaced temporarily with glucose and water, or formula.

## EXERCISE 6

■ Questions:

1. Should this infant have received an exchange transfusion for the jaundice detected at the 2-week follow-up visit?

2. What alternative therapies are available, and what are their modes of action?

## ■ Discussion:

Routine bilirubin screens (total and direct bilirubin) are costly and are not very helpful for determining an etiology for jaundice. They are also poor predictors of which infants are likely to develop kernicterus. Transcutaneous bilirubinometry can, in specific clinical settings, provide an accurate estimate of the serum bilirubin concentration. However, values provided by the bilirubinometer can vary quite considerably and before they are accepted as accurate, a correlation with serum bilirubin values must be established. At present, transcutaneous bilirubinometry should not replace standard laboratory measurements but can serve as an effective screening tool.

Some authors have advocated cry analysis as a means of detecting abnormal neuronal states due to bilirubin. The use of the Brazelton Behavioral Scale has also been employed to assess subtle changes in neurological behavior in infants with hyperbilirubinemia. Furthermore, brain stem auditory evoked responses have recently been shown to be sensitive in detecting changes in auditory nerve function and brain stem function in infants with elevated bilirubin levels. Infants in the low to moderate range of bilirubin concentrations can demonstrate alterations in these pathways, which raise concern regarding low-level bilirubin toxicity. Fortunately, the changes seen with hyperbilirubinemia are reversible after the bilirubin decreases. Therefore, it is uncertain whether low to moderate serum bilirubin concentrations increase the likelihood of long-term neurological handicaps.

Most of the follow-up studies that have evaluated full-term infants who have experienced an exaggerated physiological jaundice during the neonatal period have not demonstrated adverse effects unless bilirubin levels far exceeded 25 mg/dL. The association of kernicterus with serum bilirubin concentrations greater than 20 mg/dL exists mainly for sick infants with Rh hemolytic disease. Randomized controlled trials have not demonstrated any differences in IQ in infants undergoing exchange transfusion for high bilirubin levels compared to infants who had not received this mode of therapy. Trolle has calculated that if standard guidelines are followed more than 2,000 infants would need to receive an exchange transfusion to prevent symptomatic kernicterus in one infant. Given the published mortality rate of 0.5% to 1%, you can infer that 15 to 20 infants might die unnecessarily to prevent cerebral palsy in one infant. On the other hand, one recent study has demonstrated an association between low IQ and severe hyperbilirubinemia (>20 mg/dL) in 17-year-old males. That association held true even when corrected for factors such as prematurity, Rh hemolytic disease, and other pathological causes of jaundice. Controversy about treatment of the healthy full-term infant with hyperbilirubinemia still continues. However, in the *healthy* full-term infant, exchange transfusion should not be considered unless the serum unconjugated bilirubin concentration exceeds 25 mg/dL.

## ■ Answers:

1. Not unless bilirubin exceeds 25 mg/dL.

2. *Diet:* Early institution of feeds decreases the enterohepatic circulation, and increased fluids prevent dehydration.
   *Bezoars:* Agents such as agar and activated charcoal bind bilirubin in the gut and reduce the enterohepatic circulation.
   *Phenobarbital:* Stimulates hepatic enzymes for conjugation of bilirubin.
   *Bilirubin oxidase:* Metabolizes bilirubin to a purple pigment that is more readily excretable.
   *Metalloporphyrins:* Competitively inhibit heme oxygenase, the rate-limiting step in heme degradation.
   *Chinese herbal medicine:* Promotes bilirubin excretion.

## ■ Discussion:

We have discussed the mechanisms of action of phototherapy and discussed the risks and benefits of an exchange transfusion. Other modes of therapy are available for treating jaundiced infants. The most simple method is one of dietary changes; for example, instituting early feedings and increasing fluids to prevent dehydration. Dunn et al. investigated the early institution of hypocaloric feedings in preterm infants and noted lower peak levels of bilirubin compared to control subjects. Several studies have documented the benefits of early and frequent feedings in term infants in decreasing peak bilirubin concentrations. Nonetheless, this technique is often insufficient when the infant demonstrates rapidly increasing bilirubin values or has hemolytic disease. To further decrease the enterohepatic recirculation of bilirubin, agents can be administered that bind bilirubin in the gut. Agar, cholestyramine, and activated charcoal have all been fed to human newborn infants, but they have questionable efficacy and the potential to cause serious side effects.

In 1968, Trolle reported a diminished incidence of neonatal jaundice among offspring of epileptic mothers receiving phenobarbital. Since then, phenobarbital has been evaluated in numerous clinical trials to stimulate the hepatic enzymes required for conjugation of bilirubin. The success of this agent appears to be partially limited by its prolonged half-life. The time lag between the time of administration and the desired effect is usually 48 hours or more. Prenatal therapy with phenobarbital has been successful in decreasing peak serum bilirubin values in infants at risk for hyperbilirubinemia. The concern is that this agent is a sedative and may cause further neurological depression in very low birth weight infants or other high-risk populations. Phenobarbital might prove valuable to Third World countries, where there is limited access to other modalities for the treatment of hyperbilirubinemia. Other drugs such as nicotinamide have been investigated in the past, but this compound works best with phenobarbital. One agent, Bucolome, an anti-inflammatory, nonsedative agent with a barbiturate-like configuration, was tested in Europe and Japan in the 1970s with some success. This drug, however, leads to kernicterus in Gunn rats by displacing bound bilirubin and therefore cannot be recommended for clinical use.

Bilirubin oxidase is an endogenous enzyme that can be derived from the fungus *Myrothecium verrucaria*. It catalyzes the oxidation of bilirubin to biliverdin and to a purple pigment that is thought to be nontoxic. Bilirubin oxidase has been administered to experimental animals (orally and intravenously) and incorporated into an extracorporeal blood filter system. The primary complication noted with this latter system is a 20% reduction in circulating red blood cells, but newer approaches seem to have eliminated red cell lysis. No clinical trials have yet been performed using bilirubin oxidase. There is some concern that because this agent is derived from a fungus, allergic reactions could occur with its use.

Competitive inhibitors of heme oxygenase, the rate-limiting enzyme in heme degradation

to bilirubin, have been advocated in the treatment of neonatal jaundice. The advantage of these compounds is that they allow for decreased formation of bilirubin as well as enhanced degradation of the bilirubin that is already formed. One such compound, tin protoporphyrin, has been used in a clinical trial in Greece by Kappas and associates. Term infants with ABO incompatibility had a significant decrease in the peak bilirubin level when treated with 0.75 $\mu$mol/kg body weight tin protoporphyrin intravenously. Recently, there have been reports of photoreactivity and phototoxicity attributable to tin protoporphyrin in animals. In the Greek trial, two infants did have transient skin rashes following three doses of 0.75 $\mu$mol/kg. Although the dose used in the clinical trial was tenfold less than in the animal study, this does raise some concern about the use of this agent in infants exposed to light. Other metalloporphyrins—such as zinc, chromium, manganese, and cobalt and copper derivatives—are currently being investigated. Alterations of the porphyrin macrocycle can also modify photosensitizing properties. Though definitive studies have not yet been performed, there is hope that an agent that is less phototoxic and equally effective will be available for clinical use in the near future. Furthermore, there is reason to believe that some of these compounds might be administered orally.

Another, albeit unconventional, approach to bilirubin therapy is the use of Chinese herbal remedies containing cholegogic agents. Several reports in the Chinese literature advocate the use of these compounds, and their effectiveness has been demonstrated in infants with nonobstructive hyperbilirubinemia.

Finally, the issue has been raised of whether to treat hyperbilirubinemia at all (at least with healthy full-term infants) because bilirubin is a potent quencher of free radicals and a potentially important antioxidant. These studies, however, were done *in vitro*, and *in vivo* studies have yet to confirm the potentially beneficial effect of bilirubin. In summary, the only viable options for treating infants with hyperbilirubinemia at the current time are exchange transfusion, phototherapy, dietary intervention, and phenobarbital. Other modalities are not as yet proven and may have potentially serious side effects.

# BIBLIOGRAPHY

1. Hardy JB, Drage JS, Jackson EC: The first year of life. In *The Collaborative Perinatal Project of the National Institutes of Neurological and Communicative Disorders and Stroke.* Baltimore, Johns Hopkins University Press, 1979, p. 104.
2. Maisels MJ: Neonatal jaundice. *Semin Liver Dis* 1988; 8:148–162.
3. Hodr R: ABO haemolytic disease: Sex ratio and blood groups in the newborns requiring treatment. *Czech Med* 1989; 12:125–133.
4. Shurin S: Hematologic problems in the fetus and neonate. In Fanaroff AA, Martin RJ, eds: *Diseases of the Fetus and Infant.* St. Louis, CV Mosby, 1987, pp. 837–839.
5. Hallbrecht I: Role of hemagglutinins anti-A and anti-B in pathogenesis of jaundice of the newborn. *Am J Dis Child* 1954; 68:248.
6. Han P, Kiruba R, Ong R, et al: Haematolytic disease due to ABO incompatibility: Incidence and value of screening in an Asian population. *Aust Paediatr J* 1988; 24:35–38.
7. Linn S, Schoenbaum SC, Monson RR, et al: Epidemiology of neonatal hyperbilirubinemia. *Pediatrics* 1985; 75:770–774.
8. Brown WR, Boon WR: Ethnic group difference in plasma bilirubin levels of full-term, healthy Singapore newborns. *Pediatrics* 1965; 36:745.
9. Fischer AF, Nakamura H, Uetani Y, et al: Comparison of bilirubin production in Japanese and Caucasian infants. *J Pediatr Gastroent Nutr* 1988; 7:27–29.
10. Valaes T: Neonatal jaundice in the framework of Greek reality. *Iatriki* 1963; 3:59.
11. Cohen RS, Hopper AO, Ostrander CR, et al: Total bilirubin production in infants of Chinese, Japanese and Korean ancestry. *J Formosan Med Assoc* 1982; 81:524–529.
12. Rooney JC, Hill DJ, Danks DM: Jaundice associated with bacterial infection in the newborn. *Am J Dis Child* 1971; 122:39–41.
13. Marwaha N, Sarode R, Marwaha RK, et al: Bilirubin crystals in peripheral blood smears from neonates with unconjugated hyperbilirubinaemia. *Med Lab Sci* 1990; 47:278–281.
14. Bergstrom T, Larson H, Lincoln K, et al: Studies on urinary tract infections in infancy and childhood. XII. Eighty consecutive patients with neonatal infection. *J Pediatr* 1972; 80: 858.
15. Ng SHJ, Rawstron JR: Urinary tract infections presenting with jaundice. *Arch Dis Child* 1971; 46:173.
16. Bernstein J, Brown AK: Sepsis and jaundice in early infancy. *Pediatrics* 1962; 29:873.
17. Rajagopalan I, Katz BZ: Hyperbilirubinemia secondary to hemolysis of intrauterine intraperitoneal blood transfusion. *Clin Pediatr* 1984; 23:511–512.
18. Wright K, Tarr PI, Hickman RO, et al: Hyperbilirubinemia secondary to delayed absorption of intraperitoneal blood following intrauterine transfusion. *J Pediatr* 1982; 100:302–304.
19. Davies DP, Gomersall R, Robertson R, et al: Neonatal jaundice and maternal oxytocin infusion. *Br J Med* 1973; 3:476–477.
20. Buchan PC: Pathogenesis of neonatal hyperbilirubinemia after induction of labour with oxytocin. *Br Med J* 1979; 2:1255–1257.
21. Calder AA, Ounsted MK, Moar VA, et al: Increased bilirubin levels in neonates after induction of labour by intravenous prostaglandin E2 or oxytocin. *Lancet* 1974; 2:1339–1942.
22. Johnson DJ, Aldrich M, Angelus P, et al: Oxytocin and neonatal hyperbilirubinemia. *Am J Dis Child* 1984; 138:1047–1050.
23. Cremer RJ, Perryman PW, Richards DH: Influence of light on the hyperbilirubinaemia of infants. *Lancet* 1958; 1:1094–1097.
24. Tan KL, Boey KW: Clinical experience with phototherapy. *Ann Acad Med Singapore* 1989; 18:43–48.
25. Tan KL: Management of neonatal jaundice. *Singapore Med J* 1989; 30:393–395.
26. Polin RA: Management of neonatal hyperbilirubinemia: Rational use of phototherapy. *Biol Neonate* 1990; 58 suppl 1:32–43.
27. Pratesi R, Agati G, Fusi F: Phototherapy for neonatal hyperbilirubinemia. *Photodermatol* 1989; 6:244–257.
28. McDonagh AF, Palma LA, Lightner DA: Phototherapy for neonatal jaundice: Stereospecific and regioselective photoisomerization of bilirubin bound to human serum albumin and NMR characterization of intramolecular cyclized photoproducts. *J Am Chem Soc* 1982; 104:6867–6869.
29. Lightner DA: The photoreactivity of bilirubin and related pyrroles. *Photochem Photobiol* 1977; 26:427–436.
30. National Institute of Child Health and Human Development: Randomized controlled trial of phototherapy for neonatal hyperbilirubinemia. *Pediatrics* 1985; 75:381–441.
31. Brown AK, McDonagh AF: *Phototherapy for Neonatal Hyperbilirubinemia: Efficacy, Mechanism, and Toxicity.* St. Louis, Mosby-Year Book, 1980, pp. 341–389.
32. Scheidt PC, Bryla DA, Nelson KB, et al: Phototherapy for neonatal hyperbilirubinemia: Six-year follow-up of the National Institute of Child Health and Human Development clinical trial. *Pediatrics* 1990; 85:455–463.
33. Ennever JF: Blue light, green light, white light, more light: Treatment of neonatal jaundice. *Clin Perinatol* 1990; 17:467–481.
34. Lightner DA, Linnane WPI, Ahlfors CE: Bilirubin photooxidation products in the urine of jaundiced infants receiving phototherapy. *Pediatr Res* 1984; 19:696–799.
35. Lightner DA, Wooldridge TA, McDonagh AF: Configurational isomerization of bilirubin and the mechanism of jaundice phototherapy. *Biochem Biophys Res Commun* 1989; 86:235–243.
36. Agati G, Fusi F, Pratesi R: Configurational photoisomerization of bilirubin *in vitro.* II. A comparative study of phototherapy fluorescent lamps and lasers. *Photochem Photobiol* 1985; 41:381–392.

37. Bonnett R, Buckley DG, Hamzetash D: Photobilirubin: II. *Biochem J* 1984; 219:1053–1056.
38. Ennever JF, Costarino AT, Polin RA, et al: Rapid clearance of a structural isomer of bilirubin during phototherapy. *J Clin Invest* 1987; 79:1674–1678.
39. Ennever JF, Dresing TJ: Quantum yields for the cyclization and configurational isomerization of 4E,15Z-bilirubin. *Photochem Photobiol* 1991; 53:25–32.
40. Greenberg JW, Malhotra V, Ennever JF: Wavelength dependence of the quantum yield for the structural isomerization of bilirubin. *Photochem Photobiol* 1987; 46:453–456.
41. Tan KL: Phototherapy of neonatal jaundice. *Clin Perinatol* 1991; 18:423–439.
42. Tan KL: The pattern of bilirubin response to phototherapy for neonatal hyperbilirubinemia. *Pediatr Res* 1982; 16:670–674.
43. Ayyash H, Hadjigeorgiou E, Sofatzis J, et al: Green light phototherapy in newborn infants with ABO hemolytic disease. *J Pediatr* 1987; 111:882–887.
44. Eidelman AI, Schimmel MS: Phototherapy—1988. A green light for a new approach? *J Perinatol* 1989; 9:69–71.
45. Ennever JF: Phototherapy in a new light. *Pediatr Clin North Am* 1986; 33:603–620.
46. Jokiel K, Jahrig K, Meisel P: [Is there a green light for the use of green light in phototherapy of neonatal icterus?]. (Original: Gibt es grunes Licht fur die Verwendung von Grunem Licht in der Phototherapie des Neugeborenenikterus?) *Kinderarztl Prax* 1988; 56:369–374.
47. Tan KL: Efficacy of fluorescent daylight, blue, and green lamps in the management of nonhemolytic hyperbilirubinemia. *J Pediatr* 1989; 114:132–137.
48. Eggert P, Stick C, Swalve S: On the efficacy of various irradiation regimens in phototherapy of neonatal hyperbilirubinaemia. *Eur J Pediatr* 1988; 147:525–528.
49. Murphy MR, Oellrich RG: A new method of phototherapy: Nursing perspectives. *J Perinatol* 1990; 10:249–251.
50. McFadden EA: The Wallaby Phototherapy System: A new approach to phototherapy. *J Pediatr Nurs* 1991; 6:206–208.
51. Gale R, Dranitzki Z, Dollberg S, et al: A randomized, controlled application of the Wallaby phototherapy system compared with standard phototherapy. *J Perinatol* 1990; 10:239–242.
52. Rosenfeld W, Twist P, Concepcion L: A new device for phototherapy treatment of jaundiced infants. *J Perinatol* 1990; 10:243–248.
53. Plastino R, Buchner DM, Wagner EH: Impact of eligibility criteria on phototherapy program size and cost. *Pediatrics* 1990; 85:796–800.
54. Committee on Fetus and Newborn, American Academy of Pediatrics: Home phototherapy. *Pediatrics* 1985; 76:136–137.
55. Tyrrell RM, Keyse SM: New trends in photobiology. The interaction of UVA radiation with cultured cells. *J Photochem Photobiol B* 1990; 4:349–361.
56. Bradley MO, Sharkey NA: Mutagenicity and toxicity of visible fluorescent light to cultured mammalian cells. *Nature* 1977; 266:724–726.
57. Anderson RR, Parrish JA: The optics of human skin. *J Invest Derm* 1981; 77:13–19.
58. Messner KH: Light toxicity to newborn retina. *Pediatr Res* 1978; 12:530.
59. Moseley MJ, Fielder AR: Phototherapy: An ocular hazard revisited. *Arch Dis Child* 1988; 63:886–887.
60. Bell EF, Neidich GA, Cashore WJ, et al: Combined effect of radiant warmer and phototherapy on insensible water loss in low birth weight infants. *J Pediatr* 1979; 94:810.
61. Oh W, Karecki H: Phototherapy and insensible water loss in the newborn infant. *Am J Dis Child* 1972; 124:230.
62. Ramagnoli G, Polidori G, Catalbi L, et al: Phototherapy-induced hypocalcemia. *J Pediatr* 1979; 94:815.
63. Lucas A, Bates CJ: Occurrence and significance of riboflavin deficiency in preterm infants. *Biol Neonate* 1987; 52:113–118.
64. Zammarchi E, La Rosa S, Pierro U, et al: Free tryptophan decrease in jaundiced newborn infants during phototherapy. *Biol Neonate* 1989; 55:224–227.
65. Woody NC, Brodkey MJ: Tanning from phototherapy for neonatal jaundice. *J Pediatr* 1973; 82:1042.
66. Clark CF, Torii S, Hamamoto Y, et al: The "bronze" baby syndrome: Post mortem data. *J Pediatr* 1976; 88:461–464.
67. Wu PYK, Hodgman JE: Insensible water loss in preterm infants: Changes with postnatal development and non-ionizing radiant energy. *Pediatrics* 1974; 54:704.
68. Ahlfors CE, Dibiasio-Erwin D: Rate constants for dissociation of bilirubin from its binding sites in neonatal (cord) and adult sera. *J Pediatr* 1986; 108:295–298.
69. Esbjorner E: Albumin binding properties in relation to bilirubin and albumin concentrations during the first week of life. *Acta Paediatr Scand* 1991; 80:400–405.
70. Hayer M, Piva MT, Sieso V, de Bornier BM: Experimental studies on unconjugated bilirubin binding by human erythrocytes. *Clin Chim Acta* 1990; 186:345–350.
71. Berde CB, Benitz WE, Rasmussen LF, et al: Bilirubin binding in the plasma of newborns: Critical evaluation of a fluorescence quenching method and comparison to the peroxidase method. *Pediatr Res* 1984; 18:349–354.
72. Jahrig K, Stenger R, Meisel P: [Pathogenesis of bilirubin encephalopathy and subsequent therapeutic consequences]. *Zentralbl Gynakol* 1989; 111:1025–1032.
73. Stobie PE, Hansen CT, Hailey JR, et al: A difference in mortality between two strains of jaundiced rats. *Pediatrics* 1991; 87:88–93.
74. Gartner LM, Lee K-S: Bilirubin binding, free fatty acids and a new concept for the pathogenesis of kernicterus. *Birth Defects* 1976; 12:264.
75. Walker PC: Neonatal bilirubin toxicity. A review of kernicterus and the implications of drug-induced bilirubin displacement. *Clin Pharmacokinet* 1987; 13:26–50.

76. Amit Y, Chan G, Fedunec S, et al: Bilirubin toxicity in a neuroblastoma cell line N-115: I. Effects on Na+K+ ATPase. [3H]-thymidine uptake, L-[35S]-methionine incorporation, and mitochondrial function. *Pediatr Res* 1989; 25:364–368.

77. Andrew G, Chan G, Schiff D: Lipid metabolism in the neonate. II. The effect of intralipid on bilirubin binding *in vitro* and *in vivo*. *J Pediatr* 1976; 88:279.

78. Ebbesen F, Brodersen R: Risk of bilirubin acid precipitation in preterm infants with respiratory distress syndrome: Considerations of blood/brain bilirubin transfer equilibrium. *Early Hum Dev* 1982; 6:341–355.

79. Diamond I, Schmid R: Experimental bilirubin encephalopathy. The mode on entry of bilirubin-14C into the central nervous system. *J Clin Invest* 1966; 45:678.

80. Cashore WJ, Monin PJP, Oh W: Serum bilirubin binding capacity and free bilirubin concentration: A comparison between Sephadex G-25 filtration and peroxidation techniques. *Pediatr Res* 1978; 12:195.

81. Bratlid D, Cashore WJ, Oh W: Effects of acidosis on bilirubin deposition in rat brain. *Pediatrics* 1984; 73:431–434.

82. Hansen TW, Oyasaeter S, Stiris T, et al: Effects of sulfisoxazole, hypercarbia, and hyperosmolality on entry of bilirubin and albumin into brain regions in young rats. *Biol Neonate* 1989; 56:22–30.

83. Brann BS, Stonestreet BS, Oh W, et al: The *in vivo* effect of bilirubin and sulfisoxazole on cerebral oxygen, glucose, and lactate metabolism in newborn piglets. *Pediatr Res* 1987; 22:135–140.

84. Cronin CM, Brown DR, Ahdab BM: Risk factors associated with kernicterus in the newborn infant: Importance of benzyl alcohol exposure. *Am J Perinatol* 1991; 8:80–85.

85. Jardine DS, Rogers K: Relationship of benzyl alcohol to kernicterus, intraventricular hemorrhage, and mortality in preterm infants. *Pediatrics* 1989; 83:153–160.

86. Oie S, Levy G: Effect of sulfisoxazole on pharmacokinetics of free and plasma protein-bound bilirubin in experimental unconjugated hyperbilirubinemia. *J Pharm Sci* 1979; 68:6.

87. Rasmussen LF, Ahlfors CE, Wennberg RP: Displacement of bilirubin from albumin by indomethacin. *J Clin Pharmacol* 1978; 18:477–481.

88. Ebbesen F, Brodersen R: Comparison between two preparations of human serum albumin in treatment of neonatal hyperbilirubinemia. *Acta Paediatr Scand* 1982; 71:85–90.

89. Bratlid D, Cashore WJ, Oh W: Effect of serum hyperosmolality on opening of blood-brain barrier for bilirubin in rat brain. *Pediatrics* 1983; 71:909.

90. Brodersen R, Stern L: Deposition of bilirubin acid in the central nervous system—a hypothesis for the development of kernicterus. *Acta Paediatr Scand* 1990; 79:12–19.

91. Schmorl G: Zur kenntis des icterus neonatorum. *Verh Dtsch Ges Pathol* 1903; 6:109.

92. Kim MH, Yoon JJ, Sher J, et al: Lack of predictive indices in kernicterus: A comparison of clinical and pathologic factors in infants with or without kernicterus. *Pediatrics* 1980; 66:852.

93. Volodin NN, Chekhonin VP, Tabolin VA, et al: [Status of the blood-brain barrier in newborn infants of various gestational ages in the normal state and in pathology]. *Pediatriia* 1989; 1989:10–14.

94. Dikshit SK, Gupta PK: Exchange transfusion in neonatal hyperbilirubinemia. *Indian Pediatr* 1989; 26:1139–1145.

95. Paul SS, Thomas V, Singh D: Outcome of neonatal hyperbilirubinemia managed with exchange transfusion. *Indian Pediatr* 1988; 25:765–769.

96. Van Praagh R: Diagnosis of kernicterus in the neonatal period. *Pediatrics* 1961; 28:870–876.

97. Connolly AM, Volpe JJ: Clinical features of bilirubin encephalopathy. *Clin Perinatol* 1990; 17:371–379.

98. Byers RK, Paine RS, Crothers B: Extrapyramidal cerebral palsy with hearing loss following erythroblastosis. *Pediatrics* 1955; 15:248.

99. Volpe JJ: Neurology of the newborn. In *Neurology of the newborn*. Philadelphia, WB Saunders Co, 1987, p. 386.

100. Turkel SB: Autopsy findings associated with neonatal hyperbilirubinemia. *Clin Perinatol* 1990; 17:381–396.

101. Haymaker W, Margoles C, Pentshew A, et al: Pathology of kernicterus and posticteric encephalopathy: Presentation of 97 cases, with consideration of pathogenesis and etiology. In Thomas CC, ed: *Kernicterus and Its Importance in Cerebral Palsy*. Springfield, IL, Charles C Thomas, 1961, pp. 21–228.

102. Jew JY, Sandquist D: CNS changes in hyperbilirubinemia: Functional implications. *Arch Neurol* 1979; 36:149.

103. Ahdab-Barmada M, Moosy J: The neuropathology of kernicterus in the premature neonate: Diagnostic problems. *J Neuropathol Exp Neurol* 1984; 43:45.

104. Burgess GH, Oh W, Bratlid D: The effects of brain blood flow on brain bilirubin deposition in newborn piglets. *Pediatr Res* 1985; 19:691–696.

105. Turkel SB, Mapp JR: A ten-year retrospective study of pink and yellow neonatal hyaline membrane disease. *Pediatrics* 1983; 72:170.

106. Maisels MJ, Gifford K, Antle CE, et al: Jaundice in the healthy newborn infant: A new approach to an old problem. *Pediatrics* 1988; 81:505–511.

107. Bloomer JR, Barrett PV, Rodkey FL, et al: Studies on the mechanism of fasting hyperbilirubinemia. *Gastroenterology* 1971; 61:479–487.

108. Auerbach KG, Gartner LM: Breastfeeding and human milk: Their association with jaundice in the neonate. *Clin Perinatol* 1987; 14:89–107.

109. Stevenson DK, Bartoletti AL, Ostrander CR, et al: Effect of fasting on bilirubin production in the first postnatal week. *Clin Res* 1980; 1:126A.

110. Gartner LM, Auerbach KG: Breast milk and

breastfeeding jaundice. *Adv Pediatr* 1987; 34:249–274.

111. Rodgers PA, Cornelius CE, Vreman HJ, et al: Increased carbon monoxide excretion in Bolivian squirrel monkeys with fasting hyperbilirubinemia. *J Med Primatol* 1990; 19:485–492.

112. Dahms BB, Krauss AN, Gartner LM, et al: Breast feeding and serum bilirubin values during the first 4 days of life. *J Pediatr* 1973; 83:1049–1054.

113. De Carbalho M, Klaus MH, Merkatz RB: Frequency of breast-feeding and serum bilirubin concentration. *Am J Dis Child* 1982; 136:737–738.

114. Gale R, Dollberg S, Branski D, Stevenson D, et al: Breast-feeding of term infants. Three-hour vs. four-hour non-demand. A randomized controlled reappraisal of hospital-based feeding schedules. *Clin Pediatr (Phila)* 1989; 28:458–460.

115. Leung AK, Sauve RS: Breastfeeding and breast milk jaundice. *J R Soc Health* 1989; 109:213–217.

116. Arias IM, Gartner LM, Seifter SA: Prolonged neonatal unconjugated hyperbilirubinemia associated with breastfeeding and a steroid, pregnane-3-alpha, 20 beta-diol in maternal milk that inhibits blucoronide formation *in vitro*. *J Clin Invest* 1964; 43:2037.

117. Brooten D, Brown L, Hollingsworth A, et al: Breast-milk jaundice. *J Obstet Gynecol Neonatal Nurs* 1985; 14:220–223.

118. Poland RL, Schultz GE, Garg G: High milk lipase activity associated with breast milk jaundice. *Pediatr Res* 1980; 14:1328–1331.

119. Tazawa Y, Abukawa D, Watabe M, et al: Abnormal results of biochemical liver function tests in breast-fed infants with prolonged indirect hyperbilirubinaemia. *Eur J Pediatr* 1991; 150:310–313.

120. Stevenson DK, Bartoletti AL, Ostrander CR, et al: Pulmonary excretion of carbon monoxide in the human infant as an index of bilirubin production. IV. Effects of breastfeeding and caloric intake in the first postnatal week. *Pediatrics* 1980; 65:1170–1172.

121. Newman TB, Maisels MJ: Does hyperbilirubinemia damage the brain of healthy full-term infants? *Clin Perinatol* 1990; 17:331–358.

122. Peevy KJ: Hyperbilirubinemia in infants of diabetic mothers. *Pediatr* 1980; 66:417–419.

123. Miodovnik M, Mimouni F, Tsang RC, et al: Management of the insulin-dependent diabetic during labor and delivery. Influences on neonatal outcome. *Am J Perinatol* 1987; 4:106–114.

124. Jahrig D, Jahrig K, Stiete S, et al: Neonatal jaundice in infants of diabetic mothers. *Acta Paediatr Scand Suppl* 1989; 360:101–107.

125. Stevenson DK, Bartoletti AL, Johnson JD: Pulmonary excretion of carbon monoxide in the human infant as an index of bilirubin production. II. Infants of diabetic mothers. *J Pediatr* 1979; 94:956–958.

126. Perrine SP, Greene MF, Cohen RA, et al: A physiological delay in human fetal hemoglobin switching is associated with specific globin DNA hypomethylation. *Febs Lett* 1988; 228:139–143.

127. Newman TB, Easterling MJ, Goldman ES, et al: Laboratory evaluation of jaundice in newborns. Frequency, cost, yield. *Am J Dis Child* 1990; 144:364–368.

128. Fok TF, Lau SP, Hui CW, et al: Transcutaneous bilirubinometer: Its use in Chinese term infants and the effect of haematocrit and phototherapy on the TcB index. *Aust Paediatr J* 1986; 22:107–109.

129. Tan KL, Mylvaganam A: Transcutaneous bilirubinometry in preterm very low birthweight infants. *Acta Paediatr Scand* 1988; 77:796–801.

130. Bhardwaj HP, Narang A, Bhakoo ON: Evaluation of Minolta jaundice meter and icterometer for assessment of neonatal jaundice. *Indian Pediatr* 1989; 26:161–165.

131. Uchida K, Kaneoka T, Ichihara J, et al: [Fundamental studies on transcutaneous bilirubinometry in newborn infants using an organ scanning spectrophotometer]. *Nippon Sanka Fujinka Gakkai Zasshi* 1988; 40:167–173.

132. Vreman HJ, Rodgers PA, Gale R, et al: Carbon monoxide excretion as an index of bilirubin production in rhesus monkeys. *J Med Primatol* 1989; 18:449–460.

133. Bucalo LR, Cohen RS, Ostrander CR, et al: Pulmonary excretion of carbon monoxide in the human infant as an index of bilirubin production. IIc. Evidence for the possible association of cord erythropoietin levels and postnatal bilirubin production in infants of mothers with abnormalities of gestational glucose metabolism. *Am J Perinatol* 1984; 1:177–181.

134. Alden ER, Lyneh SR: Carboxyhemoglobin determination in evaluating neonatal jaundice. *Am J Dis Child* 1974; 127:214.

135. Stevenson DK: Personal communication. 1991.

136. Perlman M, Frank JW: Bilirubin beyond the blood-brain barrier. *Pediatrics* 1988; 81:304–315.

137. Vohr BR: New approaches to assessing the risks of hyperbilirubinemia. *Clin Perinatol* 1990; 17:293–306.

138. Koivisto M: Cry analysis in infants with Rh haemolytic disease. *Acta Paediatr Scand Suppl* 1987; 335:1–73.

139. Friedman SL, Werthman MW, Waxler M: Physiologic jaundice as a predictor of sensory, neurological and affective function in low-risk preterm infants. *Soc Res Child Dev* 1983; 4:83A.

140. Escher-Graub DC, Fricker HS: Jaundice and behavioral organization in the full-term neonate. *Helv Pediatr Acta* 1986; 41:425–435.

141. Hung KL, Wu CM: Auditory brainstem response in patients with a history of kernicterus. *Acta Paediatr Sin* 1988; 29:229–234.

142. Greenwald JL: Hyperbilirubinemia in otherwise healthy infants. *Am Fam Physician* 1988; 38:151–158.

143. Mollison PL, Cutbush M: Haemolytic disease of the newborn. In Gairdner D, ed: *Recent Advances in Pediatrics*. New York, Blakinston & Son Co, 1954, p. 110.

144. Hsia DY-Y, Allen FH, Gellis SS, et al: Erythroblastosis fetalis. VIII. Studies of serum bilirubin in relation to kernicterus. *N Engl J Med* 1952; 247:668.

145. Boggs T, Hardy J, Frazier T: Correlation of neonatal serum total bilirubin and developmental status at age eight months. *J Pediatr* 1967; 71:553.

146. Rubin RA, Balow B, Fisch RO: Neonatal serum bilirubin levels related to cognitive development at ages 4–7 years. *J Pediatr* 1979; 94:601–604.

147. Trolle D: Phenobarbitone and neonatal icterus. *Lancet* 1968; 1:251.

148. Schober PH: [Automated exchange transfusion in premature and newborn infants with hyperbilirubinemia using a peripheral arteriovenous vascular access device]. *Wien Klin Wochenschr* 1990; 102:471–475.

149. Seidman DS, Paz I, Stevenson DK, et al: Neonatal hyperbilirubinemia and physical and cognitive performance at 17 years of age. *Pediatrics* 1991; 88:828–833.

150. Dunn L, Hulman S, Weiner J, et al: Beneficial effects of early hypocaloric enteral feeding on neonatal gastrointestinal function: Preliminary report of a randomized trial. *J Pediatr* 1988; 112:622–629.

151. Poland RL, Odell GB: Physiologic jaundice: The enterohepatic circulation of bilirubin. *N Engl J Med* 1971; 284:1.

152. Odell GB, Gutcher GR, Whitington PF, et al: Enteral administration of agar as an effective adjunct to phototherapy of neonatal hyperbilirubinemia. *Pediatr Res* 1972; 17:810.

153. Nicolopoulos D, Hadjigeorgiou E, Malamitsi-Puchner A, et al: Reducing the duration of phototherapy for neonatal jaundice by cholestyramine administration. In Rubaletti FF, Jovi G, eds: *Neonatal Jaundice—New Trends in Phototherapy.* New York, Plenum Press, 1984, p. 257.

154. Ulstrom RA, Eisenblam E: The enterohepatic shunting of bilirubin in the newborn infant: I. Use of oral activated charcoal to reduce normal serum bilirubin values. *J Pediatr* 1964; 65:27.

155. Arrowsmith WA, Payne RB, Littlewood JM: Comparison of treatments for congenital nonobstructive nonhaemolytic hyperbilirubinemia. *Arch Dis Child* 1975; 50:197.

156. Halpin TF, Jones AR, Bishop HL, et al: Prophylaxis of neonatal hyperbilirubinemia with phenobarbital. *Obstet Gynecol* 1972; 40:85.

157. Blackburn MG, Orzalesi MM, Pigram P: The combined effect of phototherapy and phenobarbital on serum bilirubin levels of premature infants. *Pediatrics* 1972; 49:110.

158. Valaes T, Kipouros K, Petmezaki S, et al: Effectiveness and safety of prenatal phenobarbital for the prevention of neonatal jaundice. *Pediatr Res* 1980; 14:947.

159. Kurata N, Yoshida T, Kuroiwa Y, et al: Long-term effects of phenobarbital on rat liver microsomal drug-metabolizing enzymes and heme-metabolizing enzyme. *Res Commun Chem Pathol Pharmacol* 1989; 65:161–179.

160. Serini F, Perletti L, Marini A: Influence of diethylincotinamide on the concentration of serum bilirubin of newborn infants. *Pediatrics* 1967; 402:446.

161. Segni G, Polidori G, Romagnoli C: Bucolome in prevention of hyperbilirubinaemia in preterm infants. *Arch Dis Child* 1977; 52:549.

162. Baba K: Use of bucolome in hyperbilirubinemia. *Paediatrician* 1972; 1:109.

163. Okada K, Nagasawa K, Maruyama A, et al: Neonatal hyperbilirubinemia and bucolome. *Obstet Gynecol (Tokyo)* 1972; 31:831.

164. Semba R, Sato H, Yamamura H: Danger of bucolome in infants with hyperbilirubinemia: Experimental evidence. *Arch Dis Child* 1978; 53:503.

165. Aono S, Kashiwamata S: Patho-biochemistry of cerebellar hypoplasia in the jaundiced Gunn rat. *Med Sci Res* 1989; 17:321–324.

166. Murao S, Tanaka N: A new enzyme "bilirubin oxidase" produced by *Murothecium verrucaria* MT-1. *Agricol Biol Chem* 1981; 45:2383.

167. Levine RL, Fredericks WR, Rapoport SI: Clearance of bilirubin from rat brain after reversible osmotic opening of the blood brain barrier. *Pediatr Res* 1985; 19:1040–1043.

168. Johnson L, Dworanczyk R, Jenkins D: Bilirubin oxidase (BOX) feedings at varying time intervals and enzyme concentrations in infant Gunn rats. *Pediatr Res* 1989; 25:116A.

169. Kimura M, Matsumura Y, Miyauchi Y, et al: A new tactic for the treatment of jaundice: An injectible polymer-conjugated bilirubin oxidase. *Proc Soc Exp Biol Med* 1988; 188:364–369.

170. Kimura M: Enzymatic removal of bilirubin toxicity by bilirubin oxidase *in vitro* and excretion of degradation products *in vivo*. *Proc Soc Exp Biol Med* 1990; 195:64–69.

171. Mullon CJ, Tosone CM, Langer R: Simulation of bilirubin detoxification in the newborn using an extracorporeal bilirubin oxidase reactor [published erratum appears in *Pediatr Res* 1990; 27(2):117]. *Pediatr Res* 1989; 26:452–457.

172. Drummond GS, Kappas A: Sn-protoporphyrin inhibition of fetal and neonatal brain heme oxygenase. Transplacental passage of the metalloporphyrin and prenatal suppression of hyperbilirubinemia in the newborn animal. *J Clin Invest* 1986; 77:971–976.

173. Hamori CJ, Vreman HJ, Stevenson DK: Suppression of carbon monoxide excretion by zinc mesoporphyrin in adult Wistar rats: Evidence for potent *in vivo* inhibition of bilirubin production. *Res Commun Chem Pathol Pharmacol* 1988; 62:41–48.

174. Posselt AM, Cowan BE, Kwong LK, et al: Effect of tin protoporphyrin on the excretion rate of carbon monoxide in newborn rats after hematoma formation. *J Pediatr Gastroenterol Nutr* 1985; 4:650–654.

175. Stevenson DK, Vreman HJ: Sn-protoporphyrin: A consideration of the first clinical trial in human neonates. *Pediatrics* 1988; 81:881–882.

176. Vreman HJ, Stevenson DK: Metalloporphyrin-enhanced photodegradation of bilirubin *in vitro*. *Am J Dis Child* 1990; 144:590–594.

177. Kappas A, Drummond GS, Manola T, et al: Sn-protoporphyrin use in the management of hyperbilirubinemia in term newborns with direct Coombs-positive ABO incompatibility. *Pediatrics* 1988; 81:485–497.

178. Vreman HJ, Gillman MJ, Downum KR, et al: *In vitro* generation of carbon monoxide from organic molecules and synthetic metalloporphyrins mediated by light. *Dev Pharmacol Ther* 1990; 15:112–124.

179. Hintz SR, Vreman HJ, Stevenson DK: Mortality of metalloporphyrin-treated neonatal rats after light exposure. *Dev Pharmacol Ther* 1990; 14:187–192.

180. Keino H, Nagae H, Mimura S, et al: Dangerous effects of tin-protoporphyrin plus photoirradiation on neonatal rats. *Eur J Pediatr* 1990; 149:278–279.

181. Scott J, Quirke JM, Vreman HJ, et al: Metalloporphyrin phototoxicity. *J Photochem Photobiol B* 1990; 7:149–157.

182. Drummond GS, Galbraith RA, Sardana MK, et al: Reduction of the C2 and C4 vinyl groups of Sn-protoporphyrin to form Sn-mesoporphyrin markedly enhances the ability of the metalloporphyrin to inhibit *in vivo* heme catabolism. *Arch Biochem Biophys* 1987; 255:64–74.

183. Drummond GS, Greenbaum NL, Kappas A: Tin(Sn + 4)-diiododeuteroporphyrin; an *in vitro* and *in vivo* inhibitor of heme oxygenase with substantially reduced photoactive properties. *J Pharmacol Exp Ther* 1991; 257:1109–1113.

184. Stevenson DK, Rodgers PA, Vreman HJ: The use of metalloporphyrins for the chemoprevention of neonatal jaundice. *Am J Dis Child* 1989; 143:353–356.

185. Vreman HJ, Gillman MJ, Stevenson DK: *In vitro* inhibition of adult rat intestinal heme oxygenase by metalloporphyrins. *Pediatr Res* 1989; 26:362–365.

186. Cui NQ, Wu XZ, Zheng XL: [Effect of li dan ling in decreasing jaundice and improving liver function in patients with obstructive jaundice]. *Chung Hsi I Chieh Ho Tsa Chih* 1989; 9:137–140.

187. Chen HY: Artemisia composita for the prevention and treatment of neonatal hemolysis and hyperbilirubinemia. *J Tradit Chin Med* 1987; 7:105–108.

188. Cheng YY, Chan YS, Chuang KF, et al: [Active principle in a capillaris compound in the treatment of experimental acute jaundice in rats]. *Chung Hsi I Chieh Ho Tsa Chih* 1985; 5:356–360.

189. Sugi K, Inoue M, Morino Y: Degradation of plasma bilirubin by a bilirubin oxidase derivative which has a relatively long half-life in the circulation. *Biochim Biophys Acta* 1989; 991:405–409.

190. Wang CB, Ge AP, Song WY, et al: The jaundice-suppressing effect of blood-cooling, circulation-invigorating, viscera-dredging and cholagogic Chinese herbs in the treatment of hepatitis. *J Tradit Chin Med* 1987; 7:248–250.

191. Shi YM, Shen YJ, Fu MD, et al: The therapeutic efficacy of the choleretic mixture against the infantile hepatitis syndrome. *J Tradit Chin Med* 1989; 9:103–105.

192. Watchko JF, Oksi FA: Bilirubin 20 mg/dl = vigintiphobia. *Pediatrics* 1983; 71:660–663.

193. Stocker R, Yamamoto Y, McDonagh AF, et al: Bilirubin is an antioxidant of possible physiological importance. *Science* 1987; 235:1043–1046.

194. Stocker R, McDonagh AF, Glazer AN, et al: Antioxidant activities of bile pigments: Biliverdin and bilirubin. *Methods Enzymol* 1990; 186:301–309.

195. Stocker R: Induction of haem oxygenase as a defence against oxidative stress. *Free Radic Res Commun* 1990; 9:101–112.

196. McDonagh AF: Is bilirubin good for you? *Clin Perinatol* 1990; 17:359–369.

# Chapter 6

□

# FEEDING THE

□

# NEWBORN INFANT

□

## *Gilberto R. Pereira, M.D.*

There is no other time in a human's life during which body growth, development, and maturation proceed at a faster rate than in early infancy. Consequently, during this time nutritional deficiencies are prone to develop if feedings are inadequate in content or quantity. The ideal feeding regimen for a newborn infant is one that provides quality nutrients in amounts sufficient to permit a maximal potential for growth.

This chapter contains exercises designed to help physicians identify and solve common problems associated with feeding practices in the neonate. The first section critically examines feeding recommendations for the full-term infant. Two case histories are presented: the first describes a full-term infant fed human milk and the second a full-term infant fed formula. The second section provides a variety of exercises regarding the nutritional care of the hospitalized newborn infant. These exercises were designed to illustrate the most current recommendations for the nutritional care of the premature infant, including the use of parenteral nutrition during the neonatal period.

### CASE STUDY 1 *Feeding the Full-Term Infant: Human Milk*

The following case history contains italicized statements, numbered 1 to 18, regarding infant feedings that you are asked to identify as either correct (C) or incorrect (I). Please place a C or an I in the blank ( ) after each italicized statement.

### EXERCISE 1

Baby L was born to a healthy 25-year-old primigravida woman at term gestation after an uncomplicated pregnancy and delivery. *While in the delivery room, Mrs. L insisted on breast feeding her nude infant to stimulate breast-milk production* 1( ). *The obstetrician ordered that a radiant warmer be kept over the mother and infant* 2( ). In the nursery, *the pediatrician became aware of the mother's intention to breast feed and suggested that the infant room-in with the mother during the daytime hours with optional care during the evening* 3( ). The next feeding took place in the mother's room in the presence of a nurse. The nurse recommended *a 5- to 10-minute feeding on each breast* 4( ), *alternating breasts at the beginning of each feeding* 5( ), *and a precise feeding schedule of every 4 hours throughout the day and night* 6( ). The following day, Mrs. L asked the pediatrician whether breast feeding was beneficial in protecting her baby against infection. *She was reassured that breast feeding could be protective against respiratory, intestinal, and ear infections* 7( ).

On the third hospital day, the infant was feeding well and had a normal physical examination except for mild jaundice. The infant weighed 3,200 g (120 g below birth weight) and *was discharged on a multivitamin preparation containing fluoride* 8( ) *and iron* 9( ).

At 10 days of age, Baby L was seen at the pediatrician's office and weighed 3,220 g. Mrs.

L complained that the baby was requiring frequent feedings (at 1- to 2-hour intervals) and that he appeared to be more jaundiced. The total serum bilirubin concentration was 14.5 mg/dL (direct bilirubin = 0.5 mg/dL). *The pediatrician confirmed that milk intake was inadequate by having the baby weighed on an electronic scale immediately prior to and after breast feeding, and subsequently recommended formula supplementation after each breast-milk feeding* 10(   ).

Two days later, Baby L's total serum bilirubin level was 18.2 mg/dL (direct = 0.6) and he was then hospitalized. His admission weight was 3,300 g (20 g below birth weight). Mrs. L stated that her infant was still feeding every 2 hours and refusing formula supplementation. *Phototherapy was started and breast feeding was temporarily discontinued* 11(   ). No evidence of blood group incompatibility or infection was found. At the end of the second day of hospitalization, the serum bilirubin level declined to 10.9 mg/dL. *Phototherapy was discontinued, breast feeding was resumed, and the infant was discharged 24 hours later with a serum bilirubin level of 10.2 mg/dL* 12(   ).

One week later, Mrs. L developed mastitis on her left breast. *The obstetrician prescribed ampicillin and recommended that she feed her infant on her unaffected breast and empty her affected breast using a breast pump* 13(   ). *Mrs. L stopped taking her medication because she was concerned that the drug was being excreted in her breast milk and would adversely affect the baby* 14(   ). On the following day, she called her pediatrician, who *advised her to continue breast feeding and to observe her baby for the appearance of diarrhea and feeding intolerance while she was receiving antibiotic therapy* 15(   ).

At the age of 2 months, Baby L received his first immunizations. Mrs. L stated that her baby was feeding very well. She asked whether she should diet in order to lose some of the extra weight acquired during pregnancy. *She was discouraged from dieting* 16(   ) *and encouraged to maintain an additional intake of approximately 500 calories above her maintenance diet* 17(   ). The pediatrician further suggested that *she diet only after weaning the baby off breast milk, preferably after the baby was age 6 months* 18(   ).

### ■ Discussion

Breast milk is presently recommended as the ideal nutrient for infants based on the teleo-logical, immunologic, and psychological advantages of breast feeding over formula feeding. As such, all women inclined to breast feed should be supported and encouraged to do so by counseling. Ideally, this counseling should begin early during the pregnancy.

Breast feeding can be initiated in the delivery room soon after birth. The advantages of early institution of breast feeding for the mother include enhanced uterine contractility and early stimulation of colostrum production. However, precautions must be taken in the delivery room to prevent hypothermia in the newborn infant. Infants born prematurely, those with Apgar scores of less than 7 at 5 minutes, and infants delivered to heavily sedated mothers should not breast feed in the delivery room.

Breast-feeding mothers should be encouraged to room-in with their babies. Primigravida mothers should have the first few breast-feeding sessions supervised by the nursing staff. The duration of breast-feeding should be limited to 5 to 10 minutes on each breast to prevent trauma to the nipples. Breasts should be alternated at the beginning of each feeding to allow a more complete emptying of both breasts, a factor known to be important for further milk production. Feeding frequency should be determined by the infant's demands, and rigid schedules should be avoided. The required frequency of breast feeding in humans is higher than in other species (sometimes every 2 hours), theoretically because of the relatively low concentration of protein in human milk and the short gastric emptying time associated with the use of human milk. Therefore, the 4-hour interval breast-feeding schedule recommended by the nurse in this case history should be regarded as incorrect.

Breast milk contains white cells such as lymphocytes and macrophages and a great number of antiviral and antibacterial factors that may confer protection against several types of infection. Lower incidences of gastroenteritis, respiratory tract infection, and otitis media have been reported in breast-fed babies compared to formula-fed infants.

Although maternal infections have the potential to infect the infant, they rarely represent a contraindication to breast feeding if appropriate precautions are taken. For example, when a mother has a localized infection, breast feeding should be discontinued only until she is afebrile and has received antibiotics for at least 24 hours. The recommendation to discontinue breast feeding for the whole duration of antibiotic therapy, as presented in the case history, is often unnecessary. If mastitis occurs, the infant should feed on the unaffected breast while the affected breast "lets down." The mother should then empty the affected breast by using a breast pump. The antibiotic chosen for treatment should be well tolerated by the mother and infant. Additionally, routine hand washing prior to each breast feeding is recommended as a general prophylactic measure. Breast feeding should be discontinued if the mother is infected with cytomegalovirus, hepatitis B virus, rubella virus, or human immunodeficiency virus (HIV), because transmission of these agents through breast milk has been documented.

The nutritional composition of human milk is highly variable among individual mothers and is influenced by the mother's diet, health, and nutritional status. The nutritional adequacy of breast milk can be clinically determined by assessing the infant's growth parameters and comparing them with standard growth curves. A weekly weight gain of 20 g, as illustrated by the infant in the case history, is suggestive of inadequate milk intake. This can be confirmed by weighing the infant prior to and after breast feeding using an electronic scale. When weight gain is suboptimal (in an otherwise healthy infant), supplemental formula can be offered after each feeding. Breast milk from a healthy mother receiving a daily supplement of 500 to 600 calories should be nutritionally adequate for infants during the first 6 months of life. Nursing mothers should certainly not attempt to diet. The issue of dietary supplementation with iron, vitamin D, or fluoride for all breast-fed infants during the first 6 months of life is controversial. There is, however, general agreement that the infant's diet should be supplemented with iron as soon as solid foods are started (4 to 6 months). Furthermore, vitamin D should be provided if exposure to sunlight is reduced either from cultural customs or because of excessive cloudiness during the winter months. The recommended dose of fluoride for breast-fed babies is 0.25 mg/day. After breast feeding is discontinued, the daily dose of fluoride supplementation depends on the fluoride concentration in drinking water (Table 6-1).

Jaundice in association with breast feeding has been reported to occur in 0.5% to 2.6% of infants. In affected babies the serum bilirubin

**Table 6-1** Supplemental Fluoride Dosage Schedule (mg/day*)

| AGE | CONCENTRATIONS OF FLUORIDE IN DRINKING WATER (ppm) | | |
|---|---|---|---|
| | 0.3 | 0.3 to 0.7 | 0.7 |
| 2 weeks to 2 years | 0.25 | 0 | 0 |
| 2 to 3 years | 0.50 | 0.25 | 0 |
| 3 to 16 years | 1.00 | 0.50 | 0 |

* 2.2 mg of sodium fluoride contains 1 mg of fluoride.
*Source*: Adapted from Committee on Nutrition: Nutrition and oral health. *Pediatrics* 1979; 63:150, and American Academy of Pediatrics, *Pediatric Nutrition Handbook.* Evanston, IL, Forbes GB and Woodruff CW, eds. 1979. Adapted by permission of *Pediatrics*, vol. 63, page 150, copyright 1979.

concentration continues to rise after the fourth day of life and peaks at levels between 10 and 30 mg/dL by day 10 to day 15 of life. If breast feeding continues, bilirubin levels usually decrease slowly and gradually normalize by 3 to 12 weeks of age. Although no cases of bilirubin encephalopathy have been reported in breast-fed infants, there is no reason to believe that affected infants with breast-milk jaundice are at less risk than other infants with comparable degrees of jaundice from other causes. The temporary discontinuation of breast feeding, even without phototherapy, usually produces a prompt decline in the serum bilirubin concentration. Breast-milk jaundice rarely recurs at significant levels after reinitiation of breast feeding. Therefore, after the serum bilirubin level has declined, nursing may be continued without further concerns or blood determinations.

While most drugs taken by women who are breast feeding their children can be detected in milk specimens, breast feeding is contraindicated in only a very limited number of instances. Contraindications to breast feeding include use of chemotherapeutic agents (cyclophosphamide and amethopterin), psychotropic agents (lithium, bromocryptine, ergotamine, and cocaine), antithyroid drugs (methimazole, thyouracil), and radioactive drugs (such as gallium-69; iodine-125, -131; technetium-99m). The maternal use of antibiotics does not contraindicate breast feeding and requires only that the infant be monitored for feeding intolerance and diarrhea while the mother is treated. A recent and comprehensive report describing the excretion of drugs in breast milk and corresponding appropriate monitoring of the breast-fed infant is included in the reference list.

■ **Answers:**

1. C
2. C
3. C
4. C
5. C
6. I
7. C
8. C
9. C
10. C
11. C
12. C
13. C
14. I
15. C
16. C
17. C
18. C

---

**CASE STUDY 2** *Feeding the Full-Term Infant: Formula Feeding*

This case history presents clinical problems commonly encountered in full-term infants receiving formula feedings. As in the previous section, you are asked to evaluate a variety of italicized, numbered statements by using C for correct or I for incorrect. Similarly, a discussion on the clinical use of the infant formulas follows the case history and provides the information to evaluate your answers.

**EXERCISE 2**

---

Baby R is a healthy, full-term, newborn male infant weighing 3,300 g, delivered to a healthy 25-year-old mother by a normal spontaneous vaginal delivery. Within 1 hour of birth, the infant had a normal physical examination and a glucose test strip value ranging between 45 and 90 mg/dL. *The first feeding was given at 5 hours of life and consisted of a small volume of sterile water* 1( ), *followed by 5% dextrose and water* 2( ). *Subsequent feedings consisted of standard formula, in amounts demanded by the infant* 3( ), *at approximately 4-hour intervals* 4( ). The infant was discharged at 3 days of age *on an iron-fortified formula* 5( ) *and on a fluoride supplement* 6( ).

At 2 weeks of age, Baby R weighed 3,720 g and was doing well except for regurgitation of 5 to 15 mL of formula with each feeding. Mrs. R asked the pediatrician whether the formula should be changed to decrease the frequency of regurgitation. After learning that the infant was taking 4.5 oz. of formula (135 mL) at each feeding, the pediatrician suggested *that the volume of formula be decreased to approximately 3.5 oz. (105 mL) per feeding* 7( ). *He did not believe the formula needed changing at that time* 8( ).

One week later, Mrs. R called the pediatrician and stated that her baby was crying constantly (with colic) and that she had started the infant on a soy-based formula that morning. She further stated that her previous baby had demonstrated similar signs and that he had been diagnosed with milk allergy at 1 month of age. *The pediatrician agreed with the use of a soy formula and recommended that iron* 9( ) *and fluoride* 10( ) *supplements be continued* 10( ).

At 2 months of age, the baby weighed 4,980 g. Mrs. R reported that the infant was still waking up every 4 hours (even during evening hours). *The pediatrician then suggested that rice cereals be initiated twice a day to help the infant sleep through the night* 11( ). At 6 months of age, the infant weighed 8,200 g. Mrs. R was concerned that her baby was getting too fat. Despite the mother's request, *the pediatrician did not approve the use of skim milk during the first year of life* 12( ). When asked about the initiation of whole milk, *the pediatrician suggested waiting until fruit juices and various solid foods, including cereals and meats, were well established in the diet* 13( ).

■ **Discussion:**

During the past few decades, most nurseries have adopted the practice of providing early feedings to neonates, usually within the first few hours of life. This change in routine has proven beneficial to newborn infants by lowering the incidence of hypoglycemia, dehydration, and jaundice. Clinical studies by Desmond[22,23] have demonstrated that between 2 and 6 hours of age healthy neonates have normal cardiac and respiratory rates, active bowel sounds, and mucous membranes free of secretions. In addition, by that time, most infants are active and alert and appear ready to accept feedings.

The composition of the first feeding for the newborn infant is controversial. Sterile water, or 5% dextrose and water, or both have been recommended for the first feeding as a safe routine for babies who might vomit or aspirate the feeding. However, Olson[24] has demonstrated that the instillation of 5% dextrose or milk into the respiratory tract of rabbits causes comparable degrees of injury. Indeed, if the infant aspirates gastric contents containing hydrochloric acid, a severe chemical pneumonitis is likely to occur. Therefore, many nurseries have more recently adopted the policy of offering either breast milk or formula for the baby's first feeding.

Oral fluid and caloric requirements for healthy full-term infants have been estimated to range from 120 to 180 mL/kg/day and from 100 to 120 kcal/kg/day, respectively. Full-term infants should receive feedings on demand (time and amounts); however, because of nursery routines, feedings are commonly offered on a 4-hour interval.

With the recognition that prepared formulas contain appropriate amounts of vitamins, the practice of routine vitamin supplementation for healthy full-term infants should be strongly discouraged. Vitamin supplements should be routinely prescribed only for term infants with problems known to increase losses (e.g., fat malabsorption or chronic diarrhea), for infants receiving unusual diets (e.g., vegetarianism), and for infants receiving vitamins for metabolic disease. Fluoride supplementation beginning at 2 weeks of age is presently recommended if the concentration of fluoride in the drinking water is less than 0.3 ppm (Table 6-1).

Iron deficiency anemia is still the most widespread nutritional deficiency in the United States. Most full-term babies will deplete their iron stores between 6 and 18 months of age if the diet is not supplemented with iron in the form of iron-fortified formulas, medicinal iron, or cereals. The American Academy of Pediatrics currently recommends that iron supplementation be started before 4 months of age in full-term babies, either by using an iron-fortified formula or a medicinal iron at a dose of 1 mg/kg/day. This recommendation is further supported by the observation that formula-fed babies may experience intestinal blood loss while receiving cow's milk protein formula.

For the past several years, the American Academy of Pediatrics has recommended that the initiation of solid foods be delayed until 5 to 6 months of age. The basis for this recommendation is as follows: (1) Breast milk or iron-fortified formulas supplemented with vitamins and fluoride meet all the nutritional requirements of small infants; (2) the early introduction of allergenic foods (egg, wheat) has been implicated in the pathogenesis of inflammatory bowel disease (the result of increased permeability of the small intestine to antigens in early infancy); (3) there is a relative lack of neuromuscular readiness for solid foods in early infancy; and (4) early introduction of solid foods may lead to overfeeding. The recommendation to delay the initiation of cereals until the age of 6 months of age is supported by the finding of diminished activity of alpha-amylase in the duodenal juice of small infants. Recent studies, however, have documented that small amounts of starch can be tolerated by neonates without problems, due to well-developed activity of intestinal glucoamylase. Although it is a common belief that early feedings of semisolid foods help infants sleep through the night, careful studies have shown that this is not the case.

The nutritional adequacy of formula feedings is routinely assessed by measuring growth parameters on commonly available growth charts. As presented in the case history, overfeeding is a common problem that should be suspected when vomiting occurs in the presence of appropriate weight gain. Therefore, the pediatrician in the case history exercised good judgment in detecting excessive intake of formula and in recommending a decrease in the feeding volume rather than a change in the type of formula.

Despite being commonly implicated as a cause for colic, sensitivity to cow's milk protein (milk allergy) is rare and documented in less than 1% of symptomatic infants. The diagnosis of milk allergy cannot be confirmed by laboratory testing. It is a clinical diagnosis that relies on the disappearance of symptoms when milk products are removed from the infant's diet and recurrence of the same symptoms when milk protein is reintroduced. While soy-based formulas are commonly used to feed "milk allergic" infants, 10% to 20% of these babies also exhibit soy protein intolerance. It is well known that the majority of feeding intolerance syndromes result either from intercurrent illnesses, from the emotional distress of parents, or from transient lactase deficiency following a bout of gastroenteritis. The successful use of soy formulas in the postdiarrheal state may be attributed to the replacement of lactose for sucrose or corn syrup solids, rather than the change in protein.

A balance among calories provided by protein (10%), carbohydrate (35% to 55%), and fat (45% to 50%) is recommended for the infant's diet in order to avoid metabolic disturbances. In contrast with most infant formulas, skim milk contains excessive amounts of protein and an inadequate number of fat calories. Furthermore, even when fortified with vitamins A and D, skim milk contains inadequate amounts of essential fatty acids, vitamin C, and vitamin E. For these reasons skim milk should not be used to feed infants younger than 1 year of age. The age at which whole cow's milk can be safely introduced into the infant's diet remains controversial. However, there is general agreement that whole cow's milk can be introduced between 4.5 and 6 months of age. It is important to note that whole cow's milk has inadequate concentrations of vitamin C and iron. Therefore, infants receiving whole cow's milk should be given cereals and fruit juices or receive additional supplements of iron and vitamin C.

■ **Answers:**

1. C
2. C
3. C
4. C
5. C
6. C
7. C
8. C
9. I
10. C
11. I
12. C
13. C

## FEEDING THE PREMATURE INFANT

This section deals with the nutritional care of premature infants. The topics for discussion include immediate postnatal care, methods of providing enteral feedings, guidelines for selecting the appropriate type of infant formulas, rationale for the use of nutritional supplements, and parenteral nutrition.

### Immediate Postnatal Care

Premature infants are born with diminished hepatic glycogen stores and consequently are more susceptible to hypoglycemia than full-term babies are. Therefore, premature infants who are not expected to feed enterally within a few hours of birth should receive intravenous fluids containing dextrose until enteral feedings are established. Premature infants with birth weights of less than 1,500 g should routinely receive intravenous fluids because feedings in these tiny infants are usually started after age 12 hours and are advanced more slowly. The early introduction of feedings to premature infants has been shown to prevent malnutrition and hypoglycemia, to increase the survival rate, and to reduce long-term morbidity.

Small premature infants are also susceptible to hyperglycemia even if the amount of intravenous dextrose is not excessive. Because fluid requirements are significantly increased in premature infants weighing less than 1,000 g, the use of a 5% rather than a 10% dextrose solution is frequently indicated to prevent hyperglycemia during the first few days of life. Some of the mechanisms involved in the development of hyperglycemia in the preterm infant include a decreased serum glucose clearance rate, a diminished response to insulin, and an increase in cortisol levels mediated by stress. When the premature infant is critically ill and enteral feedings cannot be initiated by 48 hours after birth, the use of a parenteral nutrition solution containing dextrose, amino acids, minerals, vitamins, and fats is indicated. These solutions should be discontinued gradually after enteral feedings satisfy the fluid and nutritional requirements.

**Table 6-2** Methods of Feeding Premature Infants

| METHOD | INDICATIONS | COMPLICATIONS | MANAGEMENT |
|---|---|---|---|
| *Oral (nipple)* | Premature (>1,500 g)<br><br>Normal sucking and swallowing mechanism | Fatigue<br><br>Increased energy expenditure associated with sucking | Gradual transition from tube to oral feedings<br><br>Maximal nippling time per feeding: 20 min<br><br>Give remainder of feed by tube |
| *Intermittent* Gastric (gavage) | Inadequate sucking and swallowing mechanisms:<br>  Premature (1,000–1,500 g)<br>  Neurological disorders<br>  Respiratory distress<br>  (RR > 60/min) | Vomiting<br><br>Aspiration | Measure gastric residuals prior to each feeding |
| *Continuous* Gastric | Premature (<1,000 g)<br><br>Mechanical ventilation<br><br>Intolerance to intermittent gastric gavage | Vomiting<br><br>Aspiration | Measure gastric residuals every 6 to 8 hours |
| Jejunal | Intolerance to gastric feedings<br><br>Gastroesophageal reflux | Stiffened feeding tubes:<br>  GI perforation<br>  Inability to remove tubes<br><br>Decreased fat and vitamin K absorption<br><br><br>Dumping syndrome | Change feeding tubes<br><br><br><br>Use formula containing 13–50% of fat as MCT<br><br>Monitor serum electrolytes (1–2 times/wk)<br><br>Avoid hyperosmolar feedings |

## Methods of Feedings

The criteria for selecting the most appropriate method of feeding should take into account the gestational age of the infant, the presence and the type of illness, and the infant's individual tolerance. Table 6-2 summarizes the indications, complications, and important management issues for each of the feeding methods used to deliver enteral feedings to premature infants. The volume and frequency of feedings will vary with gestational age; smaller infants need smaller volumes at higher frequencies. For the extremely premature infant (less than 1,000 g), feedings ideally should be provided by continuous infusion. Recommended volumes for initiating and advancing feedings in premature infants of different birth weights are summarized in Table 6-3.

## Minimal Enteral Feedings (Trophic Feedings)

The postnatal deprivation of enteral feedings in experimental animals (even for only a few days) results in atrophic changes of the gastrointestinal tract, characterized by decreased weights of the stomach, pancreas, and small intestine, and a pronounced reduction in the

**Table 6-3** Feeding Schedule for the Low Birth Weight Infant

| | LESS THAN 1,000 g | 1,001 TO 1,500 g | 1,501 TO 2,000 g |
|---|---|---|---|
| Initial feeding (mL) | 1–2 | 3–4 | 5–10 |
| Increments, every other feeding (mL) | 1 | 2 | 5–10 |
| Feeding frequency (hour) | 1 or continuous | 2 | 2–3 |

intestinal DNA content. These observations have raised concerns about the common practice of delaying the initiation of enteral feedings in critically ill neonates, especially in premature infants whose intestines are undergoing intense maturational processes at the time of birth. During the past few years, a number of small controlled clinical trials have evaluated the effects of early administration of small volumes of enteral feedings to sick premature infants receiving parenteral nutrition compared to control infants receiving only parenteral nutrition. In these trials, continuous or intermittent enteral feedings (8 to 16 kcal/kg/day) were administered for 1 to 2 weeks through the nasogastric route. Infants who received minimal enteral feedings had higher plasma levels of intestinal hormones (gastrin, gastric inhibitory peptide) and demonstrated improved feeding tolerance, faster weight gain, a shorter length of hospitalization, a lower incidence of cholestatic jaundice, and lower levels of serum bilirubin and alkaline phosphatase compared to controls. The latter observation suggests that infants receiving trophic feeds may be at lower risk for the development of metabolic bone disease.

With the increasing popularity of trophic feeds, concerns have been raised that the use of such feedings could result in a higher incidence of necrotizing enterocolitis. Nevertheless, LaGamma et al. have studied the incidence of necrotizing enterocolitis in relation to the time of initiation of enteral feedings and found a lower incidence of this disease in premature infants who were fed early with breast milk or undiluted formula compared to those who were exclusively maintained on parenteral nutrition for the first 2 weeks of life. Although this controversy is not completely settled, it seems prudent to use minimal enteral feedings during parenteral nutrition in all sick premature infants in whom there are no contraindications to enteral feedings.

## ENERGY REQUIREMENTS

The energy requirement for premature infants nursed in a neutral thermal environment and growing at *in utero* rates approaches 148 kcal/kg/day. However, if the preterm infant is given the quantity of formula needed to provide that many calories, fat accretion rates commonly exceed *in utero* values. For this reason, the American Academy of Pediatrics presently recommends an energy intake approximating 120 kcal/kg/day, which is believed to enable most premature infants to achieve satisfactory growth. This committee also recognizes the need for higher intakes in individual low birth weight infants whose growth is inadequate at that intake. Daily energy requirements for growing premature infants can be partitioned into the portion necessary for resting metabolism (50%), the energy lost in urine and stools (12%), the energy consumed by physical activity (15%), the energy needed for tissue synthesis (8%), and the portions needed for thermoregulation (10%) and growth (25%).

Energy requirements are often modified by variations in the infant's physical activity and environmental temperature, as well as by intercurrent illnesses. Therefore, increases in caloric needs above maintenance are required for infants who have increased physical activity, are nursed at environmental temperatures outside the neutral thermal zone, and who have infections, respiratory distress, or surgical stress. Conversely, caloric requirements are decreased to levels below maintenance in infants who are physically inactive or in those whose respirations are controlled by mechanical ventilation.

### EXERCISE 3  *Initiation of Feedings and Caloric Requirements*

■ **Questions:**
Each of these questions is followed by four statements. Identify which of those statements is/are correct. (Note that more than one answer may be correct.)

1. A decision is made to institute fluid and nutritional support in a 2-hour-old, 1,200-g premature infant with severe respiratory distress. How should this support be initiated?
   (a) Begin parenteral nutrition by peripheral vein.
   (b) Begin intermittent gastric feedings with human milk.
   (c) Begin continuous nasogastric feedings with human milk.
   (d) Begin intravenous fluids with 10% dextrose and water at a rate of 80 mL/kg/day.

2. At the time of initiation of intermittent gastric feedings, what is the recommended feeding volume for an 1,800-g premature infant?
   (a) 1 to 2 mL
   (b) 5 to 10 mL
   (c) 10 to 15 mL
   (d) 20 to 25 mL
3. Of the following physiological variables, which two contribute the most to total energy requirements in a growing premature infant?
   (a) Physical activity
   (b) Growth
   (c) Resting energy expenditure
   (d) Energy lost in stools and urine
4. Which of the following statements provides a rationale for trophic feedings?
   (a) Infants receiving trophic feedings demonstrate improved feeding tolerance.
   (b) Trophic feedings decrease the incidence of cholestatic jaundice.
   (c) Infants receiving trophic feedings exhibit a diminished length of hospitalization.
   (d) Serum unconjugated bilirubin values are lower in infants receiving trophic feeds.

### ■ Answers:

1. **d.** This infant is too ill for enteral feedings. Parenteral nutrition is not generally instituted during the first 24 hours of life because of the need to make frequent changes in the composition of intravenous fluids.

2. **b.** The volume of the first feeding depends on the size of the stomach. Table 6-3 lists suggested volumes for the first feeding.

3. **b, c.** The largest contributions to caloric requirements come from resting energy metabolism (50%) and growth (25%).

4. **a, b, c, d.** All four responses are correct.

### INFANT FORMULAS FOR PREMATURE INFANTS

In comparison with full-term infants, premature infants exhibit a functional immaturity of the gastrointestinal tract. Furthermore, because of their rapid growth rates, preterm infants demonstrate increased requirements for many nutrients. These two factors must be considered when the ideal composition of infant formulas for premature infants is determined.

This section reviews several features of infant formulas with a special focus on the effect of prematurity on gastrointestinal tract function and the requirements for different nutrients. A group of questions has been prepared to test your knowledge about the nutritional composition of these formulas.

### Protein

Although pancreatic trypsin secretion and activation are depressed in premature infants (as compared to full-term infants), intestinal peptidase activity and the active transport of amino acids absorbed by the brushborder membranes are demonstrable early in gestation and appear unaffected by gestational age. The coefficient of intestinal absorption of dietary protein in premature infants approximates 87%, and recommended intakes of protein for these infants vary from 1.5 to 3 g/kg/day. Premature infants appear to require some amino acids—such as histidine, tyrosine, cysteine, and taurine—that are not essential for full-term infants. The use of proteins with a lactalbumin : casein ratio of 60 : 40 such as those found in human milk can better meet the special amino acid requirement of premature infants and cause less metabolic complications than the use of cow's milk protein with a lactalbumin : casein ratio of 18 : 82.

### Carbohydrates

Lactose, the sugar present in human milk, is also present in most infant formulas derived from cow's milk. The lactase activity in the intestinal brushborder of premature infants is known to be decreased until 34 to 38 weeks of gestation, and even full-term infants may not effectively hydrolize substantial quantities of lactose. Indeed, estimates have been made that 50% to 70% of a lactose load ingested by a 1,400-g premature infant may pass into the colon. For these reasons, the lactose content of formulas prepared for premature infants has been reduced by approximately 50% by the addition of sucrose or glucose polymers, which are effectively hydrolyzed by the immature intestine. Nevertheless, recent studies have demonstrated the presence of an active process for the salvage of malabsorbed carbohydrates by colonic bacterial flora. The by-products of this anaerobic metabolic process include $CH_4$, $H_2$, $CO_2$, and short-chain fatty acids, which can be absorbed and oxidized by the infant. These recent findings indicate that the actual enteral losses of lactose in premature infants may be far less than those previously estimated.

**Fats**

Although the full-term baby absorbs up to 90% of lipids ingested, the premature infant absorbs lipids less satisfactorily. The initial phase of fat digestion occurs in the stomach by the activity of lingual lipase. Gastric lipolysis is well preserved in premature infants and accounts for almost one-third of total fat digestion. The intestinal phase of fat digestion, however, is significantly impaired in premature infants due to several factors, including decreased activity of pancreatic lipase, decreased uptake and synthesis of bile salts, and decreased reabsorption of bile salts by the distal ileum. All of these fat absorptive mechanisms are diminished until 36 to 37 weeks of gestation and principally affect the absorption of long-chain fatty acids. Medium-chain triglycerides (MCTs) can be absorbed from the stomach and small intestine directly into the portal vein, thus bypassing the steps needed for absorption of triglyceride containing long-chain fatty acids. For this reason, formulas prepared for premature infants contain 13% to 50% of the fat blend as medium-chain triglycerides. The use of these formulas has resulted in coefficients of fat absorption in excess of 85% in premature infants.

**EXERCISE 4** *Protein Fat and Carbohydrate Requirements in Preterm Infants*

■ **Questions:**

Each of these questions is followed by four statements. Identify which of these statements is/are correct. (Note that more than one answer may be correct.)

1. In the selection of a formula for premature infants, it is important to pick one with a lactalbumin : casein ratio of 60 : 40 because that kind of ratio has been shown to do which of the following?
   (a) Improve weight gain
   (b) Cause fewer metabolic complications
   (c) Meet special amino acid requirements
   (d) Reduce the osmolality of the feeding

2. A major portion of the lactose that is malabsorbed by the small intestine of premature infants undergoes which of the following?
   (a) Complete excretion in diarrheal stools
   (b) Partial excretion in liquid stools containing a high pH
   (c) Colonic salvage by bacterial flora
   (d) Partial excretion with calcium soaps

3. Formulas designed for premature infants contain 13% to 50% of the fat blend as MCTs. The rationale for adding MCTs includes which of the following?
   (a) Fat absorptive mechanisms are diminished until 36 to 37 weeks' gestation.
   (b) Medium-chain fats can be absorbed directly from the stomach and small intestine into the portal vein.
   (c) Medium-chain triglycerides decrease the incidence of metabolic acidosis.
   (d) The digestion of long-chain fatty acids requires gastric lipolysis, which is not well developed in premature infants.

■ **Answers:**

1. **b, c.** The use of proteins with a lactalbumin/casein ratio of 60 : 40 can better meet the special amino acid requirements of premature infants. This lactalbumin/casein ratio does reduce the incidence of metabolic complications, but has no effect on weight gain or the osmolality of the formula.

2. **c.** Recent studies have demonstrated the presence of an active process for the salvage of malabsorbed carbohydrates by colonic bacterial flora. The short-chain fatty acids produced by this process are absorbed and oxidized by the infant.

3. **a, b.** Medium-chain triglyceride oil is directly absorbed from the stomach and small intestine into the portal vein circulation. Medium-chain triglycerides have no effect on the incidence of metabolic acido-

sis. Gastric lipolysis is well developed in premature infants.

## Minerals Including Trace Elements

Calcium requirements for premature infants are greater than those of term infants because of a higher rate of bone growth and mineralization and relatively poor absorption of dietary calcium (29% to 72%). The interaction between calcium and other nutrients in milk is known to alter the gastrointestinal absorption of this mineral. For example, the presence of MCT oil in feedings for low birth weight infants is believed to enhance calcium absorption by improving fat absorption. Conversely, the presence of glucose polymers may decrease calcium absorption by reducing the lactose content of the formula. (Lactose has been shown to enhance the absorption of calcium and magnesium.) Based on fetal accretion rates of calcium, it has been calculated that feedings for preterm infants should contain a minimum of 132 mg of calcium per 100 kcal. Higher intakes of calcium ranging from 200 to 250 mg/kg/day may be necessary in some infants to achieve normal bone mineralization. The concentration of phosphorus in infant formulas should be lower, but not less than one-half of the calcium concentration in order to provide a calcium : phosphorus ratio ranging between 1.1 : 1 and 2 : 1 and to prevent the syndrome of hyperphosphatemia-hypocalcemia (classical neonatal tetany).

Premature infants have a higher requirement for sodium than full-term infants because of increased growth rates and impaired mechanisms for renal conservation of sodium. The sodium concentration in premature infant feedings should range between 30 and 50 mg/100 kcal. Serum electrolytes should be monitored serially in the premature infant and sodium intakes adjusted to compensate for individual variation. Hyponatremia, either asymptomatic or clinically manifested by signs of lethargy and hypotension, has been observed in premature babies receiving formula containing less than 20 mg of sodium per 100 kcal.

Premature infants are born with decreased iron stores because most iron is accumulated toward the end of pregnancy. These iron stores are consumed by 2 to 4 months after birth. For this reason, routine iron supplementation should be initiated in premature infants before age 2 months to prevent the development of iron deficiency. However, the exact age at which iron supplementation should be started has not been clearly established. A concern has been raised about providing supplemental iron to premature infants prior to the age of 2 months because iron supplementation has been shown to increase the requirements for vitamin E (by increasing the production of free radicals). Furthermore, iron supplementation might not be needed in sick premature infants who receive frequent blood transfusions containing iron as part of hemoglobin. The American Academy of Pediatrics recommends that serum vitamin E levels be closely monitored in premature infants receiving iron supplementation prior to 2 months of age (1 to 2 mg/kg/day). Two of the three infant formulas designed for preterm infants are available with and without iron fortification (Table 6-4).

Premature infants are born with lower hepatic stores of copper than full-term infants and therefore have an increased susceptibility to copper deficiency during periods of rapid growth. Despite supplementation of infant formulas with copper (60 to 90 $\mu$g/100 kcal) copper deficiency can occur in low birth weight infants with chronic diarrhea and malabsorptive syndromes. The manifestations of copper deficiency include neutropenia, hypochromic anemia (unresponsive to iron therapy), and bone abnormalities including osteoporosis, flaring of anterior ribs with pathological fractures, flaring and cupping of the long bone metaphyses, and epiphyseal separation.

All formulas designed for low birth weight infants contain the minimal recommended daily allowance of zinc (0.5 mg/100 kcal). However, zinc deficiency commonly occurs in premature infants who either have increased enteric losses of zinc (malabsorption, short bowel syndrome) or have received a prolonged course of parenteral nutrition with inadequate zinc supplementation. Zinc deficiency may rarely result from a congenital defect of zinc metabolism (acrodermatitis enteropathica). Regardless of the etiology, zinc deficiency is clinically expressed by dry skin, perioral and perianal erythematous rash, alopecia, hair discoloration, decreased resistance to infection, and growth retardation.

**Table 6-4** Composition of Feedings Recommended for Premature Infants (per 100 mL)

| | PRETERM HUMAN MILK | PRETERM HUMAN MILK AND SIMILAC NATURAL CARE | PRETERM HUMAN MILK AND ENFAMIL FORTIFIER | PREMATURE ENFAMIL | SIMILAC SPECIAL CARE | PREMIE SMA |
|---|---|---|---|---|---|---|
| Calories/30 mL | 20.5 | 22.5 | 24.8 | 24 | 24 | 24 |
| Protein (g) | 2.1 | 2.1 | 2.8 | 2.44 | 2.2 | 1.95 |
| L : C ratio | 80 : 20 | 70 : 30 | 70 : 30 | 60 : 40 | 60 : 40 | 60 : 40 |
| Fat (g) | 3.9 | 3.7 | 3.94 | 4.15 | 4.41 | 4.4 |
| % MCT | 3.8 | 3.8 | 3.8 | 40 | 50 | 14 |
| Carbohydrate (g) | 6.5 | 7.5 | 9.2 | 9.02 | 8.62 | 8.53 |
| % GL polymers | 0 | 28 | 28 | 60 | 50 | 50 |
| Vitamin A (IU) | 280 | 415 | 1080 | 975.6 | 553 | 244 |
| Vitamin D (IU) | 2.5 | 61 | 210.5 | 219.5 | 122 | 48.8 |
| Vitamin E (IU) | 0.55 | 1.7 | 3.95 | 3.74 | 3.25 | 1.54 |
| Vitamin K ($\mu$g) | 1.5 | 5.5 | 10.6 | 10.5 | 9.7 | 7.0 |
| Vitamin $B_1$ ($\mu$g) | 70 | 103 | 194 | 203.3 | 203.3 | 81.3 |
| Vitamin $B_2$ ($\mu$g) | 30 | 265 | 280 | 284.5 | 504 | 130 |
| Vitamin $B_6$ ($\mu$g) | 44 | 102 | 197.4 | 203.3 | 203.3 | 48.8 |
| Vitamin $B_{12}$ ($\mu$g) | 0.1 | 0.25 | 0.31 | 0.24 | 0.45 | 0.24 |
| Niacin (mg) | 0.16 | 2.1 | 3.26 | 3.25 | 4.1 | 0.61 |
| Folic acid ($\mu$g) | 2.6 | 16.5 | 25.6 | 28.4 | 30.1 | 10.2 |
| Pantothenic acid (mg) | 0.19 | 0.8 | 0.9 | 0.97 | 1.5 | 0.36 |
| Biotin ($\mu$g) | 0.35 | NA | 1.1 | 1.62 | 30.1 | 1.8 |
| Vitamin C (mg) | 6.0 | 18 | 30 | 28.4 | 30.1 | 7.0 |
| Choline (mg) | NA | NA | NA | 6.2 | 8.1 | 13.0 |
| Ca (mg) | 23.5 | 97 | 111 | 134 | 146.3 | 73.1 |
| P (mg) | 14.0 | 50 | 59 | 67.5 | 73 | 40.6 |
| Mg (mg) | 2.7 | 6.4 | 6.7 | 5.53 | 9.7 | 7.0 |
| Fe (mg) | 0.1 | 0.2 | 0.1 | 0.2/1.52* | 0.3/1.46* | 0.31 |
| Na (mEq) | 2.7 | 2.2 | 3.0 | 1.4 | 1.5 | 1.4 |
| K (mEq) | 1.75 | 2.3 | 2.1 | 2.3 | 2.7 | 1.9 |
| Cl (mg) | 2.15 | 2.1 | 2.5 | 69.1 | 65.8 | 53.0 |
| Mn ($\mu$g) | 0.4 | NA | 9.4 | 10.5 | 9.7 | 13.8 |

*Contained in iron fortified formulas.

### EXERCISE 5 *Mineral and Trace Element Requirements in Preterm Infants*

■ **Questions:**

Each of these questions is followed by four statements. Identify which of these statements is/are correct. (Note that more than one answer may be correct.)

1. Formulas designed for premature infants contain a calcium : phosphorus ratio ranging from 1.1 : 1 to 2 : 1. This ratio has been shown to be important in the prevention of which of the following?
   (a) Neonatal osteopenia
   (b) Bone fractures
   (c) Neonatal tetany
   (d) Neonatal hypercalcemia

2. Two of the three infant formulas designed for premature infants are available with and without iron fortification. Which of the following statement(s) best describe(s) the rationale for selecting a formula *with or without* supplemental iron?
   (a) The need for iron supplementation in premature infants is controversial.
   (b) The age of initiation of iron supplementation is controversial.
   (c) Iron supplementation may not be necessary for sick premature infants who have received multiple blood transfusions
   (d) Iron supplementation increases vitamin E requirements.

3. The concentrations of copper and zinc are increased in preterm infant formulas. Which statement(s) best describe(s) the rationale for adding supplemental copper and zinc to these preparations?
   (a) Premature infants are born with low stores of copper and zinc.
   (b) Growing premature infants have higher requirements for copper and zinc.
   (c) Premature infants exhibit decreased gastrointestinal absorption of trace elements.
   (d) Copper deficiency may result in bony abnormalities in premature infants.

■ **Answers:**

1. **c.** The calcium : phosphorus ratio is important for prevention of classical neonatal tetany (hyperphosphatemia-hypocalcemia syndrome), which has been observed with the use of formulas with a high phosphate content.

2. **b, c, d.** All premature infants should receive routine iron supplementation. Iron supplementation is generally begun before 2 months of age.

3. **a, b, c, d.** All statements are correct.

---

## Vitamins

Ascorbic acid (vitamin C) is a water-soluble vitamin that is well absorbed in the upper small intestine of premature infants. There are no large body reserves of vitamin C and excessive intakes are excreted in the urine. Ascorbic acid has several important metabolic functions including the synthesis of collagen, the conversion of folic to folinic acid, and the hydroxylation of several amino acids such as phenylalanine and tyrosine. As a result of the diminished conversion of tyrosine to homogentisic acid, preterm neonates may experience an elevation of plasma tyrosine (and phenylalanine) levels. This disorder, designated *transient neonatal tyrosinemia*, is caused by an immaturity in the tyrosine oxidizing systems. Vitamin C has been shown to increase the levels of *p*-hydroxyphenylpyruvate hydroxylase, an important enzyme in this pathway. Although most follow-up studies have shown no adverse effect on neurological outcome, the clinical significance of transient tyrosinemia remains controversial. Severe deficiency of vitamin C (scurvy) is rare in early infancy because most infant formulas provide a minimal level of vitamin C (8 mg/100 kcal).

A daily requirement of 400 IU of vitamin D is recommended for premature infants to compensate for diminished absorption of this vitamin, to enhance gastrointestinal absorption of calcium, and to promote bone growth and mineralization. Vitamin D requirements can be even higher in infants with fat malabsorption. Generalized bone demineralization is still commonly observed in premature infants, especially babies with cholestatic liver disease receiving long-term parenteral nutrition. The etiology of osteopenia in premature infants receiving parenteral nutrition has been primarily attributed to inadequate intakes of calcium and phosphorus rather than deficiency of vitamin D.

Premature infants of less than 37 weeks of gestation have diminished stores of vitamin E at birth and a decreased ability to absorb vitamin E from their gastrointestinal tracts. The syndrome of vitamin E deficiency in premature infants is characterized by the presence of hemolytic anemia, edema, and thrombocytosis. The requirements of vitamin E are further increased in infants receiving iron supplementation and in those fed formulas with a high content of polyunsaturated fatty acids. The American Academy of Pediatrics recommends that feedings for low birth weight infants contain a minimal of 1 mg of vitamin E for each gram of polyunsaturated fatty acid in the diet.

## Osmolality

The use of formulas with an osmolality that is higher than that of the infant's serum has been associated with two complications: dumping syndrome resulting from excessive mobilization of fluid into the intraluminal space, and necrotizing enterocolitis secondary to direct injury to the intestinal mucosa. Therefore, feedings for premature infants should have an osmolality similar to, or lower than, that of the infant's serum (≤300 mOsm/L).

### Caloric Density

Feedings of high caloric density (24 kcal/30 mL) are advantageous for premature infants because these infants have a small gastric capacity, prolonged gastric emptying time, and high caloric requirements. Feedings of high caloric density are also important during the transition from tube feeding to oral feedings in order to minimize the energy spent by the premature baby during nippling. Furthermore, in infants with chronic lung disease they permit fluid restriction without restriction of calories. Feedings with a caloric density higher than 24 kcal/30 mL are usually hyperosmolar and generally provide excessive amounts of electrolytes or insufficient amounts of water. Therefore, they should not be used in the premature infant, except under special circumstances.

### EXERCISE 6 *Formulas Designed for Premature Infants*

#### ■ Questions:

Each of these questions is followed by four statements. Identify which of these statements is/are correct. (Note that more than one answer may be correct.)

1. The rationale for selecting a formula with a high caloric density for premature infants includes which of the following?
   (a) Such preparations are known to decrease the gastric emptying time.
   (b) Formulas with a high caloric density help conserve energy expended during nippling.
   (c) Formulas with a high caloric density allow for fluid restriction without caloric deprivation.
   (d) Formulas with a high caloric density provide additional calories for premature infants who have smaller gastric capacities.

2. Formulas designed for premature infants have special characteristics that make them nutritionally advantageous for the preterm population. Which GP characteristics are found in these formula preparations?
   (a) Protein with a lactalbumin : casein ratio of 60 : 40
   (b) 50% of the carbohydrates in the form of glucose polymers
   (c) 13% to 50% of the fats in the form of medium-chain triglycerides
   (d) High osmolality (>300 mOsm/L)

#### ■ Answers:

1. **b, c, d.** Feedings with a high caloric density are usually hyperosmolar and therefore increase rather than decrease gastric emptying time.

2. **a, b, c.** None of the formulas designed for premature infants is hyperosmolar (>300 mOsm/L).

### HUMAN MILK FOR PREMATURE INFANTS

Human milk is considered the preferred nutritional source for premature infants because of its unique composition and the well-established immunologic, nutritional, and psychological advantages. Milk produced by the premature infant's mother is considered the most appropriate feeding for the premature infant for a number of reasons. First, preterm human milk has a higher caloric density and higher concentrations of protein, fat, and some electrolytes than mature human milk. Second, preterm human milk can be expressed and collected in a timely fashion and refrigerated until used, precluding the need for bank processing and pasteurization. Finally, premature infants fed preterm human milk demonstrate significantly faster rates of growth in weight, length, and head circumference than control infants fed mature human milk. Furthermore, balance studies performed during the first 2 to 6 weeks of life have demonstrated that the retention rates of protein, fat, sodium, and potassium in premature infants fed preterm human milk are comparable to those of fetuses with similar postconceptional ages. More recent studies, however, have shown that the requirements of calcium, phosphorus, vitamins, and trace elements might not be met in premature infants fed preterm human milk, suggesting the need to add nutritional supplements.

Mature human milk from donors (usually processed in milk banks) is not considered appropriate for the premature infant for the following reasons: (1) it contains low concentrations of protein, minerals, and trace elements; (2) there is partial inactivation of lysozyme, lactoferrin, immunoglobulins, and lipase by the pasteurization process; and (3) there is risk of HIV transmission.

The types of products proposed for supplementation of preterm human milk include mineral preparations, protein and mineral components of skimmed milk, liquid fortifier, and powdered fortifier. Of these supplements, only the liquid and the powdered fortifiers are commercially available for general use. The composition of preterm human milk derived from published data is presented in Table 6-4. The same table also displays the final composition of preterm human milk supplemented with the liquid and the powdered fortifiers.

Supplementation of human milk with fortifiers should be considered only after feedings have been initiated and well tolerated by the infant. Liquid fortifier is mixed with human milk in a 1:1 ratio. Furthermore, since the liquid fortifier makes up 50% or more of the feeding volume, its use is suitable only when the mother's milk supply is diminished. The powdered supplement is indicated when the mother's milk supply is ample. When the powdered supplement is begun, it should be added to the mother's milk in a ratio of two packets per 100 mL of milk. If the feedings are well tolerated, this ratio should be increased to four packets per 100 mL of milk.

### EXERCISE 7   *Human Milk Feedings for Preterm Infants*

■ **Questions:**

Each of these questions is followed by four statements. Identify which of these statements is/are correct. (Note that more than one answer may be correct.)

1. Which of the following nutritional characteristics makes mature human milk *not* suitable for the premature infant?
   (a) Lower protein concentration
   (b) Lower caloric density
   (c) Excessive quantities of sodium
   (d) Lower concentration of IgA

2. Which of the following statements best describes the compositional differences between mature and preterm human milk?
   (a) There is a greater concentration of protein, energy, and electrolytes in preterm human milk.
   (b) There is a greater concentration of protein, vitamins, and trace elements in mature human milk.
   (c) There is a greater concentration of protein, fat, and carbohydrate in preterm human milk.
   (d) There is a greater concentration of energy, vitamins, and IgA in mature human milk.

■ **Answers:**

1. **a, b.**   In comparison with preterm human milk, mature human milk has a lower protein content and caloric density. It also has a *lower* concentration of sodium. The concentration of IgA is identical in preterm and mature human milk.

2. **a.**   This is the only correct statement. The concentration of minerals and vitamins is comparable in preterm and mature human milk.

---

## NUTRITIONAL SUPPLEMENTS

This section provides guidelines for the use of various supplements that are commonly added to the feeding regimen of premature infants.

### Multivitamins

While supplementation with multivitamins is generally considered unnecessary in full-term infants receiving formula, multivitamin preparations are commonly given to premature infants. The rationale for vitamin supplementation in premature infants is that the daily volume of feeding ingested by the premature infant may be insufficient to meet the recommended dietary allowance (RDA) for all vitamins. Therefore, the need for supplementation of vitamins in premature infants can be determined by knowing the vitamin concentration in the various types of feedings and the total

**Table 6-5** Vitamin Supplementation for Premature Infants

|  | SUPPLEMENT MULTIVITAMINS (1 mL/day) WHEN INTAKE IS LESS THAN | SUPPLEMENT FOLIC ACID (50 mcg/day) WHEN INTAKE IS LESS THAN |
|---|---|---|
| Similac Special Care | 330 mL/day | 170 mL/day |
| Premature Enfamil | 151 mL/day | 179 mL/day |
| Premie SMA | 780 mL/day | 500 mL/day |
| Human milk with Natural Care | 656 mL/day | 312 mL/day |
| Human milk with Enfamil Fortifier | 153 mL/day | 192 mL/day |

volume of the feeding ingested daily by the premature baby. Table 6-5 displays the minimal volume of the various feedings that provides the RDA for all vitamins in premature infants. Folic acid (50 $\mu$g/day) may need to be supplemented separately because it is not present in standard multivitamin preparations. Furthermore, daily intakes higher than 50 mcg/day may be necessary for premature infants with hemolytic anemia or chronic diarrhea.

Most vitamin preparations appropriate for enteral use contain sucrose and are hyperosmolar. It is therefore recommended that the total daily dose of these preparations be divided into several doses and administered with multiple feedings to improve feeding tolerance.

**Vitamin E**

Vitamin E is present in multivitamin preparations and in all premature infant formulas at concentrations greater than those found in full-term infant formulas. Because the intestinal absorption of this vitamin is quite variable, it is recommended that serum vitamin E levels be monitored in all premature infants receiving enteral feedings. Premature infants with serum vitamin E levels lower than 1 mg/dL (normal values range from 1 to 3 mg/dL) should receive an additional 25 to 50 IU/day in a water-soluble preparation. Higher intakes might be necessary for the maintenance of serum vitamin E levels in infants with intestinal malabsorption and cholestatic liver disease and in those receiving iron supplementation.

**Iron**

Premature infants are born with low hepatic stores of iron and are at risk of developing iron deficiency anemia if iron supplementation is not initiated by 2 months of age. Iron supplements can be provided as medicinal iron at a daily dose of 2 to 3 mg/kg/day or in a premature infant formula fortified with iron. Iron supplementation can be started as early as 2 to 6 weeks of age. However, it is recommended that infants who receive early iron fortification also receive an adequate intake of vitamin E to maintain serum levels within the normal range. Premature infants who are receiving multiple blood transfusions do not require iron supplementation.

**Energy Supplements**

It is common practice in many nurseries to augment the caloric density of feedings by adding MCT oil, emulsified long-chain triglycerides (Microlipid), or glucose polymers (Polycose). The caloric densities of these products are presented in Table 6-6. There are, however, two major disadvantages of such supplements: (1) An excessive use of these supplements will result in an unbalanced ratio between the total energy intake and the intake of protein and all other nutrients necessary for growth, and (2) use of these supplements will significantly increase the osmolality of feedings. A more suitable alternative to promote

**Table 6-6** Energy Supplements for Premature Infants

|  | WEIGHT/ VOLUME | CALORIC DENSITY |
|---|---|---|
| Glucose polymers (polycose powder) | 1 g | 3.8 kcal |
| MCT oil | 1 g (1.1 mL) | 8.3 kcal |
| Microlipid | 1 mL | 4.5 kcal |

growth in premature infants is either to increase the total volume of the feeding or to concentrate the formula. Both alternatives are preferred because neither alters the ratio between energy and nutrients.

### EXERCISE 8 *Nutritional Supplements for Preterm Infants*

■ **Questions:**

Select the *one best answer* to each of the following questions concerning the use of nutritional supplements for premature infants.

1. Select the most appropriate nutritional supplement for a 10-day-old, 1,300-g premature infant receiving 25 mL of Special Care formula with iron every 3 hours (total feeding volume = 200 mL/day) in whom the serum vitamin E level is 2.5 mg/dL?
   (a) Multivitamin preparation and vitamin E
   (b) Multivitamin preparation and folic acid
   (c) Multivitamin preparation and iron
   (d) Multivitamin preparation only
2. Premature infants should routinely receive additional vitamin E with their feedings if which of the following exist(s)?
   (a) They are exclusively fed mature human milk.
   (b) They are receiving a formula containing iron.
   (c) The serum vitamin E level is less than 1 mg/dL.
   (d) There is delayed initiation of enteral feedings.
3. Which of the following nutritional interventions is most appropriate to promote weight gain in a 3-week-old, 1,800-g premature infant receiving preterm human milk at volumes of 40 mL every 3 hours?
   (a) Add liquid or powdered fortifier to the feeding.
   (b) Increase the volume of the feeding to 45 mL every 3 hours.
   (c) Add MCT or Polycose to the feeding.
   (d) Change human milk to infant formula feeding.

■ **Answers:**

1. **b.** 200 mL of Special Care formula will not meet the RDA for most vitamins (at least 330 mL is required). Folic acid is not present in standard multivitamin preparations.

2. **b, c.** Serum levels of vitamin E of <1 mg/dL are considered low. It is controversial whether additional vitamin E should be given to infants receiving iron-fortified formulas. At Children's Hospital of Philadelphia, we administer supplemental vitamin E only if serum levels are low.

3. **a.** Adding liquid or powdered fortifier is the correct choice because it maintains human milk feedings while enhancing nutrient and caloric intake. Although the volume of each feeding might be increased, this infant is already receiving 170 cc/kg/day. Adding MCT oil or Polycose would result in an unbalanced ratio between total energy intake and the intake of protein and all other nutrients necessary for growth.

## PARENTERAL NUTRITION

Total parenteral nutrition (TPN) is indicated for neonates in whom enteral feedings are insufficient or contraindicated for prolonged periods of time. The length of time that a neonate can tolerate starvation depends on the nutritional status at the time enteral feedings are discontinued, coexisting clinical conditions, and the degree of prematurity. Neonates who are malnourished or are small-for-gestational-age, those who are hypermetabolic (sepsis/surgery), and those who are extremely premature should be routinely started on parenteral nutrition if enteral feedings are being withheld or provided in insufficient amounts.

### Mode of Delivery

Parenteral nutrition solutions can be provided by either peripheral or central vein catheters. Peripheral vein catheters are used in patients who have adequate venous access and who are expected to require parenteral nutrition for relatively short periods of time (1 to 2 weeks). TPN delivered by peripheral vein can provide up to 80 to 90 kcal/kg/day when 10% dextrose is used with intravenous fat emulsions. Solutions containing dextrose concentrations in excess of 10% should not be administered by peripheral vein because of the increased risk of phlebitis and skin injury. If the infant has poor venous access, or requires fluid restriction,

TPN for longer than 2 weeks, or energy intakes greater than that provided by peripheral vein, a central venous catheter should be electively placed for nutritional support. Although the risk of serious infection increases with the use of central catheters, aseptic techniques can reduce the incidence of infection to 2% to 5%.

### Composition

The composition of standard TPN solutions developed for use in neonates is presented in Table 6-7.

*Energy:* During parenteral nutrition, energy requirements are lower than those needed with enteral nutrition because energy is neither lost in stools nor required for absorption of nutrients by the gastrointestinal tract. Recommended energy intakes during parenteral nutrition range between 90 and 100 kcal/kg/day for full-term infants and between 90 and 110 kcal/kg/day for premature infants. The nonprotein caloric contribution to the total

**Table 6-7**  Composition of Standard TPN Solutions per 100 mL

|  | PRETERM | FULL TERM |
|---|---|---|
| Amino acid* | 1.5/2.0/2.5/3.0† | 1.5/2.0/2.5/3.0† |
| Dextrose* | 10/15/20 | 10/15/20 |
| Na (mEq) | 4 | 4 |
| K (mEq) | 2 | 2 |
| Cl (mEq) | 4.6 | 4.6 |
| Ca (mg) | 600 | 400 |
| Phos (mEq) | 1.4 | 1.4 |
| Mg (mEq) | 0.4 | 0.4 |
| Zn (mcg) | 500 | 300 |
| Cu (mcg) | 60 | 20 |
| Cr (mcg) | 0.17 | 0.17 |
| Mn (mcg) | 5 | 5 |
| Se (mcg) | 3 | 3 |
| I (mcg) | 8 | 8 |
| Fe (mg)‡ | 0.1 | 0.1 |
| Heparin (U)§ | 50 | 100 |

* Available standard amino acid and dextrose concentrations (g/100 mL).
† Trophamine or Aminosyn PF.
‡ Iron is added for all infants, including premature infants, after 8 weeks of life.
§ See text for discussion of heparin dose.

calorie intake is usually equally distributed between dextrose and fat emulsions. Calories derived from fat emulsions should generally not exceed more than 50% of the total calorie intake.

*Amino Acids:*  Table 6-8 displays the calorie concentration of various amino acid/dextrose solutions used for TPN in neonates. Recommended intakes of intravenous amino acids vary somewhat with the gestational age of the infant. Full-term infants require 2.5 to 3 g/kg/day and preterm infants require 3.0 to 3.5 g/kg/day. There are two pediatric amino acid formulations, designed for newborn infants, that use as a standard the postprandial plasma amino acid levels of breast-fed neonates. In comparison to others, these preparations have an increased ratio of essential to nonessential amino acids and an increased concentration of amino acids considered essential for premature infants, such as taurine, tyrosine, and cysteine. These amino acid preparations are recommended for infants up to the age of 6 months. The oxidation of 1 g of amino acid provides 4 kcal.

*Dextrose:*  Carbohydrates represent the major metabolic energy source during parenteral nutrition and should provide 35% to 55% of the total caloric needs. Fructose, sorbitol, and ethanol have all been suggested as alternative substrates in neonates receiving parenteral nutrition, but their use offers no clinical advantage over the use of dextrose, which remains the carbohydrate of first choice for parenteral nutrition. While dextrose concentrations in excess of 10% should not be infused through peripheral vein catheters, dextrose concentrations ranging from 20% to 30% can be safely infused through central vein

**Table 6-8**  Energy Content of Mixed Dextrose/Amino Acid Solutions* for TPN in Neonates (kcal/mL)

|  | AMINO ACID CONCENTRATION | | | |
|---|---|---|---|---|
|  | 1.5% | 2.0% | 2.5% | 3.0% |
| D10% | 0.40 | 0.42 | 0.44 | 0.46 |
| D15% | 0.56 | 0.59 | 0.61 | 0.63 |
| D20% | 0.74 | 0.76 | 0.78 | 0.80 |

* Amino acid and dextrose concentrations as g/100 mL.

**Table 6-9** Schedule for Advancement of Dextrose Solutions*

| | |
|---|---|
| ***Peripheral line TPN:***---------------------------- | (TPN panel, electrolytes) |
| Day 1 | D10W, protein as required, 2 g/kg/day fat emulsion. |
| | Check serum electrolytes, Glu, BUN, Cr, TG after 24 hours. |
| Day 2 | Increase fat emulsion to 3 g/kg/day. |
| | Check serum TG approximately 24 hours after increase in dose. |
| ***Central line TPN:***---------------------------- | (Document line placement, TPN panel, electrolytes) |
| Day 1 | D10W, protein as required, 2 g/kg/day fat emulsion. |
| | Check serum electrolytes, Glu, BUN, Cr, TG after 24 hours. |
| | If the patient was on a standard peripheral TPN solution (D10W) prior to placement of central line, the solution may be changed to D15W or D20W after line placement is confirmed. |
| | Check serum electrolytes, Glu, BUN, Cr, TG after 24 hours. |
| Day 2† | Increase to a D20W solution and increase fat emulsion to 3 g/kg/day, if additional calories are needed. |
| | Check serum electrolytes, Glu, BUN, Cr, TG after 24 hours. |

* Glu = glucose, BUN = blood urea nitrogen, Cr = creatinine, TG = triglycerides.
† For premature infants, use D15W on day 2 and D20W on day 3.

catheters. The oxidation of 1 g of dextrose yields 3.4 kcal. A schedule for the advancement of dextrose solutions in patients receiving parenteral nutrition by peripheral and central vein catheters is presented in Table 6-9.

***Fat Emulsions:*** Along with amino acids and dextrose, fats are an essential component of the TPN regimen. There are at least three major advantages to administering fats intravenously: They are the only source of essential fatty acids for infants not receiving enteral feeds, they have a high caloric density (1 g = 11 kcal), and they have a low osmolality, which makes them suitable for peripheral vein use. Despite the great number of fat emulsions currently available, they are all derived from either soybean or safflower oil. Both types of fat emulsions have been shown to be comparably effective in correcting essential fatty acid deficiency and in sparing nitrogen catabolism in neonates. While the safflower and the soybean oil emulsions both contain ample amounts of linoleic acids (75% and 50%, respectively), the concentration of linolenic acid is lower in the safflower oil emulsion than in the soybean oil emulsion (0.5% versus 9%, respectively). Furthermore, it has recently been suggested that linolenic acid is an essential fatty acid in children receiving parenteral nutrition. For that reason, it seems prudent to use soybean fat emulsions in neonates until further studies determine that minimal re-

quirements can be met with the use of safflower emulsions. Fat emulsions are available at concentrations of 10% and 20%.

***Minerals and Vitamins:*** Suggested daily intakes of minerals and vitamins are presented in Table 6-10. Higher levels of some minerals (Na, Ca, P, Zn, and Cu) are recommended for premature infants. It should be emphasized,

**Table 6-10** Intravenous Electrolyte and Mineral Requirements

| | |
|---|---|
| Sodium | 2–4 mEq/kg/day |
| Potassium | 2–4 mEq/kg/day |
| Chloride | 2–3 mEq/kg/day |
| Magnesium | 0.25–0.5 mEq/kg/day |
| Calcium | 10–40 mg/kg/day |
| Phosphorus | 0.4–0.8 mM/kg/day |
| Zinc | |
| ≤2.5 kg | 500 mcg/kg/day |
| >2.5 kg | 300 mcg/kg/day |
| Copper | |
| ≤2.5 kg | 60 mcg/kg/day |
| >2.5 kg | 20 mcg/kg/day |
| Chromium | 0.14–0.2 mcg/kg/day |
| Manganese | 2–10 mcg/kg/day |
| Selenium | 3 mcg/kg/day |
| Iodine | 5 mcg/kg/day |
| Iron | 0.1 mg–0.2 mg/kg/day |

however, that intakes of calcium and phosphorus greater than can be safely delivered in TPN solutions are necessary to promote bone mineralization in premature infants. Osteopenia, therefore, remains a nonpreventable complication in neonates dependent on long-term parenteral nutrition. Table 6-11 displays the daily requirements for vitamins administered intravenously to children. As shown in this table, 5 mL of MVI pediatric preparation (added to the hyperalimentation solution) will meet these requirements for children younger than 11 years of age.

***Heparin:*** Heparin should be provided in standard TPN solutions delivered by central vein catheters at concentrations of 1 unit/mL to maintain line patency. The presence of heparin in TPN solution leads to the detachment of endothelial lipoprotein lipases, resulting in faster lipolysis and increased release of free fatty acid. Heparin is provided at a lower dose (0.5 units/1 mL) in TPN solutions used for premature infants to prevent competition of free fatty acids and bilirubin for albumin binding sites.

**Table 6-11** Intravenous Vitamin Recommendations and Vitamin Concentrations in MVI Pediatric Preparation

| vitamin | CHILDREN <11 yr | MVI Ped (per 5 mL) |
|---|---|---|
| A (retinol) (IU) | 2,000–3,000 | 2,300 |
| D (IU) | 400 | 400 |
| E (α-tocopherol) (IU) | 7–10 | 7 |
| Ascorbic acid (mg) | 40 | 80 |
| Folate (mcg) | 100–300 | 140 |
| Niacin (mg) | 9–16 | 17 |
| Riboflavin (mg) | 0.8–1.2 | 1.4 |
| Thiamine (mg) | 0.7–1.3 | 1.2 |
| B$_6$ (mg) | 0.6–1.2 | 1.0 |
| B$_{12}$ (mg) | 1.0–2.0 | 1.0 |
| Pantothenic acid (mg) | 5.0 | 5.0 |
| Biotin (mcg) | 20 | 20 |
| K (mg) | 0.1 | 0.2 |

## EXERCISE 9  *Parenteral Nutrition*

### ■ Questions:

These questions are designed to assess your knowledge about the clinical use and composition of parenteral nutrition solutions for neonates. Select the *one best answer* to each of the following questions.

1. Baby E, a 2-kg premature infant suddenly developed feeding intolerance, abdominal distention, and bloody stools at 4 days of age. The abdominal x-ray showed mild generalized bowel dilation, but no other abnormalities. Because of the possibility of necrotizing enterocolitis, feedings were stopped and intravenous fluids and antibiotics were started.

   Which of the following parenteral nutrition regimens would you select for this infant? (Assume an infusion rate of 100 mL/kg/day, excluding fat emulsions, administered through a *peripheral vein catheter*.)
   (a) Amino acid 3%, dextrose 10%, and fat emulsion (20%, providing 2 g/kg/day)
   (b) Amino acid 2%, dextrose 12.5%, and fat emulsion (20%, providing 3 g/kg/day)
   (c) Amino acid 2.5%, dextrose 12.5%, and fat emulsion (20% providing 2 g/kg/day)
   (d) Amino acid 2%, dextrose 15%, and fat emulsion (20% providing 0.5 g/kg/day)

2. Which of the 4 TPN regimens described in Question 1 will provide Baby E with an energy intake of 83.5 kcal/kg/day?
   (a) Regimen a
   (b) Regimen b
   (c) Regimen c
   (d) Regimen d

3. On the second day of parenteral nutrition, Baby E has a serum glucose concentration of 100 mg/dL and a serum triglyceride level of 75 mg/dL. Which of the following four TPN regimens would you administer by *peripheral vein catheter* at this time? (Assume a fluid rate of 100 mL/kg/day, excluding fat emulsion.)
   (a) Amino acid 2%, dextrose 15%, and a 20% fat emulsion (providing 3 g/kg/day)
   (b) Amino acid 2.5%, dextrose 12.5%, and a 20% fat emulsion (providing 3 g/kg/day)

(c) Amino acid 3%, dextrose 10%, and a 20% fat emulsion (providing 3 g/kg/day)

(d) Amino acid 3.5%, dextrose 10%, and a 20% fat emulsion (providing 2 g/kg/day)

4. On the third day of parenteral nutrition, Baby E becomes lethargic and apneic. Marked abdominal wall redness and generalized abdominal distention are observed. The abdominal radiograph demonstrates signs of pneumatosis intestinalis and pneumoperitoneum. In the operating room 20 cm of necrosed distal ileum with two perforations is resected and a central line is placed for parenteral nutrition. Which of the following four TPN regimens would you choose to start *central vein parenteral nutrition?* (Assume a rate of fluid administration of 150 mL/kg/day, and the following laboratory values: serum glucose = 138 mg/dL; serum triglycerides = 350 mg/dL, serum albumin = 1.5 g/dL, and normal serum electrolytes.)

(a) Amino acid 3%, dextrose 15%, and 1 g/kg/day of a 20% fat emulsion

(b) Amino acid 4%, dextrose 20%, and 1 g/kg/day of a 20% fat emulsion

(c) Amino acid 3%, dextrose 25%, and 2 g/kg/day of a 20% fat emulsion

(d) Amino acid 3.5%, dextrose 10%, and 3 g/kg/day of a 20% fat emulsion

5. On the seventh day of parenteral nutrition, Baby E weighs 2.1 kg. During the preceding 3 days, Baby E received a daily energy intake of 144 kcal/kg/day and gained weight at an average rate of 35 g/day. Which of the following four parenteral nutrition regimens would you select to reduce the total energy intake to approximately 120 kcal/kg/day? (Assume the dose of intravenous fat emulsion is maintained at 2 g/kg/day.)

(a) Amino acid 3%, dextrose 20%, fluid rate = 122 mL/kg/day

(b) Amino acid 2%, dextrose 20%, fluid rate = 100 mL/kg/day

(c) Amino acid 3%, dextrose 20%, fluid rate = 150 mL/kg/day

(d) Amino acid 3%, dextrose 10%, fluid rate = 100 mL/kg/day

### ■ Answers:

1. **a.** This TPN regimen is correct because it satisfies amino acid requirements (3 g/kg/day) and maintains the dextrose concentration at 10%. It is inappropriate to infuse more than 10% dextrose through a peripheral vein.

2. **b.** Regimen "b" provides 8 kcal/kg from amino acids, 42.5 kcal/kg from dextrose, and 33 kcal/kg from fat. Total: 8 + 42.5 + 33 = 83.5 kcal/kg.

3. **c.** Regimen "c" is correct because it satisfies amino acid requirements (3 g/kg/day), maintains dextrose at a 10% concentration, and enhances the intake of fat emulsion (serum triglycerides are normal).

4. **a.** Regimen "a" provides increased quantities of amino acids (4.5 g/kg/day, which is appropriate given the low serum albumin concentration), an increased dextrose concentration (15% dextrose, the serum glucose concentration is normal), and a limited dose of fat emulsion (serum triglycerides are slightly elevated).

5. **a.** Regimen a provides 119.6 kcal/kg/day, which should permit acceptable growth.

### Monitoring

Prior to the initiation of TPN, the physician should perform an assessment of the infant's nutritional status and growth parameters and obtain baseline laboratory chemical values. This so-called TPN panel includes serum electrolytes (sodium, potassium, chloride, carbon dioxide, magnesium, calcium, and phosphorus), serum total protein, albumin, blood urea nitrogen, creatinine, triglycerides, and liver function studies. A 2-day advancement in the TPN regimen is recommended for most patients to maximize nutritional rehabilitation. A schedule for advancement and initial monitoring of peripheral and central parenteral nutrition solutions is summarized in Table 6-9.

The following parameters should be routinely monitored during TPN:

- Strict daily measurements of intake and output, urine specific gravity, and dipstick determinations for urine glucose should be obtained each shift by the patient's nurse. Serum glucose test strip determinations should be obtained whenever glycosuria is detected.

- Daily weight determinations and weekly measurements of length and head circumference should be obtained and plotted on available growth charts for neonates.
- The TPN panel should be repeated daily while the parenteral nutrition regimen is being advanced and weekly thereafter. Additional biochemical tests may need to be obtained when specific nutritional deficiencies are suspected (such as zinc, copper, selenium, vitamins).
- Central line dressings should be changed at least twice a week under aseptic conditions by trained personnel. The catheter site should be inspected for signs of swelling, redness, or discharge. If a discharge is present, the material should be sent for a Gram's stain and culture. An antiseptic solution (e.g., Betadine) should be applied to the catheter site prior to replacement of the dressing.
- Sepsis is a constant threat in all infants receiving TPN through a central vein. In babies with suspected sepsis, blood cultures should be obtained from the central line and from a peripheral vein. Central lines inserted to administer parenteral nutrition should be used solely for the delivery of these solutions to minimize the risk of infection.
- To prevent hypertriglyceridemia, lipid emulsions should be administered for prolonged times (preferably 24 hours). When serum triglyceride levels exceed 500 mg/dL, lipid emulsions should be discontinued and the level repeated 24 hours later. If the triglyceride level is still elevated, other causes of hypertriglyceridemia should be investigated. Concerns regarding the adverse effect of fat emulsions on platelet number and host defenses are not thought to be clinically significant when currently available formulations are used at recommended doses and rates of administration.

## COMPLICATIONS OF PARENTERAL NUTRITION

Complications of parenteral nutrition can be classified into three categories: those related to metabolic derangements, those related to method of delivery, and those related to infection.

### Metabolic Complications

These complications are identified by the routine biochemical monitoring of patients receiving parenteral nutrition solutions. The most common metabolic complications of parenteral nutrition in neonates include the following.

*Hypoglycemia:* This complication may occur when TPN solutions are discontinued abruptly and can be prevented or treated by immediate reinitiation of intravenous fluid solutions with appropriate concentrations of dextrose.

*Hyperglycemia:* This complication is relatively common in preterm infants and in patients with proven sepsis. When hyperglycemia occurs, it is treated either by decreasing the dextrose concentration, decreasing the rate of dextrose infusion, or administering insulin along with the TPN solution.

*Cholestatic Jaundice:* This is a common complication related to long-term administration of parenteral nutrition in neonates. It is especially common in premature infants. Cholestasis is usually observed after the second week of parenteral nutrition and is characterized by an elevation of total and direct serum bilirubin values (>2 mg/dL for both fractions). Factors associated with cholestasis include lack of enteral feedings (which decreases bile flow, alters bowel flora, decreases the bile pool size, and increases the ratio of lithocholic to taurocholic acid), direct liver toxicity from the amino acid solution, direct liver toxicity from the hypertonic dextrose concentrations, bacterial sepsis associated with the use of central lines, and production of hepatotoxic bile acids. While the majority of patients affected by this complication exhibit transient elevations of conjugated bilirubin and liver enzymes, some infants (in whom parenteral nutrition cannot be discontinued) develop progressive liver disease leading to cirrhosis. Should liver function studies deteriorate, one should attempt to advance enteral feeding and discontinue the parenteral alimentation solution. If parenteral nutrition cannot be discontinued, the dextrose and protein concentrations in the hyperalimentation fluid should be decreased to levels that satisfy minimum requirements.

*Hyperammonemia:* This complication is rarely a problem with current crystalline parenteral amino acid solutions, but it should be investigated in neonates who unexpectedly become lethargic or comatose.

*Metabolic Acidosis:* Acidosis is frequently observed in premature infants receiving amino acid solutions. Premature infants are predisposed to this complication because of impaired renal acidification mechanisms. The severity of the metabolic acidosis is related to the daily intake of amino acids, the degree of prematurity, and the postnatal age of the infant. Thus metabolic acidosis may be corrected or prevented by the addition of sodium acetate to the TPN solution.

*Osteopenia:* This complication is usually seen in premature neonates who require parenteral nutrition solutions for prolonged periods of time. Osteopenia is believed secondary to the inability of TPN solutions to deliver the amounts of calcium and phosphorus required for proper mineralization of the skeleton in growing premature infants. The administration of vitamin D intravenously does not prevent the occurrence of osteopenia in patients receiving parenteral nutrition.

*Hyperlipemia:* This term, signifying abnormally high serum concentrations of triglycerides, free fatty acids, or cholesterol, results from the infant's inability to metabolize infused fats. Serial determinations of serum triglycerides are commonly used to monitor lipid infusions during parenteral nutrition. Fasting serum triglyceride levels in excess of 250 mg/dL and a serum triglyceride level in excess of 500 mg/dL during lipid infusions indicate significant hyperlipemia and mandate a reduction in the lipid dose or a temporary discontinuation of lipid from the TPN regimen.

*Alterations in Pulmonary Function:* This complication has been observed in premature infants with respiratory distress syndrome during the first week of life and in older infants with diffuse pulmonary disease who received lipid emulsions over short periods of time (4–6 h). The administration of fat emulsions should be temporarily discontinued in patients who exhibit a deterioration of pulmonary function (as evidenced by a change in oxygenation) during the administration of fat

emulsions. Fortunately, this complication is rarely seen anymore because of the current practice of administering lipid emulsions over prolonged infusion periods (15–24 h).

*Bilirubin Displacement:* An elevation in the serum concentration of free fatty acids results from the hydrolysis of infused fat emulsions. In jaundiced infants, elevated levels of free fatty acids may compete with bilirubin for albumin binding and therefore increase the risk of kernicterus by increasing the serum level of free bilirubin. In jaundiced premature infants <30 weeks' gestation who require phototherapy, the maximal rate of fat infusion should be 1 g/kg/day; jaundiced premature infants >30 weeks' gestation can receive up to 2 g/kg day. If an infant requires an exchange transfusion for the treatment of hyperbilirubinemia, the fat infusion should be discontinued.

## Complications Resulting from the Method of TPN Delivery

These complications are usually associated with placement or use of central vein catheters for the delivery of TPN solutions. The incidence of central vein catheter complications ranges from 4% to 9.2%. Common complications include pneumothorax, pneumomediastinum, arterial puncture, hemorrhage, arrythmias, superior vena cava syndrome, chylothorax, and pericardial tamponade. Broken catheters at the site of connection with the plastic TPN tubing are frequently noted in patients who require placement of a Broviac catheter for long-term parenteral nutrition. Patients receiving parenteral nutrition by peripheral vein catheters are at risk of skin slough in the event of accidental infiltration of TPN solutions. Therefore, the dextrose concentration in TPN solutions administered by peripheral vein catheters should not exceed 10%.

## Infectious Complications

The reported incidence of sepsis in neonates receiving parenteral nutrition varies from 21% to 45%; however, in recent years the incidence of sepsis has plummeted (to the 2% to 5% range) because of the broader acceptance of aseptic techniques. Predisposing factors for the development of sepsis in neonates receiving parenteral nutrition include the adverse effects of prematurity and or malnutrition on the immune system and the contamination of the central catheter by skin pathogens at the insertion site. In addition, both parenteral nutrition solutions and fat emulsions can easily become contaminated during the process of preparation because they are known to support the growth of staphylococcal and candidal species as well as other gram-negative organisms. The most common organisms causing sepsis in patients receiving parenteral nutrition include coagulase positive and negative *Staphylococcus, Streptococcus viridans, Escherichia coli, Pseudomonas sp, Klebsiella sp,* and *Candida albicans.* Aseptic preparation of infusates by trained pharmacists working under laminar-flow hoods is known to minimize the preadministration risk of contamination of parenteral nutrition solutions. Furthermore, the risk of infection can be decreased further if the central vein catheter is not used for the administration of blood products or medications, blood sampling, and monitoring of central venous pressure. Sepsis must be ruled out in any patient receiving TPN by a central vein catheter who develops fever or other signs compatible with infection. When sepsis is suspected, blood cultures should be obtained from the central line and peripheral vein catheters. The central vein catheter should be removed in patients with catheter-related sepsis only if blood cultures remain positive after 48 hours of appropriate antibiotic therapy administered through the central line.

### EXERCISE 10  *Complications of TPN and Monitoring Infants Receiving TPN*

■ **Questions:**

These questions are designed to assess your knowledge of the kinds of monitoring required for infants receiving TPN and the complications associated with its use. (Note that more than one answer may be correct.)

1. Which of these complications have been associated with the prolonged use of parenteral nutrition?
   (a) Increased serum unconjugated bilirubin
   (b) Candidiasis
   (c) Osteopenia
   (d) Vitamin D deficiency
2. Routine clinical and laboratory monitoring of neonates during the first week of

parenteral nutrition therapy should include which of the following measurements?
   (a) Daily weight
   (b) Fluid intake and output
   (c) Daily blood glucose
   (d) Daily urinary specific gravity
3. Which one of the following complications of TPN is *not* associated with the use of fat emulsions in premature infants?
   (a) Bilirubin displacement
   (b) Hypertriglyceridemia
   (c) Cholestatic jaundice
   (d) Impaired respiratory function
4. A 1,200-g infant receiving TPN through a central vein catheter develops catheter-related sepsis with *S. epidermidis.* How should this infant be managed?
   (a) Parenteral nutrition should be continued.
   (b) Initiate antibiotic therapy through the central catheter.
   (c) Remove the central catheter.
   (d) Initiate antibiotic therapy through a peripheral venous line.

■ **Answers:**

1. **a, b, c.** Vitamin D deficiency should not occur in infants receiving TPN because the multivitamin preparations contain ample amounts of vitamin D.

2. **a, b, d.** Blood glucose levels should not be measured on a daily basis, except when glycosuria occurs or when glucose test strip values are elevated.

3. **c.** The use of intravenous fat emulsions is not thought to cause cholestatic jaundice.

4. **a, b.** *S. epidermidis* sepsis can usually be treated successfully by administering antibiotics through the central line. The central line should not be removed.

### BIBLIOGRAPHY

**Breastfeeding**

1. American Academy of Pediatrics, Committee on Nutrition: Breastfeeding. *Pediatrics* 1978; 62:591.
2. Lawrence RA: Management of the mother-infant nursing couple. In Lawrence R, ed: *Breastfeeding: A Guide for the Medical Profession.* St. Louis, CV Mosby Co, 1980, p. 109.
3. Lozoff B, Brittenham GM, Trause MA, et al: The mother newborn relationship: Limits of adaptability. *J Pediatr* 1977; 91:1.

4. Hayes K, Danks DM, Gibas H, et al: Cytomegalovirus in human milk. *N Engl J Med* 1972; 287:177.

5. Linnemann C, Goldberg S: Hepatitis B antigen in breast milk. *Lancet* 1974; 2:155.

6. Boxall EH, Flewett TH, Dane DS, et al: Hepatitis B surface antigen in breast milk. *Lancet* 1974; 2:1997.

7. Lawrence RA: Medical complications of the mother. In Lawrence R, ed: *Breastfeeding: A Guide for the Medical Profession*. St. Louis, CV Mosby Co, 1980, p. 221.

8. Lawrence RA: Appendix F: Drugs in breast milk and the effect on the infant. In Lawrence R, ed: *Breastfeeding: A Guide for the Medical Profession*. St. Louis, CV Mosby Co, 1980, p. 315.

9. National Center for Health Sciences: NCHS growth charts—1976. *Monthly Vital Statistics Report*. 1976; 25(3)suppl(HRA):76–120.

10. Saarinen UM, Siimes MA: Iron absorption from breast milk, cow's milk and iron supplemented formula. An opportunistic use of changes in total body iron determined by hemoglobin ferritin and body weight in 132 infants. *Pediatr Res* 1979; 13:143.

11. Woodruff CW: The science of infant nutrition and the art of infant feeding. *JAMA* 1978; 240:657.

12. American Academy of Pediatrics, Committee on Nutrition: Fluoride supplementation: Revised dosage schedule. In Forbes GB, ed: *Pediatric Nutrition Handbook*. Evanston, IL, American Academy of Pediatrics, 1979, p. 373.

13. Gartner LM, Lee KS: Jaundice and liver disease. In Behrman BE, ed: *Neonatal-Perinatal Medicine*. St. Louis, CV Mosby Co, 1977, p. 294.

14. Maisels MJ, Gifford K: Neonatal jaundice and breastfeeding. *Pediatr Res* 1975; 9:308.

15. Gartner LM, Arian I: Studies of prolonged neonatal jaundice in the breast fed infant. *J Pediatr* 1966; 68:54.

16. Bevan BR, Holten JB: Inhibition of bilirubin conjugation in rat liver slices by free fatty acids, with relevance to the problem of breast-milk jaundice. *Clin Chim Acta* 1972; 41:101.

17. Cole AP, Hargreaves T: Conjugation inhibitors in early neonatal hyperbilirubinemia. *Arch Dis Child* 1972; 47:451.

18. Hargreaves T: Effect of fatty acids on bilirubin conjugation. *Arch Dis Child* 1973; 48:446.

19. Foloit TA, Ploussard JP, Housset E, et al: Breast milk jaundice: In vitro inhibition of rat liver bilirubinuridine diphosphate glucuronyl transferase activity and Z proteinbromosulfophthalein binding by human breast milk. *Pediatr Res* 1976; 10:594.

20. Poland RL, Schultz GE, Garg G: High milk lipase activity associated with breast milk jaundice. *Pediatr Res* 1980; 14:1328.

**Formula Feeding**

21. Fanaroff A, Klaus M: The gastrointestinal tract. Feeding and selected disorders. In Klaus M and Famaroff A, eds: *Care of the High Risk Neonate*. Philadelphia, WB Saunders Co, 1979, p. 113.

22. Desmond M, Rudolph A: Progressive evaluation of the newborn. *Postgrad Med* 1965; 37:207.

23. Desmond M, Franklin R, Vallabona C, et al: Clinical behavior of the newly born. I. The term baby. *J Pediatr* 1965; 62:307.

24. Olson M: Effects of water, 5% glucose or milk on rabbit lungs. *Pediatrics* 1970; 46:538.

25. Engle WD, Baumgart S, Schwartz JC, et al: Combined effect of radiant warmer and phototherapy on insensible weight loss in the critically ill infant. *Am J Dis Child* 1981; 135:516.

26. Oh W, Karecki H: Phototherapy and insensible water loss in the newborn infant. *Am J Dis Child* 1972; 124:230.

27. Wu PYC, Moosa A: Effect of phototherapy on nitrogen and electrolyte levels and water balance in jaundiced full term infants. *Pediatrics* 1978; 6:193.

28. Bakken AF: Temporary intestinal lactase deficiency in light treated jaundiced infants. *Acta Pediatr Scand* 1977; 66:91.

29. Oski FA, Pearson HA: Iron nutrition revisited. In Oski FA and Pearson HA, eds: *Report of the 82nd Ross Conference on Pediatric Research*. Columbus, OH, Ross Laboratories, 1981, p. 1.

30. American Academy of Pediatrics, Committee on Nutrition: Iron supplementation for infants. *Pediatrics* 1976; 58:765.

31. Sandstead HH, Burk RF, Booth EH Jr, et al: Current concepts on trace minerals. *Med Clin North Am* 1970; 54:1509.

32. McMillan JA, Landau SA, Oski FA: Iron sufficiency in breast fed infants and the availability of iron from human milk. *Pediatrics* 1976; 58:686.

33. Saarinen VM, Siimes MA, Dallmann PR: Iron absorption in infants. High bioavailability of breast milk iron as indicated by the extrinsic tag method of iron absorption and by the concentration of serum ferritin. *J Pediatr* 1977; 91:36.

34. Sarrinen VM: Need for iron supplementation in infants on prolonged breastfeeding. *J Pediatr* 1978; 93:177.

35. Forman SJ, Filer LJ Jr, Anderson TA, et al: Recommendation for feeding normal infants. *Pediatrics* 1979; 63:52.

36. Glaser J, Johnstone DE: Soy bean milk as a substitute for mammalian milk in early infancy, with special reference to prevention of allergy to cow's milk. *Ann Allergy* 1952; 10:433.

37. Glaser J: The dietary prophylaxis of allergic disease in infancy. *J Asthma Res* 1966; 3:199.

38. Johnstone DE, Dutton AM: Dietary prophylaxis of allergic disease in children. *N Engl J Med* 1966; 274:715.

39. Walker WA: Antigen absorption from the small intestine and gastrointestinal disease. *Pediatr Clin North Am* 1975; 22:731.

40. Anderson AS, Purvis GA, Chopra JG: The introduction of mixed feeding in infancy. In Forbes GB, ed: *Pediatric Nutrition Handbook*. Evanston, IL, American Academy of Pediatrics, Committee on Nutrition, 1979, p. 139.

41. Husband J, Husband P, Mallison CN: Gastric emptying of starch meals in the newborn. *Lancet* 1970; 2:290.

42. Anderson DH: Pancreatic enzymes in the duodenal juice in the celiac syndrome. *Am J Dis Child* 1942; 63:643.

43. Beyress K: Resorption and Umsatz von Fruktose bei Neugeborenen und Sauglingen. *Acta Biol Med Germ* 1972; 29:404.

44. Auricchio S, Della Pietra D, Vegnente A: Studies on intestinal digestion of starch in man. II. Intestinal hydrolysis of amylopectin in infants and children. *Pediatrics* 1967; 39:853.

45. Beal VA: Termination of night feeding in infancy. *J Pediatr* 1969; 75:690.

46. Grunwaldt E, Bates T, Guthrie D Jr: The onset of sleeping through the night in infancy: Relation to introduction of solid food in the diet, birthweight and position in the family. *Pediatrics* 1960; 26:667.

### Premature Infant

47. Lubchenco LO, Delivoria-Papadopoulos M, Butterfield LJ, et al: Long-term followup studies of prematurely born infants. I. Relationship of handicaps to nursery routines. *J Pediatr* 1972; 80:501.

48. Dweck HS, Brans YW, Summers JE, et al: Glucose intolerance in infants of very low birth weight. II. Intravenous glucose tolerance tests in infants of birth weight of 500–1380 grams. *Biol Neonate* 1976; 30:261.

49. Cornblath M, Wybregt SH, Baens GS, et al: Studies of carbohydrate tolerance in premature infants. *Pediatrics* 1963; 32:1007.

50. Sherwood WG, Hill DW, Chance GW: Glucose homeostasis in preterm Rhesus monkey neonates. *Pediatr Res* 1977; 11:874.

51. Cashore WJ, Sedaghatian MR, Usher RN: Nutritional supplements with intravenously administered lipid, protein hydrolysate and glucose in small premature infants. *Pediatrics* 1975; 56:8.

52. Pildes RS, Ramamurthy RS, Cordero GV, et al: Intravenous supplementation of L-amino acids. *J Pediatr* 1973; 82:945.

53. Pereira GR, Lemons JA: Comparative study between transpyloric and gavage feeding in preterm infants. *Pediatrics* 1981; 67:68.

54. Pereira GR, Herold R, Ziegler M, et al: Sustained flexibility in infant tubes containing nonmigrating plasticizers. *J Parent Ent Nutr* 1982; 6:64.

55. Roy RN, Pollnitz RP, Hamilton JR, et al: Impaired assimilation of nasojejunal feedings in healthy and low birthweight newborn infants. *J Pediatr* 1977; 90:431.

56. Reichman BL, Chessex P, Putet G, et al: Partition of energy metabolism and energy cost of growth in the very low birthweight infant. *Pediatrics* 1982; 69:446.

57. Lemons JA, Moye L, Hall D, et al: Differences in composition of preterm and term human milk during early lactation. *Pediatr Res* 1982; 16:113.

58. Mehta NR, Jones JB, Hamosh M: Bile salt stimulated lipase in preterm human milk—Its role in neonatal fat digestion. *Pediatr Res* 1981; 15:540.

59. Williams ML, Shotts RJ, O'Neal PL, et al: Role of dietary iron and fat on vitamin E deficiency anemia of infancy. *N Engl J Med* 1975; 292:887.

60. Oski FA: Nutritional anemias. *Semin Perin* 1979; 3:381.

61. Gaull GE, Rassin DK, Raiha NCR, et al: Milk protein quantity and quality in low birthweight infants. III. Effects of sulfur aminoacids in plasma and urine. *J Pediatr* 1977; 90:348.

62. Hittner HM, Godio LB, Rudolph AJ, et al: Retrolental fibroplasia: Efficacy of vitamin E in a double blind clinical study of preterm infants. *N Engl J Med* 1982; 305:1365.

63. British Pediatric Association, Committee on Hypercalcemia: Hypercalcemia in infants and vitamin D. *Br Med J* 1956; 2:149.

64. Greer FR, Steichen JJ, Tsang RC: Effects of increased calcium, phosphorus and vitamin D intake on bone mineralization in very low birthweight infants fed formulas with polycose and medium chain triglycerides. *J Pediatr* 1982; 100:951.

65. Steichen JJ, Gratton TL, Tsang RC: Osteopenia of prematurity: The cause and possible treatment. *J Pediatr* 1980; 96:528.

66. American Academy of Pediatrics, Committee on Drugs and Committee on Nutrition: The use and abuse of vitamin A. *Pediatrics* 1971; 48:655.

67. American Academy of Pediatrics, Committee on Nutrition: Iron balance and requirements in infancy. *Pediatrics* 1969; 43:134.

68. American Academy of Pediatrics, Committee on Nutrition: Nutritional needs of low birthweight infants. *Pediatrics* 1977; 60:519.

69. Slagle TA, Gross SJ: Effect of early low volume enteral substrate on subsequent feeding tolerance in very low birthweight infants. *J Pediatr* 1988; 133:526.

70. Dunn L, Hulman S, Weiner J, et al: Beneficial effects of early hypocaloric enteral feeding on neonatal gastrointestinal function: Preliminary report of a randomized trial. *J Pediatr* 1988; 112:622.

71. La Gamma EF, Ostertag SG, Birenbaum H: Failure of delayed oral feedings to prevent necrotizing enterocolitis: results of a study in very low birth weight neonates. *Am J Dis Child* 1985; 139:385.

### Parenteral Nutrition

72. Pereira G, Glassman M: Parenteral nutrition in the neonate. In Rombeau J, Caldwell M, eds: *Parenteral Nutrition*, vol 2. Philadelphia, WB Saunders Co, 1986.

73. Winters RW, Heird WC, Dell RB, et al: Plasma amino acids in infants receiving parenteral nutrition. In Green HL, Holliday MA, Munro HN, eds: *Clinical Nutrition Update*. Chicago, American Medical Association Publishing Co, 1977, pp. 147–157.

74. Heird WC, Dell RB, Driscoll JN Jr, et al: Metabolic acidosis resulting from intravenous alimentation mixtures containing synthetic amino acids. *N Engl J Med* 1972; 287:943.

75. Veleisis RA, Inwood R, Hunt CR: Prospective controlled study of parenteral nutrition associated cholestatic jaundice: Effect of protein uptake. *Pediatrics* 1980; 96:893.

76. Cornblath M, Wybright SH, Baens GS: Studies on carbohydrate metabolism in the newborn in-

fant. VII. Tests on carbohydrate tolerance in premature infants. *Pediatrics* 1963; 32:1007.

77. Kaye R, Williams ML, Barbero G: A comparative study of the metabolism of glucose and fructose in infants. *Am J Dis Child* 1957; 93:85.

78. Van den Berghe G, Hers HG: Dangers of intravenous fructose and sorbitol. *Acta Pediatr Belg* 1978; 31:115.

79. Pereira GR, Yudkoff M, Moskowitz S: Effect of Intralipid therapy on nitrogen retention in premature infants. *J Parent Enter Nutr* 1981; 4:112.

80. Holman RT, Johnson SB, Hatch TF: A case of human linolenic acid deficiency involving neurological abnormalities. *Am J Clin Nutr* 1982; 35:617.

81. Shennan AT, Bryan MH, Angel A: The effect of gestational age on Intralipid tolerance in newborn infants. *J Pediatr* 1977; 91:134.

82. Dhainreddy R, Hamosh M, Sivasubramanian KN, et al: Post-heparin lipolytic activity and Intralipid clearance in very low birthweight infants. *J Pediatr* 1981; 98:617.

83. Filer RM, Takada Y, Carreras T, et al: Serum Intralipid levels in neonates during parenteral nutrition: The relation to gestational age. *Pediatr Surg* 1980; 15:1405.

84. Pereira GR, Fox WW, Stanley CA, et al: Decreased oxygenation and hyperlipemia during intravenous fat infusions in premature infants. *Pediatrics* 1980; 66:26.

85. Pereira GR, Sherman MS, DiGiacomo J, et al: Hyperalimentation induced cholestasis: Increased incidence and severity in premature infants. *Am J Dis Child* 1981; 135:842.

86. Shennan AT, Bryan MH, Angel A: The effect of gestational age on Intralipid tolerance in newborn infants. *J Pediatr* 1977; 91:134.

87. Zlotkin SH, Bryan MH, Anderson GH: Cysteine supplementation to cysteine-free intravenous feeding regimens in newborn infants. *Am J Clin Nutr* 1981; 34:914.

88. Zlotkin SH, Buchanan BE: Meeting zinc and copper intake requirements in the parenterally fed preterm and full-term infant. *J Pediatr* 1983; 103:441.

89. American Medical Association, Department of Foods and Nutrition: Multivitamin preparations for parenteral use—A statement by the Nutrition Advisory Group. *J Parent Enter Nutr* 1979; 3:258.

90. Gillis J, Jones G, Penchaz P: Delivery of vitamins A, D, and E in parenteral nutrition solutions. *J Parent Enter Nutr* 1983; 7:11.

91. Heird WC, Hay W, Helms RA, et al: Pediatric parenteral amino acid mixture in low birthweight infants. *Pediatrics* 1988; 81:41.

92. Stahl GE, Spear ML, Hamosh M, et al: The intravenous administration of lipid emulsions in premature infants. *Clin Perinatol* 1986; 13:133.

# Chapter 7

# ANEMIA IN

# THE NEWBORN

## James A. Stockman III, M.D.

No single entity reflects the rapid developmental changes associated with growth and age than the remarkable variations in normative hematologic data in the newborn. This makes the care provider's task of evaluating an infant for anemia more difficult because the breadth of understanding of what is *normal* is greater than at any other time of life.

As you progress through this chapter, you will encounter clinical data from six newborn infants; these data are presented in Table 7-1. We would like you to read each set of data carefully at that point, determine what additional information would be helpful, and make a tentative "diagnosis." Each case represents an infant with a different diagnosis illustrative of how one must understand what is considered normal before one can approach the differential diagnosis of anemia at this age.

The first part of this chapter reviews what is meant by *normal* and the factors that can affect various hematologic parameters. The middle of the chapter provides an overall diagnostic approach to anemia in the neonate. Finally, the chapter concludes with a discussion of each of the six infants presented in Table 7-1, using the normative data and diagnostic approaches suggested earlier in the chapter.

### WHAT IS NORMAL?

#### Hemoglobin

The normal range for hemoglobin concentration is greater in the newborn period than any other time of life. *In utero,* the hemoglobin concentration varies with postconceptional age (Table 7-2). At 10 weeks' postconceptional age, the hemoglobin concentration is normally about 9 g/dL, while at term gestation hemoglobin rises to a mean value of 16.5 g/dL (Table 7-3). Values of hemoglobin below 14.3 g/dL in cord blood (at term gestation) should be considered low and are worthy of evaluation. Some of the variation seen in individual infants with respect to hemoglobin values is due to artifacts of the method used to collect the blood sample as well as the timing of umbilical cord clamping at the moment of birth.

Hemoglobin determinations obtained by capillary techniques are likely to be higher than those obtained by venopuncture. Although this statement applies at all ages, it is more of a problem in neonates because of stasis of blood in the extremities and the resultant hemoconcentration. Errors of 100% or more may occur when the capillary technique is used. For this reason, venopuncture is preferred to capillary specimens, if at all possible. If a venopuncture cannot be performed, a reasonably accurate capillary specimen can be obtained by warming the area to be sampled, which permits a free flow of blood.

Some of the wide variation seen in hemoglobin values during the first few days of life is related to the time of cord clamping. Delayed cord clamping can result in significant rises in hemoglobin concentration (Table 7-4). For example, holding a baby slightly below the mother's perineum and delaying clamping of the cord for 30 to 60 seconds can result in a transfusion of placental and cord blood that will increase the baby's blood volume by as much as 25% to 35%. Delayed cord clamping can result in transient tachypnea and other potentially serious problems associated with

Table 7-1 Six Cases of "Anemia" in the Neonate*

CASE STUDY

| | 1 | 2 | 3 | 4 | 5 | 6 |
|---|---|---|---|---|---|---|
| Age | 6 hours | 30 minutes | 2 days | 6 weeks | 3 days | 1 day |
| Sex | M | F | M | M | F | F |
| Race | W | W | B | W | W | B |
| Hgb | 17.1 | 15.1 | 14.9 | 7.5 | 14.1 | 8.5 |
| Hct % | 52 | 46 | 45 | 22 | 44 | 25 |
| MCV | 110 | 107 | 93 | 89 | 106 | 118 |
| MCHC | 31.6 | 32.0 | 33.0 | 33.2 | 38.0 | 33.0 |
| RBC | 5.0 | 4.9 | 5.7 | 3.0 | 4.4 | 2.7 |
| RDW | 13.5 | 14.1 | 14.0 | 14.1 | 16.1 | 20.5 |
| NRBC | 10 | 220 | 0 | 0 | 110 | 220 |
| Retic. % | 3.5 | 4.0 | 2.1 | 1.0 | 8.2 | 15.1 |
| Platelets | 220.0 | 390.0 | 210.0 | 190.0 | 250.0 | 240.0 |
| Smear | Mild anisocytosis/poikilocytosis | Mild anisocytosis/poikilocytosis | Mild anisocytosis/poikilocytosis Occasional target cells | Mild anisocytosis/poikilocytosis | Moderate anisocytosis Occasional spherocytes | Moderate anisocytosis polychromasia |
| Spleen size | 0.5 cm | Not palpable | Not palpable | Not palpable | 3.5 cm | 6.0 cm |
| Clinical features | GA = 39.5 wk Normal vaginal delivery | GA = 40 wk Pale, heart rate 200 BPM, with weak pulses Cesarean section | GA = 40 wk Normal vaginal delivery Bilirubin 4.3 mg% | GA = 28 wk BW = 1,000 g Vaginal delivery preterm, incompetent cervix | GA = 39 wk Family history of early gallstones Bilirubin 18 mg% | GA = 34 wk 3rd born Moderate hydrops at birth |
| What other studies are needed? | | | | | | |
| Diagnosis? | | | | | | |

* Hgb = hemoglobin, Hct = hematocrit, MCV = mean corpuscular volume, MCHC = mean corpuscular hemoglobin concentration, RBC = red blood cell, RDW = red blood cell distribution width, NRBC = nucleated red blood cell, GA = gestational age, BW = birth weight.

**Table 7-2**  Mean Red Blood Cell Values During Gestation

| AGE (WEEKS) | Hgb (g/dL) | HEMATOCRIT (%) | RBC (10 U/mm³) | MEAN CORPUSC. VOLUME (fL) | MEAN CORPUSC. Hgb (pg) | MEAN CORPUSC. Hgb CONC. (g/dL) | NUCLEATED RBCS (% OF RBCS) | RETICULOCYTES (%) | DIAMETER (U) |
|---|---|---|---|---|---|---|---|---|---|
| 12 | 8.0–10.0 | 33 | 1.5 | 180 | 60 | 34 | 5.0–8.0 | 40 | 10.5 |
| 16 | 10.0 | 35 | 2.0 | 140 | 45 | 33 | 2.0–4.0 | 10–25 | 9.5 |
| 20 | 11.0 | 37 | 2.5 | 135 | 44 | 33 | 1.0 | 10–20 | 9.0 |
| 24 | 14.0 | 40 | 3.5 | 128 | 38 | 31 | 1.0 | 5–10 | 8.8 |
| 28 | 14.5 | 45 | 4.0 | 120 | 40 | 31 | 0.5 | 5–10 | 8.7 |
| 34 | 15.0 | 47 | 4.4 | 118 | 38 | 32 | 0.2 | 3–10 | 8.3 |

*Source:* Modified from Oski FA: Normal blood values in the newborn period. In Oski FA, Naiman JL, eds: *Hematologic Problems in the Newborn*, 3rd ed. Philadelphia, WB Saunders Co, 1982, p. 4. Modified with permission of W.B. Saunders Company.

**Table 7-3**  Normal Cord Hemoglobin Values

| GESTATIONAL AGE (WEEKS) | Hgb (g/100 mL) | |
|---|---|---|
| | MALE | FEMALE |
| 28 to 29 | 15.00 ± 2.45 | 13.60 ± 2.16 |
| 30 to 31 | 15.91 ± 1.34 | 14.73 ± 1.07 |
| 32 to 33 | 16.29 ± 1.86 | 15.21 ± 2.64 |
| 34 to 35 | 16.29 ± 2.05 | 15.82 ± 2.43 |
| 36 to 37 | 16.20 ± 2.20 | 15.88 ± 2.45 |
| 38 to 39 | 16.22 ± 2.24 | 16.68 ± 2.23 |
| 40 to 41 | | 16.56 ± 1.65 |

*Source:* Modified from Burman D, Morris AF: Cord hemoglobin in low birth weight infants. *Arch Dis Child* 1974; 49:382. Modified with permission of the British Medical Association.

polycythemia and hyperviscosity. Because little, if any, benefit is derived from this method of delivery, delayed cord clamping is generally no longer recommended. It is, in fact, contraindicated in situations in which it would not be desirous for a baby to have greater quantities of his or her own red blood cells (RBCs). For example, infants with red cell sensitization may exhibit higher degrees of hyperbilirubinemia if they are permitted to be born with higher hemoglobin concentrations as a result of delayed cord clamping.

The cord hemoglobin concentration of infants born prematurely may be slightly lower than that of infants born at term, as noted earlier. These differences, however, are negligible beyond 28 weeks' gestation. Male infants might have slightly higher hemoglobin values, at least until the 38th week of pregnancy.

Rapid postnatal changes in hemoglobin concentration occur in most infants during the first day or so of life. The magnitude of the increase is a reflection of the amount of blood received from the umbilical cord and placenta at delivery and is a result of hemoconcentration. After this initial rise, the hemoglobin will begin to fall fairly rapidly, reaching a low value by 6 to 12 weeks of age in the term infant and earlier in preterm infants. Tables 7-5 and 7-6 illustrate the serial changes that occur in the normal hematologic values of term infants during the first 12 weeks of life. A normal term infant should not experience a decrease in hemoglobin levels below 9.8 g/dL at any time during the first 3 months of life. After 12 weeks of age, all healthy term infants will exhibit a gradual rise in hemoglobin concentration equal to or greater than 11.0 g/dL by 4 to 5 months of age.

This situation, however, is very different in preterm infants. Such infants experience a more rapid and greater decline in hemoglobin levels during the first few weeks of life. Hemoglobin values in the range of 7 to 8 g/dL are common in small preterm babies by several weeks of age. The smaller the infant, the greater the expected fall in hemoglobin concentration. Table 7-7 and Figure 7-1 demonstrate the changes in serial hemoglobin values in low birth weight infants and are indicative of the marked variations that are dependent on gestational age and birth weight.

An excessive decrease in hemoglobin concentration during the first week of life indicates either increased red cell destruction or blood loss. It has been suggested that any venous hemoglobin concentration less than 13.0

**Table 7-4**  Effect of Cord Clamping on Hemoglobin Concentration

| STUDY | EARLY CLAMPING Hgb (g/dL) | DELAYED CLAMPING Hgb (g/dL) | TIME OF STUDY |
|---|---|---|---|
| 1. Phillips (1941)* | 15.6 | 19.3 | 20–30 hours of age |
| 2. DeMarsh et al. (1948)† | 17.4 | 20.8 | 3rd day |
| 3. Colozzi (1954)‡ | 14.7 | 17.3 | 72 hours |
| 4. Lanzkowsky (1960)§ | 18.1 | 19.7 | 72–96 hours |
| | 11.1 | 11.1 | 3 months of age |

* Phillips AGS: Haptoglobins in the newborn. I. Full-term infants. *Biol Neonate* 1941; 19:185.
† DeMarsh QB, Alt HL, Windle WF: Factors influencing the blood picture of the newborn: Studies on sinus blood on the first and third days. *Am J Dis Child* 1948; 75:860.
‡ Colozzi AE: Clamping of the umbilical cord; its effect on the placental transfusion. *N Engl J Med* 1954; 250:629.
§ Lanzkowsky P: Effects of early and late clamping of umbilical cord on infant's hemoglobin level. *Br Med J* 1960; 2:1777.

**Table 7-5**  Normal Hematologic Values During the First 2 Weeks of Life in the Term Infant*

| VALUE | CORD BLOOD | DAY 1 | DAY 3 | DAY 7 | DAY 14 |
|---|---|---|---|---|---|
| Hgb (g/dL) | 16.8 | 18.4 | 17.8 | 17.0 | 16.8 |
| Hematocrit (%) | 53.0 | 58.0 | 55.0 | 54.0 | 52.0 |
| Red cells (mm³) | 5.25 | 5.8 | 5.6 | 5.2 | 5.1 |
| MCV (fL) | 107 | 108 | 99.0 | 98.0 | 96.0 |
| MCH (pg) | 34 | 35 | 33 | 32.5 | 31.5 |
| MCHC (g/dL) | 31.7 | 32.5 | 33 | 33 | 33 |
| Reticulocytes (%) | 3–7 | 3–7 | 1–3 | 0–1 | 0–1 |
| Nucleated RBCs (mm³) | 500 | 200 | 0–5 | 0 | 0 |
| Platelets (1,000s/mm³) | 290 | 192 | 213 | 248 | 252 |

* During the first 2 weeks of life, a venous hemoglobin less than 13.0 g/dL or a capillary hemoglobin less than 14.5 g/dL should be regarded as anemia.
*Source:* Modified from Oski FA, Naiman JL: *Hematologic Problems in the Newborn,* 2nd ed. Philadelphia, WB Saunders Co, 1972, p. 12. Modified with permission of W.B. Saunders Company.

g/dL in the first 2 weeks of life should be regarded as evidence of anemia. A capillary hemoglobin concentration less than 14.5 g/dL is regarded as evidence of anemia as well.

### Hematocrit

Changes in hematocrit should parallel variations in hemoglobin concentration. With electronic cell counting, the hematocrit is merely a derived number. Because the hemoglobin is directly measured with such equipment, it is rarely useful to take note of the hematocrit except when there is a discrepancy between the manually measured spun hematocrit and the electronically computed hematocrit. With electronic counting equipment, the hematocrit is extrapolated by computation [hematocrit = mean corpuscular volume (MCV) × RBC]. Thus, any time there is marked variation in size and shape (anisocytosis and poikilocytosis), you may anticipate a discrepancy between the computed hematocrit obtained with electronic counting equipment and a manually spun hematocrit.

### Mean Corpuscular Volume

The red cells of the newborn infant are, in general, much larger than the cells of the normal adult, although considerable variation in size can be observed in any individual infant.

The developmental changes in MCV from cord blood samples (28 weeks to term) and from term infants to 6 months postnatal age are shown in Figure 7-2. As might be expected, the cord MCV is greatest in the most immature infants and decreases with advancing gestational age. All newborn infants, however, exhibit macrocytic RBC indices in comparison with adult values for MCV.

Table 7-6 provides information on the serial changes in red cell indices including the MCV of erythrocytes. The latter is estimated to range from 104 to 118 fL, compared to the

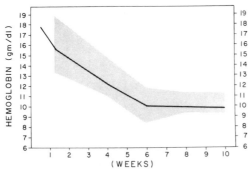

**Figure 7-1**  The relationship between hemoglobin concentration and age from birth in a group of 40 infants with birth weights of less than 1,500 g. Dark line indicates mean value; shaded area includes all values observed. All infants were vitamin E–iron sufficient.
From Nathan D, Oski FA: *Hematology of Infancy and Childhood,* 3rd ed. Philadelphia, WB Saunders Co, 1987, p. 39. Reprinted with permission of W.B. Saunders Company.

**Table 7-6** Postnatal Changes in Hemoglobin and RBC Indices in Term Infants

| | AGE OF INFANTS | | | | | | | | |
| | DAYS | | | WEEKS | | MONTHS | | | |
| RBC PARAMETERS | 1 | 3 | 7 | 2 | 4 | 2 | 3 | 4 | 6 |
|---|---|---|---|---|---|---|---|---|---|
| **Hemoglobin (g/dL)** | | | | | | | | | |
| x̄ | 19.4 | 18.6 | 18.7 | 17.6 | 13.9 | 11.2 | 11.4 | 12.0 | 12.1 |
| ±2 SD | 17.2 | 16.5 | 16.5 | 13.9 | 10.6 | 9.3 | 9.5 | 10.7 | 10.4 |
| (N) | (78) | (66) | (78) | (275) | (272) | (271) | (73) | (123) | (114) |
| **MCV (fL)** | | | | | | | | | |
| x̄ | 114 | 110 | 108 | 106 | 101 | 95 | 88 | 84 | 77 |
| ±2 SD | 101–128 | 104–116 | 102–114 | 88–125 | 90–112 | 83–107 | 78–98 | 74–95 | 67–87 |
| (N) | (78) | (66) | (78) | (275) | (272) | (271) | (73) | (123) | (114) |
| **MCH (pg)** | | | | | | | | | |
| x̄ | 36.6 | 36.7 | 36.2 | 33.6 | 32.5 | 30.4 | 30.4 | 28.1 | 26.4 |
| (N) | (59) | (47) | (66) | (232) | (240) | (241) | (60) | (123) | (114) |
| **MCHC (%)** | | | | | | | | | |
| x̄ | 33.0 | 33.1 | 33.9 | 31.7 | 32.1 | 32.0 | 34.6 | 33.3 | 34.2 |
| (N) | (78) | (66) | (78) | (275) | (272) | (271) | (73) | (123) | (114) |

*Source:* Modified from Guest GM, Brown EW: Erythrocytes and hemoglobin of the blood in infancy and childhood. III. Factors in variability, statistical studies. *Am J Dis Child* 1957; 93:486–509; Saarinen UM, Siimes MA: Developmental changes in red blood cell counts and indices of infants after exclusion of iron deficiency by laboratory criteria and continuous iron supplementation. *J Pediatr* 1978; 92:412–416; and Matoth Y, Zaizov R, Varsano I: Postnatal changes in some red cell parameters. *Acta Paediatr Scand* 1971; 60:317–323.

**Table 7-7**  Serial Hemoglobin Values in Low Birth Weight Infants

| BIRTH WEIGHT (g) | AGE (WEEKS) | | | | |
|---|---|---|---|---|---|
| | 2 | 4 | 6 | 8 | 10 |
| 800–1,000 | 16.0 (14.8–17.2) | 10.0 (6.8–13.2) | 8.7 (7.0–10.2) | 8.0 (7.1–9.8) | 8.0 (6.9–10.2) |
| 1,001–1,200 | 16.4 (14.1–18.7) | 12.8 (7.8–15.3) | 10.5 (7.2–12.3) | 9.1 (7.8–10.4) | 8.5 (7.0–10.0) |
| 1,201–1,400 | 16.2 (13.6–18.8) | 13.4 (8.8–16.2) | 10.9 (8.5–13.3) | 9.9 (8.0–11.8) | 9.8 (8.4–11.3) |
| 1,401–1,500 | 15.6 (13.4–17.8) | 11.7 (9.7–13.7) | 10.5 (9.1–11.9) | 9.8 (8.4–12.0) | 9.9 (8.4–11.4) |
| 1,501–2,000 | 15.6 (13.5–17.7) | 11.0 (9.6–14.0) | 9.6 (8.8–11.5) | 9.8 (8.4–12.1) | 10.0 (8.6–11.8) |

*Source:* Modified from Williams ML, Shott RJ, O'Neal PL, et al: Dietary iron and fat in vitamin E deficiency anemia of infancy. *N Engl J Med* 1975; 292:877. Modified with permission from *The New England Journal of Medicine*, vol. 292, page 877, 1975.

normal adult value of 82 to 92 fL. More precisely, the normal MCV of a term infant is 106.4 ± 5.7 fL. Values of 94 fL or less are indicative of microcytosis. The differential diagnosis of microcytosis is discussed later in this chapter.

As noted, the MCV is considerably higher in the preterm infant. In a group of infants with an average birth weight of approximately 1,300 g, the MCV was found to be 115 ± 5.0 fL on the first day of life and declined to a mean value of 95 ± 5 fL by the seventh week postnatally. The MCV can be an important clue in the differential diagnosis of certain forms of anemia in the neonate.

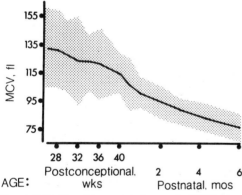

**Figure 7-2**  Developmental changes in MCV from cord measurements in premature infants to 38 weeks and term infants to 6 months postnatal age. Line and hatched areas represent mean and ±2 SD of combined means and pooled variances.
Reprinted with permission from Zaizov R, Matoth Y: Red cell values on the first postnatal day during the last 16 weeks of gestation. *Am J Hematol* 1976; 1:275–278; Saarinen UM: Need for iron supplementation in infants on prolonged breast feeding. *J Pediatr* 1978; 93:177–180; and Matoth Y, Zaizov R, Varsano I: Postnatal changes in some red cell parameters. *Acta Paediatr Scand* 1971; 60:317–323.

## Mean Corpuscular Hemoglobin

The mean corpuscular hemoglobin (MCH) is slightly higher in the newborn period than at other times of life (Table 7-5). Again, recall that the MCH is a derived number when electronic counting equipment (MCH = hemoglobin/RBC) is used. The MCH rarely assists in the establishment of a differential diagnosis of anemia in the neonatal period.

## Mean Corpuscular Hemoglobin Concentration

The mean corpuscular hemoglobin concentration (MCHC) in the newborn is quite similar to that of the normal adult (Table 7-6). Elevations in the MCHC are usually indicative of circumstances in which the red cell has been so altered as to compress hemoglobin within a smaller red cell volume. The MCHC, therefore, is a clue to disorders characterized by the presence of spherocytes. These disorders would include hereditary spherocytosis, ABO incompatibility, and microangiopathic hemolytic anemia (such as may be seen in infants and older children with disseminated intravascular coagulation, severe vasculitis, or hemangiomas). In these disorders, the red cell is affected in such a manner that it exhibits the least surface area for any given volume (the geometric definition of a sphere), which accounts for an elevation in the MCHC.

## Red Cell Distribution Width

The red cell distribution width (RDW) is the coefficient of variation in red cell volume distribution. Similar distribution values may be obtained for white blood cells and platelets. Figure 7-3 shows a normal distribution of red

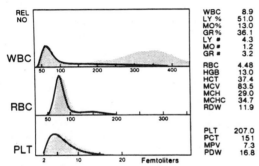

| WBC | 8.9 |
| LY % | 51.0 |
| MO% | 13.0 |
| GR% | 36.1 |
| LY # | 4.3 |
| MO # | 1.2 |
| GR # | 3.2 |
| RBC | 4.48 |
| HGB | 13.0 |
| HCT | 37.4 |
| MCV | 83.5 |
| MCH | 29.0 |
| MCHC | 34.7 |
| RDW | 11.9 |
| PLT | 207.0 |
| PCT | 151 |
| MPV | 7.3 |
| PDW | 16.8 |

**Figure 7-3** Typical histogram and other information produced by the instrument for leukocytes, erythrocytes, and platelets. The shaded areas represent the normal range obtained from a study of 70 normal subjects. The ordinate is the relative number of cells, and the abscissa is the size range of the cells in femtoliters (fL).
Modified from Cox CJ, Haberman TM, Payne BA, et al: Distribution patterns of cellular blood elements. *Am J Clin Pathol* 1985; 84:297–306. Modified with permission of J.B. Lippincott Company.

cell size. The more homogeneous the red cell size, the lower the RDW. The more heterogeneous (often reflecting anisocytosis or reticulocytosis), the greater the RDW.

The average value of the RDW in a newborn infant is 13.0 ± 1.5. Table 7-8 illustrates the expected variations in RDW based on age.

Table 7-9 lists the changes in RDW in a variety of common and not so common childhood anemias, most of which occur beyond the neonatal period. In general, infants and children with microcytosis due to iron deficiency have high RDWs. Children with thalassemia trait syndromes have normal RDWs.

**Table 7-8** Age-Appropriate Values for RDW

| AGE | NUMBER OF PATIENTS | RBC DISTRIBUTION WIDTH (MEAN ± SD) |
| --- | --- | --- |
| 1–6 months | 68 | 13.0 ± 1.5 |
| 7–12 months | 84 | 13.7 ± 0.9 |
| 13–24 months | 108 | 13.4 ± 1.0 |
| 2–3 years | 119 | 13.2 ± 0.8 |
| 4–5 years | 151 | 12.7 ± 0.9 |
| 6–8 years | 106 | 12.6 ± 0.8 |
| 9–11 years | 98 | 12.8 ± 1.0 |

*Source:* Modified from Novak RW: Red blood cell distribution width in pediatric microcytic anemias. *Pediatrics* 1987; 80:251. Modified by permission of *Pediatrics*, vol. 80, page 251, copyright 1987.

These principles would be expected to apply to newborns as well. By comparing the MCV to the RDW, you can quickly characterize various forms of anemia, as is illustrated in the diagnostic approach to anemia later in this chapter.

## Red Blood Cell Count

The red blood cell count (RBC) shows great variability at the time of birth (Table 7-5). The mean red blood cell count in a newborn is approximately $5.0 \times 10^9/mm^3$. The RBC value is rarely of diagnostic importance in assisting in the differential diagnosis of anemia in the newborn.

## Nucleated Red Blood Cell Count

The presence of nucleated red blood cells (NRBCs) should cause no alarm if present at birth or observed during the first few days of life. NRBCs may be observed in the peripheral blood of almost all infants at the time of birth and certainly throughout the first day of life. Many laboratories express the number of NRBCs as a percentage of white blood cells (WBCs). Because of the marked variability in the number of white blood cells normally present at birth, it is more helpful to express the NRBC in absolute numbers, or as a percentage of the red cells, as can be done for an absolute reticulocyte count. If this approach is used, the term infant has approximately 500 $NRBC/mm^3$ of blood at birth, which represents 0.1% of the red cell population. By the time the infant is 12 hours of age, this number has decreased by half. When the infant is 2 days of age, the NRBC value should be only 20 to 30. Any NRBC seen in a peripheral blood smear beyond the fourth to fifth day of life should be considered abnormal and a cause for the increase should be sought.

Preterm infants have higher NRBC values than term infants. In the preterm infant, 1,000 to 1,500 $NRBC/mm^3$ may be present at the time of birth. The younger the infant, the greater this number. As with term infants, these values tend to decline rapidly during the first week of life, although it would not be unusual to see an occasional NRBC in the peripheral blood smear of an infant as old as 6 to 8 weeks of age.

If the NRBC is expressed in terms of numbers of white blood cells, the term infant has

**Table 7-9** Proposed Classification of Anemic Disorders Based on Red Blood Cell Mean (MCV) and Heterogeneity (RDW)

| MCV LOW RDW NORMAL (MICROCYTIC HOMOGENEOUS) | MCV LOW RDW HIGH (MICROCYTIC HETEROGENEOUS) | MCV NORMAL RDW NORMAL (NORMOCYTIC HOMOGENEOUS) | MCV NORMAL RDW HIGH (NORMOCYTIC HETEROGENEOUS) | MCV HIGH RDW NORMAL (MACROCYTIC HOMOGENEOUS) | MCV HIGH RDW HIGH (MACROCYTIC HETEROGENEOUS) |
|---|---|---|---|---|---|
| Heterozygous thalassemia | Iron deficiency | Normal | Mixed deficiency | Aplastic anemia | Folate deficiency |
| Chronic disease | S $\beta$-thalassemia | Chronic disease or chronic liver disease | Early iron or deficiency | Preleukemia | Vitamin $B_{12}$ deficiency |
| | Hemoglobin H | Nonanemic hemoglobinopathy (e.g., AS, AC) | Anemic hemoglobinopathy (e.g., SS, SC) | Diamond-Blackfan syndrome | Immune hemolytic anemia |
| | Red cell fragmentation | Transfusion | Myelofibrosis | Acute leukemia (some) | Cold agglutinins |
| | | Chemotherapy | Sideroblastic | Down's syndrome | Chronic lymphocytic leukemia, high count |
| | | Chronic lymphocytic leukemia | | | Liver disease |
| | | Chronic myelocytic leukemia | | | Hypothyroidism |
| | | Hemorrhage | | | Reticulocytosis |
| | | Hereditary spherocytosis | | | Normal newborns |

*Source:* From Bessman JD, Hughes EN, Skinner J, et al: Improved classification of anemias by MCV and RDW. *Am J Clin Pathol* 1983; 80:322–326. Reprinted with permission of J.B. Lippincott Company.

an average of 7.3 NRBC/100 WBC at birth with a range of 0 to 24. In the preterm infant, the average figure is 21 NRBC/100 WBC.

Increased numbers of NRBCs are observed in hemolytic disease states, following hemorrhage, during hypoxic periods, and in disorders associated with abnormal erythropoiesis (for example, as in the dyshematopoietic syndromes that may occur in infants with Down's syndrome).

## Reticulocyte Count

The mean reticulocyte count on the first day of life in term infants is 5.5% with a range of 4.2% to 7.2% (absolute value = 300,000 reticulocytes/mm³). The reticulocyte count *in utero* decreases from a value of approximately 80% at 12 weeks' gestation to the lower values seen at term. For these reasons, infants born prematurely would be expected to have higher reticulocyte counts at birth. Values between 6% and 10% are commonly noted in infants whose gestational ages range between 28 and 36 weeks' gestation.

Whether an infant is born preterm or at term gestation, the reticulocyte count decreases rapidly. Postnatally, evidence of very active erythropoiesis (as reflected in an elevated reticulocyte count) persists for the first 3 days of life. By the end of the first week of life, however, the reticulocyte count should drop to values of about 1%, equal to the normal adult reticulocyte count.

Persistence of reticulocytosis suggests the presence of blood loss, hemolysis, or ongoing hypoxemia. An increased reticulocyte count may again be observed at 4 to 8 weeks of age (Fig. 7-4) in preterm infants, shortly after the physiological nadir in hemoglobin levels.

## Peripheral Blood Smear

Just as there is much variation in sizes of newborn red cells, there is much variation in shape. Increased numbers of irregularly shaped cells and target cells can be observed during the neonatal period as compared with the normal adult. If the blood of neonates is examined in a wet preparation, 43% of neonatal red cells appear as discocytes and 40% are stomatocytes. In adults, the equivalent percentages are 78% and 18%, respectively. The remainder of neonatal cells consist of various irregularly shaped forms. The red blood cell morphology

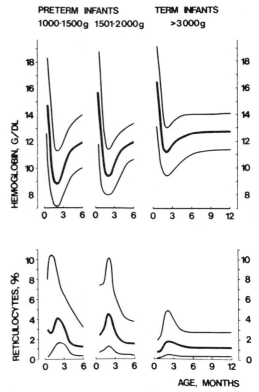

**Figure 7-4** The mean and range of normal values for hemoglobin concentration and reticulocyte count of preterm and term infants.
From Dallman PR: Anemia of prematurity. *Annu Rev Med* 1981; 32:143. Reproduced, with permission, from the *Annual Review of Medicine*, Vol. 32, © 1981 by Annual Reviews Inc.

of preterm infants shows even greater variability. Figure 7-5 highlights the wide variety of red blood cell shapes that may be seen in preterm and term neonates in comparison with adults.

One unique characteristic of the neonatal red cell is the presence of membrane surface pits (Fig. 7-6). These are most easily demonstrated by means of interference contrast microscopy. While only 2.5% of erythrocytes in adults appear to have surface pits or craters, 47% of the erythrocytes of preterm infants and 24% of the erythrocytes of term infants have pits. Red cell surface pits most likely represent the formation of endocytic vacuoles. These pits are virtually identical in appearance with pits that are visible on the surfaces of cells from splenectomized subjects. It has long been presumed that the hypofunctional and immature neonatal spleen does not remodel the red cell membrane, nor does it remove these vacuoles to the same degree as is seen in older children or adults.

In conclusion, the peripheral blood smear of a neonate should be expected to show significant variation in RBC size and shape. The peripheral blood smear of a neonate is, therefore, somewhat more difficult to interpret in comparison to the older child or adult. Such interpretations must be made in the context of what is normal for the neonate.

## Summary of What is Normal

Normal term and preterm infants are slightly more polycythemic and display hemoglobin values that are slightly higher than older infants, children, and adults. The size of the RBCs is increased in neonates (versus the adult); however, only minor differences exist in the other red cell indices. The presence of NRBCs or an elevated reticulocyte count is not unusual for the first few days of life. The

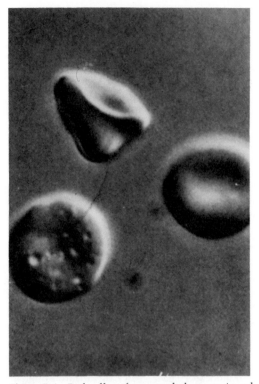

**Figure 7-6** Red cell surface morphology as viewed with an interference contrast microscope. Courtesy of Christopher P. Holroyde, MD.

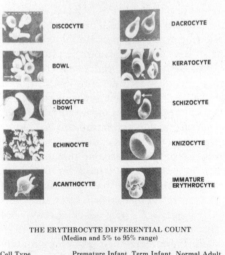

THE ERYTHROCYTE DIFFERENTIAL COUNT
(Median and 5% to 95% range)

| Cell Type | Premature Infant | Term Infant | Normal Adult |
|---|---|---|---|
| Discocyte | 39.5 (18-57) | 43 (18-62) | 78 (42-94) |
| Bowl | 29.0 (13-53) | 40 (14-58) | 18 ( 4-50) |
| Discocyte-Bowl | 3.0 ( 0-10) | 2 ( 0-5 ) | 2 ( 0-4 ) |
| Spherocyte | 0.0 ( 0-3 ) | 0 ( 0-1 ) | 0 ( 0-0 ) |
| Echinocyte | 5.5 ( 1-23) | 1 ( 0-4 ) | 0 ( 0-3 ) |
| Acanthocyte | 0.0 ( 0-2 ) | 1 ( 0-2 ) | 0 ( 0-1 ) |
| Dacrocyte | 1.0 ( 0-5 ) | 1 ( 0-3 ) | 0 ( 0-1 ) |
| Keratocyte | 3.0 ( 0-7 ) | 2 ( 0-5 ) | 0 ( 0-1 ) |
| Schizocyte | 2.0 ( 0-5 ) | 0 ( 0-2 ) | 0 ( 0-1 ) |
| Knizocyte | 3.0 ( 0-11) | 3 ( 0-8 ) | 1 ( 0-5 ) |
| Immature erythrocyte | 1.0 ( 0-6 ) | 0 ( 0-2 ) | 0 ( 0-0 ) |

**Figure 7-5** The variety of morphological abnormalities of the erythrocyte observed in premature infants, term infants, and normal adults. Photomicrographs courtesy of Zipursky, Brown, and Brown. Adapted from *Am J Pediatr Hematol Oncol;* The erythrocyte differential count in newborn infants; A. Zipursky, E. Brown, A. Brown, et al.; vol. 5; 1983; pages 48–49. Adapted with permission of Raven Press, Ltd.

peripheral blood smear would be considered abnormal by any standard in comparison with older children and adults. Therefore, extreme caution must be used in the interpretation of RBC shape abnormalities in the neonate.

With this background information, the chapter now focuses on the differential diagnosis and diagnostic approach to anemia in the neonate.

## APPROACH TO THE DIFFERENTIAL DIAGNOSIS OF ANEMIA IN THE NEWBORN

As with the diagnosis of any disorder, a careful history and physical examination, along with a minimum amount of laboratory information permits a logical approach to the differential diagnosis of anemia.

In the neonate, the differential diagnosis of anemia is somewhat more perplexing because of the wide variety of disorders that can result in anemia at this age. Certainly, the presence of anemia in other family members may be a clue to various congenital forms of hemolytic anemia. Similarly, a maternal drug history may be critically important with regard to disorders such as glucose-6-phosphate dehydrogenase deficiency, which can be exacerbated by a variety of drugs taken by the mother.

Severe anemia presenting at birth is almost always due either to hemorrhage or severe red cell isoimmunization. In contrast, anemia manifesting itself during the first day of life is generally caused by internal or external hemorrhage. Anemia appearing after 48 hours of life is usually due to a hemolytic process and is generally associated with jaundice.

Appropriate laboratory testing of an anemic newborn includes determination of hemoglobin concentration, hematocrit, red cell indices, a reticulocyte count, an NRBC count, a review of the peripheral blood smear, maternal and fetal RBC typing, a direct and an indirect Coombs test, and, if indicated, an examination of maternal blood for the presence of fetal erythrocytes.

With just this minimum amount of history and laboratory data, you can initiate a logical approach to the differential diagnosis of anemia in the newborn. For older infants and children, the differential diagnosis is usually first approached by using the value provided by the MCV. This is not true in newborn infants because most anemias do not reflect themselves in abnormalities of the MCV. The reticulocyte count, on the other hand, provides the first and most valuable laboratory clue to anemia as illustrated in Figure 7-7.

A depressed reticulocyte count suggests a bone marrow failure state. The differential diagnosis of anemia in the newborn period associated with reticulocytopenia includes congenital hypoplastic anemia, drug-induced red cell suppression, refractory sideroblastic anemia, and a rare disorder known as *transcobalamin II deficiency*. Additionally, bone marrow infiltrative disorders such as congenital leukemia or myelofibrosis can result in a reticulocytopenic state in association with anemia. Any infant with significant anemia and a low reticulocyte count warrants a bone marrow examination and perhaps (if possible) a bone marrow biopsy.

If an anemia is the result of either hemorrhage or hemolysis, the reticulocyte count is usually (but not always) elevated. Patients with anemia and reticulocytosis should be as-

sumed to have either experienced a recent hemorrhage or to have an active hemolytic process. All such infants should have a careful history and physical examination to determine if recent blood loss has occurred. The next most logical test to perform if there is little or no possibility of recent hemorrhage is a Coombs test.

A direct Coombs test is likely to be positive in all cases of Rh incompatibility. With ABO incompatibility a weakly positive Coombs test is usually seen; however, a negative reaction may occur as well. A positive Coombs test can, of course, be seen with minor blood group incompatibilities and may be observed in association with maternal autoimmune hemolytic anemia.

A patient with an elevated reticulocyte count who has a negative Coombs test should then have a careful determination of the MCV. The MCV will either be low, normal, or elevated, and at this point in the diagnostic workup it becomes an extremely valuable tool in the differential diagnosis of anemia in the neonate.

A neonate with a low MCV has a very limited differential diagnosis. The major diagnostic possibilities include prenatal blood loss resulting in iron deficiency and the presence of the α-thalassemia trait. Other causes of microcytosis occur only rarely during the newborn period. Table 7-10 lists the types of blood loss that can occur prior to or at the time of birth. Although physical examination can be helpful in suggesting a diagnosis of acute hemorrhage (when signs of cardiovascular instability are present), it is not very useful for detecting chronic hemorrhage. In that circumstance, a complete obstetric history will often help pinpoint the diagnosis. The passage of fetal cells into the maternal circulation occurs commonly during pregnancy; in approximately 50% of pregnancies, some fetal cells can be demonstrated in the maternal circulation. A chronic fetomaternal hemorrhage has been described in association with placental chorioangioma and choriocarcinoma. Furthermore, approximately 70% of monozygous twin pregnancies have monochorial placentas, which can be associated with twin-to-twin transfusions. With dichorionic placentas, vascular anastamoses are uncommon.

Infants who have experienced chronic intrauterine blood loss from any cause can readily develop iron deficiency. As might be ex-

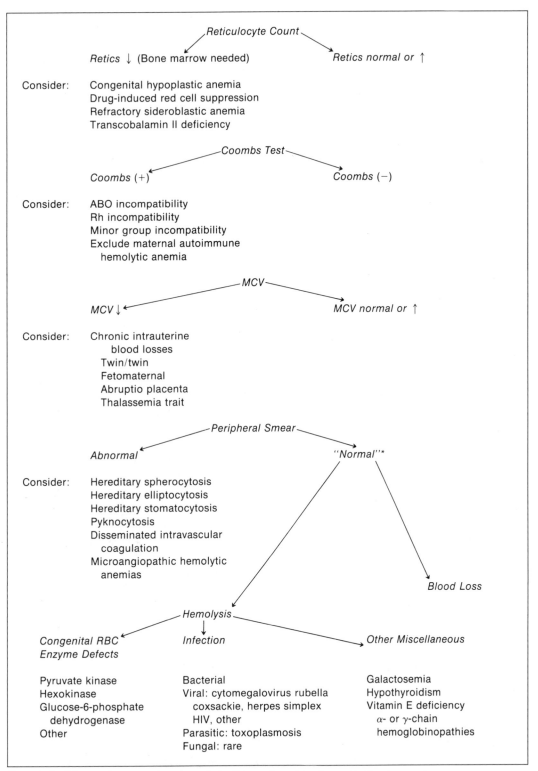

**Figure 7-7** Diagnostic approach to anemia in the newborn based on reticulocyte count.
Modified from Oski FA: The erythrocyte and its disorders. In Nathan DG, Oski FA, eds: *Hematology of Infancy and Childhood*, 3rd ed. Philadelphia, WB Saunders Co, 1987, p. 38. Modified with permission of W.B. Saunders Company.
* Indicates a peripheral blood smear with no specifically diagnostic abnormalities.

**Table 7-10** Types of Hemorrhage in the Newborn

*Obstetric accidents, malformations of the placenta and cord*------------------------------------------

Rupture of a normal umbilical cord
   Precipitous delivery
   Entanglement
Hematoma of the cord or placenta
Rupture of an abnormal umbilical cord
   Varices
   Aneurysm
Rupture of anomalous vessels
   Aberrant vessel
   Velamentous insertion
   Communicating vessels in multilobed placenta
Incision of placenta during cesarean section
Placenta previa
Abruptio placentae

*Occult hemorrhage prior to birth*------------------------

Fetoplacental
   Tight nuchal cord
   Cesarean section
   Placental hematoma
Fetomaternal
   Traumatic amniocentesis
   Following external cephalic version, manual
     removal of placenta, use of oxytocin
   Spontaneous
   Chorioangioma of the placenta
   Choriocarcinoma
Twin-to-twin
   Chronic
   Acute

*Internal hemorrhage*-------------------------------------

Intracranial
Giant cephalohematoma, subgaleal, caput
   succedaneum
Adrenal
Retroperitoneal
Ruptured liver, ruptured spleen
Pulmonary

*Iatrogenic blood loss*-------------------------------------

Source: Modified from Oski FA: Anemia in the neonatal period. In Oski FA, Naiman JL, eds: *Hematologic Problems in the Newborn*, 3rd ed. Philadelphia, WB Saunders Co, 1982, p. 57. Modified with permission of W.B. Saunders Company.

pected, these infants develop a microcytic form of anemia similar to older children and adults. Although microcytosis due to iron deficiency is unusual in the newborn period, it can occur. Note that most infants with chronic blood loss are quite vigorous despite the presence of profound pallor.

All infants born with microcytic indices should have further evaluation for intrauterine blood loss. A diagnosis of fetomaternal hemorrhage may be made by any one of sev-

eral techniques, the most common procedure being the acid-elution method (the Kleihauer-Betke technique), which identifies cells containing fetal hemoglobin in the maternal circulation. After the maternal blood smear is stained, the number of cells containing fetal hemoglobin can be counted, permitting a rough estimate of the degree of hemorrhage that has occurred. The acid-elution technique can be relied on with certainty for diagnosis only when other conditions capable of producing elevations in maternal fetal hemoglobin levels are absent. Thus, in the presence of maternal thalassemia minor, sickle-cell anemia, or hereditary persistence of fetal hemoglobin, other techniques based on differential agglutination may be needed to detect fetal cells in the maternal circulation. In addition, remember that the maternal concentration of fetal hemoglobin normally increases during pregnancy. Finally, the diagnosis of a fetomaternal hemorrhage may be missed in situations in which the mother and infant are incompatible in the ABO or Rh blood group systems. In such instances, the infant's A, B, or Rh positive cells are rapidly cleared from the maternal circulation by maternal anti A, anti B, or anti D antibody and, therefore, are unavailable for staining.

A search for fetomaternal hemorrhage should be made in all anemic newborn infants in whom no previous blood loss has occurred and in whom isoimmunization has been excluded. As noted previously, it is important to exclude a maternal-infant blood group incompatibility by determining the ABO/Rh blood types of the mother and child and performing a direct Coombs test on the infant's cells. This information will permit the interpretation of tests such as the Kleihauer-Betke that are used to diagnose chronic or acute intrauterine blood loss.

If blood loss is excluded as a cause of microcytosis in a newborn infant, the infant is likely to have the $\alpha$-thalassemia trait. Alpha-thalassemia syndromes are particularly common in individuals of Oriental background and can also be observed in black infants. Indeed, the most common cause of microcytosis in a newborn black infant is the $\alpha$-thalassemia trait. In the absence of blood loss, a black infant with an MCV of less than 95 fL can be assumed to have the $\alpha$-thalassemia trait. Such infants are rarely anemic and are diagnosed only by the presence of a low MCV.

In a patient who has a normal or elevated reticulocyte count, in whom the Coombs test is negative, and in whom the MCV is *not* decreased, the peripheral blood smear becomes extremely helpful in the diagnostic approach to anemia. In this circumstance, the peripheral blood smear will either be abnormal or normal. *Normal* refers to a peripheral blood smear that does not demonstrate a particular morphological abnormality suggestive of a specific diagnosis. Examples of *abnormal* peripheral blood smears include those showing evidence of spherocytes, elliptocytes, stomatocytes, pyknocytes, or red cells affected by a microangiopathic process. Such abnormal blood smears should lead you toward a specific confirmatory test for these disorders.

If the peripheral blood smear is normal (in the presence of a normal or elevated MCV and a negative Coombs test), you should pursue the possibility of acute blood loss (Table 7-10) or a nonimmune hemolytic anemia. Acute blood loss will not result in microcytosis because it does not cause iron deficiency. If acute blood loss is not a likely possibility, the various causes of hemolysis must be sought.

The causes of hemolytic anemia in an infant are extremely varied and are usually divided into extrinsic or intrinsic RBC disorders. Isoimmunization, drugs and toxins, infections, and disseminated intravascular coagulation are common causes of *extrinsic* hemolytic anemias. *Intrinsic* RBC disorders are generally caused by enzymatic defects of the red cell, hemoglobin abnormalities (structural or synthetic defects), or defects of the red cell membrane. The various causes of hemolytic disease in the newborn are listed in Table 7-11. The detailed evaluation of the many varied causes of hemolytic anemia in the newborn period is beyond the scope of this chapter. The reader is referred to any one of several textbooks of hematology (listed in the references) dealing with infancy and childhood.

The clinician will often find the infant who has an anemia in association with a non-specific peripheral blood smear to be most challenging. In this instance, the presence of jaundice or splenomegaly is an important consideration in formulating a differential diagnosis. The significantly jaundiced infant or the infant with splenomegaly is unlikely to have external blood loss as a cause of anemia and is more likely to have one of the varieties of hemolytic anemia.

**Table 7-11**   Causes of Hemolytic Disease in the Newborn

*Isoimmunization (erythroblastosis fetalis) enzymatic deficiencies of the red cell*‒‒‒‒‒‒‒‒‒‒‒‒‒‒‒‒‒‒

Glycolytic enzymes
  Hexokinase
  Glucose phosphate isomerase
  Phosphofructokinase
  Aldolase
  Triose phosphate isomerase
  2,3-DPG mutase
  Phosphoglycerate kinase
  Pyruvate kinase
  Glucose-6-phosphate dehydrogenase
  Galactose-1-phosphate uridyltransferase
    deficiency-galactosemia
Nonglycolytic enzymes
  Glutathione peroxidase
  Glutathione synthetase
  γ-glutamylcysteine synthetase
  ATPase
  Adenylate kinase
  Adenosine deaminase
  Pyrimidine-5'-nucleotidase
Drugs and Toxins
  Heinz body anemia

*Defects characterized by abnormalities of red cell morphology*‒‒‒‒‒‒‒‒‒‒‒‒‒‒‒‒‒‒‒‒‒‒‒‒‒‒‒‒‒‒‒‒‒‒‒‒‒‒‒‒‒

Cell membrane disorders
  Hereditary spherocytosis
  Hereditary elliptocytosis
  Hereditary stomatocytosis
  Infantile pyknocytosis
  Pyropoikilocytosis
Infections
  Bacterial
  Viral (cytomegalic inclusion disease, hepatitis)
  Toxoplasmosis
  Syphilis
Defects in Hemoglobin Synthesis
  Hemoglobin barts (α-thalassemia)
  Unstable hemoglobins (congenital Heinz body anemias)
Miscellaneous
  Erythropoietic porphyria
  Disseminated intravascular coagulation

*Source:* Modified from Oski FA: Disorders of red cell metabolism. In Oski FA, Naiman JL, eds: *Hematologic Problems in the Newborn*, 3rd ed. Philadelphia, WB Saunders Co, 1982, p. 98. Modified with permission of W.B. Saunders Company.

## CASE STUDIES

With the background information provided, you should now be able to evaluate the six case studies presented in Table 7-1. Each case study was carefully selected to illustrate a specific point concerning the developmental hematology of the newborn infant or to apply the principles of the approach to anemia in the newborn as outlined. Each case study will be discussed separately, but taken together they present a spectrum of the various causes of anemia that present during the neonatal period.

## EXERCISE

*Please carefully review each set of data from Table 7-1 at this point. Determine what additional information would be helpful and formulate a differential diagnosis.*

### ■ Discussion of Case Study 1:

You should conclude that Case Study 1 is an example of a perfectly healthy term neonate with normal age-appropriate hematologic values. Because this infant is already 6 hours old, his hemoglobin concentration already reflects the consequences of a placental transfusion. By age 6 hours, hemoconcentration has already taken place and you should expect to see the maximal postnatal hemoglobin values. In the case of infant 1, a hemoglobin of 17.1 g/dL is near the mean value of normal, as are the values for MCV, the MCH, the RBC count, and the RDW.

The observation that this infant has 10 NRBCs on peripheral smear at this age is expected as is the mild reticulocytosis. The mild anisocytosis and poikilocytosis are commonly observed on the peripheral blood smear in an infant of this age.

Last, it is quite normal to be able to palpate the spleen tip easily in a neonate. Thus, finding a spleen tip that is palpable 0.5 cm below the left costal margin would not be remarkable in itself.

Because all the hematologic data in this infant appear within normal limits and the infant appears otherwise well, no other studies are needed and the diagnosis is that of a normal infant.

### ■ Answer:

What other studies are needed?   None

Diagnosis?   Normal infant

### ■ Discussion of Case Study 2:

This is an interesting infant. Following a term gestation and delivery by cesarean section, Baby 2 rapidly became pale and tachycardic and exhibited diminished pulses.

In this case, the differential diagnosis includes those disorders capable of causing pallor in the immediate newborn period. More careful questioning of the obstetrician indicates that infant 2 had a tight nuchal cord at the time of delivery by cesarean section. Infants with tight nuchal cords can develop profound hypovolemia during labor and delivery because of compression of the umbilical vein and inhibition of blood flow from the placenta to the infant. The umbilical arteries, in contrast, are not readily compressible because of their differing anatomy and more rigid structure.

Furthermore, blood is delivered through the umbilical arteries under much higher systolic and diastolic pressures. Therefore, during deliveries in which cord compression occurs, an infant can literally exsanguinate through the umbilical arteries into the placenta, at the same time demonstrating poor venous return (from the umbilical vein). These infants will appear pale with thready pulses and a tachycardia.

By the time the infant is 30 minutes of age, there has not been sufficient time to experience a fall in hemoglobin concentration, which can result only from reexpansion of the plasma volume (either from fluids given intravenously or from the transfer of fluid from the extravascular space). *Because the hemoglobin level itself is unremarkable, it does not assist the clinician in detecting the etiology of the pallor.* In this situation, you must recognize that the infant's clinical signs and symptoms are consistent with hypovolemic shock.

Table 7-12 provides an approach to the differential diagnosis of pallor in the neonate. Any cause of acute prepartum or intrapartum hemorrhage can present with a similar clinical picture and should be easily distinguishable from the causes of chronic blood loss (Table 7-13). One clue that this infant was not normal hematologically was the markedly elevated NRBC count, which indicates either early compensation in response to hypovolemia or a response to tissue hypoxia resulting from the shock-like state. After a clinical diagnosis of acute blood loss is made in infant 2, this infant should receive volume expansion. With adequate reconstitution of the plasma volume, the true fall in hemoglobin and hematocrit will become evident.

### ■ Answer:

What other studies are needed?   Quantify fetal cells in maternal circulation

Diagnosis?   Acute blood loss

**Table 7-12**  Differential Diagnosis of Pallor in the Newborn

| ASPHYXIA | ACUTE SEVERE BLOOD LOSS | HEMOLYTIC DISEASE |
|---|---|---|
| 1. Respiratory findings: retractions, response to oxygen, cyanosis | 1. Decrease in venous and arterial pressure | 1. Hepatosplenomegaly, jaundice |
| 2. Moribund appearance | 2. Rapid shallow respirations | 2. Positive Coombs test |
| 3. Bradycardia | 3. Acyanotic | 3. Anemia |
| 4. Stable hemoglobin | 4. Tachycardia | |
| | 5. Drop in hemoglobin | |

*Source:* Adapted from Kirkman HN, Riley HD Jr: Differential diagnosis of anemia in the newborn. *Pediatrics* 1959; 24:97. Adapted by permission of *Pediatrics*, vol. 24, page 97, copyright 1959.

### ■ Discussion of Case Study 3:

Infant 3 is a 2-day-old black male, delivered following a full-term gestation, who has hemoglobin and hematocrit values that are within normal ranges. The bilirubin level of 4.3 mg% is well within the limits of normal for his age. In fact, only one abnormality is found among this infant's laboratory data; the low value for MCV.

A black newborn infant with microcytosis has the $\alpha$-thalassemia trait until proven otherwise because the likelihood of iron deficiency at this age is relatively remote. Unlike $\alpha$-thalassemia, $\beta$-thalassemia trait does not produce abnormalities in red cell indices at birth because $\beta$-globin chain production is not suffi-

ciently developed in comparison to $\gamma$-globin chain production. Therefore, neither structural defects of the $\beta$-chain (such as sickle-cell anemia) nor synthetic defects in production (such as the $\beta$-thalassemia syndromes) would normally be apparent at birth.

Some clinicians have suggested that all black neonates should have a complete blood count (which includes RBC indices) in order to detect the presence of the $\alpha$-thalassemia trait. Because the differential diagnosis of microcytosis at this age is principally that of the $\alpha$-thalassemia trait, the newborn period is clearly the best time of life to establish this diagnosis. Beyond a few months of life, iron deficiency is a much more common cause of

**Table 7-13**  Characteristics of Acute and Chronic Blood Loss in the Newborn

| CHARACTERISTIC | ACUTE BLOOD LOSS | CHRONIC BLOOD LOSS |
|---|---|---|
| Clinical | Acute distress; pallor; shallow, rapid, and often irregular respiration; tachycardia; weak or absent peripheral pulses; low or absent blood pressure; no hepatosplenomegaly | Marked pallor disproportionate to evidence of distress; on occasion signs of congestive heart failure may be present, including hepatomegaly |
| Venous pressure | Low | Normal or elevated |
| Laboratory | | |
|   Hemoglobin concentration | May be normal initially then drops quickly during first 24 hours of life | Low at birth |
|   Red cell morphology | Normochromic and macrocytic | Hypochromic and microcytic Anisocytosis and poikilocytosis |
|   Serum iron | Normal at birth | Low at birth |
| Course | Prompt treatment of anemia and shock necessary to prevent death | Generally uneventful |
| Treatment | Intravenous fluids and whole blood; iron therapy later | Iron therapy; packed red cells may be necessary on occasion |

*Source:* Modified from Oski FA: Anemia in the neonatal period. In Oski FA, Naiman JL, eds: *Hematologic Problems in the Newborn*, 3rd ed. Philadelphia, WB Saunders Co, 1982, p. 62. Modified with permission of W.B. Saunders Company.

microcytosis. The "early" diagnosis of the α-thalassemia trait is particularly important for the older infant or child because the presence of microcytosis later in life is frequently equated with the diagnosis of iron deficiency. In fact, some individuals with the α-thalassemia trait have been incorrectly treated with iron for years, occasionally to the point of hemosiderosis. In addition, the α-thalassemia trait is a more difficult diagnosis to establish in the older infant or child because it requires the exclusion of iron deficiency. The hemoglobin electrophoresis in the α-thalassemia trait is normal (unlike the β-thalassemia trait in the older infant or child in whom an elevation of hemoglobin $A_2$ and/or hemoglobin F would be suggestive or confirmatory). Therefore, it is much simpler (and potentially important) to make this diagnosis by the observation of a low MCV in the newborn period.

Alpha-thalassemia syndromes are relatively common in black infants. The α-thalassemia syndromes are gene deletion disorders, involving up to four genes. Four genes are necessary to make the total complement of α-globin. Twenty-eight percent of black children and adults lack a single gene. This condition is known as the silent carrier state of α-thalassemia. The silent carrier state is not detectable by any routine laboratory study. A two-gene deletion state, seen in about 3% of American blacks, is known as the α-thalassemia trait (i.e., the diagnosis in Case Study 3). A three-gene deletion disorder is known as hemglobin H disease, which results in the production of large quantities of γ-chains unpaired with α-globin chains (Bart's hemoglobin). The four-gene deletion state causes hydrops fetalis and is incompatible with life.

Table 7-14 highlights the clinical and laboratory features of the α-thalassemia syndromes at birth and in later life.

With respect to Case Study 3, no other studies are needed at this time to confirm the diagnosis of the α-thalassemia trait.

### ■ Answer:

What other studies are needed?   None

Diagnosis?   Alpha-thalassemia trait

### ■ Discussion of Case Study 4:

This infant, although born prematurely, had normal hematologic values at birth. Within 2 weeks, the hemoglobin concentration had fallen dramatically as a consequence of repeated phlebotomy for laboratory blood sampling. This initial anemia is known as the early anemia of prematurity and often requires transfusion.

Later, however (usually between 4 and 8 weeks of age), a secondary period of anemia develops. In infant 4, the hemoglobin has declined to 7.5 g/dL. This latter anemia is known as the true *anemia of prematurity*. As noted in Figure 7-4, hemoglobin values as low as 7 g/dL are not uncommon in such low birth weight infants. Additionally an MCV of 89 is appropriate for an infant of this age and is consistent with the normal decline in MCV.

With few exceptions, infants born prematurely will experience a decline in hemoglobin concentration during the first 1 to 3 months of life. Although this decline also occurs in term infants (at approximately the same postgestational age), the magnitude of the decline in preterm infants is remarkably greater and may, in fact, be seen earlier. The actual decline may be so great as to raise concern regarding the need for transfusion. In contrast with the situation in older children and adults, the indications for transfusion in the nursery setting are not well defined. Indeed, many infants seem to tolerate remarkably low levels of hemoglobin concentration with no clinical difficulties. This is the origin of the frequently used term *physiological anemia of prematurity*. Nonetheless, some infants will manifest a variety of signs and symptoms of anemia, including apnea and bradycardia, tachycardia, poor weight gain, and pallor.

Plasma erythropoietin levels have recently been established to be relatively low in preterm infants with physiological anemia of prematurity during these early weeks of life. This suggests that these infants may not respond appropriately to decreasing levels of hemoglobin. Historically, infants who develop signs or symptoms in association with the late anemia of prematurity have been transfused. It is possible that with the availability of recombinant erythropoietin, this agent may become an alternative to transfusion for some of these infants.

### ■ Answer:

What other studies are needed?   None

Diagnosis?   Anemia of prematurity

**Table 7-14** Features of α-Thalassemia Syndromes

| SYNDROME | CLINICAL FEATURES | | HEMOGLOBIN PATTERN | | $B : x$ RATIO | NUMBER OF GENES AFFECTED BY THAT MUTATION |
|---|---|---|---|---|---|---|
| | BIRTH | LATER LIFE | BIRTH | LATER LIFE | | |
| Silent carrier | No anemia or microcytosis | No anemia or microcytosis | 1%–2% Hgb Bart's | Normal | S.I. > 1 | 1 |
| Thalassemia trait | Mild anemia and microcytosis | Mild anemia and microcytosis | 3%–10% Hgb Bart's | Normal | 1.2 : 1 | 2 |
| Hb H disease | Moderate microcytic hypochromic hemolytic anemia | Same | 20%–40% Hgb Bart's | 5%–30% Hb H | 2.5 : 1 | 3 |
| Fetal hydrops syndrome | Moderate to severe hypochromic microcytic anemia | Lethal | ~80% Hgb Bart's 0–20% Hgb H Small amount of Hgb Portland | — | x | 4 |

*Source:* From Oski FA, Naiman JL, eds: *Hematologic Problems in the Newborn,* 3rd ed. Philadelphia, WB Saunders Co, 1982, p. 266. Reprinted with permission of W.B. Saunders Company.

145

■ **Discussion of Case Study 5:**

The 3-day-old female, infant 5, demonstrates several hematologic abnormalities. Her hemoglobin concentration is just below the lower limit of normal for a full-term baby. Her reticulocyte count is very slightly elevated when adjusted for age. The same is true of her nucleated RBC count. In addition a modest elevation in the RDW is suggestive of some variation in the size and shape of the RBCs on the peripheral blood smear.

These hematologic findings (in association with a positive family history for gallstones and an abnormal elevation in the serum bilirubin concentration) suggest that this infant is experiencing a hemolytic anemia.

This child's problem can be approached in any one of several ways. Table 7-15 lists the causes of jaundice in the first week of life. Given the laboratory abnormalities, the degree of hyperbilirubinemia, the age of the infant and the well being of the infant, it is unlikely that this infant has any cause for the hyperbilirubinemia other than a hemolytic disorder.

The peripheral smear in infant 5 demonstrates occasional spherocytes. The presence of these spherocytes was predicted based on an abnormality in the MCHC (a value of 38 is significantly elevated). As discussed previously, an elevated MCHC is seen in relatively few disorders, one of which is hereditary spherocytosis. This child was ultimately determined to have a negative Coombs test, which lessened the probability of ABO incompatibility (another cause of spherocytes on peripheral blood smears). For this reason, the most likely cause of this infant's hemolytic anemia would be hereditary spherocytosis.

Confirmation of a diagnosis of hereditary spherocytosis is made by a determination of the osmotic fragility of the infant's red blood cells. Note that under normal circumstances neonatal red cells have an increased osmotic resistance. When an osmotic fragility is obtained in a neonate, reference values for neonatal osmotic fragility curves should be used. It should also be emphasized that erythrocytes in other hemolytic states may demonstrate a similar abnormality in osmotic fragility, so a positive diagnosis of hereditary spherocytosis should *never* be made by this means alone. Any cell that is spherocytic may have increased osmotic fragility. For this reason, some confusion may exist between the abnormal osmotic fragilities seen with ABO incom-

**Table 7-15** Causes of Jaundice During the First Week of Life

*Hemolytic diseases* ----------------------------------------

Erythroblastosis fetalis: Rh or ABO incompatibility, etc.
Inherited red cell defects
    Hereditary spherocytosis
    Enzyme deficiencies (±drugs); glucose-6-phosphate dehydrogenase, pyruvate kinase, etc.
    Drugs and toxins: vitamin $K_3$ (excessive doses), naphthalene (moth balls), oxytocin

*Infections* ------------------------------------------------

Bacterial: sepsis, congenital syphilis
Viral: cytomegalic inclusion disease, disseminated herpes simplex, congenital rubella syndrome, echovirus 11
Protozoal: congenital toxoplasmosis

*Enclosed hemorrhage* ------------------------------------

*Polycythemia* --------------------------------------------

*Metabolic disorders* ------------------------------------

Galactosemia
Crigler-Najjar syndrome
Breast-milk jaundice
Transient familial neonatal hyperbilirubinemia
Hypothyroidism and hypopituitarism
α-1-antitrypsin deficiency
Infants of diabetic mothers

*Increased enterohepatic absorption* -------------------

Bile stasis due to restricted intake, upper GI obstruction
Swallowed blood

*Neonatal (giant-cell) hepatitis* --------------------------

*Physiological jaundice* ----------------------------------

*Miscellaneous* -------------------------------------------

Asphyxia
Reduced calorie intake

*Source:* Modified from Naiman JL: Erythroblastosis fetalis. In Oski FA, Naiman JL, eds: *Hematologic Problems in the Newborn*, 3rd ed. Philadelphia, WB Saunders Co, 1982, p. 294. Modified with permission of W.B. Saunders Company.

patibility in comparison with those noted in hereditary spherocytosis. Further testing may be necessary to distinguish these two disorders. Generally, the autohemolysis test is abnormal in both hereditary spherocytosis and ABO incompatibility. The increased autohemolysis of hereditary spherocytosis, however, can be reduced by the addition of glucose (glucose has no beneficial effect in infants with hemolytic disease as a consequence of ABO incompatibility). Thus an infant with a hemolytic anemia and spherocytes on the peripheral blood smear can be distinguished by the use of the autohemolysis test. The differentiation between hereditary spherocytosis and ABO incompatibility, however, may sometimes be problematic, particularly in the infant whose Coombs reaction is either negative or so weakly positive as to not suggest ABO incompatibility. Table 7-16 illustrates the distinguishing characteristics between ABO incompatibility and hereditary spherocytosis.

### ■ Answer:

What other studies are needed?   Osmotic fragility

Diagnosis?   Hereditary spherocytosis

### ■ Discussion of Case Study 6:

Severely anemic newborn 6 was born with hydrops fetalis. In the evaluation of any anemic newborn infant, maternal and fetal blood group typing and Coombs testing of the newborn would be performed. With this information, the cause of the hydrops fetalis can be immediately divided into immune and nonimmune causes. Table 7-17 presents the differential diagnosis of nonimmune hydrops fetalis. In the case of infant 6, the blood type of the mother was A⁻ and that of the baby A⁺. The direct Coombs test was positive with the baby's cells. This mother had not received prenatal care and had become sensitized in an earlier pregnancy to the Rh antigen system. The baby, therefore, represents a case of alloimmune hemolytic anemia, a cause of immune-associated hydrops fetalis. The antibody was defined as anti D antibody, representing the most common form of alloimmune sensitization.

Under ordinary circumstances, routine blood samples are sent for testing at the first prenatal visit for each pregnant woman. If she is Rh negative and already Rh sensitized (presence of Rh antibodies in the serum), antibody specificity and titers are determined. Another sample is obtained at 18 weeks' gestation and approximately every 2 weeks thereafter (the interval is dependent on the antibody titer). A history of the clinical course of previous pregnancies is obtained and the zygosity of the husband for Rh antigen status is determined. Based on the past history and level of antibody titer, amniocentesis and amniotic fluid spectrophotometry are carried out. Figure 7-8 illustrates the amniotic fluid optical density spectrum reading by the Liley method in a typical infant with severe erythroblastosis. The optical density is proportionate to the degree of bilirubin pigment and bilirubin breakdown products and, therefore, to the degree of hemolytic anemia *in utero*. Significantly affected infants will require percutaneous umbilical cord blood sampling for determination of hemoglobin concentration. If the fetus is severely anemic, packed cells may be administered through the umbilical cord.

Infant 6, therefore, represents one end of a

**Table 7-16**   Comparison Between ABO and Rh Hemolytic Diseases of the Newborn

| CLINICAL PARAMETERS | ABO HEMOLYTIC DISEASE | Rh HEMOLYTIC DISEASE |
| --- | --- | --- |
| Value of maternal screening | None | Important |
| Subsequent pregnancies affected | Variable | Usually worse |
| Cord blood direct Coombs | + or − | ++ |
| Cord blood indirect Coombs | + or − | ++ |
| Cord hemoglobin | Normal | Normal or decreased |
| Blood-smear spherocytes | +++ | + |
| Hepatosplenomegaly | + or − | ++ |
| Jaundice | Variable | Severity predictable from early bilirubin rise |
| Prevention | None | RhoGAM administration to the mother during pregnancy or after birth of Rh⁺ infant |
| Early anemia | + or − | ++ |
| Late anemia | Rare | Common |

*Source:* Modified from Brown MS: Physiologic anemia of infancy: Nutritional factors and abnormal states. In Stockman JA III, Pochedly C, eds: *Developmental and Neonatal Hematology.* New York, Raven Press, 1988, p. 286. Modified with permission of Raven Press, Ltd.

**Table 7-17** Nonimmune Hydrops Fetalis
Causes and Associations

*Fetal*................................................................

Hematologic
  Homozygous α-thalassemia
  Chronic fetomaternal transfusion
  Twin-to-twin transfusion (recipient or donor)
  Multiple gestation with "parasitic" fetus
Cardiovascular
  Severe congenital heart disease (atrial septal
    defect, ventricular septal defect, hypoplastic
    left heart, pulmonary valve insufficiency,
    Ebstein's subaortic stenosis)
  Premature closure of foramen ovale
  Myocarditis
  Large arteriovenous malformation
  Tachyarrhythmias: paroxysmal supraventricular
    tachycardia (SVT), atrial flutter
  Bradyarrhythmias: heart block
  Fibroelastosis
Pulmonary
  Cystic adenomatoid malformation of lung
  Pulmonary lymphangiectasia
  Pulmonary hypoplasia (diaphragmatic hernia)
Renal
  Congenital nephrosis
  Renal vein thrombosis
Intrauterine infections
  Syphilis
  Toxoplasmosis
  Cytomegalovirus
  Leptospirosis
  Chagas disease
  Congenital hepatitis
Congenital anomalies
  Achondroplasia
  E trisomy
  Multiple anomalies
  Turner's syndrome
Miscellaneous
  Meconium peritonitis
  Fetal neuroblastomatosis
  Dysmaturity
  Tuberous sclerosis
  Storage disease
  Small bowel volvulus
Placental
  Umbilical vein thrombosis
  Chorionic vein thrombosis
  Chorioangioma
Maternal
  Diabetes mellitus
  Toxemia
Idiopathic

*Source:* From Etchers PC, Lemons JA: Nonimmune hydrops. *Pediatrics* 1979; 64:326. Reproduced by permission of *Pediatrics*, vol. 64, page 326, copyright 1979.

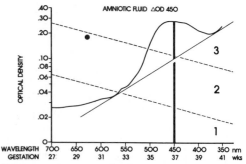

**Figure 7-8** Amniotic fluid spectrophotometric reading by means of the Liley method: $\Delta OD_{450}$ (0.200 in this example) falls high in zone II at 29.5 weeks of gestation, indicating severe Rh erythroblastosis.

Modified from Bowman JM: Haemolytic disease of the newborn, Vol 19 Part IV. In Robertson NRC, ed: *A Textbook of Neonatology.* Edinburgh, Churchill Livingstone, 1986, pp. 469–483. Modified with permission of Churchill Livingstone.

molytic anemia. Unlike Rh disease, ABO incompatibility is seen as often as not during a first pregnancy. There is no way to predict severity for ABO incompatibility in subsequent pregnancies; whereas, each subsequently affected fetus with Rh disease is generally more severely compromised. Infant 6 is unlikely to have ABO incompatibility simply based on the fact that the baby was severely anemic and hydropic, two very unusual circumstances with ABO incompatibility. Unlike infants with Rh disease, those affected in the ABO system may have weakly positive or negative Coombs tests. Spherocytes are seen frequently with ABO incompatibility, but rarely with Rh disease. Table 7-18 also describes the differences in management for infants with Rh disease and those with ABO incompatibility.

■ **Answer:**

Diagnosis?   Rh incompatibility

## SUMMARY

A careful review of these six cases presents a spectrum of red cell abnormalities in newborns, ranging from a normal infant (Case Study 1), an infant who is not anemic but who, in fact, has had a severe hemorrhage (Case Study 2), an infant who also is not anemic but who by virtue of a low MCV was readily diagnosed in the newborn period as having the α-thalassemia trait (Case Study 3), a 6-week-old preterm infant with the typical physiological

spectrum of alloimmunization of a fetus *in utero*. The most common causes of alloimmune hemolytic anemia are ABO and Rh incompatibility. Table 7-18 compares the laboratory and clinical aspects of Rh alloimmune hemolytic anemia and ABO alloimmune he-

**Table 7-18**  Comparison of Rh and ABO Incompatibility

| | Rh | ABO |
|---|---|---|
| Blood group setup | | |
|   Mother | Negative | O |
|   Infant | Positive | A or B |
| Type of antibody | Incomplete (IgG) | Immune (IgG) |
| Clinical aspects | | |
|   Occurrence in firstborn | 5% | 40%–50% |
|   Predictable severity in subsequent pregnancies | Usually | No |
|   Stillbirth and/or hydrops | Frequent | Rare |
|   Severe anemia | Frequent | Rare |
|   Degree of jaundice | +++ | + |
|   Hepatosplenomegaly | +++ | + |
| Laboratory findings | | |
|   Direct Coombs test (infant) | + | (+) or O |
|   Maternal antibodies | Always present | Not clear-cut |
|   Spherocytes | 0 | + |
| Treatment | | |
|   Need for antenatal measures | Yes | No |
|   Value of phototherapy | Limited | Great |
|   Exchange transfusion | | |
|     Frequency | Approx. 2/3 | Approx. 1% |
|     Donor blood type | Rh negative | Rh same as infant |
| | Group-specific, when possible | Group O only |
| Incidence of late anemia | Common | Rare |

*Source:* Modified from Naiman JL: Erythroblastosis fetalis. In Oski FA, Naiman JL, eds: *Hematologic Problems in the Newborn* 3rd ed. Philadelphia, WB Saunders Co, 1982, p. 333. Modified with permission of W.B. Saunders Company.

anemia of prematurity (Case Study 4), an infant with a congenital hemolytic anemia, prototypical of other nonimmune hemolytic anemias (Case Study 5), and, finally, to a typical case of Rh hemolytic anemia in a newborn (Case Study 6).

A knowledge of what is normal and an orderly approach to diagnosis should enable you to institute management techniques quickly where needed in such infants. Because an infant's clinical condition can rapidly change, a working knowledge of how to approach anemia at this age can often prevent more serious problems from occurring.

**BIBLIOGRAPHY**

1. Stockman JA III, Pochedly C, eds: *Developmental and Neonatal Hematology. Pediatric Hematology/Oncology Series.* New York, Raven Press, 1988.
2. Rodeck CH, Nicholaides KH, Warsof SL, et al: The management of severe rhesus isoimmunization by fetoscopic intravascular transfusions. *Am J Obstet Gynecol* 1984; 150:769–774.
3. Bowman JM, Manning FA: Intrauterine fetal transfusions. Winnipeg 1982. *Obstet Gynecol* 1983; 61:203–209.
4. Bowman JM: Haemolytic disease of the newborn, V 19 Part IV. In Robertson NRC, ed: *A Textbook of Neonatology.* Edinburgh, Churchill Livingstone, 1986, pp. 469–483.
5. Rudolph N, Preis O, Bitzos EI, et al: Hematologic and selenium status of low-birth-weight infants fed formulas with and without iron. *J Pediatr* 1981; 99:57–62.
6. Saarinen UM: Need for iron supplementation in infants on prolonged breast feeding. *J Pediatr* 1978; 93:177–180.
7. Zaizov R, Matoth Y: Red cell values on the first postnatal day during the last 16 weeks of gestation. *Am J Hematol* 1976; 1:275–278.
8. Matoth Y, Zaizov R, Varsano I: Postnatal changes in some red cell parameters. *Acta Paediatr Scand* 1971; 60:317–323.
9. Saarinen UM, Siimes MA: Developmental changes in serum iron, total iron-binding capacity, and transferrin saturation in infancy. *J Pediatr* 1977; 91:875–877.
10. Kanto WP, Marino B, Goodwin AS, et al: ABO hemolytic disease: A comparative study of clinical severity and delayed anemia. *Pediatrics* 1978; 62:365–369.
11. Baumann R, Rubin H: Autoimmune hemolytic anemia during pregnancy with hemolytic disease in the newborn. *Blood* 1973; 41:293–297.
12. Stockman JA III: Physical properties of the neonatal red blood cell. In Stockman JA III, Pochedly C, eds: *Developmental and Neonatal Hematology.* New York, Raven Press, 1988, pp. 297–323.
13. Schmaier AH, Maurer HM: Alpha-thalassemia screening in neonates by mean corpuscular volume and mean corpuscular hemoglobin concentration. *J Pediatr* 1983; 83:794.

14. Stockman JA III, Oski FA: Red blood cell values in low birth weight infants during the first seven weeks of life. *Am J Dis Child* 1980; 134:945.

15. Zipursky A, Brown E, Palko J, et al: The erythrocyte differential count in the newborn infant. *Am J Pediatr Hematol Oncol* 1983; 5:45.

16. Holyrode CP, Oski FA, Gardner FH: The "pocked" erythrocyte. *N Engl J Med* 1969; 281:516.

17. Schröter W, Kahsnitz E: Diagnosis of hereditary spherocytosis in newborn infants. *J Pediatr* 1983; 103:460.

18. Stockman JA III: Principles of electronic red blood cell counting: Helpful clues to the interpretation of data. *The Child's Doctor* 1991; 8:4–11.

19. Bessman JD, Gilmer PR, Gardner FH: Classification of red cell disorders by MCV and RDW. *Am J Clin Pathol* 1983; 80:322.

20. Cox CJ, Habermann TM, Payne BA, et al: Evaluation of the Coulter Counter Model S-Plus IV. *Am J Clin Pathol* 1985; 84:297.

21. Meloni T, Solinas L, Erre S, et al: The unreliability of mean corpuscular volume and mean cellular hemoglobin determinations in the diagnosis of α-thalassemia in newborn infants. *Eur J Pediatr* 1980; 135:165.

22. Andrews BF, Thompson JW: Materno-fetal transfusion. A common phenomenon. *Pediatrics* 1962; 29:500.

23. Dannon Y, Kleinman A, Canon D: The osmotic fragility and density distribution of erythrocytes in the newborn. *Acta Haemat* 1970; 43:242.

24. Garn SM, Shaw HA, McCabe KD: Effect of maternal smoking on hemoglobins and hematocrits of the newborn. *Am J Clin Nutr* 1978; 31:557.

25. Lanzkowsky P: Effects of early and late clamping of umbilical cord on infant's hemoglobin level. *Br Med J* 1980; 2:1777.

26. Luzzatto L, Esan GJF, Ogiemudia SE: The osmotic fragility of red cells in newborns and infants. *Acta Haemat* 1970; 43:248.

27. Marsh WL, Allen FH Jr: Erythrocyte blood groups in humans. In Nathan DG, Oski FA, eds: *Hematology of Infancy and Childhood*, 2nd ed. Philadelphia, WB Saunders Co, 1981, pp. 1411–1437.

28. Pearson HA, McIntosh S, Rooks Y, et al: Interference phase microscopic enumeration of pitted RBC and splenic hypofunction in sickle cell anemia. *Pediatr Res* 1978; 12:471.

29. Zipursky A: The erythrocytes of the newborn infant. *Semin Hematol* 1965; 2:167.

30. Zipursky A: Erythrocyte morphology in newborn infants. A new look. *Pediatr Res* 1977; 11:843.

31. Zipursky A, Chintu C, Brown E, et al: The quantitation of spherocytes in ABO hemolytic disease. *J Pediatr* 1979; 94:965.

32. Oski FA, Naiman JL, eds: *Hematologic Problems in the Newborn*, 3rd ed. Philadelphia, WB Saunders Co, 1982.

# Chapter 8

# RESPIRATORY

# DISTRESS SYNDROME

*Alan R. Spitzer,* M.D.

*John Stefano,* M.D.

The maturation of the lung is a primary concern for the physician responsible for the care of the newborn infant. Although the past two decades have produced many advances in our understanding and the treatment of lung disease, respiratory distress syndrome (RDS) remains the leading cause of neonatal morbidity and mortality. The purpose of this chapter is to review lung development, the pathophysiology of RDS, and the clinical problems associated with this disease in order to provide the neonatologist, neonatal nurse practitioner, pediatrician, family physician, and obstetrician with the fundamental information necessary to manage this common problem. You are asked to attempt to answer the questions throughout the chapter prior to reading the descriptive text. These questions introduce the topics to be covered and enable you to determine adequacy of knowledge in each area. The answers for each of the questions are provided at the end of each exercise.

## DEVELOPMENT OF THE LUNG

Throughout fetal life, the placenta acts as the organ of gas exchange. After birth, a complex series of changes must occur in the lungs and the circulation so that the processes of oxygen uptake and carbon dioxide elimination can be initiated. The capacity for such gas transfer within the lungs and the ultimate viability of the baby are directly related to the degree of lung maturation present at birth. The infant with inadequate lung development will usu-

ally demonstrate the clinical signs of RDS. Thus, an understanding of the process of fetal lung maturation is essential if one is to treat RDS appropriately.

### EXERCISE 1

#### ■ Questions:

1. Which of the following statements regarding the timing of fetal lung development is true?
   (a) Fetal lung development can be divided into glandular, canalicular, saccular, and alveolar stages.
   (b) Alveolar development begins at approximately 36 weeks' gestation.
   (c) Surface active phospholipids are not produced until 36 weeks' gestation.
2. The adequacy of gas exchange in the lung is the principal determinant of extrauterine fetal viability. Select the minimal gestational age at which the lungs are mature enough to permit efficient exchange of oxygen and carbon dioxide.
   (a) 20 weeks
   (b) 22 weeks
   (c) 24 weeks
   (d) 26 weeks

#### ■ Discussion:

Prior to approximately 23 to 24 weeks of gestation, airway and capillary proliferation are insufficient for gas exchange. As a result, this gestational age remains the lower limit of viability for the human neonate at the present time. The development of the lung begins in the 24- to 25-day-old embryo as an outpouching of the gut (Fig. 8-1). Within 2 days, primary branches appear and ultimately become the right and left mainstream bronchi. During the remainder of the first trimester, lung growth consists of further branching of the endodermal tube into surrounding mesenchyme. This period (8 to 16 weeks postconception) is referred to as the *glandular* or *pseudoglandular* stage of lung development. At approximately 16 weeks, the *canalicular* stage of lung development begins. During this stage, canalization of the primitive airways progresses. Throughout this stage, the terminal air spaces are lined by simple cuboidal epithelium. At about 28 weeks of gestation, the penultimate stage of prenatal lung development (the *saccular* stage) begins. During this stage, preparation for air breathing occurs. The cuboidal epithelium begins to attenuate, connective tissue decreases, and capillaries proliferate in number, surrounding the terminal air spaces. Starting at 36 weeks, true alveoli begin to arise from alveolar ducts, and the potential for viability increases substantially.

Midway through the canalicular stage of lung development, at 18 to 20 weeks of gestation, two distinct types of cells can be distinguished in the terminal air spaces: a nonvacuolated cell similar to that found in other connective tissue (Type I cell) and a larger vacuolated cell containing lipoidal material (Type II cell). These latter cells can also be distinguished by cytoplasmic inclusion bodies, which appear concurrently with secretion of pulmonary surfactant. Macklin first suggested in 1954 that the Type II cell, or granular pneumonocyte, was a secretory cell, and subsequent studies have confirmed its role in the synthesis and secretion of surface-active phospholipids. The function of these materials at the alveolar lining layer is discussed later in the section under "Surface-Active materials in man."

Continued airway division, growth of the lung, and biochemical maturation proceeds steadily until birth. Lung growth, however, continues throughout childhood and into adulthood. As seen in Table 8-1, alveoli increase in number until approximately 8 years of age. After this time, although the alveolar

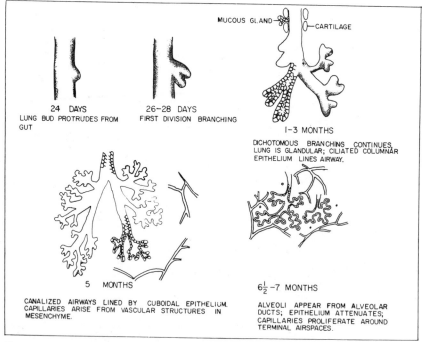

**Figure 8-1** Diagrammatic respresentation of the stages of lung development during gestation.
Adapted from Avery ME, Fletcher BD, Williams RG (eds): *The Lung and Its Disorders.* Philadelphia, WB Saunders Co, 1981, p. 5.

**Table 8-1**  The Effect of Age on Lung Size

| AGE | NUMBER OF ALVEOLI ($\times 10^8$) | NUMBER OF AIRWAYS ($\times 10^6$) | AIR-TISSUE INTERFACE ($m^2$) | BODY SURFACE AREA ($m^2$) |
|---|---|---|---|---|
| Birth | 24 | 1.5 | 2.8 | 0.21 |
| 3 months | 77 | 2.5 | 7.2 | 0.29 |
| 7 months | 112 | 3.7 | 8.4 | 0.38 |
| 13 months | 129 | 4.5 | 12.2 | 0.45 |
| 4 years | 257 | 7.9 | 22.2 | 0.67 |
| 8 years | 280 | 14.0 | 32.0 | 0.92 |
| Approximate fold-increase birth to adult | 10 | 10 | 21 | 9 |

*Source:* From Dunhill MS: Postnatal growth of the lung. *Thorax* 1962; 17:329. Reprinted with permission of the British Medical Association.

surface continues to expand, no increase in cell number occurs. It is very important for lung development to continue after birth, especially for the child who has had lung disease during the perinatal period. Whereas damaged portions of the lung may ultimately become fibrotic, healthy lung tissues can still subdivide, hypertrophy, and provide the infant with adequate surface area for gas exchange.

■ **Answers:**

1. a, b.

2. c.

## The Role of Surfactant

### EXERCISE 2

■ **Question:**

1. Which of the following statements regarding surfactant is true?
   (a) Surfactant is produced by Type II alveolar cells.
   (b) Surfactant is completely absent from lungs of infants dying from RDS.
   (c) Surfactant is primarily protein.
   (d) Surfactant decreases alveolar surface tension.

■ **Discussion:**

Since Macklin's description of the granular pneumonocyte, now referred to as the Type II cell of the lung, numerous investigators have pursued the role of these cells in lung function. In 1955, Pattle described the existence of a surface-active material in the lung that re-

sulted in reduced surface tension. Clements, in 1957, isolated an extract from lung tissue, which he called *surfactant*, and demonstrated that this preparation had surface-active properties. Finally, in 1959, Avery and Mead showed that infants dying from RDS had decreased amounts of surfactant in their lungs. Subsequent studies have shown that surfactant is produced by the Type II cell, and that surfactant *reduces alveolar surface tension.*

To understand clearly the role of surfactant in the development of respiratory distress syndrome, the concept of surface tension must be considered. Surface tension refers to the sum of the cohesive forces that hold a liquid together. Within a liquid, the forces exerted on a single molecule are equal in all directions because each molecule attracts, and is in turn attracted by, other molecules with identical strength. At the interface of the liquid with air, however, the liquid molecules exert a net force that is directed inward, reducing the surface to its minimum area. This force is expressed per unit length (dynes per centimeter) and is called *surface tension.*

Within the lung itself, a similar situation exists, with an air/liquid interface at the lining of the terminal air spaces, or alveoli (Figs. 8-2 and 8-3). The net tendency of the lung therefore is to reduce the alveolar surface to its minimum area or, in other words, to collapse (to become atelectatic). To prevent atelectasis, the design of the lung must be such that the net force tending to collapse the alveoli (surface tension) is reduced to zero. This reduction of surface tension is brought about at air/liquid interfaces by substances referred to as *surface-active materials.* Surface-active materials

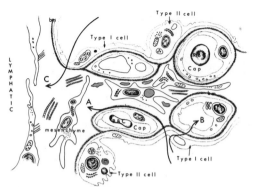

**Figure 8-2** Schemmatic representation of the relationships of the cells of the distal air spaces. The Type I cell is the cell across which gas exchange occurs. The Type II cell is the cell responsible for surfactant synthesis, storage, and release. Also illustrated in this representation are the pathways of fetal lung fluid reabsorption. Arrow A shows a pathway across the basement membrane; arrow B points to a capillary entrance; arrow C enters a lymphatic. RBC = red blood cell; Cap = capillary; and bm = basement membrane.
From F. Gonzalez-Crussi, R.W. Boston, *Lab Invest,* vol. 26, page 114, 1972, © by The U.S. and Canadian Acad. of Pathology, Inc. Reprinted with permission.

lower surface tension by forming an insoluble surface film that expands spontaneously on the liquid surface. The molecules of the surface-active materials have a lower surface tension than the bulk of the molecules of the liquid to which they are added, and usually consist of a polar and a nonpolar group. The polar group, possibly through hydrogen bonding, is drawn toward the liquid, while the nonpolar group turns toward the gas phase. The dispersion of surface-active molecules thus reduces the surface tension at the air/liquid interface, and the liquid no longer has a tendency to shrink to a minimum area.

In the lung, the presence of surfactant counteracts the tendency of the lung to collapse at the end of a breath, allowing a functional volume of gas to remain in the lung at the end of expiration (functional residual capacity). Subsequent breaths therefore require far less effort to inflate the lung. The child with RDS, however, who has an inadequate amount of surface-active material, continues to have atelectasis. This collapse of the lung is progressive with time as the moist alveolar surfaces become increasingly adhesive.

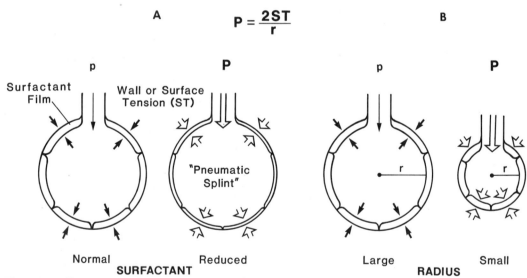

**Figure 8-3** Illustration of the role of surface tension within the lung. Surfactant acts as a surface-active material, decreasing the surface tension within the alveolus. CPAP can also decrease surface tension by acting as a pneumatic splint. In addition, from the LaPlace relationship, it is evident that surface tension will be greatest in alveoli with the smallest radii.
Adapted from Harris TR: Physiological principles. In Karotkin E, Goldsmith J eds: *Assisted Ventilation of the Neonate.* Philadelphia, WB Saunders Co, 1988, p. 35. Adapted with permission of W.B. Saunders Company.

**Table 8-2** Composition of Surfactant from Adult and Fetal Lungs

| | SURFACTANT FROM ADULT LUNGS (%) | | SURFACTANT FROM IMMATURE LUNGS (%) | |
|---|---|---|---|---|
| Protein | 10 | | 10 | |
| Neutral lipids | 10 | | 10 | |
| Phospholipids | 80 | | 80 | |
| Total phosphatidylcholine | | 80* | | 70** |
| Phosphatidylethanolamine | | 3 | | 5 |
| Sphyngomyelin | | 2 | | 15 |
| Phosphatidylinisitol | | 5 | | 10 |
| Phosphatidylglycerol | | 10 | | 0 |
| Totals | 100 | 100 | 100 | 100 |

* = 70% saturated, ** = 60% saturated.
*Source*: Adapted from Jobe A: Surfactant and the developing lung. In Thibeault DW, Gregory GA, eds: *Neonatal Pulmonary Care*. Norwalk, CT, Appleton-Century-Crofts, 1986, p. 77.

■ **Answer:**

1. a, d.

***Surface-Active Materials in Man:*** The main components of surfactant are dipalmitoyl phosphatidylcholine (DPPC) and, to a lesser extent, phosphatidylglycerol (PG) and protein (Table 8-2). Other phospholipid compounds, such as phosphatidylethanolamine, are also present. It appears that this mixture of phospholipids and protein ensures the optimal capability for stability, spreading, and reuptake of the surfactant molecules.

During the past decade, much work has focused on the isolation or development of both natural and artificial surfactants (Table 8-3). At the present time, two preparations of surfactant have been approved by the FDA for use in neonates. Exosurf® (Burroughs Wellcome, Research Triangle, North Carolina) and Survanta® (Ross Laboratories, Columbus, Ohio) are both commercially available. Exosurf® is an artificial surfactant composed of phosphatidylcholine, tyloxapol, and hexadecanol. The latter two components, not found in natural surfactant, are included for stability and spreading of the phosphatidylcholine. Survanta® is a natural surfactant prepared from calf lung. Human surfactant, while extensively studied, has not yet been made available commercially. The difficulty in harvesting adequate amounts from human amniotic fluid has thus far been prohibitive. It appears, however, that genetically engineered human surfactant will soon be available and may replace the current preparations. All exogenous surfactants have been shown to reduce the incidence and severity of neonatal respiratory distress syndrome. Furthermore, the complications of RDS, such as pulmonary air leak and bronchopulmonary dysplasia (BPD), also appear to be substantially lessened. Unfortunately, the incidence of patent ductus arteriosus (PDA) and intraventricular hemorrhage (IVH) do not appear to be dramatically altered. To date, no comparative large-scale studies have demonstrated superiority of one surfactant preparation over another. The clinical use of surfactant is discussed in Case Study 5.

**Table 8-3** Available Surfactant Preparations

1. Modified natural or semisynthetic
   (a) Survanta® (bovine lung extract with hydrophobic proteins, added lecithin, and palmitic acid)
   (b) Curosurf® (porcine extract with hydrophobic proteins)
   (c) Calf lung surfactant extract (with protein)
   (d) Human surfactant (from amniotic fluid)

2. Synthetic surfactant
   (a) Exosurf® (dipalmitoyl phosphatidylcholine, tyloxapol, and cetyl alcohol)

## Fetal Lung Fluid

### EXERCISE 3

■ **Question:**

1. Which of the following statements about fetal lung fluid is true?
   (a) Fetal lung fluid is produced by the fetus throughout gestation.
   (b) Fetal lung fluid has a composition identical to amniotic fluid.
   (c) Fetal lung fluid is completely removed at the time of birth.
   (d) Fetal lung fluid contains surfactant.

■ **Discussion:**

In 1948, Jost and Policard performed a series of studies on fetal rabbits; these studies demonstrated that lung volume increased after tracheal ligation. This led them to postulate that the fetal lung contributed to the volume of amniotic fluid. Prior to that time, lung fluid, as found in an autopsy of a stillborn fetus, was believed to be the result of *in utero* aspiration. Subsequent studies corroborated Jost and Policard's observations and confirmed that the fetal lung is one of several sites that eventually form the composite volume of amniotic fluid. Fetal lung fluid has a unique composition that distinguishes it from amniotic fluid. The volume of fetal lung fluid that contributes to the amniotic fluid is relatively small compared to the contribution from the fetal genitourinary system. The net outward flow of fetal lung fluid into the uterine cavity is augmented by the process of fetal breathing. It has been known for nearly a century that the fetus demonstrates respiratory activity of a rapid, irregular nature beginning at the end of the first trimester. These activities have been precisely categorized and are thought to be crucial to the development of respiratory muscle tone, preparing the chest wall and diaphragm for air breathing. Infants who fail to exhibit such respiratory movements (as in the case of congenital absence of the diaphragm) demonstrate severe lung hypoplasia, a diaphragm deficient in muscle fibers, and a decreased fetal lung fluid volume.

At term gestation, the amount of fetal lung fluid present within the lung is approximately 20 to 30 mL/kg of body weight, which is equal to the functional residual capacity in the healthy term infant postnatally. Fetal lung fluid is partially removed at the time of birth through circumferential chest wall compression by the birth canal, an important, but not critical, event. Hormonal factors appear equally important. Approximately two-thirds of lung fluid is expressed upward through the trachea and one-third is absorbed by the pulmonary capillaries and lymphatics. The child born by cesarean section may have delayed reabsorption of lung fluid and demonstrate respiratory symptoms for some time after birth. This syndrome is referred to as *transient tachypnea of the newborn* (TTN). Infants with TTN typically demonstrate rapid, shallow respirations, with few retractions. In some cases, however, the child with TTN can be very sick and require mechanical ventilator support.

These investigations into the nature of fetal lung fluid have provided the obstetrician with valuable tools for assessing lung maturation. Because the net flow of fetal lung fluid is outward into the amniotic cavity, biochemical determination of surfactant adequacy can rapidly be made to determine the risk of RDS for the premature baby. In 1971, Gluck and coworkers demonstrated that a lecithin to sphingomyelin (L : S) ratio of greater than 2 : 1 was associated with pulmonary maturity and very low risk of respiratory distress syndrome. They have subsequently developed an expanded "lung profile," which looks at additional factors and provides a more complete estimate of lung maturation (Fig. 8-4). An alternative test with almost the same reliability as the L : S ratio is the "shake," or fluid-foam, stability test devised by Clements et al. This test is a rapid bedside evaluation that involves diluting amniotic fluid with 95% ethanol in 1 : 1, 1 : 1.2, and 1 : 2 dilutions in a test tube while shaking the tube. The ring of bubbles at the surface of the fluid is observed to obtain an estimate of surfactant present with amniotic fluid. Infants who are positive in the highest dilutions have a lower incidence of RDS than those babies who are negative. Recently, commercial variations of these tests (Amniostat) have become available for rapid bedside assessments of lung maturation. This approach tests for the presence of phosphatidylglycerol, which is the last phospholipid to appear in the surfactant profile. Therefore, a "positive" Amniostat is highly specific for a mature (phospholipid sufficient) lung.

You can see that a complex series of developmental changes must occur in preparation for breathing at the moment of birth. Failure

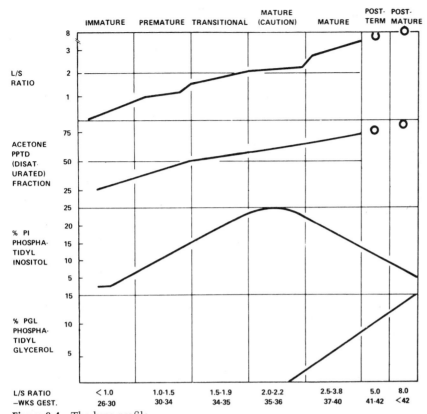

**Figure 8-4** The lung profile.
From Kulovich M, Hallman MB, Gluck L: The lung profile. *Am J Obstet Gynecol* 1979; 135:57.
Reprinted with permission of Mosby-Year Book, Inc.

to accomplish these preparatory steps, as in the case of the prematurely born infant, can markedly impair the baby's ability to initiate respiration and, in the case of insufficient surfactant, lead to the development of respiratory distress syndrome.

■ **Answer:**

1. a, d.

## MANAGEMENT OF THE PRETERM INFANT: PRACTICAL PERINATAL CONSIDERATIONS

The woman who presents in premature labor poses numerous management difficulties for both the obstetrician and the neonatologist. Exercises 4 through 6 illustrate some of the important decisions commonly encountered in high-risk perinatology in relationship to respiratory distress syndrome.

**CASE STUDY 1**

Mrs. E has a 24-week gestation fetus by dates. Upon arising in the morning, she feels a sudden fullness in her lower abdomen, followed by a brisk gush of fluid from her vagina. She calls the hospital to report that her membranes have ruptured and she is told to go to the hospital immediately.

**EXERCISE 4**

■ **Question:**
What should be done for Mrs. E and her baby?

■ **Discussion:**
The management of the extremely premature infant is fraught with hazards and complications, not to mention the profound ethical

problems posed. The baby born at 23 to 24 weeks' gestation is at the lower limit of viability and has approximately a 25% chance of survival in the best nurseries. This infant, however, is potentially viable and should be approached as such. The ethical dilemma in such infants is confounded by the fact that gestational age estimation is accurate only within a 2-week margin of error. Therefore, the fetus estimated at 24 weeks' gestation may actually be nonviable (22 weeks' gestation) or substantially more viable at 26 weeks' gestation.

An attempt to enhance labor with oxytocin is not appropriate at this time. The infant's prognosis will improve substantially with each additional day it remains *in utero*. Thus, in the absence of any complications, such as evidence of infection, maternal bleeding, or fetal asphyxia, efforts should be made to prolong the pregnancy, even in the face of ruptured membranes. Care of this baby will require a close working relationship between the obstetrician and the neonatologist and is best carried out in a specialized perinatal center. The initial consideration for the obstetrician should be confirmation of the infant's gestational age. This is best done by performing an ultrasound determination of the fetal biparietal diameter (Fig. 8-5). A carefully performed ultrasound examination will reliably estimate the baby's age within 8 days before 20 weeks' gestation and within 15 days after 24 weeks' gestation. Manual estimation of fetal weight is notoriously unreliable and should not be used as the primary method for estimation of fetal maturity. After the gestational age is confirmed, the mother should be placed at bed rest to prevent onset of labor. Pelvic examinations should be restricted because the risk of chorioamnionitis increases with frequent examinations. Whenever there is evidence of infection, as manifested by maternal fever, increased maternal white blood cell count, or fetal tachycardia, delivery of the fetus can no longer be safely delayed. Frequent or daily white blood counts and fetal heart rate monitoring, therefore, should be undertaken in this mother's pregnancy at this stage.

One of the most difficult management decisions pertaining to pregnancy at this stage is whether or not to use glucocorticoids to accelerate maturation of the lung and reduce the risk of RDS. In 1972, Liggins and Howie reported their results on a large series of women

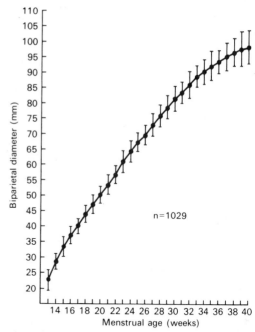

**Figure 8-5** Mean ± SD fetal biparietal diameter. Reprinted with permission from Campbell S: Fetal growth. In Beard R, Nathanielsz P, eds: *Fetal Physiology and Medicine.* Philadelphia, WB Saunders Co, 1976, 288.

who presented in premature labor and received glucocorticoids. The women were prospectively assigned to either treatment or control groups, with the treatment group receiving betamethasone in two doses. Labor was delayed for 48 hours after the initial dose. In the group of babies ranging from 26 to 34 weeks of gestation, there was a marked reduction in the incidence of respiratory distress syndrome.

Animal studies performed by Liggins, Kotas, and other investigators have confirmed the maturational effects of steroids on the lung. These effects appear to be both anatomic (thinning of alveolar septa, decreased connective tissue) and biochemical (increased release and synthesis of surfactant). In humans, however, more recent evaluations of the effects of corticosteroids are less clear. Most reports have confirmed Liggins's original data, but a national collaborative study among five perinatal centers in the United States suggested that corticosteroids may be effective primarily in female infants. Because it is not always possible to predict the gender of the offspring (unless prior karyotyping has been performed, or if male genitalia have been visualized on ultrasound), many centers currently use cortico-steroids in the hope that the risk of respiratory distress syndrome can be reduced. To date, adverse effects of this therapy have not materialized, although few long-term follow-up studies have been published. Standard practice has been to administer 12 mg of betamethasone or dexamethasone every 12 hours and delay labor for a minimum of 48 hours after the initial dose. This therapy should be initiated in infants less than 34 weeks' gestation unless there are contraindications to its use such as chorioamnionitis, maternal hypertension, pre-eclampsia, or severe intrauterine growth retardation. Furthermore, recent evidence indicates that the use of corticosteroids along with postnatal surfactant administration may be the most effective treatment for the very premature neonate.

In addition to bed rest, intravenous fluids, and sedation, the pharmacological inhibition of premature labor should be considered in this case. Intravenous ethanol was one of the first agents shown to inhibit labor. Ethanol, however, has largely been replaced by beta-adrenergic drugs such as isoxsuprine, and, more recently, ritodrine, salbutamol, and terbutaline, which have been shown to stimulate myometrial beta receptors in smooth muscle and decrease uterine activity. Beta-adrenergic therapy may, however, produce fetal tachycardia and hyperglycemia and increase the incidence of neonatal hypoglycemia and hypotension. Magnesium sulfate is also an effective tocolytic agent in many instances. The use of tocolytic agents is contraindicated in cases of active vaginal bleeding, dilatation of the cervix beyond 4 to 5 cm, abruptio placenta, chorioamnionitis, and fetal distress. The inhibition of premature labor in the presence of premature rupture of membranes is still not agreed on. Note that an increase in uterine activity in the mother described after a period of quiescence may be an indication of infection or fetal asphyxia. Before continuing beta-adrenergic therapy, ultrasound studies, fetal heart rate monitoring, and a complete blood count should be obtained. In the case of Mrs. E, if delivery can be delayed for 2 to 3 weeks, survival rate in most neonatal intensive care units will more than double. The question of whether premature rupture of membranes by itself will accelerate lung maturation is unclear. Some studies have suggested that this maturation occurs after 24 hours of rupture of membranes, but other studies suggest no significant benefits.

### ■ Answer:
The gestational age of the infant should be confirmed using ultrasound. After the gestational age is confirmed, the mother should be placed at bed rest to prevent the onset of labor. Frequent or daily white blood counts (to detect an incipient infection) and fetal heart rate monitoring should be performed. If there is no evidence of infection, corticosteroids can be administered. The use of pharmacological agents to inhibit labor is controversial, but probably indicated in selected cases.

### CASE STUDY 2
Mrs. R is a 26-year-old gravida 1, para 0 woman in her 31st week of pregnancy. For several hours today, she has been having crampy abdominal pain and decides to call her obstetrician. He asks her to come to his office where he examines her and finds her to be in active labor. Her cervix is dilated 3 cm and fully effaced. Membranes are intact.

### EXERCISE 5

### ■ Question:
Which actions from the following list would you take in this case?

(a) Amniocentesis

(b) Corticosteroids

(c) Bed rest and intravenous fluid

(d) Pitocin to stimulate labor

(e) Fetal heart rate monitoring

### ■ Discussion:
There are two important differences between this case and the previous one. First, this infant is significantly more mature at 31 weeks' gestation compared to the previous baby with a gestational age of 24 weeks. Second, Mrs. R has intact membranes, a major advantage for her infant because the risk of infection is substantially reduced. Consequently, the approach to this more mature baby is different in many respects from the case of the extremely immature fetus. The initial approach to this infant should again involve confirmation of gestational age by ultrasound assessment of biparietal diameter. Evaluation of the mater-

nal-fetal well-being is also important as is determination of why premature labor has occurred. You should determine if urinary tract infection, abruptio placenta, or any other factor has been responsible for the initiation of labor. The fetal heart rate should be monitored to determine if fetal compromise is present. Typical patterns of fetal heart rate changes are demonstrated in Figure 8-6. The most common type of deceleration (decrease in the fetal heart rate), usually seen during labor, is referred to as an early, or Type I, deceleration, resulting from compression of the infant's head against the cervix. Type II, or late decel-

erations, most often result from uteroplacental insufficiency and are evidence of fetal distress. Delivery in such cases should generally not be delayed. The final pattern, referred to as *variable decelerations*, signifies umbilical cord compression and can usually be resolved by repositioning the mother or by administering oxygen. In addition to decelerations, the baseline fetal heart rate and the variability of the heart rate should be noted. The baseline heart rate refers to the number of beats per minute calculated for a period of 10 minutes and is the stable heart rate that reappears following a contraction. The baseline heart rate

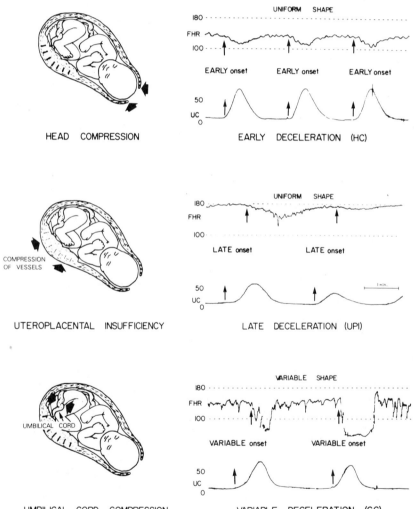

**Figure 8-6** Fetal heart rate patterns. UC = uterine contraction, FHR = fetal heart rate.

may be classified as normocardia (120 to 160 BPM), bradycardia (less than 120 BPM), or tachycardia (more than 160 BPM). Persistent bradycardia not varying with contraction is most commonly seen in association with cardiac malformations or impending fetal demise. Tachycardia may reflect prematurity, maternal hyperthermia, sepsis, use of medications (atropine, catecholamines), or fetal hypotension. Variability refers to beat-to-beat changes in heart rate as evidenced by alterations in the R-R interval on the electrocardiogram. Variability is a normal finding and is thought to reflect the integrity of the autonomic nervous system and fetal well-being. Diminished variability therefore has potentially serious implications for fetal status.

Many methods of determining fetal well-being have been developed. These investigations include assessment of fetal movement, fetal breathing, fetal heart rate accelerations in response to fetal movements (nonstress testing, NST), or decelerations with induced uterine contractions (contraction stress testing, CST). Although each of these individual tests has been shown to predict a normal birth outcome accurately, there is approximately a 50% false-positive rate when the results of a single test suggest a compromised fetus. For this reason, a scoring system has been developed that uses a combination of tests to assess fetal well-being. This system is the biophysical profile (Table 8-4). The biophysical profile was devised by Manning and co-workers in 1980. By combining both acute (fetal heart rate, breathing, and movements) and chronic (amniotic fluid volume) markers of fetal well-being, the sensitivity of the test is greatly improved compared to a single outcome variable.

Fetal heart rate testing is most commonly performed by ultrasound based on the Doppler principle. A transducer is applied to the maternal abdomen in the direction of the fetal heart and the difference in frequency between transmitted and reflected waves with each systole and diastole is amplified and filtered. The fetal heart rate may be examined with the mother at rest (nonstress test) or receiving a controlled infusion of oxytocin (stress test). Evidence of significant fetal distress (e.g., sudden onset of bradycardia that does not recover) should lead to rapid delivery by either the vaginal route or by cesarean section. If late decelerations are present and membranes are ruptured, fetal scalp sampling to determine the pH of fetal blood may help with the decision of when to deliver the infant. After gestational age and fetal status are ascertained, amniotic fluid should be obtained to determine fetal lung maturity. In this case, further management will depend on the results of lung profile and the degree of lung maturity found. If the L : S ratio

**Table 8-4** The Biophysical Profile

| VARIABLE | SCORE 2 | SCORE 0 |
|---|---|---|
| Fetal breathing movements (FBM) | The presence of at least 30 seconds of sustained FBM in 30 minutes of observation. | <30 seconds of FBM in 30 minutes. |
| Fetal movements | Three or more gross body movements in 30 minutes of observation. Simultaneous limb and trunk movements are counted as a single movement. | Two or fewer gross body movements in 30 minutes of observation. |
| Fetal tone | At least one episode of movement of a limb from a position of flexion to extension and a rapid return to flexion. | Fetus in a position of semi- or full-limb extension with no return to flexion with movement. Absence of fetal movement is counted as absent tone. |
| Fetal reactivity | The presence of two or more fetal heart rate accelerations of at least 15 BPM and lasting at least 15 seconds and associated with fetal movement in 40 minutes. | No accelerations or less than two accelerations of the fetal heart rate in 40 minutes of observation. |
| Qualitative amniotic fluid volume | A pocket of amniotic fluid that measures at least 1 cm in two perpendicular planes. | Largest pocket of amniotic fluid <1 cm in two perpendicular planes. |

Maximal score = 10, minimal score = 0.

is immature and there is no evidence of infection or fetal distress, most obstetricians would attempt to inhibit labor with the techniques previously discussed in order to allow progression of fetal lung maturation. The administration of corticosteroids at this point in time may be beneficial and should be considered. If the lung is found to be mature, however, prolongation of pregnancy may not be in the best interest of either mother or fetus, especially if the cause of premature labor is infection or fetal distress.

■ **Answer:**

The gestational age of the infant should be confirmed using ultrasound. It is also important to evaluate maternal-fetal well-being and to determine why premature labor has occurred. The fetal heart rate should be carefully monitored using an electronic fetal monitor. Amniotic fluid should be obtained to assess fetal lung maturity. If the L : S ratio is immature, corticosteroids are indicated.

---

### CASE STUDY 3

Mrs. J has been followed in a high-risk obstetric clinic since 22 weeks of gestation, when her uterine growth was observed to be below expected size. Her dates were confirmed on two subsequent occasions by B-scan ultrasound. She is now at 32 weeks' gestation and having occasional contractions. Uterine growth has been minimal and, at present, is of a 25-week size. Examination reveals the cervix to be dilated 2 to 3 cm.

### EXERCISE 6

---

■ **Question:**

What should be done at this time?

■ **Discussion:**

The unique feature of this pregnancy is that the fetus has not experienced the expected intrauterine growth. The pregnancy therefore can be classified as one in which there is intrauterine growth retardation. This fetus has several risk factors that are somewhat different from those present in the previous case discussions. The decision, therefore, must be made whether to suppress labor or to allow this

mother to deliver. Underlying this decision is the urgent need to confirm the well-being of the fetus. As noted previously, fetal heart rate monitoring is one test that enables the physician to assess intrauterine well-being. Thus, nonstress testing, in which the fetal heart rate pattern is examined while the mother is at rest, is very helpful in this situation. As long as heart rate variability is within previously determined limits and no significant heart rate decelerations are observed, fetal asphyxia is not likely and the pregnancy can continue. If there is uncertainty as to fetal status, the stress or oxytocin challenge test should be carried out. Evidence of abnormal decelerations or a decrease in variability may indicate fetal compromise.

If either the nonstress or stress test prove equivocal, additional information regarding fetal well-being is necessary. In this clinical situation, the biophysical profile can be of great value in assessing overall fetal status.

In recent years, Doppler ultrasonography has been used to evaluate placental and umbilical blood flow in normal and high-risk pregnancies. The umbilical artery peak systolic to nadir diastolic ratio (S : D ratio) has been the most frequently used index. In normal pregnancies, this value decreases as gestation progresses. An elevated value is thought to represent an impairment of placental perfusion. Absent or reverse diastolic flow (S : D ratio approaches infinity) is associated with a poor prognosis. Abnormalities in the S : D ratio may precede the onset of intrauterine growth retardation. After growth retardation has been identified, umbilical artery S : D ratios can be followed to determine if delivery of the premature infant is indicated.

In Mrs. J, if these investigations are normal, the physician should consider delaying delivery (at least until the degree of lung maturation can be determined). Considerations regarding the causes of both the growth retardation (Table 8-5) and the premature labor should be undertaken. Fortunately, small-for-gestational-age (SGA) infants appear to have a lower risk for development of respiratory distress syndrome than appropriate-for-gestational-age infants born at equivalent ages.

■ **Answer:**

The gestational age of the infant should be confirmed using ultrasound. An assessment of

**Table 8-5** Etiology of Growth Retardation

*Fetal*

   Chromosomal abnormalities
   Multiple congenital anomalies
   Intrauterine infections (TORCH)
   Dwarfing syndromes
   Primordial short stature
   Skeletal disorders
   Syndromes associated with retarded growth
   Endocrinopathies (Laron dwarfism, thyroid
     deficiency)
   Oligohydramnios

*Placental*

   Malformations (hemangioma, chorangioma)
   Chronic villitis
   Placenta previa
   Multiple infarcts, premature aging (placental
     insufficiency)
   Circumvallate placenta
   Twin-to-twin transfusion syndrome (placental
     arteriovenous anastomoses)

*Maternal*

   Short mother
     Low pregnancy weight
     Low weight gain during pregnancy
   Maternal environment (high altitude)
   Maternal habits/conditions
     Smoking
     Drug abuse (heroin, cocaine) or use (steroids,
      antimetabolites)
     Poor nutrition
   Low socioeconomic status
   Maternal status
     Hypertensive disorders
      Toxemia (pregnancy-induced hypertension)
      Essential hypertension
     Renal
      Chronic renal disease
      Asymptomatic bacteriuria (with reduced
       creatinine clearance)
      Diabetes mellitus (class D, F, R with vascu-
       lar disease)
      Sickle hemoglobinopathies
      Folate deficiency anemia
     Cardiac disease
      Cyanotic congenital heart disease
      Symptomatic mitral stenosis
     Collagen vascular disease
     Gastrointestinal disease
      Ulcerative colitis
      Crohn's disease
      Pancreatitis
     Severe psychiatric disorders (with impaired
      body image and leading to faulty nutrition)
     Uterine abnormalities leading to fetal con-
      straint
      Fibroids
      Bicornuate uterus
      Small uterus

*Source:* From Crawford C: The growth-retarded newborn. In Bolognese RJ, Schwarz RH, Schneider J, eds: *Perinatal Medicine.* © 1982, the Williams & Wilkins Co., Baltimore. Reprinted with permission of R.J. Bolognese and the Williams & Wilkins Co.

fetal well-being should occur using electronic fetal heart rate monitoring and Doppler ultrasonography. The etiology of the intrauterine growth retardation should be determined. If there is no evidence of fetal compromise and the lungs are immature, delivery should be delayed.

## THE INFANT WITH RESPIRATORY DISTRESS SYNDROME (RDS): PRACTICAL MANAGEMENT PROBLEMS

### CASE STUDY 4

Baby S is born by precipitous vaginal delivery to a 19-year-old, gravida 1, para 0 mother following a 32-week gestation. Mrs. S received no prenatal care during her pregnancy and arrived at the hospital in active labor. Physical examination revealed the cervix to be completely dilated and fully effaced. Delivery occurred within 30 minutes of arrival at the hospital. Apgar scores for this infant were 5 and 8 at 1 and 5 minutes, respectively. The baby was sent to the observation nursery, where 1 hour later he was noted to be breathing at a rate of 80 per minute, cyanotic, and audibly grunting at the end of each breath.

### EXERCISE 7

■ **Questions:**

1. What is the most likely diagnosis for this infant?

2. What other diagnoses should be considered?

3. Which laboratory studies would you order at this time?

■ **Discussion:**

One of the primary maxims of medicine is first diagnosis, then treatment. In the case of the newly born premature infant, this approach is critical. *Not every infant with respiratory symptoms has respiratory disease.* Thus, the practicing physician must approach each child with a healthy skepticism regarding the differential diagnosis, so that the proper investigations can be performed and the optimal therapy initiated. It is imperative to know the primary signs of respiratory disease in the newborn infant (tachypnea, cyanosis, retractions, grunting, apnea, nasal flaring, and decreased activity—Table 8-6) in order to formulate a differential diagnosis (Fig. 8-7) based on the gestational age of the child, the history of the pregnancy, labor and delivery, and the physical findings.

Some of the diagnoses listed, while very appropriate for term infants, rarely occur in premature babies, and therefore can be immediately dismissed if one is dealing with a premature infant. Meconium aspiration and primary pulmonary hypertension of the neonate (PPHN, also referred to as persistence of the fetal circulation), for example, are diseases almost always noted in term infants. In contrast, respiratory distress syndrome and pulmonary hemorrhage primarily affect the preterm baby. Thus, the differential diagnosis can rapidly be narrowed by performing an assessment of gestational age. The time of onset of signs and symptoms is also a critical factor in helping one to arrive at a diagnosis. Respiratory distress syndrome almost always becomes apparent within 1 to 2 hours of birth, usually within minutes in the very immature neonate. The child who first becomes symptomatic at 8 to 12 hours of age probably has a different etiology for respiratory distress, such as pneumonia or hypoglycemia.

After a complete differential diagnosis has been generated based on the factors outlined here, appropriate studies should be ordered either to confirm or to eliminate certain diagnoses. Table 8-7 lists studies that should be part

**Table 8-6** Respiratory Signs in the Newborn Period and Their Interpretation

| SIGN | INTERPRETATION |
| --- | --- |
| 1. Tachypnea (RR > 60) | Increase in respiratory rate usually means that either oxygenation or ventilation is inadequate. The infant responds to the decreased $PaO_2$ or increased $PaCO_2$ by breathing more rapidly. |
| 2. Cyanosis | Reflects an increase in desaturated hemoglobin in the blood, usually greater than 3 to 5 g/dL in the neonate. May occur in cardiac, respiratory, neurological, and metabolic diseases. |
| 3. Retractions | May occur in any muscle group of, or attached to, the thorax: intercostal muscles, supraclavicular muscles, subxiphoid muscles, etc. Retractions are usually evidence that respiratory inadequacy exists. The infant attempts to compensate for this inadequacy by using all available respiratory muscles to augment ventilation. Retractions are most common in diseases that reduce alveolar ventilation, usually from atelectasis. |
| 4. Grunting | Audible grunting at the end of a breath is caused by the infant's breathing against a closed or partially closed glottis. The effort by the baby represents a physiological response that attempts to increase residual volume of the lung. It is most commonly seen in RDS but can occur whenever there is volume loss in the lung. |
| 5. Apnea | A respiratory pause of 15 seconds or longer, or less than 15 seconds but with bradycardia below 100 BPM or oxygen desaturation. Although it is a common event in most premature infants, apnea in the first 24 to 48 hours of life may indicate severe disease. An etiology must be determined if apnea is present early in prematurity, or if present in a term infant. |
| 6. Nasal flaring | Widening of the nares during inspiration, representing an increased effort on the part of the infant. |
| 7. Decreased activity | Often overlooked as a respiratory sign is the fact that many neonates with pulmonary disease will divert all effort into breathing if lung disease is severe and all extraneous activity ceases. An early sign of improvement is increased activity level. This sign, however, is nonspecific and may accompany problems such as sepsis or CNS injury. |

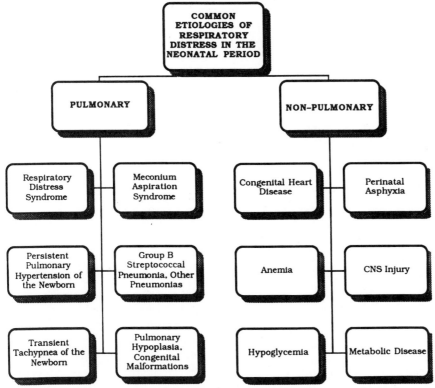

**Figure 8-7** Common etiologies of respiratory distress during the neonatal period, divided by pulmonary and nonpulmonary causes.

of the evaluation of any newborn infant who presents with respiratory distress. Blood cultures should always be obtained prior to the initiation of antimicrobial therapy, and are included in the category of essential studies because group B streptococcal disease can masquerade as RDS radiographically. In such instances, it is likely that the preterm infant

**Table 8-7** Initial Studies for the Infant with Respiratory Disease During the Neonatal Period

| ESSENTIAL STUDIES | PURPOSE OF STUDY |
|---|---|
| 1. Chest radiograph | Diagnose respiratory, cardiac abnormalities. |
| 2. Complete blood count (CBC) | Diagnose anemia, polycythemia, infection. |
| 3. Blood glucose | Diagnose hypoglycemia. |
| 4. Blood culture | Diagnose septicemia, pneumonia. |
| 5. Arterial blood gas | Measure oxygenation, acid-base status. |
| OPTIONAL STUDIES (depends on clinical situation) | |
| 1. Head ultrasound | Evaluate brain for hemorrhage, injury, structural abnormality. History will determine need for this study early. |
| 2. Echocardiogram | Evaluate structural heart disease, cardiac function (may be abnormal in many disease states during the newborn period). |
| 3. Hyperoxia test | Differentiate respiratory from cardiac disease. |
| 4. Pulmonary function tests | Evaluate clinical status. Can be used to follow infant's progress and assist in weaning. Also can be used to evaluate appropriateness of ventilator settings. |

may actually have both disease entities, since pneumonia may interfere with surfactant synthesis and release. Because this disease is often so rapidly fatal, it has been standard practice to obtain blood cultures on all infants with respiratory symptoms and initiate antibiotic therapy pending culture results. If cultures are negative at 48 to 72 hours, antibiotics are stopped. Positive cultures are an indication for 2 to 3 weeks of therapy, depending on the organism isolated, antibiotic sensitivity, and body site involved.

Arterial blood gases are very useful for assessing the status of an infant with respiratory distress syndrome, especially if performed serially. Serial blood gases can be most easily obtained through an indwelling umbilical artery catheter. Umbilical artery catheterization has many potential complications and should be undertaken only by someone skilled in the technique and in a nursery where the procedure is commonly used. Some of the problems associated with umbilical catheters include hemorrhage, thrombosis, infection, renal and mesenteric infarction, and microembolization into distal vessels. The preferred location for the arterial catheter tip is between the third and fourth lumbar vertebrae, below the origin of renal and mesenteric arteries and above the aortic bifurcation. Umbilical vein catheterization also has potentially serious complications such as liver necrosis, portal vein thrombosis, and spontaneous perforation of the colon. In most infants, use of an umbilical artery catheter is preferable for blood gas and blood pressure determination and a peripheral intravenous line for infusion of medications.

To distinguish neonatal cardiac disease from pulmonary disease, it is helpful to place the infant in 100% oxygen, the so-called *hyperoxia test*. In general, the child with cyanotic congenital heart disease will not be able to generate a $PaO_2$ greater than 100 mm Hg because of fixed intracardiac shunting that bypasses the pulmonary circulation. The child with severe lung disease, however, will be able to improve oxygenation substantially greater than 100 mm Hg, especially if given positive pressure ventilation (PPV). This test should be carried out for only a very brief period of time (less than 5 minutes) because of the risk of retinopathy of prematurity when the infant's eyes are immature.

■ **Answers:**

1. Respiratory distress syndrome.

2. Hypothermia, pneumonia, sepsis, hypoglycemia, pneumothorax, congenital heart disease.

3. Complete blood count and differential, chest x-ray, arterial blood gas, blood culture, blood glucose.

**CASE STUDY 4 continued**

The initial studies on baby S reveal the following:

Chest x-ray: bilateral reticulogranular pattern with air bronchograms

Complete blood count: hemoglobin 16.2 g/dL

White blood cell count: 18,000/mm³ with a normal differential count

Platelet count: 265,000/mm³

Blood cultures: results pending

Percutaneous arterial blood gases: pH 7.22/ $PaO_2$ 43 mm Hg/$PaCO_2$ 52 mm Hg/BE − 8

**EXERCISE 8**

Place a check mark next to each of the following statements that is true.

_____1. The description of the x-ray in this case is typical for respiratory distress syndrome.

_____2. Air bronchograms are caused by an increased amount of air in the small airways.

_____3. If this child receives no ventilatory support, it is likely that his lung fields will become progressively more radiopaque during the next few hours.

_____4. The reticulogranular appearance on chest radiographs reflects diffuse pulmonary atelectasis.

_____5. Most babies with respiratory distress syndrome have a mixed respiratory acidosis and metabolic acidosis.

_____6. This infant needs to be observed for only 6 hours.

## ■ Discussion:

The clinical findings in this infant together with the radiological and blood gas studies suggest that this child has respiratory distress syndrome. The classic findings of this disease are listed in Table 8-8. The pathophysiology of the disease, as noted in the initial section of this chapter, begins with surfactant deficiency. Surfactant deficiency leads to a progressive loss in alveolar volume, resulting in profound ventilatory, metabolic, and histologic changes (Fig. 8-8). It is evident from Figure 8-8 that not only does surfactant deficiency produce physiological disturbances, but these changes feed back at several levels to create progressively more severe disease. After respiratory distress syndrome occurs, therefore, symptoms tend to worsen unless some intervention occurs. The infant who presents with RDS shortly after birth will often deteriorate during the first hours of life. Radiographically, this deterioration is seen as a decrease in lung aeration. As the atelectasis increases, the reticulogranular pattern, which represents microatelectasis (Fig. 8-9), becomes increasingly confluent, leading to a ground glass appearance ("white-out"). Air bronchograms, which are simply the major airways surrounded by airless lung parenchyma, become increasingly prominent. Few infants who demonstrate this progression will survive untreated. The arterial blood gas results in this child are characteristic of the infant with respiratory distress syndrome. The physiological changes outlined

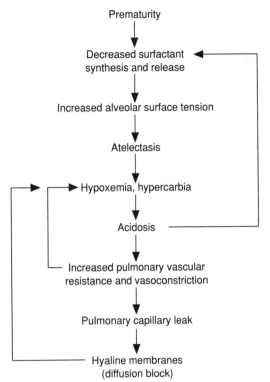

**Figure 8-8**  The pathogenesis of RDS.

**Table 8-8**  Classic Signs of Respiratory Distress Syndrome

Prematurity

Onset of symptoms prior to 6 hours of life, usually before 2 hours

Tachypnea

Retractions

Cyanosis

Expiratory grunting

Hypotension*

Generalized edema*

Reticulogranular alveolar infiltrate with air bronchograms, progressing to ground glass appearance on chest radiograph

---

* Less common.

in Figure 8-8 commonly result in alterations of pulmonary function (Table 8-9). These alterations in pulmonary function ultimately produce hypoxia (fall in $PaO_2$) and hypercapnia (increase in $PaCO_2$). Thus, early blood gas determinations in an infant with respiratory distress syndrome often reveal a decreased $PaO_2$ and an increased $PaCO_2$. As the progressive hypoxia continues, metabolism becomes increasingly anaerobic, and lactic acid accumulates in body tissues, leading to a metabolic acidosis. In the very premature infant, these changes may take place very rapidly, literally during minutes, resulting in profound respiratory symptoms within a very short time after birth. It is not uncommon to see arterial blood gas values such as those seen in this baby. Continued observation at this stage is no longer indicated and intervention must occur immediately.

## ■ Answers:

Statements 1, 3, 4, and 5 are true.

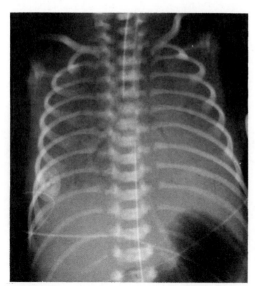

**Figure 8-9**   An infant with classic RDS. The lung shows diffuse microatelectasis, producing a generalized "haziness" or "white-out" appearance. Air bronchograms, which reflect the airways surrounded by gasless lung are also noted.
Courtesy of George Gross, M.D.

### EXERCISE 9

See the chart on page 169 and match each of the therapies with the rationale for that therapy.

■ **Discussion:**
The management of the neonate with respiratory distress syndrome can be divided into three distinct phases: initial therapy during the first hours of life, the phase of continued acute care, and chronic therapy. Not all infants enter the third phase. On the contrary, the majority recover after the phase of continued acute care. An important decision that must be made early during the infant's disease

**Table 8-9**   Pulmonary Function Changes During RDS

1. Decreased lung compliance
2. Normal inspiratory resistance
3. Increased expiratory resistance
4. Decreased functional residual capacity (FRC)
5. Increased respiratory rate
6. Decreased tidal volume
7. Decreased alveolar ventilation

is whether adequate personnel and facilities exist for undertaking the phase of continued acute care. If not, transport of the baby to a center that provides this level of care must be made promptly.

■ **Answers:**

1. Improve hydration
2. $R_x$ metabolic acidosis
3. Maintain functional residual capacity, reduce hypoxia, and $R_x$ respiratory failure
4. $R_x$ respiratory failure
5. Reduce hypoxia
6. Maintain temperature
7. $R_x$ respiratory failure and secure airway
8. Monitor blood gases and blood pressure

### Initial Care and Stabilization

**CASE STUDY 5**
Baby girl F is born after 22 hours of labor to a gravida 1, para 0 mother at 26 weeks' gestation. Her birth weight is 760 g. Initially, she makes some feeble attempts at respiration, but soon becomes apneic. Her heart rate falls below 100 BPM, and she is rapidly becoming cyanotic.

### EXERCISE 10

■ **Question:**
What would you do immediately?

■ **Discussion:**
The initial care of the premature infant begins prenatally. The obstetrician and pediatrician or neonatologist should carefully evaluate the mother and fetus in order to determine the best way to manage the final stages of labor and delivery. After the premature baby is delivered, however, a series of decisions must be made quickly to ensure optimal care for the infant. In the delivery room, the physician in attendance at the birth of a premature baby should be experienced in intubation and resuscitation. Ideally, either two physicians, or a physician and a nurse, should have direct re-

**Exercise 9**

RATIONALE

| THERAPY | MAINTAIN FUNCTIONAL RESIDUAL CAPACITY | REDUCE HYPOXIA | IMPROVE HYDRATION | $R_x$ METABOLIC ACIDOSIS | MAINTAIN TEMPERATURE | $R_x$ RESPIRATORY FAILURE | SECURE AIRWAY (PERMIT MECHANICAL VENTILATION) | MONITOR BLOOD GASES AND BLOOD PRESSURE |
|---|---|---|---|---|---|---|---|---|
| 1. Intravenous fluids | | | | | | | | |
| 2. NaHCO$_3$ | | | | | | | | |
| 3. Cont. positive airway pressure | | | | | | | | |
| 4. Mechanical ventilation | | | | | | | | |
| 5. Increased inspired oxygen | | | | | | | | |
| 6. Radiant heater | | | | | | | | |
| 7. Endotracheal intubation | | | | | | | | |
| 8. Umbilical artery catheterization | | | | | | | | |

sponsibility for the infant alone. They should not be distracted from the task of resuscitation. Any other tasks that must be performed in the delivery room should be carried out by additional personnel. Equipment should be ready and thoroughly checked prior to the delivery (see Chapter 1).

The primary decisions facing the physician in the delivery room, however, are very basic. First, what is the extent of resuscitation needed by this infant and, second, does this baby have respiratory distress syndrome? After these questions have been resolved, therapy can be appropriately directed. It has been estimated that approximately 10% of term deliveries require some resuscitation. The incidence increases in less mature infants. At most large hospitals, it is standard practice to resuscitate the premature baby vigorously. Resuscitation should be initiated within seconds after birth, as opposed to waiting for Apgar scores, in order to prevent asphyxia and resulting acidosis. Once acidosis ensues, production of surfactant decreases rapidly and the likelihood and severity of respiratory distress syndrome are enhanced. The acidotic infant is ultimately far more difficult to treat than the child who receives vigorous initial resuscitation and stabilization. Therapy may be withdrawn as improvement is observed.

While the physician is initiating resuscitation and determining the Apgar scores, the likelihood of respiratory distress syndrome in the baby must be estimated. You should look for the signs of neonatal respiratory disease previously discussed. It is essential that adequate warmth be provided because a sudden fall in the infant's body temperature may lead to acidosis, pulmonary vasoconstriction, and respiratory distress with grunting. In the symptomatic infant with respiratory distress syndrome who weighs less than 2 kg, it has been standard practice to place the baby on 5 cm $H_2O$ of continuous positive airway pressure (CPAP) with 40% to 50% oxygen as a starting point, either with nasal prongs or an endotracheal tube (Fig. 8-10). The baby weighing more than 2 kg can initially be placed in an oxygen hood (30% to 40%) and closely observed. The larger premature infant with greater energy reserves and surfactant stores may tolerate oxygen therapy alone. Ideally, an umbilical artery catheter should be used whenever the inspired oxygen concentration ($FiO_2$) is greater than 30%. The smaller infant

(less than 2 kg) is much more likely to develop increasingly severe disease during the first 24 to 48 hours of life. Early intubation and institution of CPAP or mechanical ventilation will lessen acidosis and progressive atelectasis.

### ■ Answer:

Resuscitation should be initiated immediately. Apgar scores should then be assigned. An assessment should then be made to determine whether the infant has RDS. An infant of this size with respiratory distress syndrome is generally intubated and placed on CPAP or a mechanical ventilator.

---

### CASE STUDY 5 continued

After intubation of Baby Girl F and institution of CPAP, her color improves and you hear adequate breath sounds. A pulse oximeter reading, however, is 88% saturation. There is no retention of carbon dioxide and the base excess is zero.

### EXERCISE 11

Place a check next to each of the steps you would consider now.

_____(a) Increasing CPAP

_____(b) Increasing $FiO_2$

_____(c) Increasing frequency of ventilation

_____(d) Surfactant administration

_____(e) Administration of $NaHCO_3$

### ■ Discussion:

At this point, it is also important to consider whether the infant is a candidate for surfactant replacement therapy. Although surfactant deficiency has been recognized as the basis for lung disease in the premature infant for many years, only during the past decade has surfactant administration become a practical adjunct to ventilatory care. As mentioned earlier, currently, two preparations are available in the United States for neonatal administration, Exosurf®, an artificial surfactant, and Survanta®, a natural surfactant from cow lung. Porcine surfactant (Curosurf®) is available in Europe. These drugs represent the most extensively studied drugs ever developed for the newborn infant. All surfactants have been shown to be highly effective in reducing death from RDS and may decrease the incidence of air leak and bronchopulmonary dysplasia.

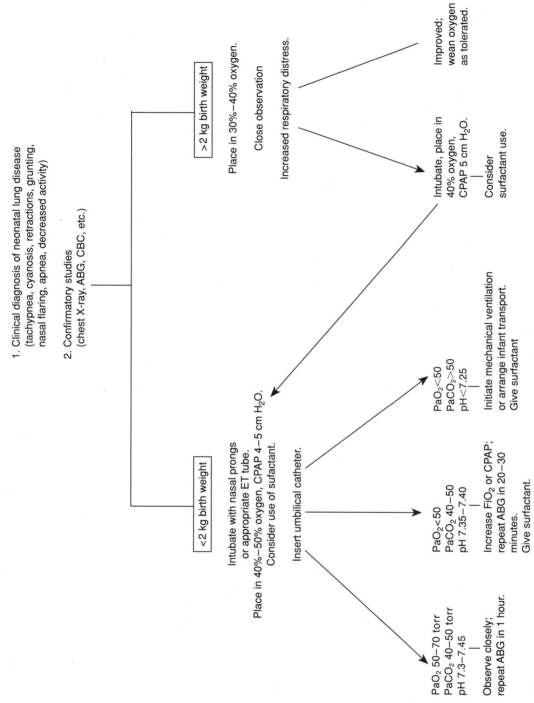

1. Clinical diagnosis of neonatal lung disease (tachypnea, cyanosis, retractions, grunting, nasal flaring, apnea, decreased activity)

2. Confirmatory studies (chest X-ray, ABG, CBC, etc.)

> 2 kg birth weight

Place in 30%–40% oxygen.

Close observation

Increased respiratory distress.

Improved; wean oxygen as tolerated.

Intubate, place in 40% oxygen, CPAP 5 cm H₂O.

Consider surfactant use.

< 2 kg birth weight

Intubate with nasal prongs or appropriate ET tube.
Place in 40%–50% oxygen, CPAP 4–5 cm H₂O.
Consider use of sufactant.

Insert umbilical catheter.

PaO₂ < 50
PaCO₂ > 50
pH < 7.25

Initiate mechanical ventilation or arrange infant transport.
Give surfactant

PaO₂ < 50
PaCO₂ 40–50
pH 7.35–7.40

Increase FiO₂ or CPAP; repeat ABG in 20–30 minutes.
Give surfactant.

PaO₂ 50–70 torr
PaCO₂ 40–50 torr
pH 7.3–7.45

Observe closely; repeat ABG in 1 hour.

**Figure 8-10** Initial management plan for the neonate with respiratory disease.

171

They represent the most important addition to neonatal therapy in recent years. Surfactant use is not without complications, however. Some studies have suggested an increased incidence of pulmonary hemorrhage and patent ductus arteriosus (PDA) following surfactant use.

If a decision is made to use surfactant, it should be administered as early as possible in the illness. Surfactant should be given to all infants with RDS; however, it does not need to be used prophylactically before it has been established that a given infant has RDS. In the extremely low birth weight infant (<1,000 g), surfactant should be given as soon as the infant is sufficiently stable to tolerate the procedure. Delay in administration has been shown to make treatment less effective. The dosage of surfactant varies from preparation to preparation. Exosurf® is usually given in a dose of 5 mL/kg. Half is given to the infant through the endotracheal tube while the baby's head is turned to the right, and the remainder is given when the child's head is turned to the left. Survanta® (4 mL/kg) is administered in four aliquots, in four different body positions. At our institution, we have some concern with administration techniques as currently suggested because they may enhance the likelihood of atelectasis in an already compromised infant. Furthermore, the spreading effects of surfactant should not require these positioning attempts to enhance its effects. Further work is needed, both with respect to technique and dosage, for all surfactants currently in use.

The immediate stabilization of the infant with respiratory distress syndrome is unquestionably one of the most critical phases of treatment of this disease. Initial management of ventilatory assistance will depend on the infant's arterial blood gas values (Fig. 8-10). Ideally, however, the obstetrician and the pediatrician should recognize that some infants cannot be cared for at their institution because of an inability to perform certain procedures or a lack of skilled nursing staff. *Maternal transport is always preferable to infant transport if the mother can be safely moved.* If maternal transport is not possible, an important decision must be made: Should the infant remain at the birth hospital or be transferred to an intensive care nursery facility? It is difficult to give specific guidelines because each hospital is different, each infant is different, and the

physician must carefully analyze the situation to determine where the baby will get optimal care. In general, you should always transfer to level III nurseries babies who fall into the following categories:

1. Infants weighing less than 1,500 g with respiratory distress syndrome.

2. Infants who require early intubation and mechanical ventilation, regardless of size.

3. Asphyxiated infants with respiratory distress syndrome.

4. Large-for-gestational-age (LGA) infants with respiratory distress syndrome.

5. Infants who appear to have suffered complications associated with respiratory distress syndrome—pneumothorax, PDA, intraventricular hemorrhage, infection, necrotizing enterocolitis.

This listing includes only those infants with respiratory distress syndrome. Babies with other neonatal problems unrelated to respiratory distress syndrome, such as surgical problems, congenital heart disease, and seizures, should also be transferred to a perinatal center. Again, the decision to refer an infant must take into account the capabilities of the birth hospital, the potential risks to the infant during the first several days of life, and the recognized capabilities of the intensive care nursery at the transfer hospital. After the decision to transport has been made, the physician responsible for the care of the infant should follow the guidelines outlined in Table 8-10. The ability of the primary care physician to carry out these procedures can substantially reduce the time spent on neonatal transport. You should be aware that it is not always possible to intubate an individual baby, nor can umbilical catheters always be easily inserted. In such instances, alternative therapies are available and appropriate until the transport team arrives. Virtually all infants can be adequately ventilated for prolonged periods of time by bag and mask inflation. Oxygenation can be judged by the point at which one barely abolishes cyanosis. If arterial blood gases cannot be obtained, peripheral venous or capillary blood gas determination will give reasonable estimates of pH and $PaCO_2$. You can then adjust bag and mask inflation accordingly. If this method of airway management is used, an orogastric or nasogastric tube is essential to re-

**Table 8-10** Guidelines for
Neonatal Transport

1. Obtain transport permission from family.
2. Copy available prenatal and perinatal records.
3. Copy available infant radiographs.
4. Obtain a specimen of maternal blood for cross-matching.
5. Secure endotracheal tube well prior to moving infant.
6. Secure catheters and peripheral IVs.
7. Obtain Dextrostik® (Miles Inc., Elkhart, IN).
8. Check hematocrit.
9. Obtain arterial blood gas; readjust ventilator support if necessary (see Figures 8-10 and 8-11).
10. Place an adequately sized nasogastric tube (6 to 8 Fr.).
11. Be sure vitamin K has been administered.
12. Remain with infant until transport team has left with baby.

move swallowed gastric air and avoid perforation of the stomach. It is critical, however, that a physician or nurse skilled in these techniques remain with the infant at all times. Because the potential for complications and deterioration is so great, you must be poised to act instantly should problems arise (Table 8-11).

■ **Answer:**
a, b, d (in some cases, c and e may also be of value).

**Advanced Study of Continuing Acute Care and Chronic Care in Respiratory Distress Syndrome**

**EXERCISE 12**

1. List five potentially life-threatening complications that may occur during the care of an infant with respiratory distress syndrome.

2. Place a check next to each of the following statements that is true.

_____1. One should initiate mechanical ventilation only when ventilatory failure occurs and the infant requires 100% inspired oxygen.

_____2. A pneumothorax should be observed for at least 2 hours before therapy is instituted.

_____3. High fluid volume administration is preferred to fluid restriction in the therapy of respiratory distress syndrome.

_____4. Appearance of a PDA will significantly affect recovery from respiratory distress syndrome.

**Table 8-11** Complications of
Mechanical Ventilation

Airway Injury
  Tracheal inflammation
  Tracheobronchomalacia
  Subglottic stenosis
  Granuloma formation
  Palatal grooving
  Nasal septal injury
  Necrotizing tracheobronchitis

Endotracheal Tube Complications
  Dislodgement
  Obstruction
  Accidental extubation
  Airway erosion

Chronic Lung Injury
  Bronchopulmonary dysplasia (BPD)
  Acquired lobar emphysema

Air Leaks
  Pulmonary interstitial emphysema (PIE)
  Pneumothorax
  Pneumomediastinum
  Pneumopericardium
  Pneumoperitoneum
  Hyperinflation

Cardiovascular
  Decreased cardiac output
  Patent ductus arteriosus (PDA)
  IVH

Miscellaneous
  Retinopathy of prematurity
  Apnea
  Infection
  Feeding intolerance
  Developmental delay

_____5. In weaning an infant from the ventilator, it is preferable to make frequent small changes as opposed to occasional larger changes.

_____6. Infants with respiratory distress syndrome should be frequently evaluated for the possibility of intraventricular hemorrhage.

## ■ Discussion:

After initial stabilization of the child with respiratory distress syndrome, the primary goal of the continued care of the child is intense monitoring and one-to-one nursing care. Any intensive care nursery that assumes responsibility for infants with respiratory inadequacy must provide monitoring of heart rate, cardiac rhythm, respiratory rate, arterial pressure, venous pressure, and transcutaneous oxygen, oxygen saturation, and carbon dioxide concentrations with accurate electronic devices. Essential in the use of such equipment is a knowledgeable, highly trained nursing staff, who must not only be skilled in the care and calibration of the monitors, but know how to respond quickly and appropriately to the various alarms. *It is sufficient to say that an intensive care nursery is only as good as its nursing staff.*

After the child has been stabilized in the delivery room and returned to the nursery or transported to a tertiary care center, anticipation of problems (such as those listed in Table 8-11) becomes the hallmark of care. Table 8-12 lists a series of suggested routine orders that attempts to prevent and anticipate many of the complications commonly noted in premature infants with respiratory distress syndrome. As mentioned previously, the nurse at the infant's bedside is the cornerstone of care. Vital signs, blood pressure, fluid intake and urine output, and assessment of the infant's overall condition should be performed hourly at first. As the baby improves, frequency of noted observation can be reduced, but any alteration in the baby's status may require reinstitution of frequent monitoring of vital signs. A physical examination, a simple procedure that is too often overlooked after the initial evaluation, should be done at least twice a day in the early days of therapy. Of special importance are infant activity, appearance of the fontanelles, breath sounds, cardiac examination, and abdominal findings. Such examinations may make the physician aware of prob-

**Table 8-12**   Routine Procedures in the Care of the Infant with RDS

1. Frequent vital signs and nursery observation, initially hourly; later this may be decreased.

2. Repeat physical examination at least twice daily during initial few days of life.

3. Frequent arterial blood gases. Every 1 to 2 hours during initial phases; less frequently thereafter. A blood gas should be obtained approximately 20 minutes after any ventilator or oxygen change.

4. Careful determination of fluid intake and output. Hourly during intensive care.

5. At least daily determinations of Na, K, Cl, $CO_2$, hemoglobin/hematocrit, white blood count, calcium, and glucose.

6. Bilirubin determinations as indicated. Every 6 to 8 hours at time of peak of hyperbilirubinemia.

7. Daily nutritional assessment.

8. Cultures as indicated for possible sepsis.

9. Ophthalmologic examination for retinopathy of prematurity. Beginning at 4 weeks of age, every other week; thereafter until maturation of the retinal vessels.

10. Ultrasound examination of the central nervous system. Upon admission to nursery; every 2 to 3 days thereafter until 1 week of age.
    If an intraventricular hemmorhage has occurred:
    Weekly thereafter until 1 month of age, and then biweekly until 3 months of age. Repeat studies should be obtained for sudden clinical deteriorations or an accelerated head growth rate.

11. Daily chest x-ray while on ventilatory support. Repeat chest roentgenograph should be obtained if a sudden change occurs in infant status.

lems long before they manifest as major complications.

Ongoing care of the baby with respiratory distress syndrome presents the physician with a large number of problems and decisions that must be made on an hour-to-hour basis. Follow-up data of babies with respiratory distress syndrome indicate that successful management of these problems results in a highly favorable outcome. Therefore, the physician caring for such an infant must have such a well-devised approach to the difficulties invariably encountered. Mechanical ventilation, in particular, is one of the most difficult aspects of the care of the infant with respiratory distress syndrome.

## ■ Answers:

1. Pneumothorax, pulmonary hemorrhage, intraventricular hemorrhage, infection, bronchopulmonary dysplasia.

2. The true statements are 4, 5, and 6.

## Mechanical Ventilation

After you are certain that mechanical ventilation is necessary, the scheme outlined in Figure 8-11 may be used to provide optimal ventilation and avoid complications of therapy. Certain points of this therapy deserve emphasis. No infant should be placed directly on a respirator before hand ventilation with a bag and pressure manometer is used to determine appropriate ventilator settings. The risk of sudden tension pneumothorax is substantial if a child is placed directly on a ventilator. Manual inflation starting points are listed in Table 8-13, but experience will demonstrate that these may be excessive in some very small (less than 750 g) babies, or inadequate in larger (more than 2 kg) infants. Adjustments should be made very quickly in those cases.

**Table 8-13** Initiation of Mechanical Ventilation in Neonatal Lung Disease

1. Intubate infant, secure endotracheal tube adequately.

2. Place pressure manometer in gas flow line to determine appropriate pressures for ventilation.

3. Begin manual inflation with:
   $FiO_2 \geq 0.5$
   Rate at 40–50 BPM
   Initial PIP at 15 cm $H_2O$
   Initial PEEP at 4–5 cm $H_2O$
   Inspiration : expiration ratio at 1 : 1 to 1 : 2

4. Observe infant for:
   Cyanosis
   Chest wall excursion
   Capillary perfusion
   Breath sounds

5. If ventilation is inadequate, increase PIP by 1 cm $H_2O$ every few breaths, until air entry seems adequate.

6. If oxygenation is poor and cyanosis remains, increase $FiO_2$ by 5% every minute until cyanosis is abolished.

7. Draw an arterial blood gas.

8. Adjust ventilation as indicated by arterial blood gas results (Figure 8-11).

**Table 8-14** Treatment of Pneumothorax in the Neonate

1. Determination of the presence of a pneumothorax under tension (decreased breath sounds, shift of heart and mediastinum, confirmatory x-ray).

2. Insert a 23-gauge butterfly needle attached to a 20-cc syringe anteriorly in the third interspace in the midclavicular line.

3. Evacuate air until none can be removed. Recheck periodically.

4. Insert a 10- to 14-Fr. catheter in the fourth to fifth interspace in the midaxillary line, or in the second interspace in the midclavicular line. The catheter should be advanced for a total of 4 to 6 cm.

5. Attach to suction drainage system; set at an initial negative pressure of 10 cm $H_2O$. Increase as needed.

6. Continue suction until no air is bubbling in the second chamber to indicate continued air leak.

7. When no bubbling has been observed for at least 24 hours, place chest tube to water seal only (no suction) for 24 hours and obtain chest x-rays at 2 and 24 hours. Do not clamp tube!

8. Remove tube and cover opening with ointment seal. Tube should be removed at the end of a positive pressure breath to prevent air from entering pleural space.

Chest wall excursion should be approximately 0.25 to 0.5 cm in the infant who is adequately ventilated. At the time of initiation of mechanical ventilation, you should auscultate the chest and attempt to achieve breath sounds that mimic faint inspiratory rales, indicating the opening of terminal air spaces. If you ventilate at this stage to achieve good breath sounds, you will commonly find that the baby is being excessively ventilated 1 to 2 hours later. Thus, the minimal settings that achieve adequate oxygenation and ventilation are the desired goal. Overventilation may quickly result in pulmonary interstitial emphysema, pneumomediastinum, or pneumothorax. The treatment of pneumothorax is outlined in Table 8-14.

Ventilator therapy for the infant with respiratory distress syndrome continues to be a source of controversy. Numerous techniques of ventilation have been devised to treat RDS, but few controlled studies have been performed. All techniques of mechanical ventilation attempt to provide adequate oxygenation

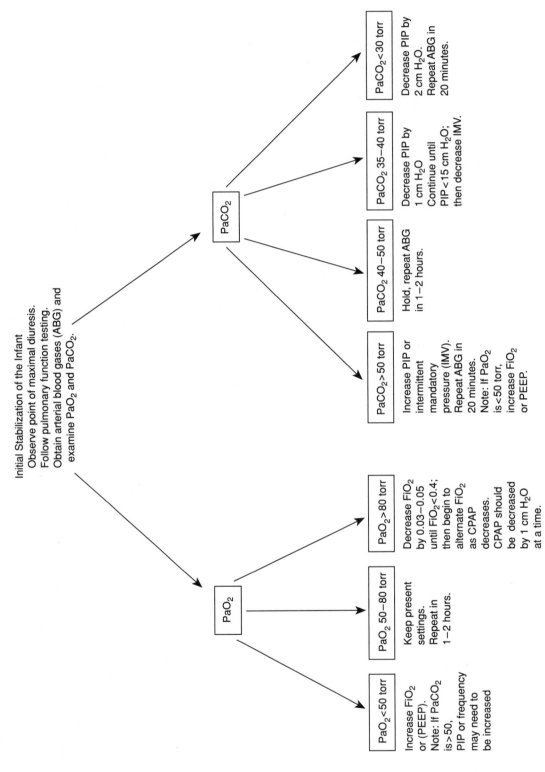

**Figure 8-11** Ventilator therapy during neonatal lung disease.

176

and ventilation at the least pulmonary cost. Barotrauma to the lungs, which can result in permanent disability, is the primary adverse effect of mechanical respirators. During the past few years, techniques such as high-frequency ventilation and flow synchronized mechanical ventilation have been developed to try to reduce lung injury. Unfortunately, to date there is little scientific evidence to demonstrate that these newer techniques result in major advantages for the premature infant with RDS.

At Thomas Jefferson University Hospital, we currently use the approach outlined in Figure 8-11. These recommendations are only guidelines and should not be adhered to blindly. In general, the approach to stabilization of the infant with respiratory distress syndrome, as described in Figure 8-11, commonly leads to initial ventilator rates of 40 to 60 breaths per minute, and an inspiratory to expiratory (I : E) ratio of 1 : 1 to 1 : 2. Our practice is to avoid increasing (reversing) this ratio because of the risk of overdistending the lung and impeding central venous return to the heart, particularly as recovery is initiated. In addition, we limit inspiration to a maximum of 0.5 to 0.6 second so that inspiratory time does not become excessively prolonged as ventilator rate is reduced.

In weaning from the ventilator, frequent small changes are preferable to occasional

**Table 8-15**  Ventilator Variables in Neonatal Respiratory Care: Advantages and Disadvantages

| VARIABLE | ADVANTAGES | DISADVANTAGES |
|---|---|---|
| Oxygen | Prevent hypoxemia and lactic acidosis. Essential in preventing perinatal asphyxia, which may occur with many neonatal lung diseases. | Excessive or prolonged oxygen use may contribute to the development of chronic lung disease (bronchopulmonary dysplasia) and retinopathy of prematurity. |
| Continuous positive airway pressure (CPAP) | Maintain alveolar volume; recruit atelectatic areas of the lung; improve distribution of ventilation and V/Q matching; assist in weaning phases; may enhance surfactant release. | High CPAP may overdistend lung and cause air leaks; reduce compliance; reduce venous return and cardiac output, leading to IVH; increase pulmonary vascular resistance (PVR); cause $CO_2$ retention. |
| Peak inspiratory pressure (PIP) Relative PIP level depends on size of the infant, the basic lung disease, compliance, resistance, and lung volume. | Improve tidal volume and minute ventilation; decrease $PaCO_2$; increase $PaO_2$; prevent atelectasis and recruit alveoli. May also reduce pulmonary hypertension. | Prolonged or elevated PIP may overdistend the lung and cause air leaks; impede venous return and cardiac output; enhance the probability of BPD developing; increase PVR. |
| Rate or Frequency For the neonate, high rate usually refers to frequencies above 60 BPM. Low rate usually refers to rates of 40 BPM and below. | Low rates appear to improve $CO_2$ elimination at normal I : E ratios. Oxygenation may improve with low rates and reversed I : E, or at high rates, if air trapping occurs. Gradual rate reduction useful in weaning (IMV). High rates may reduce pulmonary hypertension with hyperventilation. Increased frequency may allow a decrease in $V_T$ and PIP. | With low rate, $V_T$ must be increased to achieve adequate ventilation and oxygenation. Often increased MAP is needed as well, increasing chances of BPD. High rate may increase air trapping and lead to air leaks. Respiratory alkalosis can also occur with too rapid a ventilatory rate. |
| Inspiratory to expiratory ratio (I : E) | Prolonging inspiration increases mean airway pressure and improves oxygenation. Prolonging expiration enhances $CO_2$ removal and decreases risk of air trapping. Prolonged expiration is also useful during weaning phases and helpful during hyperventilation for pulmonary hypertension. | Prolonged inspiration may impede venous return and increase IVH risk; result in air trapping and air leaks; reduce pulmonary blood flow in pulmonary hypertension syndromes. Prolonged expiration may reduce oxygenation; increase dead space ventilation if tidal volume is too low. |

large changes. This latter type of weaning often results in sudden deterioration, which necessitates a large increase in the inspired oxygen concentration or ventilator settings. Such errors in weaning inevitably increase the ultimate amount of time spent on the ventilator, since the infant will usually have increasing periods of instability. The use of small decrements as noted in Figure 8-11 usually prevents this difficulty. In addition, the physician using mechanical ventilation should have a clear understanding of the pros and cons of changing ventilator controls in the infant with respiratory distress (Table 8-15).

While on a ventilator, an infant may suddenly deteriorate or fail to oxygenate and ventilate adequately. In these circumstances, the physician must rapidly evaluate whether the baby is having a clinical problem (such as a pneumothorax) that requires immediate intervention, or whether the ventilator is malfunctioning. The child should be removed from the mechanical ventilator during such periods and be hand ventilated with a bag and mask. The thought processes outlined in Table 8-16 should then be followed. If, after this approach has been carried out, it appears that the severity of the infant's lung disease is progressing to the point where conventional mechanical ventilation is inadequate, then you should consider the use of high-frequency ventilation for the further management of the infant.

**Table 8-16** The Response to Acute Deterioration of a Ventilated Infant

---

**Acute Deterioration of Clinical Status**
(cyanosis, hypotension, hypercapnea, bradycardia)

1. Remove infant from ventilator and hand ventilate with bag and mask.

2. Check ventilator:
   Occlude outlet.
   Check movement of pressure gauge.
   Check hoses.
   Check humidification system.
   Check internal machine function.

3. Observe infant:
   Are breath sounds adequate?
   If not, increase inspiratory pressure.
   If pressure fails to improve situation, child may have tube malposition, obstruction, or tension pneumothorax.
   Also consider nonpulmonary causes such as patent ductus arteriosus or intraventricular hemorrhage.

---

# HIGH-FREQUENCY VENTILATION

## CASE STUDY 5 continued

Baby F continues to do poorly after 48 hours on conventional mechanical ventilation. Her respiratory settings are as follows: frequency, 50 BPM; peak inspiratory pressure (PIP), 38 cm $H_2O$; positive end-expiratory pressure (PEEP), 6 cm $H_2O$; inspiratory oxygen concentration ($FiO_2$), 0.86; inspiratory time (*Ti*), 0.6 seconds. Her latest arterial blood gas reveals the following: pH, 7.22; $PaCO_2$, 56 mm Hg; $PaO_2$, 48 mm Hg; BE −5. Her chest radiograph reveals bilateral pulmonary interstitial emphysema.

## EXERCISE 13

### ■ Question:
What would you do now?

### ■ Discussion:
High-frequency ventilation (HFV) is a form of mechanical ventilation that uses extremely small tidal volumes and high frequencies to provide gas exchange. The theoretical advantage of this form of therapy is that it can potentially reduce pulmonary barotrauma while maintaining oxygenation and ventilation. The mechanism by which HFV produces gas exchange is not understood at the present time. One of the primary difficulties in describing the physiological effects of HFV derives from the fact that with most forms of HFV, tidal volume is near or less than dead space volume. Because alveolar ventilation equals the product of ventilatory frequency and tidal volume minus the dead space volume, alveolar ventilation would seem to approach zero! Alternative mechanisms (e.g., spike formation, augmented diffusion, or helical diffusion) must, therefore, operate during high frequency to enable adequate gas exchange.

The two basic types of HFV available at the present time are *high-frequency oscillatory ventilation* (HFOV) (Fig. 8-12), in which a piston or a vibrating diaphragm creates a bidirectional sine wave movement of gas within the airway, and *high-frequency jet ventilation* (HFJV) (Fig. 8-13) in which a positive-pressure gas flow to the patient is intermittently interrupted, followed by a passive expiratory relaxation of the lung. Entrainment appears to as-

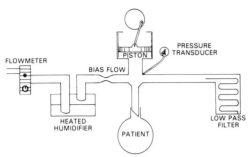

**Figure 8-12** Diagrammatic representation of high-frequency oscillatory ventilation.
From Bancalari E, Goldberg RN: High frequency ventilation in the neonate. *Clin Perinatol* 1987; 14:585. Reprinted with permission of W.B. Saunders Company.

**Table 8-17** Indications for High-Frequency Ventilation

Demonstrated Efficacy
1. Severe RDS
2. RDS complicated by pulmonary air leak
3. Bronchopleural fistula

Occasional Efficacy
1. Persistent pulmonary hypertension
2. Meconium aspiration syndrome
3. Neonatal pneumonia (group B streptococcus)
4. Pulmonary hypoplasia

Undetermined Efficacy
1. Surfactant delivery in RDS
2. Congenital diaphragmatic hernia
3. Cystic malformations of the lung
4. HFV in combination with extracorporeal membrane oxygenation (ECMO) (to reduce pulmonary injury)

sist in gas exchange in both forms of HFV. Entrainment refers to the process by which vacuum effects in the vicinity of the orifice of the high-frequency device draw additional gas molecules into the airway. Thus, an additional gas volume is delivered beyond what is directly injected by the high-frequency ventilator. As a result, gas exchange at a given level of airway pressure seems to be greater with high-frequency ventilation than with more conventional modes of ventilatory support.

Studies with HFJV indicate that improved gas exchange occurs at lower peak inflating pressures and lower mean airway pressures when compared to conventional ventilation. In particular, carbon dioxide elimination is more effective at lower peak pressures, so theoretically HFJVs may provide a safer modality of therapy in the infant with severe neonatal lung disease. To date, HFJV has not produced a significant reduction in the incidence of chronic lung injury, although resolution of

pulmonary air leaks does appear to be enhanced with HFJV. In addition, infants with respiratory failure refractory to treatment with conventional mechanical ventilation often appear to improve on HFJV (Table 8-17).

High-frequency oscillatory ventilation, in contrast to HFJV, appears to require higher mean airway pressures to achieve similar degrees of effectiveness. In a major prospective collaborative trial using HFOV for the treatment of neonatal lung disease in preterm infants, no benefit of HFOV could be shown. In addition, pulmonary air leaks and severe degrees of neonatal intracranial hemorrhage were more common in infants treated with HFOV compared to infants treated with conventional mechanical ventilation. These results suggest that the higher mean airway pressures needed with HFOV may result in overdistention of airways and impedance of venous return to the heart, leading to the noted complications. In contrast to those findings, however, several recent more limited studies have indicated that HFOV may ventilate infants with RDS more effectively and result in less chronic lung disease.

■ **Answer:**
Initiate HFJV.

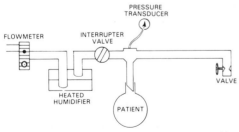

**Figure 8-13** Diagrammatic representation of high-frequency jet ventilation (HFJV).
From Bancalari E, Goldberg RN: High frequency ventilation in the neonate. *Clin Perinatol* 1987; 14:583. Reprinted with permission of W.B. Saunders Company.

**The Technique of High-Frequency Jet Ventilation**

HFJV has proved to be a valuable addition to the treatment modalities available to the neonatologist. Preliminary evidence indicates that some infants who no longer respond to conventional modes of mechanical ventilation can be effectively managed with HFJV. In addition, pulmonary air leak syndromes appear to resolve more rapidly with HFJV. At present, only one jet ventilator is FDA approved in the United States, the Bunnell Life Pulse® (Bunnell, Salt Lake City, Utah). The Bunnell Life Pulse® is a pressure-driven, servo-controlled, solenoid-based device that uses several unique designs to achieve effectiveness.

The Life Pulse is designed to be used in parallel with a conventional mechanical ventilator. To accomplish this synchronization, a specially designed endotracheal (ET) tube needs to be inserted into the infant's airway. This ET tube, referred to as the Hi-Lo tube® (Mallinckrodt, St. Louis, Missouri) must be placed before HFJV is started. The tube is a triple-lumen tube. The main port is connected to the conventional ventilator. The remaining two ports are used for sensing pressure (near the tip of the ET tube) and delivery of jet gas flow (in the midportion of the tube). Distal tracheal airway pressure is constantly sensed through the pressure port, resulting in real-time adjustment of PIP during treatment. Jet pulsations are delivered by the opening and closing of a solenoid valve on a piece of plastic tubing, which lies in a box near the infant's head. This interruption of flow produces spike-like jets of gas in the airway, resulting in *jet ventilation.*

If the patient to be treated with HFJV does have a pulmonary air leak, HFJV is usually started alone (without background ventilation). PEEP is provided through the main port, which connects to the conventional ventilator. For infants with RDS, the starting PIP on HFJV is approximately 80% of the peak pressure used on the conventional mechanical ventilator. For infants with diseases other than RDS, or if pulmonary hypertension is a significant component of the child's illness, the same initial PIP is used on the HFJV. The Life Pulse ventilator starts with a rate of 420 BPM. Empirical observations and animal studies have indicated that rates of 400 to 500 BPM are optimal for this particular ventilator. We have noted that each type of high-frequency ventilator appears to have its own optimal frequency. This frequency is an inherent characteristic of the unit and not related to the underlying disease. Following initiation of HFJV

in the presence of an air leak, we allow 6 to 24 hours before adding background ventilation with the conventional ventilator.

In the neonate, one of the common complications of HFJV is atelectasis. As a result, failure to provide background positive-pressure conventional breaths usually results in a deterioration in the infant's status. The rate for such background ventilation is usually 5 to 10 breaths per minute. This technique improves oxygenation and reduces the incidence of atelectasis. Pressures dissipate rapidly with this approach, so that the airway is not exposed to unusually high pressures.

The *jet valve on-time* (equivalent to inspiratory time) on the jet ventilator is set at 0.02 seconds, the shortest possible. Prolonging inspiration during HFJV does not improve oxygenation and it appears that the jet ventilator is most effective when the "jet" is sharpest. The primary ways to improve oxygenation during HFJV are (1) increasing the inspiratory oxygen concentration, (2) increasing the PEEP, and (3) increasing the rate of background sighing to 15 to 20 BPM or higher.

Carbon dioxide elimination is extremely effective during HFJV and it is not uncommon to see $PaCO_2$ levels in the range of 20 to 35 torr when an infant is first placed on the HFJV. In practice, there is often a need to raise the $PaCO_2$ because of theoretical risk of cerebral ischemia, which is mediated by a fall in the blood carbon dioxide concentration. $PaCO_2$ can be increased by (1) increasing the PEEP, (2) decreasing the background sigh rate, (3) increasing the background sigh (peak) pressure, or (4) reducing the PIP on the jet ventilator. In some cases, prolonging the background sigh time may also help raise the $PaCO_2$. Decreasing the jet ventilator rate can potentially increase the $PaCO_2$. However, it also typically decreases oxygenation (as ventilator effectiveness is reduced) and is therefore not recommended as an initial approach.

Weaning from HFJV again concentrates on reducing the factors primarily responsible for bronchopulmonary dysplasia. The inspiratory oxygen concentration and PIP are usually reduced first. With HFJV, you must be extremely cautious during the weaning process. The most common mistake made is to wean too rapidly, leading to clinical deterioration and a need to increase settings. This weaning error is often difficult to pick up because it occurs several hours after a change has been made in ventilatory support. It appears that decreasing the PIP in a child on HFJV may lead to a gradual, progressive atelectasis that is not reflected in arterial blood gases for several hours. To reinflate the lung, increased pressure is needed. Weaning should therefore be approached cautiously, and changes should not be made more frequently than every 1 to 2 hours.

The complications of HFJV do not appear to be any different from conventional mechanical ventilation. Necrotizing tracheobronchitis (NTB), a severe airway injury that results in sloughing of the tracheal mucosa, was once thought to be a problem specific to HFJV. It has since been demonstrated that NTB occurs with all forms of ventilation and is far less common with the current modes of HFJV. You should be sure, however, that humidification is adequate during HFJV treatment. Earlier prototypes of the Life Pulse® ventilator had a less effective method for humidifying gas, so that airway injury may have occurred not only from the shear forces on the airway, but also from the dryness of the gases as well.

### Fluid Therapy

Fluid therapy during mechanical ventilation is also of critical importance. This subject is reviewed in detail in Chapter 2. In general, however, fluids should be kept at the minimum level that adequately supports blood pressure and tissue perfusion. Excessive fluid administration in the form of sodium bicarbonate, fresh frozen plasma, or crystalloid solution may contribute to development of PDA, intraventricular hemorrhage, and bronchopulmonary dysplasia. One should not, however, restrict fluids to the point where the infant begins to demonstrate lactic acidosis from circulatory compromise.

A clinical sign that we have found particularly useful in the management of infants with RDS is that of maximum diuresis. In general, infants with respiratory distress syndrome demonstrate a brisk diuresis exceeding 100% of fluid intake for an 8- to 16-hour period between 24 and 60 hours of life. Improvement in ventilator settings rarely occurs before this time, but often changes quickly after the diuresis has been initiated. You can therefore anticipate improved oxygenation and ventilation, and an attempt to wean should be made at this time using frequent blood gases. Babies who demonstrate a diuresis after 72 hours of age have a greater likelihood of developing bronchopulmonary dysplasia.

### Nutrition

Adequate nutrition is essential for the recovery of all critically ill infants. Initiation of early peripheral intravenous alimentation will prevent significant protein breakdown and enhance the overall nutritional status. Parenteral nutrition with peripheral alimentation should be started on the second or third day of life. Central alimentation is used only when it is evident that the infant will have a prolonged period during which enteral feeding is contraindicated. In general, enteral feedings of low volume and reduced concentration (quarter-strength premature formulas) are started when the respiratory disease has diminished.

In very low birth weight infants who require prolonged intubation, you should proceed with feedings even when the endotracheal tube is still in place. A cautious approach to feeding is urged. For the small infant, either continuous or intermittent nasogastric or continuous nasotranspyloric feedings are used. You should ultimately strive to provide 120 cal/kg/day in these babies. Increased caloric intake may be necessary for infants with increased work of breathing or evidence of malabsorption. The reader is referred to Chapter 6 for a more complete discussion of nutritional requirements.

### CNS and Ultrasound Examination

Ultrasound evaluation of the central nervous system (CNS) has become an essential part of neonatal care. The risk of intraventricular hemorrhage is considerable in the baby with respiratory distress syndrome, and critical therapeutic decisions will commonly arise based on whether a substantial intraventricular hemorrhage exists. Our current practice is to obtain an ultrasound examination of the head during the acute phases of the illness (days 3 and 7) and less frequently thereafter. Most CNS injury in the premature infant occurs during the first 24 hours of life, again highlighting the importance of initial care and stabilization. During this period in particular, rapid changes in respiratory status or ventilator therapy can have major long-term implications for the infant with respiratory distress syndrome. A sudden increase or decrease in $PaCO_2$, the development of pneumothorax, and the use of excessive PIP all contribute to the development of neurological injury and intraventricular hemorrhage.

### Retinopathy of Prematurity

Retinopathy of prematurity (ROP), formerly called retrolental fibroplasia, is a common complication of prematurity. Although oxygen exposure has been implicated in its pathogenesis, there is a great deal of variability in the relationship between ROP and the duration of time spent in oxygen. Some investigators have therefore suggested that it is not only the high levels of oxygen, but the variability of oxygen levels and carbon dioxide levels that may be important in the etiology of ROP. In fact, a newly proposed study will attempt to maintain higher than normal oxygen levels in infants who reach threshold ROP in an attempt to limit progression of the disease. Any infant who has been exposed to oxygen for even brief periods should be periodically examined by an ophthalmologist beginning at 4 weeks of age and intermittently thereafter until the retina has matured. Infants with evidence of ROP will need frequent examinations throughout the first year of life.

### Chronic Care Following RDS

### EXERCISE 14

Select the one most appropriate answer for each of the following questions.

1. Bronchopulmonary dysplasia:
   (a) Is invariably fatal
   (b) Usually results in little functional limitation
   (c) Requires constant oxygen therapy
   (d) Responds to administration of trace metals
2. Tracheostomy in the chronically ventilated infant:
   (a) Should not be performed before 6 months of age
   (b) Is indicated for subglottic stenosis
   (c) Can never be removed
   (d) Should be routinely performed after 4 weeks of intubation

### ■ Discussion:

Most infants with respiratory distress syndrome successfully recover from their initial illness and ultimately do well. The value of follow-up studies in such children cannot be overemphasized, and they have contributed significantly to the improvements in care that have occurred during the past decade. A small number of infants, however, fail to recover from initial problems and survive with chronic respiratory disease. Although many of these babies have neurological problems and nutritional and feeding difficulties, the problem that causes the greatest management difficulty is the ventilator-dependent baby with bronchopulmonary dysplasia. This chapter ends with a brief discussion of some of the management issues involved in the care of these babies. The reader is referred to Chapter 9 for a more detailed discussion.

### ■ Answers:

1. b.

2. b.

### BRONCHOPULMONARY DYSPLASIA

Bronchopulmonary dysplasia was first described by Northway et al. in 1967. Four stages of the disease were described:

*Stage 1:* acute hyaline membrane disease (2 to 3 days of life)
*Stage 2:* stage of lung regeneration (4 to 10 days)
*Stage 3:* bronchial metaplasia, interstitial fibrosis, alveolar emphysema (10 to 20 days)
*Stage 4:* obstructive bronchiolitis with extensive interstitial fibrosis and increased focal emphysema (more than 1 month of age)

Numerous etiological factors have been evaluated, but at present it appears that PPV, oxygen administration, and increased pulmonary lung water are the elements that produce bronchopulmonary dysplasia (BPD) in a susceptible baby. Typically, these infants often have an insidious course during which the physician recognizes that there is increasing radiological evidence of lung injury, while the baby clearly demonstrates that continued rapid ventilator weaning is not possible. Most of these infants weigh less than 1,500 g at birth and have had a more severe course of respiratory distress syndrome. Growth is often poor as the caloric expenditure for increased work of breathing is increased. Attempts to give additional calories often lead to deterioration in pulmonary status because of the added fluid delivered. Thus, physicians find themselves with infants who have severe lung disease, who are ventilator dependent, and who are malnourished. Despite the need to maximize caloric intake, unlimited fluid intake is not advised. Fluid intake, in general, should rarely exceed 150 mL/kg/day because of the risk of aggravating interstitial lung edema (necessitating a 24 or 27 cal/oz. formula). If greater fluids are needed to provide calories for growth, diuretics may be useful in limiting interstitial edema.

Ventilator weaning is often very difficult in the child who has required intubation for more than 1 month. A simple approach that we have used successfully is outlined in Table 8-18. The error most commonly made in caring for these children is to wean them too rapidly. The chronically ventilator-dependent baby must have changes made that are almost imperceptible. Sudden decreases in ventilatory support may lead to retention of carbon dioxide, increased pulmonary artery pressure, and acute decompensation. Bronchodilators (theophylline, caffeine, metoproterenol, albuterol) are useful adjuncts during the weaning process. Infants should not be kept in a borderline hypoxic state because this tends to retard growth and may result in right-sided congestive heart failure. In that regard, it is important to remember that oxygen delivery depends not only on the degree of oxyhemoglobin saturation, but also on the amount of hemoglobin present. In addition, it has recently been demonstrated that infants with BPD exhibit decreased erythropoietin levels, which undoubtedly accentuates their anemia. Therefore, it is our recommendation that infants with BPD who are ventilator (and oxygen) dependent and who have hemoglobin concentrations less than 12 to 14 g/dL should receive packed red blood cell transfusions. Care during transfusion should be taken, since this volume load has the ability to worsen pulmonary compliance. Diuretic therapy may be valuable under such circumstances immediately following the transfusion.

Constant surveillance for septicemia and pneumonia is of critical importance in these infants. Lukens aspirates of the endotracheal tube 2 times per week will identify potential pathogens that are colonizing the upper respiratory tract. If pneumonia does occur, appropriate antimicrobial therapy should be initiated immediately.

After the infant has been intubated for more than 6 to 8 weeks, tracheostomy should be considered. There are no specific guidelines for this surgical intervention, although infants

**Table 8-18**  Approach to Ventilator Management in Infants with BPD

1. Note current ventilator settings. This approach is designated for the child who is more than 1 month of age, who has reached a plateau in weaning with little recent progress.

2. Estimate the probable number of days of ventilatory assistance that may be needed until extubation. A simple method is to allow 1 day for each breath per minute and each cm $H_2O$ PIP that is currently needed. For example, a child receiving a rate of 30 and a PIP of 24 will probably not be extubated for approximately 50 days.

3. Establish a predetermined weaning pattern that is likely to get the child to a point of extubation in that time period. The changes that are made should be almost imperceptible to the infant, i.e., each wean should be approximately one breath per minute, 1 cm $H_2O$ of PIP, or 1% to 2% oxygen. Faster weaning in BPD patients is usually not tolerated. *It is important to note that these children may tolerate larger weans for a period of time but often are unable to sustain the added respiratory effort that may be required.*

4. Use computerized pulmonary function testing (PFT) frequently to assess the effect of weaning, particularly in the child with tracheobronchomalacia. Excessively rapid pressure weaning in such infants may result in evidence of airway collapse on flow-volume loops on the PFT. The effects of bronchodilators, diuretics, and other therapy should also be assessed with PFT.

5. Flexible fiber optic bronchoscopy should be performed in any infant who fails to show progress after several weeks. In many instances, airway injury or granuloma formation may be present and interfere with successful weaning.

6. Pulse oximetry, transcutaneous $CO_2$ monitoring, end-tidal $CO_2$ monitoring, and occasional arterial blood gases can assist greatly in weaning.

7. The use of corticosteroids is controversial in these infants. Although some children with BPD may have a dramatic response to treatment, careful surveillance for infection is essential. One must also be aware of the fact that some children, particularly those treated after 1 month of age, can have a serious rebound deterioration in pulmonary status that typically occurs about 10 to 14 days after steroids are stopped. This rebound can be a life-threatening complication.

rarely can remain intubated for more than 3 months without developing subglottic stenosis. Unfortunately, this complication of intubation is typically not recognized until an initial attempt at extubation fails because of airway obstruction. Once subglottic stenosis is recognized, tracheostomy is a necessity. A discussion of parental involvement in care during chronic hospitalization is beyond the scope of this chapter. It is essential, however, for both parent and infant that a strong relationship be maintained, and parents should be urged to participate actively in the care of these infants. Infant stimulation programs, designed to involve parents as well as nursing staff, can help immeasurably in guiding the chronically ventilated child through prolonged hospitalization.

The prognosis for the infant with severe BPD from a respiratory standpoint is good. Because of the capacity of the lung to generate new tissue, once barotrauma is reduced and infant growth ensues, recovery occurs over a period of several months. The majority of infants are no longer oxygen dependent by a year of age, even with the most severe forms of the disease. However, infants with congestive heart failure on the basis of cor pulmonale tend to do less well and may not survive.

## BIBLIOGRAPHY

### Development of the Lung

1. Adams FH, Fujiwara T, Rowshan G: The nature and origin of the fluid in the fetal lamb lung. *J Pediatr* 1963; 63:881–888.
2. Baycroft J, Barron DH: The genesis of respiratory movements in the foetus of sheep. *J Physiol* 1937; 88:56–61.
3. Clements JA, Brown ES, Johnson RP: Pulmonary surface tension and the mucous lining of the lungs: Some theoretical considerations. *J Appl Physiol* 1958; 12:262.
4. Stahlman MT, Gray ME: Anatomic development and maturation of the lungs. *Clin Perinatol* 1978; 5:181.
5. Torday JS, Nielsen HC, Montserrat DeM, et al: Sex differences in fetal lung maturation. *Am Rev Resp Dis* 1981; 123:205.

### Surfactant

6. Avery ME, Mead J: Surface properties in relation to atelectasis and hyaline membrane disease. *Am J Dis Child* 1959; 97:517–523.
7. Clements JA, Platzker ACG, Tierney DF, et al: Assessment of the risk of respiratory distress syndrome by a rapid test for surfactant in pulmonary fluid. *N Engl J Med* 1972; 286:1077–1081.
8. Clements JA: Surface tension of lung extracts. *Proc Soc Exp Biol Med* 1957; 95:170–172.
9. Collaborative European Group: Surfactant replacement therapy for severe neonatal respiratory distress syndrome: An international randomized clinical trial. *Pediatrics* 1988; 82:683–691.
10. Enhorning G, Shennon A, Possmayer F, et al: Prevention of neonatal respiratory distress syndrome by tracheal instillation of surfactant: A randomized clinical trial. *Pediatrics* 1985; 76:145–153.
11. Farrell PM, Hamosh M: The biochemistry of fetal lung development. *Clin Perinatol* 1978; 5:197.
12. Fujiwara T, Chida S, Watobe Y, et al: Artificial surfactant therapy in hyaline membrane disease. *Lancet* 1980; 1:55–58.
13. Hennes HM, Lee MB, Raimm AA, et al: Surfactant replacement therapy in respiratory distress syndrome. *Am J Dis Child* 1991; 145:102–104.
14. Kwong M, Egan E, Notter RH, et al: Double-blind clinical trial of calf lung surfactant extract for the prevention of hyaline membrane disease in extremely premature infants. *Pediatrics* 1985; 76:585–592.
15. Merritt TA, Hallman M, Bloom BT, et al: Prophylactic treatment of very premature infants with human surfactant. *N Engl J Med* 1986; 315:785–790.

### Obstetric Considerations

16. Berkowitz ES, Mehalek KE, Chithara U, et al: Doppler umbilical velocimetry in the prediction of adverse outcome in pregnancies at risk for intrauterine growth retardation. *Obstet Gynecol* 1988; 71:742–746.
17. Clements JA, Platzker ACG, Tierney DF, et al: Assessment of the risk of respiratory distress syndrome by a rapid test for surfactant in pulmonary fluid. *N Engl J Med* 1972; 286:1077.
18. Evertson LR, Gauthier RJ, Schifrin BS, et al: Antepartum fetal heart rate testing: I. Evolution of the nonstress test. *Am J Obstet Gynecol* 1979; 29:133.
19. Gluck L, Kulovich MV, Borer RC Jr: Estimates of fetal lung maturity. *Clin Perinatol* 1974; 1:125.
20. Gluck L, Kulovich MV, Borer RC Jr, et al: Diagnosis of the respiratory distress syndrome by amniocentesis. *Am J Obstet Gynecol* 1971; 109:440.
21. Huddleston JF, Freeman RK: Assessment of fetal well-being by antepartum fetal heart rate testing. In Bolognese RJ, Schwarz RH, Schneider J, eds: *Perinatal Medicine*. Baltimore, Williams and Wilkins, 1982, pp. 129–152.
22. Manning FA, Platt LD, Sipos L: Antepartum fetal evaluation. Development of a fetal biophysical profile score. *Am J Obstet Gynecol* 1980; 136:787.
23. Morrow R, Ritchie K: Doppler ultrasound fetal velocimetry and its role in obstetrics. *Clin Perinatol* 1989; 16(3):771.

24. Patrick J, Challis J: Measurement of human fetal breathing movements in healthy pregnancies using a real-time scanner. *Semin Perin* 1980; 4:275.
25. Patrick JE, Featherson W, Vick H, et al: Human fetal breathing and gross body movements at weeks 34–35 of gestation. *Am J Obstet Gynecol* 1978; 130:693.
26. Ray M, Freeman R, Pine S, et al: Clinical experience with the oxytocin challenge test. *Am J Obstet Gynecol* 1972; 114:1.
27. Rochard F, Schefrin BS, Guilan C: Non-stressed fetal heart rate monitoring in the antepartum period. *Am J Obstet Gynecol* 1976; 126:669.
28. Roy M, Freeman RK, Pine S, et al: Clinical experience with the oxytocin challenge test. *Am J Obstet Gynecol* 1972; 114:1.
29. Schleuter MA, Phibbs RH, Creasy RK, et al: Antenatal prediction of graduated risk of hyaline membrane disease by amniotic fluid from test for surfactant. *Am J Obstet Gynecol* 1979; 134:671.
30. Usher RH, McLean F, Maughan GB: Respiratory distress syndrome in infants delivered by cesarean section. *Am J Obstet Gynecol* 1964; 88:806.
31. Vintzileos AM, Campbell WA, Rodis JF: Fetal biophysical profile scoring: Current status. *Clin Perinatol* 1989; 16(3):661.
32. Yoon JJ, Kohl S, Harper RG: The relationship between maternal hypertensive disease of pregnancy and the incidence of idiopathic respiratory distress syndrome. *Pediatrics* 1980; 65:735.

### Prevention of Respiratory Distress Syndrome

33. Bauer CR, Stein L, Colle E: Prolonged rupture of membranes associated with a decreased incidence of respiratory distress syndrome. *Pediatrics* 1974; 53:7.
34. Collaborative Group on Antenatal Steroid Therapy: Effect of antenatal dexamethasone administration on the prevention of respiratory distress syndrome. *Am J Obstet Gynecol* 1981; 141:276.
35. Kotas RV, Avery MD: Accelerated appearance of pulmonary surfactant in the fetal rabbit. *J Appl Physiol* 1971; 30:358.
36. Liggins GC, Howie RN: A controlled trial of antepartum glucocortoid treatment for prevention of the respiratory distress syndrome in premature infants. *Pediatrics* 1972; 50:515.

### Differential Diagnosis of Respiratory Distress Syndrome

37. Ablow RC, Driscoll SG, Effman EL, et al: A comparison of early onset of group B streptococcal neonatal infection and the respiratory distress syndrome of the newborn. *N Engl J Med* 1976; 294:65.
38. Avery ME, Gatewood OB, Brumley G: Transient tachypnea of the newborn. *Am J Dis Child* 1966; 111:380.
39. Edwards DK, Jacob J, Gluck L: The immature lung. *Am J Roentgenol* 1980; 131:1009.

### Pathophysiology of Respiratory Distress Syndrome

40. Avery ME, Mead J: Surface properties in relation to atelectasis and hyaline membrane disease. *Am J Dis Child* 1959; 97:517.
41. Chu J, Clements B, Colten E, et al: The pulmonary hypoperfusion syndrome. *Pediatrics* 1967; 35:733.
42. Spitzer AR, Fox WW, Delivoria-Papadopoulos M: Maximum diuresis—A factor in predicting recovery from respiratory distress syndrome and the development of bronchopulmonary dysplasia. *J Pediatr* 1981; 98:476.

### Management of Respiratory Distress Syndrome

43. Bell EF, Warburton D, Stonestreet BS, et al: Effect of fluid administration on the development of symptomatic patent ductus arteriosus and congestive heart failure in premature infants. *N Engl J Med* 1980; 302:598.
44. Berman LS, Fox WW, Raphaely RC, et al: Optimum levels of CPAP for tracheal extubation of newborns. *J Pediatr* 1976; 89:109.
45. Friedman WF, Hirschklan MR, Printz MP, et al: Pharmacologic closure of patent ductus arteriosus in the premature infant. *N Engl J Med* 1976; 295:526.
46. Fujiwara T, Chida S, Watobe Y, et al: Arterial surfactant therapy in hyaline membrane disease. *Lancet* 1980; 1:55.
47. Gregory GA, Kitterman JA, Phibbs RH, et al: Treatment of the idiopathic respiratory distress syndrome with continuous positive airway pressure. *N Engl J Med* 1971; 284:1333.
48. Heaf DP, Belik J, Spitzer AR, et al: Changes in pulmonary function during the diuretic phase of respiratory distress syndrome. *J Pediatr* 1982; 101:103.
49. Heymann MA, Rudolph AM, Silverman NH: Closure of the ductus arteriosus in premature infants by inhibition of prostaglandin synthesis. *N Engl J Med* 1976; 295:530.
50. Peabody JL, Gregory GA, Willis MM, et al: Transcutaneous oxygen tension in sick infants. *Am Rev Resp Dis* 1978; 118:83.
51. Reynolds EOR: Management of hyaline membrane disease. *Br Med Bull* 1975; 31:18.

### Mechanical Ventilation in Respiratory Distress Syndrome

52. Bancalari E: Inadvertent positive end-expiratory pressure during mechanical ventilation. *J Pediatr* 1986; 108:567–569.
53. Bland RD, Kim MH, Nyak MJ, et al: High frequency mechanical ventilation of low birthweight infants with respiratory failure from hyaline membrane disease: 92% survival. *Pediatr Res* 1977; 11:531.
54. Bonta BW, Vavy R, Warshaw JB, et al: Determination of optimal continuous positive airway

pressure for the treatment of RDS by measurement of esophageal pressure. *J Pediatr* 1977; 91:449.

55. Boros SJ: Variations in inspiratory-expiratory ratio and air pressure waveform during mechanical ventilation: The significance of mean airway pressure. *J Pediatr* 1979; 94:114–117.

56. Boros SJ, Bing BR, Mammel MC, et al: Using conventional ventilators at unconventional rates. *Pediatrics* 1984; 74:487–492.

57. Boros SJ, Mabaln SV, Ewald R, et al: The effect of independent variations in inspiratory-expiratory ratio and end expiratory pressure during mechanical ventilation in hyaline membrane disease: The significance of mean airway pressure. *J Pediatr* 1977; 91:794.

58. Butler WJ, Bohn DJ, Mujaska K, et al: Ventilation of humans by high frequency oscillations. *Anesthesiology* 1979; 51:J368.

59. Field D, Milner AD, Hopkins IE: Effects of positive end expiratory pressure during ventilation of the preterm infant. *Arch Dis Child* 1985; 60:843–847.

60. Field D, Milner AD, Hopkin IE: Inspiratory-to-expiratory ratio during ventilation for idiopathic respiratory distress syndrome. *Pediatr Pulmonol* 1989; 7:2–7.

61. Frantz D, Start AR, Dorbun HL: Ventilation of infants at frequencies up to 1,800/minute. *Pediatr Res* 1980; 14:642.

62. Gluck L, Kulovich MV, Borer RC Jr, et al: Diagnosis of respiratory distress syndrome by amniocentesis. *Am J Obstet Gynecol* 1971; 109:440–445.

63. Haman S, Reynolds EOR: Methods of improving oxygenation in infants mechanically ventilated for severe hyaline membrane disease. *Arch Dis Child* 1973; 48:612–617.

64. Stark AR, Bascom R, Frantz ID: Muscle relaxation in mechanically ventilated infants. *J Pediatr* 1979; 94:439.

### High-Frequency Ventilation

65. Bland RD, Kim MH, Light MJ, et al: High frequency mechanical ventilation in severe hyaline membrane disease. An alternative treatment? *Crit Care Med* 1980; 8:275–280.

66. Boros SJ, Mammel MC, Coleman JM, et al: Neonatal high-frequency jet ventilation: Four years experience. *Pediatrics* 1985; 75:657–663.

67. Carlo WA, Siner B, Chatburn RL, et al: Early randomized intervention with high frequency jet ventilation in respiratory distress syndrome. *J Pediatr* 1990; 117:765–770.

68. Carter JM, Gerstmann DR, Clark RH, et al: High frequency oscillatory ventilation and extracorporeal membrane oxygenation for the treatment of acute neonatal respiratory failure. *Pediatrics* 1990; 85:159–164.

69. Fredberg JJ: Augmented diffusion in the airways can support pulmonary gas exchange. *J Appl Physiol* 1980; 49:232–238.

70. Fredberg JT, Glass GM, Boynton BR, et al: Factors influencing performance of neonatal high frequency ventilators. *J Appl Physiol* 1987; 62:2485–2490.

71. Hanson JB, Waldstein G, Hernandez JA, et al: Necrotizing tracheobronchitis: An ischemic lesion. *Am J Dis Child* 1988; 142:1094–1098.

72. HiFi Study Group: High frequency oscillatory ventilation compared with conventional intermittent mechanical ventilation in the treatment of respiratory failure in preterm infants: Neurodevelopmental follow-up at 16 to 24 months post-term age. *J Pediatr* 1990; 117:939–946.

73. HiFi Study Group: High frequency oscillatory ventilation compared with conventional mechanical ventilation in the treatment of respiratory failure in preterm infants. *N Engl J Med* 1989; 320:88–93.

74. HiFi Study Group: Pulmonary follow-up of children treated with high frequency oscillatory ventilation compared to conventional mechanical ventilation. *J Pediatr* 1990; 116:933–941.

75. Keszler M, Donn SM, Bucciarelli RL: Controlled multicenter trial of high frequency jet ventilation vs. conventional ventilation in newborns with pulmonary interstitial emphysema. *Pediatr Res* 1990; 27:309A.

76. McCullough PR, Forkert PG, Froese AB: Lung volume maintenance prevents lung injury during high frequency oscillatory ventilation in surfactant deficient rabbits. *Am Rev Resp Dis* 1988; 137:1185–1192.

77. Spitzer AR, Butler S, Fox WW: Ventilatory response of combined high-frequency jet ventilation and conventional mechanical ventilation for the rescue treatment of severe neonatal lung. disease. *Pediatr Pulmonol* 1989; 7:244–249.

### Complications of Respiratory Distress Syndrome

78. Berg TJ, Pagatkhan RD, Reed MH, et al: Bronchopulmonary dysplasia and lung rupture in hyaline membrane disease: Influence of continuous distending pressure. *Pediatrics* 1975; 55:51.

79. Brown ER, Start AR, Sosenko I, et al: Bronchopulmonary dysplasia: Possible relationship to pulmonary edema. *J Pediatr* 1978; 92:982.

80. Davis JM, Bhutani VK, Stefano JL et al: Changes in pulmonary mechanics following caffeine administration in infants with bronchopulmonary dysplasia. *Pediatr Pulmonol* 1989; 6:49–52.

81. Edwards DK: Radiographic aspects of bronchopulmonary dysplasia. *J Pediatr* 1979; 95:823.

82. Edwards DK, Wayne MD, Northway WH: Twelve years' experience with bronchopulmonary dysplasia. *Pediatrics* 1977; 59:839.

83. Fox WW, Spitzer AR, Rozycki HJ: Clinical assessment and management of bronchopulmonary dysplasia. In Guthrie R, ed: *Neonatal Intensive Care*. Edinburgh, Churchill Livingstone, 1988, pp. 75–90.

84. Hall RT, Rhodes PG: Pneumothorax and pneumomediastinum in infants with idiopathic respiratory distress syndrome receiving

continuous positive airway pressure. *Pediatrics* 1975; 55:493–499.

85. Jacob J, Gluck L, DeSessa T, et al: The contribution of PDA in the neonate with severe RDS. *J Pediatr* 1980; 96:79.

86. Kazzi NJ, Brans YW, Poland RL: Dexamethasone effects on the hospital course of infants with bronchopulmonary dysplasia who are dependent on artificial ventilation. *Pediatrics* 1990; 86:722–727.

87. Kushnamoorthy KS, Shannon DC, DeLong GR, et al: Neurologic sequelae in the survivors of neonatal intraventricular hemorrhage. *Pediatrics* 1979; 64:233.

88. Lipscomb AP, Thorburn RJ, Reynolds EOR, et al: Pneumothorax and cerebral hemorrhage in preterm infants. *Lancet* 1981; 1:414.

89. Modanoky DL, Lawson EE, Chernick V, et al: Pneumothorax and other forms of pulmonary air leak in newborns. *Am Rev Resp Dis* 1979; 120:729.

90. Northway WH, Rosan RC, Porter DY: Pulmonary disease following respiratory therapy of hyaline membrane disease. *N Engl J Med* 1967; 276:375.

91. Ogata ES, Gregory GA, Kitterman JA, et al: Pneumothorax in the respiratory distress syndrome: Incidence and effect on vital signs, blood gases and pH. *Pediatrics* 1976; 58:177.

92. Philip AGS: Oxygen plus pressure plus time: The etiology of bronchopulmonary dysplasia. *Pediatrics* 1975; 55:44–50.

93. Sotomayor JL, Godinez RI, Borden S, Wilmott RW: Large airway collapse due to acquired tracheobronchomalacia in infancy. *Am J Dis Child* 1986; 140:367–371.

94. Spitzer AR, Fox WW, Delivoria-Papadopoulos M: Maximum diuresis—a factor in predicting recovery from respiratory distress syndrome and the development of bronchopulmonary dysplasia. *J Pediatr* 1981; 98:476–491.

95. Stefano JL, Abbasi S, Pearlman SA, et al: Closure of the ductus arteriosus with indomethacin in ventilated neonated with respiratory distress syndrome. *Am Rev Resp Dis* 1991; 143:236–239.

96. Stefano JL, Bhutani VK: Role of furosemide therapy after booster-packed erythrocyte transfusions in infants with bronchopulmonary dysplasia. *J Pediatr* 1990; 117(6):965–968.

97. Stefano JL, Bhutani VK, Fox WW: A randomized placebo-controlled study to evaluate the effects of oral albuterol on pulmonary mechanics in ventilator-dependent infants at risk of developing BPD. *Pediatr Pulmonol* 1991; 10:183–190.

98. Taghezadek A, Reynolds EOR: Pathogenesis of bronchopulmonary dysplasia following hyaline membrane disease. *Am J Pathol* 1976; 82:241.

99. Van Marter LJ, Leviton A, Kuban KCK, et al: Maternal glucocorticoid therapy and reduced risk of bronchopulmonary dysplasia. *Pediatrics* 1990; 86:331–336.

## Long-Term Outcome

100. Cryotherapy for retinopathy of prematurity cooperative group. Multicenter trial of cryotherapy for retinopathy of prematurity. *Arch Opthal* 1988; 106:471–479.

101. Heldt GP, McIlroy MB, Haveen TN, et al: Exercise performance of the survivors of hyaline membrane disease. *J Pediatr* 1980; 96:996.

102. Lucey JF, Dangman B: A re-examination of the role of oxygen in retrolental fibroplasia. *Pediatrics* 1984; 73:82–96.

## General

103. Farrel PM, Avery MD: Hyaline membrane disease. *Am Rev Resp Dis* 1975; 111:657.

## Pulmonary Function Testing

104. Bhutani VK, Sivieri EM, Abbasi S, et al: Evaluation of neonatal pulmonary mechanics and energetics: A two factor least mean square analysis. *Pediatr Pulmonol* 1988; 4:150–158.

105. Bhutani VK, Shaffer TH, Vidyasagar D: *Neonatal Pulmonary Function Testing.* Ithaca, New York, Perinatology Press, 1988.

106. England SJ: Current techniques for assessing pulmonary function in newborn and infant: Advantages and limitations. *Pediatr Pulmonol* 1988; 4:48–53.

107. Greenspan JS, Abbasi S, Bhutani VK: Sequential changes in pulmonary mechanics in the very low birthweight (≤1000 grams) infant. *J Pediatr* 1988; 113:732–737.

108. Philips JB III, Beale EF, Howard JE, et al: Effect of positive end-expiratory pressure on dynamic respiratory compliance in neonates. *Biol Neonate* 1980; 38:270–275.

109. Richardson P, Bose CL, Carlstrom JR: The functional residual capacity of infants with respiratory distress syndrome. *Acta Paediatr Scand* 1986; 75:267–271.

110. Shaffer TH, Delivoria-Papadoupolos M: Alteration in pulmonary function of premature lambs due to PEEP. *Respiration* 1978; 36:183–188.

111. Sly PD, Brown KA, Bates JHT, et al: Noninvasive determination of respiratory mechanics during mechanical ventilation of neonates: A review of current and future techniques. *Pediatr Pulmonol* 1988; 4:39–47.

112. Teague WG, Darnall RA, Suratt PM: A noninvasive constant-flow method for measuring respiratory compliance in newborn infants. *Crit Care Med* 1985; 13(11):965.

113. Tooley WH, Clements JA, Muramatsu K, et al: Lung function in prematurely delivered rabbits treated with synthetic surfactant. *Am Rev Resp Dis* 1987; 136:651–656.

# Chapter 9

# BRONCHOPULMONARY DYSPLASIA

*Jeffrey S. Gerdes*, M.D.

Bronchopulmonary dysplasia (BPD) is a chronic lung disorder, which follows an acute pulmonary disease such as respiratory distress syndrome (RDS) and affects both preterm (most commonly) and term newborn infants. Although the definition of BPD is in transition, the infant classically considered to have BPD exhibits respiratory symptoms, an abnormal chest radiograph, and the need for supplemental oxygen at 28 days of age. The hallmark pathological findings in this disorder are a chronic inflammatory and reparative cellular response to unresolved acute lung injury. Infants with BPD are characterized clinically by chronic respiratory distress, retention of carbon dioxide (hypercapnia), a diminished blood oxygen concentration (hypoxemia), and an abnormal chest radiograph. BPD is a unique phenomenon in pulmonary medicine in that it is a disease in which simultaneous lung injury and repair are superimposed on a system of ongoing organ growth and development. While BPD is recognized in approximately 15% of preterm births, as many as 69% of babies of birth weight less than 1,000 g may develop the condition. More significantly, 18% of those babies exhibit a severe form of the disease. These infants require a high level of care, and they often develop long-term pulmonary and neurodevelopmental complications. The etiology of BPD is multifactorial and includes inherent factors such as lung underdevelopment secondary to prematurity, as well as factors ensuing from therapies provided to the preterm neonate, such as oxygen administration and mechanical ventilation. The methods of prevention and treatment are as varied as the many possible etiologies, providing one of the greatest challenges in modern neonatal-perinatal medicine.

## PREDISPOSING FACTORS AND ETIOLOGIC MECHANISMS

Prematurity is one of the major factors predisposing to the development of BPD. The smaller, more premature infant is more likely to develop the disease than the infant born at or near term gestation. However, as noted earlier, BPD is a multifactorial disease (Table 9-1).

You will be presented with the case of TJ from birth through 50 days of age. You will be asked to analyze a variety of problems related to this infant's condition.

### CASE STUDY 1

Baby boy TJ was born after 25 weeks of gestation, weighing 725 g. His mother had premature cervical dilatation, premature labor, and asthma; the latter two conditions were treated with terbutaline. She was given two doses of betamethasone three days before delivery to promote lung maturation. Labor progressed despite the addition of indomethacin and resulted in a spontaneous vaginal delivery. TJ had Apgar scores of 4 at 1 minute and 8 at 5 minutes. He was intubated immediately after birth and placed on a ventilator with an inspiratory pressure (IP) of 20 cm $H_2O$, a positive end-expiratory pressure (PEEP) of 5 cm $H_2O$, a rate of 40, and an inspired oxygen concentration ($FiO_2$) of 0.80. He was treated prophylactically with surfactant and transported on the ventilator to the intensive care nursery (ICN).

**Table 9-1** Factors Predisposing
to the Development of
Bronchopulmonary Dysplasia

Anatomic lung immaturity

Biochemical lung immaturity (surfactant deficiency)

Genetic predisposition

Fluid overload

Patent ductus arteriosus

Pneumothorax

Pulmonary interstitial emphysema

Barotrauma from mechanical ventilation

Oxygen therapy and anti-oxidant insufficiency

Early development of increased airway resistance

Malnutrition

Lung inflammation and disordered fibrosis

### EXERCISE 1

■ **Question:**

What three factors predispose TJ to develop
BPD?

1.

2.

3.

■ **Discussion:**

*Anatomic immaturity of the lung structures is
a major risk factor for the development of
BPD.* At 25 weeks' gestation, the lungs are still
in the canalicular phase of development and
are just beginning the saccular phase when respiratory saccules appear from the transitional
ducts. Interruption of lung development may
occur simply by preterm birth and air breathing, when the lung is meant to be fluid-filled,
and is certainly disrupted by mechanical ventilation and oxygen therapy. In addition, the
immature lung is characterized by an altered

collagen composition and decreased elastin
concentration compared to the mature lung,
resulting in diminished elasticity, which reduces pulmonary compliance on an anatomic
basis. Fortunately, the preterm lung has a remarkable potential for remodeling and
growth, and undergoes an increase in surface
area from 0.5 m² at 24 weeks' gestation to 4.5
m² at term (Fig. 9-1). This growth potential

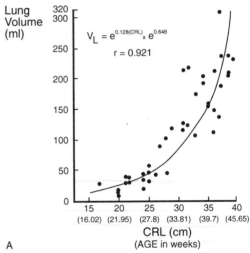

A

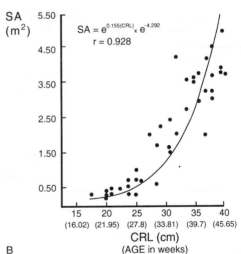

B

**Figure 9-1** Graphic representation of fetal and
early neonatal lung growth. (A) The exponential
increase in lung volume between 16 and 45 weeks
of gestation, with the corresponding crown-rump
length (CRL) at each gestation. (B) A similar
growth pattern for internal surface area of the lung
(SA) as a function of gestational age and crown-
rump length.
From Langston C, Kida K, Reed M, et al: Human lung
growth in late gestation and in the neonate. *Am Rev Resp
Dis* 1984; 129:610–611. Reprinted with permission of the
American Lung Association.

makes the development of chronic lung disease less likely in the preterm baby and also makes possible recovery from BPD.

*Surfactant deficiency is an important cause of RDS and contributes to lung injury on a primary basis.* Surfactant deficiency may also occur on a secondary basis due to therapies administered for acute lung diseases and can further contribute to the development of BPD. Neonates who have RDS are more likely to develop BPD than those who do not, although it is important to recognize that BPD has developed in preterm neonates who never received oxygen or ventilator treatment. Although surfactant replacement therapy reduces the severity of RDS and the incidence of air leak, it has not been shown to decrease the incidence of BPD in the very tiny premature infant (*micropremie*). However, synthetic surfactant replacement has been proven to reduce the incidence of BPD in infants of birth weights greater than 1,350 g in controlled clinical trials. Further, a meta-analysis of five rescue trials of synthetic surfactants has also demonstrated a reduction in the incidence of BPD. In contrast, maternal treatment with corticosteroids has not been shown to alter the incidence of BPD.

The history of asthma in TJ's mother is also an important consideration in this case. *BPD is more likely to develop in babies with a family history of reactive airway disease.* However, the pathophysiological basis for this observation remains uncertain.

---

## CASE STUDY 1 continued

TJ was continued on mechanical ventilation in the ICN. In the first 12 hours of life, he stabilized well, and the ICN staff was able to wean the FiO$_2$ to 0.40, the ventilator pressures to 17/5 (IP/PEEP), and the rate to 30 per minute. He was given one infusion of normal saline to maintain a mean blood pressure greater than 30 mm Hg. The initial chest radiograph showed low lung volumes with bilateral haziness and air bronchograms, consistent with RDS. Second and third doses of surfactant were given at 12 and 24 hours of age, with continued slow but steady improvement in gas exchange and clinical status. Intravenous fluid therapy was given at the rate of 100 to 130 cc/kg/day to maintain serum sodium in the range of 138 to 145 MEq/L, and to allow a weight loss of 10% to 15% from birth weight. At 48 hours of age, TJ developed car-

bon dioxide (pCO$_2$) retention to 50 mm Hg, and a blood pressure of 43/18; however, there was no change in the physical examination or chest radiograph. No heart murmur was auscultated, but a suspected patent ductus arteriosus (PDA) with left-to-right shunting was confirmed by color Doppler echocardiography. A course of indomethacin was administered, with resolution of the PDA. After PDA closure, TJ continued to improve, but he was unable to be extubated because of poor chest wall stability and apnea, which was unresponsive to theophylline. Pulmonary function testing on day 5 showed a modestly reduced compliance and significant elevation of pulmonary airway resistance.

## EXERCISE 2

### ■ Question:
Which elements of *this* case further increased the probability that TJ would develop BPD?

### ■ Discussion:
The presence of a PDA with left-to-right shunting increases interstitial lung water, decreases lung compliance, elevates lung airway resistance, and ultimately results in an increase in the degree of ventilatory support. *Even though the PDA was treated aggressively in this case, the presence of a PDA does increase the likelihood that BPD will ensue.*

Given the presence of severe RDS and a PDA with left-to-right shunting, fluid therapy is a major issue for this infant. *This patient was given appropriate intravenous fluid therapy for his weight and gestational age.* A larger preterm infant should be restricted to fluids in the range of 80 cc/kg/day, but the tiny micropremie often requires fluids greater than 100 cc/kg/day to compensate for insensible water loss (see Chapter 2). Retrospective studies have demonstrated an increased incidence of BPD in neonates who received higher fluid volumes than were necessary to maintain euhydration. Excess fluid administration increases interstitial lung water in patients with RDS because of the capillary leak that accompanies the disease. Further evidence that excess lung fluid is deleterious is the finding of an increased rate of BPD in RDS patients who do not exhibit the expected diuresis on days 2 to 3 versus patients whose RDS resolves without BPD. This concept of overhydration predisposing to BPD is tempered, however, by a prospective trial in which fluid restriction in neonates with RDS did not prevent development of BPD.

Fortunately, TJ did not show signs of air leak such as pulmonary interstitial emphysema (PIE) or pneumothorax. These complications can be difficult to manage acutely, and their management often dictates an increase in oxygen and ventilator support. Furthermore, air leak syndromes clearly increase the risk of developing BPD.

*Barotrauma from mechanical ventilation can cause direct mechanical injury to the developing lung, and the incidence of BPD is higher in babies who are ventilated with high inspiratory pressures (IP >30 mm Hg) or who are exposed to high inspiratory oxygen concentrations (>80% FiO2) for an excessive period of time.* In this case, TJ was not treated with high ventilator pressures or a particularly high FiO2; however, as noted in Exercise 1, even low levels of artificial positive pressure support are very foreign to the immature lung and may lead to lung injury. Similarly, even low levels of inspired oxygen and arterial pO2 levels of 50 to 80 mm Hg are certainly higher than levels the fetus is exposed to *in utero* and may be toxic to the pulmonary epithelial cell.

There are a variety of reasons why the lung of the premature newborn infant may be particularly susceptible to oxidant injury. First, the immature lung's defense against oxygen toxicity is diminished relative to the lung activity of the term baby or adult. Not only are there reduced levels of intracellular antioxidant enzymes (superoxide dismutase, catalase, and glutathione peroxidase), but the usual developmental increase in these enzymes prior to term birth may not occur in the preterm lung. Extracellular substances that protect against oxidant injury such as vitamin E, ceruloplasmin, and trace element cofactors are also deficient in the preterm lung. Second, the metabolism of alveolar macrophages and surfactant secretion by Type II pneumocytes is also adversely affected by hyperoxia. In addition to inducing lung cell cytotoxicity, hyperoxic exposure of experimental animals during the early critical periods of lung development has been shown to disrupt normal alveolar development. Finally, note that the acute pathological changes of BPD are very similar to those of experimental oxygen toxicity in animals.

*Pulmonary inflammation contributes to the pathophysiology of pulmonary microvascular injury and altered membrane permeability that occurs with oxygen toxicity.* While polymorphonuclear neutrophil recruitment is a normal phase of lung healing, persistence of neutrophils and the neutrophil secretory products (e.g., elastase and arachidonic acid metabolites) is poorly tolerated by the injured immature lung. These inflammatory mediators cause connective tissue damage, pulmonary vasoconstriction, pulmonary capillary leak, bronchoconstriction, and further amplification of the inflammatory response.

*Babies with RDS who exhibit high airway resistance during the first week of life are predisposed to the development of BPD.* Whether the elevated resistance is etiologic or just symptomatic is unclear. However, investigators have begun to use pulmonary function testing (measurements of lung resistance and compliance) during the first week of life, along with gestational age, to predict which infants are likely to develop BPD.

## CASE STUDY 1 continued

TJ remained ventilator dependent, although he could be maintained on an FiO2 of 0.30 to 0.35, very low rates, and ventilator pressures of <20 cm H2O. During the third week of life, he gradually developed an increased need for respiratory support, with an oxygen requirement up to 75% and increased retractions and work of breathing. A chest radiograph showed bilateral infiltrates, and a tracheal aspirate Gram's stain demonstrated many polymorphonuclear neutrophils and gram-negative rods. Cultures were taken, and vancomycin and cefotaxime were administered with improvement in the presumed pneumonia. However, after antibiotic treatment his baseline oxygen requirement remained at 50%. Also, a higher ventilator rate and pressures were needed. Attempts were made to introduce enteral feedings by the orogastric route, but the patient's poor gut motility and general condition did not allow for advancement of feedings above 2 mL every 2 hours. Enteral nutrition was supplemented by intravenous hyperalimentation with Intralipid, but poor glucose tolerance permitted a total intake of only 70 cal/kg/day. By 28 days of age, TJ weighed 860 g, and he still required assisted ventilation and an inspired oxygen concentration of 0.38. His chest radiograph was abnormal with characteristic small cystic changes consistent with BPD.

## EXERCISE 3

### ■ Question:

From the preceding case history, what three factors predisposed TJ to develop BPD?

### ■ Discussion:

Rapid weight gain and organ growth take place in the fetus between 26 weeks' gestation (when TJ was born) and term gestation. Unfortunately, once an infant is born prematurely, our ability to provide adequate nutrition is limited and usually cannot match the effectiveness of the *in utero* environment. *If the poor postnatal nutrition is not corrected, it ultimately leads to nutritional deficiencies that interfere with lung repair and lung growth.* In a general sense, malnutrition leads to a catabolic state, which inhibits cell and organ growth. More specifically, however, malnutrition is believed to lead to impaired surfactant production, decreased lung cell replication, and decreased structural alveolar development. It has recently been suggested that vitamin A may be critically important for infants born prematurely. Vitamin A is necessary for epithelial integrity and healing of the airways. Furthermore, preterm neonates who develop BPD are often deficient in vitamin A, and early supplementation of vitamin A may ameliorate the development and progression of the disorder.

Malnutrition may also impair the ability of the newborn infant to defend against oxidant injury by limiting both antioxidant enzyme synthesis and the availability of vitamin E. Attempts to replace these deficiencies have not reduced the incidence or severity of BPD, but they are likely to be important in the pathogenesis of the disease. Sosenko et al. have recently suggested that provision of intravenous lipid emulsions may help ameliorate oxygen toxicity by providing intracellular polyunsaturated fatty acids that act as free radical scavengers, although early administration of Intralipid did not prevent BPD in one clinical study. Very low birth weight infants are also prone to develop a deficiency of zinc, an important cofactor for many enzymes, including the antioxidant enzyme superoxide dismutase.

Malnutrition can further compromise the already deficient immune system in the neonate. Deleterious effect of malnutrition have been demonstrated on both cellular and humoral immunity. These immune deficiencies predispose to development of intercurrent infections and pneumonia.

*Nosocomial pneumonia often causes a clinical deterioration, from which neonates with evolving BPD may have difficulty recovering.* The infection may result in increased lung injury because the influx of polymorphonuclear neutrophils release elastase and presumably other proteolytic enzymes that cause lung injury. Viral infections such as adenovirus may cause an obliterative bronchiolitis even in healthy infants, and so may exacerbate the small airway disease that is part of BPD. Recent evidence has implicated *Ureaplasma urealyticum* colonization and/or infection with the development of BPD, but the extent of this potential problem is not yet understood.

As noted in the introduction, lung injury and repair in the neonate are superimposed on an immature respiratory system that is undergoing a rapid process of normal growth and development. *These developmental changes along with an immature and diminished response to lung injury, lead to structural and biochemical changes favoring lung repair with fibrosis, a response not commonly observed in the lung healing of adult patients.* In uncomplicated RDS that resolves without lung scarring, normal lung reparative phases include transient inflammation, proliferation of Type II pneumocytes, and restoration of lung growth and differentiation. When BPD develops, however, the acute inflammatory phase of RDS evolves into a persistent inflammatory exudative phase. During this time, a period of extensive fibroblast proliferation occurs with deposition of collagen and lung scarring. Because the ventilator cannot be discontinued, the lung continues to be exposed to injurious agents such as oxygen and barotrauma, which inhibit the proliferation and biosynthetic functioning of many cells in the lung. Interestingly, however, fibroblast proliferation is not suppressed by hyperoxia and may go unchecked. In fact, hyperoxia stimulates alveolar macrophage release of fibronectin and insulin growth factor-1, which stimulate fibroblast migration into the lung. The acute lung injury also damages the pulmonary epithelial-capillary basement membrane and intercellular matrix architecture as indicated by the release of elastin degradation products and fibronectin. Finally, the collagen composition of the lung of the BPD infant is abnormal. Whereas the Type I : Type III collagen ratio is 2 : 1 in the lung of a normal adult, and 1 : 6 in the non-BPD immature lung of a preterm infant, the ratio in the lungs of infants who died from BPD is greater than 3 : 1. Because Type I collagen is less elastic than Type III collagen, the lungs of infants with BPD are inappropriately stiff.

## THE CLINICAL PICTURE—AN EVOLVING PROCESS

As is evident from the previous discussion, the development of BPD is an evolving process. As such, it is difficult to determine exactly when BPD starts. From the pathophysiological point of view, BPD starts as soon as the acute lung injury of RDS fails to resolve, and the abnormal exudative and reparative processes begin. Biochemical studies of lung inflammation and physiological studies of pulmonary function suggest that the process begins as soon as 5 to 7 days of age. However, from an operational point of view, many neonates who show these early signs of chronic lung disease resolve their symptoms within several weeks, and so would not be considered to have chronic lung disease. The traditional operational or epidemiological definition of BPD is (1) the need for supplemental oxygen, (2) the presence of an abnormal chest radiograph, and (3) clinical symptoms of respiratory distress at 28 days of age. Most studies of BPD have used this definition, and it remains the standard clinical definition at many centers. However, because very few micropremies will escape BPD by this definition (simply on the basis of anatomic lung immaturity), a more recent, and perhaps more reasonable, definition of BPD is the need for supplemental oxygen and an abnormal chest radiograph at 36 weeks' postconceptional age (Table 9-2). These definitions

**Table 9-2** Diagnostic Criteria for BPD

The presence at day of life 28 *or* at 36 weeks postconceptional age of the following:

1. Supplemental oxygen requirement
2. Abnormal chest radiograph
3. Clinical symptoms of respiratory distress

have been further modified in different studies to exclude those infants who have very mild, clinically insignificant disease. For instance, in the clinical trials of Exosurf Neonatal®, the definition of BPD was the presence at 28 days of age of an oxygen requirement, clinical symptoms of respiratory distress, and at least a moderately abnormal chest radiograph, defined as an Edwards score of greater than or equal to 4, as discussed next.

BPD was first described in 1967 by Dr. Northway, a radiologist. Then, as now, the chest radiograph is an important factor in the diagnosis and staging of BPD. The radiographic appearance of BPD evolves slowly during the first weeks of life, analogous to the pathophysiological and clinical evolution noted earlier. In Northway's description, Stage I BPD is indistinguishable from RDS, with hazy lung fields, a ground-glass appearance, and air bronchograms (Fig. 9-2A). Stage II BPD (Fig. 9-2B) shows continued or advancing homogeneous opacity of the lung fields, at 4 to 10 days of age, when acute RDS should be resolving. The histopathological correlate of Stage II BPD is the development of alveolar and airway epithelial necrosis, with early repair, and exudation into the airways. Cystic change begins in Stage III BPD (Fig. 9-2C) in association with early changes of interstitial fibrosis. These changes tend to be diffuse and homogeneous, without gross distortion of lung architecture. The histopathological findings of Stage III BPD are mucosal metaplasia, obliterative bronchiolitis, and microscopic atelectasis and emphysema (Fig. 9-3). Stage IV disease (Fig. 9-2D) occurs beyond 1 month of age, and is characterized radiographically by gross distortion of lung architecture, interstitial fibrosis, large cystic areas, hyperinflation, shifting atelectasis, and emphysema. Cardiomegaly is occasionally an associated finding. Edwards devised a radiographic scoring system for BPD that has been helpful in stan-

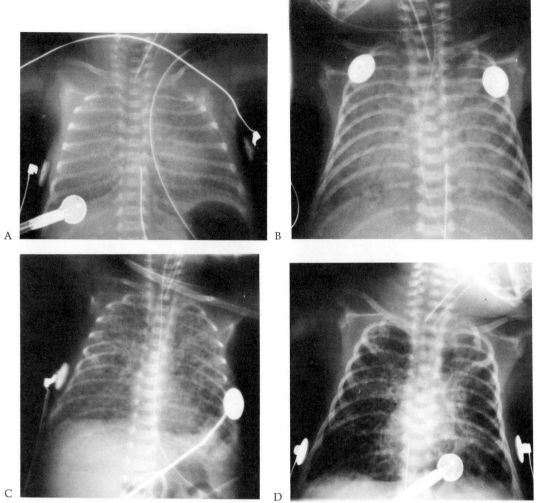

**Figure 9-2** (A) Northway Stage I BPD, as indistinguishable from acute RDS. (B) Stage II BPD with continued or advancing homogeneous opacity of the lung fields at 4 to 10 days of age, when RDS should be resolving. (C) Stage III BPD exhibits diffuse cystic changes, with early interstitial fibrosis. (D) The findings of Stage IV BPD include gross distortion of lung architecture, with interstitial fibrosis, large cystic change, shifting atelectasis, and emphysema.

dardizing diagnosis and data validity for research. Points are assigned for varying degrees of cardiomegaly, hyperinflation, cystic change or emphysema, interstitial fibrosis, and a subjective severity assessment, with a final score ranging from 1 to 10.

The symptoms and signs of BPD also undergo a developmental process. The classic early signs of RDS (grunting and retractions), which are secondary to a diminished lung compliance and functional residual capacity, are gradually replaced with a more chronic respiratory distress characterized by tachypnea, hypoxemia, hypercarbia, wheezing, and retractions secondary to increased airway resistance. These infants have increased work of breathing related both to continued poor compliance and increased airway resistance. Most of them appear chronically ill and fatigued, and may require prolonged ventilatory support to lessen work of breathing. Even if a given patient can maintain gas exchange, the metabolic cost of breathing may be too high to allow that infant to breathe spontaneously.

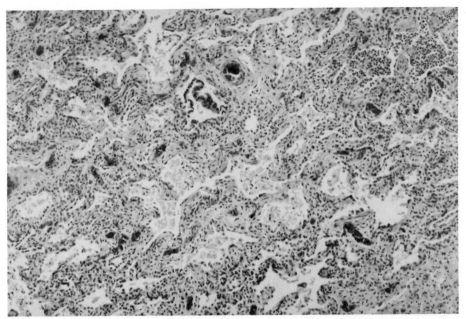

**Figure 9-3** The histopathological findings of Stage III BPD include mucosal metaplasia, obliterative bronchiolitis, and microscopic atalectasis and emphysema.

## CASE STUDY 1 continued

TJ continued to be a management problem in the ICN during the second month of life. He remained on the ventilator and required inspired oxygen concentrations of 35% to 40%. His pulmonary function tests demonstrated a low specific compliance of 0.5 mL/cm $H_2O$/kg, and a high airway resistance of 110 cm $H_2O$/L/sec. His flow-volume loops exhibited early signs of expiratory flow limitation (Fig. 9-4B). He had occasional episodes of wheezing with a concomitant increase in retractions. He did not exhibit excess weight gain, edema, or other obvious signs of fluid overload. His nutritional status improved, with gradual tolerance of enteral feedings and weaning of his intravenous hyperalimentation. A vitamin A level was 12 $\mu$g/mL.

## EXERCISE 4

One of the fundamental tenets of neonatal intensive care is to make sure every infant is adequately oxygenated. There is, however, a wide range of arterial $pO_2$ values that can achieve that goal and can satisfy tissue oxygen needs.

## ■ Question 1:

If you were managing this infant's ventilator, what range of arterial $pO_2$ values would you try to maintain?

(a) $pO_2$ range of 40 to 60 mm Hg to minimize further oxygen toxicity.

(b) $pO_2$ range of 90 to 120 mm Hg to provide plenty of oxygen to the healing tissues of this chronically ill baby

(c) $pO_2$ range of 60 to 85 mm Hg to provide adequate tissue oxygenation and to help avoid future complications of BPD

## ■ Discussion:

Choice (a) is incorrect. Although oxygen toxicity may be operative in the pathogenesis of BPD, it is unlikely that continued provision of 35% to 40% oxygen as seen in this case will cause significant further damage. To the contrary, there is evidence suggesting that any degree of chronic hypoxemia may be deleterious for the recovery of the BPD patient. Weight gain is better for those infants with BPD who are maintained normoxemic than for those who are allowed to have lower levels of oxygenation. Adequate oxygenation may help forestall the development of pulmonary hyper-

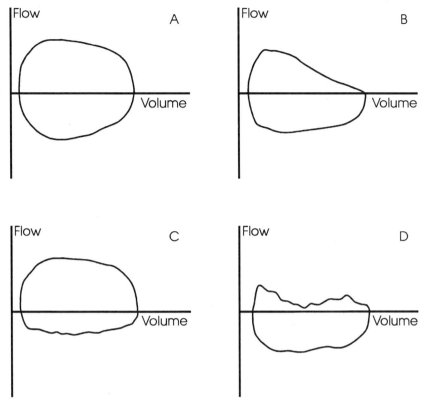

**Figure 9-4** Representative pulmonary function flow-volume loops. (A) Normal tracing, with even flow characteristics on inspiration and expiration. (B) Infants with BPD often demonstrate limitation of expiratory flow because of small airway damage and bronchospasm. (C) Subglottic stenosis produces an inspiratory, extrathoracic obstruction on flow-volume loop. (D) Tracheobronchomalacia exhibits an intrathoracic obstructive pattern, with intermittent airway closure during the expiratory phase.

tension and right heart strain (cor pulmonale), one of the most feared complications of BPD. The propensity for high pulmonary vascular resistance in these patients is due to a combination of factors including (1) anatomic distortion with an associated decreased cross-sectional area of the pulmonary vasculature, (2) hypoxic pulmonary vasoconstriction, and (3) pulmonary artery vasoconstriction from elaboration of inflammatory mediators such as leukotrienes. Many infants with BPD exhibit sensitivity to $O_2$ administration and exhibit an acute decrease in pulmonary vascular resistance when the arterial $pO_2$ value is increased. Recurrent hypoxemia is also likely to be harmful to the developing brain. Babies with chronic BPD and recurrent hypoxic spells are at significant risk for developmental delay.

Choice (b) is also incorrect. There is no evidence to indicate that hyperoxia is beneficial to the infant with BPD. Furthermore, hyperoxia is one of many factors implicated in the pathogenesis of retinopathy of prematurity.

*Choice (c) is correct.* As noted previously, there are several cogent reasons for maintaining relative normoxemia in the patient with BPD. This level of oxygen supplementation should be continued for as long as needed, even if some infants remain on low levels of inspired oxygen (0.23 to 0.25) for long periods of time. Home use of oxygen should be used if the infant is otherwise ready for discharge but cannot yet maintain normoxemia in room air.

An equally important issue, but one that is considerably more controversial, is how to regulate this infant's blood carbon dioxide concentration. Some clinicians believe that the chronically ill BPD infant should be aggressively ventilated to lessen work of breathing and permit better nutritional recovery. Others feel that it is important to always minimize barotrauma by keeping ventilator pressures low and allowing modest $CO_2$ retention, as long as the pH is compensated by renal mechanisms. At our institution we try to keep the $pCO_2$ between 45 and 55 mm Hg.

### ■ Question 2:

What other medications would you consider using at this time to hasten this infant's recovery?

### ■ Discussion:

*Of the wide variety of drugs used in infants with chronic lung disease, bronchodilators* are selected most frequently (Table 9-3). As many as 60% of infants with BPD have reactive airway disease as defined by the presence of wheezing, by an increase in airway resistance after bronchoprovocation, or by the response to bronchodilating agents. Bronchiolar smooth muscle hyperplasia and bronchospasm may begin at a very young postnatal age and have been observed in infants with BPD whose postconceptional age is only 26 weeks. Theophylline, caffeine, albuterol, and terbutaline have all been shown to provide acute therapeutic relief for bronchospasm in these babies. Albuterol is the $\beta$-agonist of choice because it has better $\beta$-selectivity than terbutaline. Inhalation is the preferred route of administration of $\beta$-agonists because the acute response is better than with oral dosing and side effects are less because of the selective effect on the bronchi with inhalation. In in-

**Table 9-3** Drug Therapy and Dosages for Neonates with BPD

| DRUG | DOSAGE | COMMENTS |
|---|---|---|
| ***Bronchodilators*** | | |
| 1. Theophylline | Load 6 mg/kg | Maintain serum level of 10 to 15 $\mu$g/mL for bronchodilation. |
| | Maintenance 1.1 mg/kg/day q. 80 | |
| 2. Caffeine citrate | Load 20 mg/kg | Maintain serum level of 10 to 25 $\mu$g/mL for bronchodilation. |
| | Maintenance 5 mg/kg/day q. 120 | |
| 3. Albuterol inhalation | Nebulize 0.1 to 0.15 mL/kg q. 6 hours *or* metered dose inhaler 1 puff q. 6 hours | |
| 4. Oral albuterol | 0.1 to 0.5 mg/kg/q. 8 hours | |
| ***Diuretics*** | | |
| 1. Furosemide (IV or IM) | 1.0 mg/kg once daily *or* q.o.d (po dose, 1 to 5 mg/kg) | Monitor electrolytes; give KCl supplement. |
| 2. Chlorothiazide | 20 to 40 mg/kg/day, divide B.I.D. | Monitor electrolytes; give KCl supplement. |
| 3. Spironolactone | 1 to 3 mg/kg/day, divide B.I.D. | Monitor electrolytes. |
| ***Nutritional supplements*** | | |
| 1. Vitamin A | 2,500 to 5,000 U/kg/day po or IM | Maintain serum level of 20 to 50 $\mu$g/mL. |
| 2. Vitamin E | 25 U/day po | Change as needed to maintain serum level of 1.0 to 2.0 $\mu$g/mL. |
| 3. Zinc sulfate | 1.0 mg/kg/day po | Maintain serum level of 70 to 100 $\mu$g/mL. |
| ***Anti-inflammatory agent*** | | |
| 1. Dexamethasone | 0.25 to 0.5 mg/kg/day divide B.I.D. | Starting dose; then taper every 3 days for a 14- to 42-day period. |

fants with severe recurrent bronchospasm, theophylline is commonly used as well.

*The majority of babies with BPD will benefit from the use of diuretics, even if there are no obvious signs of systemic fluid overload (Table 9-3).* Interstitial water accumulation occurs in the lung of the BPD infant for a variety of reasons including capillary leak from the damaged epithelium, increased pulmonary capillary pressure, impaired lymphatic drainage due to the distorted architecture, and decreased plasma oncotic pressure from malnutrition or fluid overload. Furosemide has been the most frequently studied diuretic in BPD. The administration of furosemide results in a diuresis that minimizes total lung water and raises plasma oncotic pressure. However, furosemide also has important nonrenal effects on pulmonary function, which are evident soon after the dose and well before the effect of diuresis could have taken place. Furosemide causes venodilation, which increases venous capacitance and therefore decreases right ventricular end-diastolic volume and pulmonary capillary pressure. There are also direct effects of furosemide on airway epithelium, which may result in decreased chloride and water transport across the epithelium, as well as diminished airway reactivity. Studies of pulmonary mechanics have demonstrated improvement in both lung compliance and lung resistance. Most studies have used a dose of 1 mg/kg/day, but a recent investigation suggested that a 1 mg/kg/dose every other day led to a sustained improvement with fewer side effects. The side effects of furosemide include fluid and electrolyte imbalance (chloride depletion and metabolic alkalosis, hyponatremia), hypercalciuria and nephrolithiasis, osteopenia, and ototoxicity.

The combination of chlorothiazide and spironolactone results in a diuresis similar to that of furosemide, but the effects on pulmonary mechanics are less clear-cut. Whereas earlier studies showed improvement in lung compliance and airway resistance with this therapy, more recent works have demonstrated an adequate diuresis but no improvement in pulmonary function or oxygenation. The safety profile of these drugs is an advantage, however, because fewer side effects (e.g., nephrolithiasis, ototoxicity) have been noted.

At Pennsylvania Hospital our current approach is to initiate therapy with furosemide in the early stages of BPD when weaning from the ventilator is a goal. When the infant is tolerating enteral feedings and is more stable, therapy is changed to chlorothiazide/spironolactone; intermittent doses of furosemide are administered if respiratory deterioration or signs of fluid retention occur. Supplemental potassium chloride should be administered to prevent chloride and potassium depletion. Diuretics are generally continued until the infant no longer requires oxygen therapy.

*The use of dexamethasone in infants with BPD is controversial.* Numerous studies have shown that the administration of high-dose dexamethasone to ventilator-dependent infants with BPD facilitates weaning from respiratory support, with improvement in pulmonary function and attenuation of lung inflammation. These same studies indicate an acceptable level of side effects, ranging from no side effects in some studies to manageable degrees of hyperglycemia or hypertension in others. The theoretical risk of immune suppression and increased risk of infection has not been borne out in the prospective studies; however, clinicians often withhold corticosteroid therapy from patients who are already infected. Of concern and controversy still are the unanswered questions regarding the possible effects of corticosteroid treatment on long-term neurological and pulmonary development. Furthermore, it is not yet clear whether the improvement in respiratory status of these babies translates into decreased mortality, morbidity, or hospital length of stay.

The commonly used dexamethasone treatment protocols start with 0.25 to 0.5 mg/kg/day for 3 days, followed by a reduction in dosage every 3 days. Initiation of dexamethasone therapy is usually considered between 2 and 4 weeks of age in the ventilator-dependent infant, although some recent studies are examining the possible benefits of commencing therapy in the first week of life. Therapy is usually continued for 14 to 42 days. The literature is controversial as to the most beneficial course of treatment. Our usual approach is to start steroid therapy by 2 weeks of age only in the most severely ill infants. When the infants are 1 month of age, we use dexamethasone in most ventilator-dependent BPD babies, even at low levels of support, if they are not making progress despite optimal medical and respiratory management. On the other hand, if the patient is progressing and weaning (even slowly), we reserve treatment and allow the infant to heal on his own.

As discussed previously, there is enough evidence to suggest that vitamin A deficiency is an important factor in the development of BPD. Therefore, it probably makes good clinical sense to maintain vitamin A levels in a normal range. Vitamin A levels greater than 20 $\mu$g/mL can be achieved with daily oral supplementation of 2,500 to 5,000 U of Aquasol A, or with several doses per week of parenteral vitamin A (2,000 U IM). Therapeutic response should be monitored with serum levels.

## ■ Question 3:
What are three important nutritional considerations for this patient?

## ■ Discussion:
*Because of the increased work of breathing and increased metabolic rate, many infants with BPD will require 120 to 150 cal/kg/day to maintain an adequate weight gain of 15 to 30 g/day.* While this caloric intake is not possible when the infant is on hyperalimentation, enteral feedings should consist of 24 cal/oz. preterm infant formulas, which have added nutrients such as calcium, phosphorus, zinc, and vitamin E. *Adequate mineral intake is necessary to prevent osteopenia, or "rickets" of prematurity, which may occur in those chronically ill infants with BPD who do not have an adequate intake of calcium and phosphorus.* Older infants with BPD can be given infant formulas designed for term infants that are concentrated up to 30 cal/oz. *Additional calories can also be supplied by additives such as medium-chain triglyceride (MCT) oil, microlipids, vegetable oil, or baby cereal. Carbohydrate additives such as polycose should be used with caution, since the high respiratory quotient of carbohydrates generates more $CO_2$ per unit of oxygen consumption, which may lead to hypercarbia or increased work of breathing.*

Mechanical problems may also interfere with adequate intake. *Some BPD infants use too much energy trying to suck, swallow, and breathe, while other infants are unable to suck because of neurological deficits.* These kinds of babies should be given orogastric feedings as needed to minimize the work of breathing and maximize weight gain. Gastroesophageal reflux is also a common problem in the older BPD infant, which may require treatment with antireflux positioning, cereal-thickened feedings, metoclopramide, or fundoplication in the most recalcitrant cases.

## CASE STUDY 1 continued
TJ was started on furosemide 1 mg/kg/day, continued on theophylline, and given supplemental vitamin A. He gained weight at a rate of 15 g/day. However, he remained on the same level of ventilatory support, and his chest radiograph persisted with mild Stage III BPD. A 40-day tapering course of dexamethasone was instituted, with improvement of oxygenation ($FiO_2$ at 0.25) and ventilation (IP weaned to 15 cm $H_2O$ and the rate to 10). He could not be extubated, however, because whenever the PEEP was reduced to less than 5 cm $H_2O$, he would exhibit spells characterized by increased retractions and cyanosis.

## EXERCISE 5

## ■ Question:
What diagnostic workup should be performed at this time?

## ■ Discussion:
**BPD spells** are sudden episodes of hypoxemia and agitation, which may occur in the older BPD infant, especially those who are ventilator dependent. The etiology for these spells is often unclear, and their diagnosis and management can be frustrating to the clinician. However, an attempt should be made to find a treatable cause and thereby minimize the undesired exposure to hypoxemia.

*Sepsis or pneumonia should always be considered in the ventilator-dependent infant with any type of instability or deterioration in baseline need for support.* In TJ's case, the chest x-ray showed no infiltrates, the white blood cell count was normal, and blood and tracheal aspirate cultures were negative.

*The clinical description of these spells (retractions and cyanosis) appears to indicate an airway problem.* However, episodes of hypoxemia could also be due to right-to-left shunting at the atrial level related to right heart strain and pulmonary hypertension, which are symptoms of cor pulmonale. In infants with BPD, normal pulmonary vascular development is disrupted. Chronic hypoxia leads to hypertrophy of the pulmonary artery smooth muscle, and the anatomic distortion of lung architecture leads to a decreased total cross-sectional area of the pulmonary vasculature. The resulting pulmonary hypertension causes right heart strain, as well as a secondary strain on the left ventricle. Infants with cor pulmonale may have an increase in oxygen and ventilator requirements, a single second heart sound, and hepatomegaly. The ECG usually shows right atrial enlargement and right ventricular hypertrophy. An ECG should be obtained at 2 months of age in the infant with chronic BPD, and then every 1 to 2 months until the patient is off supplemental oxygen and shows no further signs of respiratory distress. Echocardiography has not been shown to be of consistent value in affected infants, although the information gained is of some use in following progression of this life-threatening complication. Infants with cor pulmonale are administered oxygen to achieve pulmonary vasodilation and diuretics to reduce filling pressure in the right heart. Inotropic agents have not been useful in treating this complication of BPD.

As many as 25% of infants with BPD may have systemic hypertension, the exact etiology of which is unclear. Antihypertensive medications are indicated if the systolic blood pressure is consistently greater than 115 mm Hg.

*The presence of retractions during the hypoxic spells and the inability to wean the PEEP despite a low inspired oxygen concentration suggest that airway collapse is occurring during the spells.* Tracheobronchomalacia is fairly common in infants with BPD and is likely due to the inherent weakness of the cartilaginous airways of the the preterm infant, along with damage to the supporting parenchymal structure of the lung. The diagnosis can be made by demonstrating a characteristic flow-volume loop on pulmonary function tests (Fig. 9-4D), by fluoroscopy or bronchoscopy, during which the airways can be observed to collapse on inspiration as the distending pressure is lowered. There is no specific treatment for this condition. Most infants will improve with time as the major airways increase in diameter. An occasional infant will require a tracheostomy if tra-

cheomalacia persists as the major respiratory problem.

*Another potential airway problem for the chronically ventilated BPD infant is subglottic stenosis, secondary to prolonged endotracheal intubation.* This complication can be suspected by demonstrating an extrathoracic obstruction on flow-volume loops during pulmonary function testing (Fig. 9-4C). Subglottic stenosis is confirmed by bronchoscopy. Treatment may require a cricoid split procedure, or a tracheostomy in severe cases.

*Infants with BPD are very prone to development of shifting atelectasis because of anatomic distortion of the airways, mucosal inflammation and edema, and exudative plugging.* Treatments include chest physiotherapy and positioning of the infant with the atelectatic side dependent. Fiber optic bronchoscopy may demonstrate airway obstruction by inflammatory granulomas, which may respond to short-term corticosteroid treatment.

## LONG-TERM FOLLOW-UP

### CASE STUDY 1 continued

By 50 days of age, TJ demonstrated regular weight gain and an increase in respiratory muscle strength. The PEEP was weaned to 4 cm $H_2O$, and TJ was eventually weaned to a nasal cannula. Oxygen therapy was discontinued at 70 days of age, and he was discharged home on diuretics and theophylline. Diuretics were discontinued after 1 month at home. Following an upper respiratory infection at age 5 months, wheezing developed, requiring a brief hospitalization and treatment with nebulized albuterol. When TJ was 6 months of age, pulmonary function testing showed residual abnormalities of compliance, resistance, and expiratory flow limitation (Fig. 9-4C), but he appeared to be clinically well and thriving, without dyspnea or noticeable respiratory symptoms.

### EXERCISE 6

#### ■ Question:
What are the long-term pulmonary and neurodevelopmental problems that TJ faces?

## ■ Discussion:

As noted earlier in this chapter, the neonatal lung has a remarkable growth potential. Structural remodeling and physiological improvements in pulmonary function can occur in infants with chronic lung disease for as long as 10 years. The decreased compliance observed in acute RDS persists in those infants who develop the early stages of BPD. Dynamic compliance tends to be reduced more than static compliance because of the concomitant airflow abnormalities in BPD. *Airway abnormalities are a more significant long-term problem in these infants, with persistence of increased total pulmonary resistance and expiratory flow limitation up to 3 years of age.* The expiratory flow limitation, indicating abnormal airway growth and function, can even be documented in those infants who do not exhibit respiratory symptoms. *Fifty percent to 75% of infants with BPD have bronchoreactivity demonstrated by methacholine, exercise, or cold-air challenge, and many of these infants have wheezing requiring acute or chronic bronchodilator therapy. At 10 years of age, children with BPD tend to have evidence of hyperinflation. Pulmonary function tests in these children demonstrate an increased residual volume, an improving but still slightly low FEV$_1$, and abnormal forced expiratory flows.* It should be emphasized that most of these children have normal exercise tolerance, although aerobic exercise in the BPD children occurs at the expense of a drop in oxygen saturation and a rise in transcutanous $CO_2$. *In summary, most infants with BPD can be expected to "outgrow" the disease from the point of view of symptoms, except for wheezing in some infants.* The residual pulmonary function abnormalities although not often noticed by the child or his parents, may persist into adolescence or young adulthood. At the extreme severity range of BPD, however, are those few infants (less than 1% of ventilated preterm neonates) who do not exhibit good lung growth and repair, and who remain ventilator dependent for months to years.

*Infants with BPD are at risk for poor neurodevelopmental outcome* because of (1) recurrent episodes of hypoxia in those infants with chronic disease and lability with BPD spells, (2) the association of BPD with intraventricular hemorrhage and periventricular leukomalacia, (3) poor nutrition during periods of critical brain growth, and (4) prolonged hospitalization and illness, which may preclude normal stimulation and parent-infant interaction. *The incidence of developmental delay as measured by low Bayley Mental Developmental scores ranges from 10% to 45%. Cerebral palsy may occur in 7% to 28% of BPD infants, and those infants may also exhibit a high incidence of early, but transient, neuromotor problems.*

## SUMMARY—A MULTIFACTORIAL APPROACH TO A MULTIFACTORIAL DISEASE

Bronchopulmonary dysplasia is a disease with many underlying etiologies and predispositions, including immature lung anatomy,

**Table 9-4**  Complications of BPD and Recommended Therapies

| COMPLICATION OF BPD | THERAPY |
|---|---|
| 1. Fluid retention | Fluid restriction; diuretics |
| 2. Bronchospasm | Bronchodilators; diuretics |
| 3. Intercurrent infection | Antibiotics |
| 4. Acute respiratory failure | Ensure patient airway<br>Increase ventilatory support<br>Increase bronchodilation and diuresis |
| 5. Tracheobronchomalacia | Maintain end-distending pressure |
| 6. Cor pulmonale | Oxygen and diuretic therapy |
| 7. Neurodevelopmental delay | Ongoing neurodevelopmental assessment,<br>with physical and occupational therapy |
| 8. Malnutrition | Maximize balanced caloric intake at a<br>minimum of 120 cal/kg/day<br>Optimize trace element and vitamin intake |

physiology, and cell biology; toxicities related to the use of oxygen and ventilators; nutritional deprivation; and infection. Prevention of the disease is not yet within our grasp. However, it is the hope of all clinicians who care for these infants that a multifactorial approach using different ventilator strategies, improved surfactant replacement, new antioxidant and anti-inflammatory agents, and prevention of prematurity will lead to a reduction in the incidence of chronic lung disease in preterm neonates (Table 9-4).

Once BPD develops, the primary goal of therapy is to provide an environment that will permit lung growth and repair and eventual resolution of the major abnormalities in lung function. The therapies for these babies must include an integrated approach that provides sufficient oxygen, adequate calories for growth, vitamins and minerals for antioxidant defense and repair processes, diuretics and bronchodilators to improve lung function, aggressive therapy of intercurrent infection, treatment of the airway and inflammatory process with corticosteroids, and constant attention to appropriate levels of infant stimulation and neurodevelopmental support.

## BIBLIOGRAPHY

1. Northway WH Jr, Rosan RC, Porter DY: Pulmonary disease following respirator-therapy of hyaline membrane disease: Bronchopulmonary dysplasia. *N Engl J Med* 1967; 276:357–368.
2. Bancalari E, Abdenour GE, Feller R: Bronchopulmonary dysplasia: Clinical Presentation. *J Pediatr* 1979; 95:819–822.
3. Shennan AT, Dunn MS, Ohlsson A, et al: Abnormal pulmonary outcomes in premature infants: Prediction from oxygen requirement in the neonatal period. *Pediatrics* 1988; 82:527.
4. Gerdes JS, Abbasi S, Bhutani VK, et al: Improved survival and short-term outcome of inborn "Micropremies." *Clin Pediatr* 1986; 25:391–394.
5. Langston C, Kida K, Reed M, et al: Human lung growth in late gestation and in the neonate. *Am Rev Resp Dis* 1984; 129:607–613.
6. Shoemaker CT, Reiser KM, Goetzman BW, et al: Elevated ratios of type I/III collagen in the lung of chronically ventilated neonates with respiratory distress. *Pediatr Res* 1984; 18:1176–1180.
7. Mandl I, Kuller S, Frerer J, et al: The role of proteolytic enzyme inhibitors and connective tissue proteins in the maturation of the lung. In Villee CA, et al, eds: *Respiratory Distress Syndrome.* New York, Academic Press, 1973, pp. 99–115.
8. Nickerson BG, Taussig LM: Family history of asthma in infants with bronchopulmonary dysplasia. *Pediatrics* 1980; 65:1140–1144.
9. Long W, Corbet A, Cotton R, et al: A controlled trial of synthetic surfactant in infants weighing 1,250 g or more with respiratory distress syndrome. *N Engl J Med* 1991; 325:1696–1703.
10. Soll RF: Synthetic surfactant treatment of RDS. In Chalmers I, ed: *Oxford Database of Perinatal Trials,* Version 1.2, Disk Issue 6, Record 5252, Autumn 1991.
11. Van Marter LJ, Leviton A, Kuban KCK, et al: Maternal glucocorticoid therapy and reduced risk of bronchopulmonary dysplasia. *Pediatrics* 1990; 86:331–336.
12. Brown ER: Increased risk of bronchopulmonary dysplasia in infants with patent ductus arteriosus. *J Pediatr* 1979; 95:865–866.
13. Brown ER, Stark A, Sosenko I, et al: Bronchopulmonary dysplasia: Possible relationships to pulmonary edema. *J Pediatr* 1978; 92:982–984.
14. Van Marter LJ, Leviton A, Allred EN, et al: Hydration during the first days of life and the risk of bronchopulmonary dysplasia in low birth weight infants. *J Pediatr* 1990; 116:942–949.
15. O'Brodovich H, Coates G: Pulmonary clearance of TcDTPA in infants who subsequently develop bronchopulmonary dysplasia. *Am Rev Resp Dis* 1988; 137:210–212.
16. Spitzer AR, Fox WW, Delivoria-Papadopoulos M: Maximum diuresis—a factor in predicting recovery from respiratory distress syndrome and the development of bronchopulmonary dysplasia. *J Pediatr* 1981; 98:476–479.
17. Lorenz J, Kleinman L, Kotagal U, et al: Water balance in very low birth weight infants; relationship to water and sodium intake and effect on outcome. *J Pediatr* 1982; 101:423–432.
18. Moylan FMB, Walker AM, Krammer SS, et al: Alveolar rupture as an independent predictor of bronchopulmonary dysplasia. *Crit Care Med* 1978; 6:10–13.
19. Rhodes PG, Graves GR, Patel DM, et al: Minimizing pneumothorax and bronchopulmonary dysplasia in ventilated infants with hyaline membrane disease. *J Pediatr* 1983; 103:634–637.
20. Autor AP, Frank L, Roberts RJ: Developmental characteristics of pul superoxide dismutase: Relationships to idiopathic respiratory distress syndrome. *Pediatr Res* 1976; 10:154–158.
21. Frank L, Sosenko IRS: Development of the lung antioxidant enzyme system in late gestation: Possible implications for the prematurely born infant. *J Pediatr* 1987; 110:9–14.
22. Saldanha RL, Capeda EE, Poland RL: The effect of vitamin E prophylaxis on the incidence and severity of bronchopulmonary dysplasia. *J Pediatr* 1982; 101:89–93.
23. Rosenfeld W, Concepcion L, Evans H, et al: Serial trypsin inhibitory capacity and ceruloplasmin levels in prematures at risk for bronchopulmonary dysplasia. *Am Rev Resp Dis* 1986; 134:1229–1232.
24. Sherman MP, Evans MJ, Campbell LA: Prevention of pulmonary alveolar macrophage proliferation in newborn rabbits by hyperoxia. *J Pediatr* 1988; 112:782–786.

25. Ward JA, Roberts RJ: Effect of hyperoxia on phosphatidylcholine synthesis, secretion, uptake and stability in the newborn rabbit lung. *Biochem Biophys Acta* 1984; 796:42–50.

26. Crapo JD, Barry BE, Fascise HA, et al: Structural and biochemical changes in rat lungs occurring during oxygen exposures to lethal and adaptive doses of oxygen. *Am Rev Resp Dis* 1978; 122:123–143.

27. Roberts RJ, Weisner KM, Bucker JR: Oxygen-induced alterations in lung vascular development in the newborn rat. *Pediatr Res* 1983; 17:368–375.

28. Merritt TA, Cochrane CG, Holcomb K, et al: Elastase and alpha-1-proteinase inhibitor activity in tracheal aspirates during respiratory distress syndrome. Role of inflammation in the pathogenesis of bronchopulmonary dysplasia. *J Clin Invest* 1983; 72:656–666.

29. Ogden Be, Murphy SA, Saunders GC, et al: Neonatal lung neutrophils and elatase/proteinase inhibitor imbalance. *Am Rev Resp Dis* 1984; 130:817–821.

30. Bruce MC, Wedig KE, Jentoft N, et al: Altered urinary excretion of elastin cross-links in premature infants who develop bronchopulmonary dysplasia. *Am Rev Resp Dis* 1985; 131:568–572.

31. Stenmark KR, Eyzaguine M, Westcott JY, et al: Potential role of lipid mediators of inflammation in bronchopulmonary dysplasia. *Am Rev Resp Dis* 1987; 136:770–772.

32. Goldman SL, Gerhardt T, Sonni R, et al: Early prediction of chronic lung disease by pulmonary function testing. *J Pediatr* 1983; 102:613–617.

33. Bhutani VK, Abbasi S: Relative likelihood of bronchopulmonary dysplasia based on pulmonary mechanics in preterm neonates during the first week of life. *Pediatr J* 1992; 120:605–613.

34. Gross I, Ilic I, Wilson CM, et al: The influence of postnatal nutritional deprivation on the phospholipid content of developing rat lung. *Biochem Biophys Acta* 1976; 441:412–422.

35. Frank L, Groseclose EE: Oxygen toxicity in newborn rats: The adverse effect of undernutrition. *J Appl Physiol* 1982; 53:1248–1256.

36. Shenai JP, Kennedy KA, Chytil F, et al: Clinical trial of vitamin A supplementation in infants susceptible to bronchopulmonary dysplasia. *J Pediatr* 1987; 111:269–277.

37. Sosenko IR, Innis SM, Frank L: Polyunsaturated fatty acids and protection of newborn rats from oxygen toxicity. *J Pediatr* 1988; 112:630.

38. Sosenko RS, Rodriquez MP, Bean J, et al: Intralipid administration beginning at 12 hours of life fails to protect 600–1,000 g premature infants from chronic lung disease. *Pediatr Res* 1992; 31:1338A.

39. Gordon EF, Gordon RC, Passal DB: Zinc metabolism; basic, clinical, and behaviorial aspects. *J Pediatr* 1981; 99:341–349.

40. Chandra RK: Influence of nutrition–Immunity axis on perinatal infections. In Ogra PL, ed: *Neonatal Infections*, vol 14. Orlando, Florida, Grune & Stratton, Inc., 1984, pp. 229–245.

41. Harris MC, Douglas SD, Lee JC, et al: Diminished polymorphonuclear leukocyte adherence and chemotaxis following protein-calorie malnutrition in newborn rats. *Pediatr Res* 1987; 21:542–546.

42. Gerdes JS, Harris MC, Dworznczyk R, et al: Effect of dexamethasone and intercurrent infection on tracheal lavage elastase and proteinase inhibitor in bronchopulmonary dysplasia. *Pediatr Res* 1986; 20:429A.

43. Cassell GH, Waites KB, Crouse DT, et al: Association of Ureaplasma urealyticum infection of the lower respiratory tract with chronic lung disease and death in very-low-birth-weight infants. *The Lancet* 1988; 2:240–245.

44. Wang EEL, Frayha H, Watts J, et al: Role of Ureaplasma urealyticum and other pathogens in the development of chronic lung disease of prematurity. *Pediatr Infect Dis J* 1988; 7:547–551.

45. Adamson IYR, Bowden DH: The type 2 cell as progenitor of alveolar epithelial regeneration: A cytodynamic study in mice after exposure to oxygen. *Lab Invest* 1974; 30:35–42.

46. Northway WH Jr, Petriceks R, Shabinian L: Quantitative aspects of oxygen toxicity in the newborn: Inhibition of lung DNA synthesis in the mouse. *Pediatrics* 1972; 50:67–72.

47. Bowman CM, Lloyd CL, Scanlon KL, et al: Mechanisms of pulmonary vascular injury and repair: Hyperoxia decreases endothelial cell synthesis of DNA and protein. *Am Rev Resp Dis* 1986; 133:A298.

48. Kirpalani H, Jordana M, Irving L, et al: Effects of oxygen exposure on human neonatal pulmonary fibroblast proliferation. *Pediatr Res* 1988; 23:512A.

49. Davis WB, Rennard SI, Bitterman PB, et al: Pulmonary oxygen toxicity. Early reversible changes in human alveolar structures induced by hyperoxia. *N Engl J Med* 1983; 309:878–883.

50. Bruce MC, Wedig KE, Jentoft N, et al: Altered urinary excretion of elastin cross-links in premature infants who develop bronchopulmonary dysplasia. *Am Rev Resp Dis* 1985; 131-568-572.

51. Gerdes JS, Yoder MC, Douglas SD, et al: Tracheal lavage and plasma fibronectin: Relationship to respiratory distress syndrome and development of bronchopulmonary dysplasia. *J Pediatr* 1986; 108:601–606.

52. Greenspan JS, Abbasi S, Bhutani VK: Sequential changes in pulmonary mechanics in the very low birthweight (1,000 gms) infants. *J Pediatr* 1988; 113:732–737.

53. Long W, Thompson T, Sundell H, et al: Effects of two rescue doses of a synthetic surfactant on mortality rate and survival without bronchopulmonary dysplasia in 700- to 1,350-gram infants with respiratory distress syndrome. *J Pediatr* 1991; 118:595–605.

54. Edwards DK: Radiology of hyaline membrane disease, transient tachypnea of the newborn, and bronchopulmonary dysplasia. In Farrell PM, ed: *Lung Development: Biological and Clinical Perspectives*, vol 2. New York, Academic Press, 1982, pp. 47–89.

55. Bernbaum JC, Williamson-Hoffman M: Chronic lung disease of infancy; bronchopulmonary dysplasia. *Prim Care Preterm Infant* 1991; 5:87–119.

56. Tay-Uyboco JS, Kwiatkowski K, Cates DB, et al:

Hypoxic airway constriction in infants of very low birth weight recovering from moderate to severe bronchopulmonary dysplasia. *J Pediatr* 1989; 115:456–459.

57. Abman SH, Wolfe RR, Accurso FJ, et al: Pulmonary vascular response to oxygen in infants with severe bronchopulmonary dysplasia. *J Pediatr* 1985; 75:80–84.

58. Motoyama EK, Fort MD, Klesh KW, et al: Early onset of airway reactivity in premature infants with bronchopulmonary dysplasia. *Am Rev Resp Dis* 1987; 136:50–57.

59. Greenspan JS, DeGiulio PA, Bhutani VK: Airway reactivity as determined by a cold air challenge in infants with bronchopulmonary dysplasia. *J Pediatr* 1988; 114:452–454.

60. Mirmanesh SJ, Abbasi S, Bhutani VK: Alpha-adrenergic bronchoprovocation in neonates with bronchopulmonary dysplasia. *J Pediatr* 1992; 121:622–625.

61. Motoyama EK, Fort MD, Klesh WK, et al: Early onset of airway reactivity in premature infants with bronchopulmonary dysplasia. *Am Rev Resp Dis* 1987; 136:50–57.

62. Rotschild A, Solimano A, Puterman M, et al: Increased compliance in response to salbutamol in premature infants with developing bronchopulmonary dysplasia. *J Pediatr* 1989; 115:984–991.

63. Davis JM, Bhutani VK, Stefano JL, et al: Changes in pulmonary mechanics following caffeine administration in infants with bronchopulmonary dysplasia. *Pediatr Pulmonol* 1989; 6:49–52.

64. Stefano JL, Bhutani VK, Fox WW: A randomized placebo-controlled study to evaluate the effects of oral albuterol on pulmonary mechanics in ventilator-dependent infants at risk of developing BPD. *Pediatr Pulmonol* 1991; 10:183–190.

65. Sosulski R, Abbasi S, Bhutani VK, et al: Physiologic effects of terbutaline on pulmonary function of infants with bronchopulmonary dysplasia. *Pediatr Pulmonol* 1986; 2:269–273.

66. Walker SR, Evans ME, Richards AJ: The clinical pharmacology of oral and inhaled salbutamol. *Clin Pharmacol Ther* 1971; 13:861–867.

67. O'Brodovich HM, Mellins RB: Bronchopulmonary dysplasia: Unresolved neonatal acute lung injury. *Am Rev Resp Dis* 1985; 132:694–709.

68. Rush MG, Engelhardt B, Parker RA, et al: Double-blind, placebo-controlled trial of alternate-day furosemide therapy in infants with chronic bronchopulmonary dysplasia. *J Pediatr* 1990; 117:112–118.

69. Engelhardt B, Gerhardt T: Short and long-term effects of furosemide on lung function in infants with bronchopulmonary dysplasia. *J Pediatr* 1986; 109:1034–1039.

70. Kao LC, Warburton D, Cheng MH, et al: Effect of oral diuretics on pulmonary mechanics in infants with chronic bronchopulmonary dysplasia: Results of a double-blind crossover sequential trial. *J Pediatr* 1984; 73:509–514.

71. Engelhardt B, Blalock WA, DonLevy S, et al: Effect of spironolactone-hydrochlorothiazide on lung function in infants with chronic broncho-pulmonary dysplasia. *J Pediatr* 1989; 114:619–624.

72. Harkavy KL, Scanlon JW, Chowdhry PK, et al: Dexamethasone therapy for chronic lung disease in ventilator- and oxygen-dependent infants: A controlled trial. *J Pediatr* 1989; 115:979–983.

73. Kazzi NJ, Brans YW, Poland RL: Dexamethasone effects on the hospital course of infants with bronchopulmonary dysplasia who are dependent on artificial ventilation. *Pediatrics* 1990; 86:722–727.

74. Collaborative Dexamethasone Trial Group: Dexamethasone therapy in neonatal chronic lung disease: An international placebo-controlled trial. *Pediatrics* 1990; 88:421–427.

75. Mammel MC, Green TP, Johnson DE, et al: Controlled trial of dexamethasone therapy in infants with bronchopulmonary dysplasia. *Lancet* 1983; 1:1356–1358.

76. Avery GB, Fletcher AB, Kaplan M, et al: Controlled trial of dexamethasone in respirator-dependent infants with bronchopulmonary dysplasia. *Pediatrics* 1985; 75:106–111.

77. Cummings JJ, D'Eugenio DB, Gross SJ: A controlled trial of dexamethasone in preterm infants at high risk for bronchopulmonary dysplasia. *N Engl J Med* 1989; 320:1505–1510.

78. Kao LC, Durand DJ, Nickerson BG: Improving pulmonary function does not decrease oxygen consumption in infants with bronchopulmonary dysplasia. *J Pediatr* 1988; 112:616–621.

79. Sindel BD, Maisels MJ, Ballantine VN: Gastroesophageal reflux to the proximal esophagus in infants with bronchopulmonary dysplasia. *Am J Dis Child* 1989; 143:1103–1106.

80. Giuffre R, Rubin S, Mitchell I: Antireflux surgery in infants with BPD. *Am J Dis Child* 1987; 141:648–651.

81. Bonikos DS, Bensch KC, Northway WH: Bronchopulmonary dysplasia: The pulmonary pathologic sequel of necrotizing bronchiolitis and pulmonary fibrosis. *Hum Pathol* 1976; 7:643.

82. Tomashefski JF Jr, Oppermann HC, Vawter GF, et al: Bronchopulmonary dysplasia: A morphometric study with emphasis on the pulmonary vasculature. *Pediatr Pathol* 1984; 2:469–487.

83. Sherman FS: Cor pulmonale. In Merritt TA, Northway WH Jr, Boynton BR, eds: *Contemporary Issues in Fetal and Neonatal Medicine. Bronchopulmonary Dysplasia*, vol 14. Boston, Blackwell Scientific Publications, 1985, pp. 251–262.

84. Berman W, Katz R, Yabek SM, et al: Long-term follow-up of bronchopulmonary dysplasia. *J Pediatr* 1986; 109:45–50.

85. Abman SH, Warady BA, Lum GM, et al: Systemic hypertension in infants with bronchopulmonary dysplasia. *J Pediatr* 1984; 104:928–931.

86. Sotomayor JL, Godinez RI, Borden S, et al: Large airway collapse due to acquired tracheobronchomalacia in infancy. *Am J Dis Child* 1986; 140:367–371.

87. Rajagopalan L, Abbasi S, Gerdes JS, et al: Tracheobronchomalacia evaluated by airflow me-

chanics and direct bronchoscopy. *Pediatr Res* 1988; 23:521A.

88. Blayney M, Kerem E, Whyte H, et al: Bronchopulmonary dysplasia: Improvement in lung function between 7 and 10 years of age. *J Pediatr* 1991; 118:201–206.

89. Heldt GP: Pulmonary status of infants and children with bronchopulmonary dysplasia. In Merritt TA, Northway WH Jr, Boynton BR, eds: *Contemporary Issues in Fetal and Neonatal Medicine*, vol 25. Boston, Blackwell Scientific Publications, 1985, pp. 421–438.

90. Mallory GB, Chaney H, Mutich RL, et al: Longitudinal changes in lung function during the first three years of life in premature infants with moderate to severe bronchopulmonary dysplasia. *Pediatr Pulmonol* 1991; 11:8–14.

91. Tepper RS, Morgan WA, Cata K, et al: Expiratory flow-limitation in infants with broncho-pulmonary dysplasia. *J Pediatr* 1986; 109:1040–1046.

92. Bader D, Ramos AD, Lew CD, et al: Childhood sequelae of infant lung disease: Exercise and pulmonary function abnormalities after bronchopulmonary dysplasia. *J Pediatr* 1987; 110:693–699.

93. Smyth JA, Tabachnik E, Duncan WJ, et al: Pulmonary function and bronchial hyperreactivity in long-term survivors of bronchopulmonary dysplasia. *Pediatrics* 1981; 68:336–340.

94. Northway WH, Moss RB, Carlisle KB, et al: Late pulmonary sequelae of bronchopulmonary dysplasia. *N Engl J Med* 1990; 323:1793–1799.

95. Byrne PJ, Piper MC, Darrah J: Motor development at term of very low birth weight infants with BPD. *J Perinatol* 1989; 9:301–306.

# Chapter 10

# BREATHING DISORDERS IN THE NEWBORN INFANT

*Douglas A. Dransfield*, M.D.

This chapter deals with those conditions that cause episodic interruption of breathing in premature and newborn term infants. You will note that this section begins with a brief discussion of normal respiratory physiology. This material has been included because an understanding of the mechanisms responsible for normal breathing is fundamental to managing infants with abnormal breathing patterns (i.e., apnea, excessive periodic breathing, etc.). The remainder of the chapter focuses on the clinical management of apnea with sections on recognition, clinical significance, diagnosis, and treatment. Because the causes, overall significance, and appropriate treatment for apnea in premature and newborn infants still remain controversial, some opinions presented may be slightly different than you have previously encountered. It is hoped that the approach presented in this chapter can be justified, and that the evidence presented will provide you with an appreciation of why differences in management philosophy exist.

## CONTROL OF RESPIRATION

Rhythmic regular respirations occur because of central nervous system activity, which is influenced by peripheral, chemical, and mechanical receptors. Control of respiration begins during fetal life and continues to develop postnatally. As might be anticipated, the fine control of respiration is still somewhat immature at the time of birth. Furthermore, the pre-

term infant exhibits a greater degree of immaturity in respiratory control than the term baby. Therefore, while short apneas (3 to 15 seconds) occur in both term and preterm infants, they are more frequent in the latter population (Fig. 10-1). With increasing postconceptional age (gestational age plus postnatal age), apnea frequency has been shown to decrease. The immaturity in control of breathing observed in newborn infants is likely to at least partially reside within the central nervous system. In that regard, Henderson-Smart et al. demonstrated that premature infants with apnea exhibited delays in acoustic brain stem responses, which were not present when the infants no longer had apnea. This suggests that a change in central nervous system function is associated with development in control of respiration. Many respiratory responses in newborns, particularly premature infants, differ from those of adults. Exercise 1 addresses some of these differences and how they may contribute to the apnea seen in newborns.

## EXERCISE 1

1. *Response to hypoxemia:* The minute ventilation of a 38-week gestation, healthy, 1-day-old infant is measured for 5 minutes in room air [0.21 inspired oxygen fraction ($FiO_2$)] and then for 5 minutes while the infant breathed a gas mixture with only 0.15 $FiO_2$.

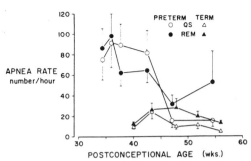

**Figure 10-1**  The central apnea rate (3- to 15-seconds duration) for term and preterm infants followed sequentially until 56 weeks' postconceptional (gestational plus postnatal) age. Apnea decreased for preterm infants with increasing gestational age. The apnea in quiet sleep (QS) and rapid eye movement (REM) sleep is plotted, and more apnea in REM compared to QS is seen after 44 weeks.
From Lee D, Caces R, Kwiatkowski K, et al: A developmental study on types and frequency distribution of short apneas (3 to 15 seconds) in term and preterm infants. *Pediatr Res* 1987; 22(3):348. Reprinted with permission.

■ **Questions:**

What is the expected change in minute ventilation in response to inhaled carbon dioxide?

What differences in the responses of the two infants might be expected?

How does the concentration of oxygen in the infant's blood modify the response to increased carbon dioxide?

Does the adult behave in a similar fashion?

■ **Questions:**

What would be the expected change in minute ventilation during the 5-minute exposure to a lowered $FiO_2$?

How would the response differ in an adult?

2. *Response to carbon dioxide:* The minute ventilation of a preterm infant (30-week gestation) *without clinical apnea* is measured while he is breathing room air and then while he is breathing a gas mixture containing an increased concentration of carbon dioxide. A second infant of the same gestational age *who has episodes of apnea* has measurements taken under the same two conditions.

3. *Sensory reflexes:* A variety of sensory stimuli have been reported to affect respirations in newborn infants.

■ **Question:**

What changes in respiration would be expected with the following stimuli?

(a) A sudden increase in the air temperature inside the incubator of a premature infant

(b) Pooling of water at the level of the glottis or larynx in a premature infant with apnea

(c) Stimulation of the pharynx with a suction catheter

4. *Mechanical receptor reflexes:* Proprioceptive nerves in the lung and respiratory muscles of the chest provide afferent input to the nervous system. One method of studying these reflexes is to measure the response to airway occlusion during the respiratory cycle. If the airway is occluded at end-expiration in an older child, the inspi-

ratory duration for the next breath is prolonged.

### ■ Question:

How do the responses differ in newborn infants with and those without apnea?

5. *Muscles controlling respiration and airway patency:* In normal individuals, contraction of the diaphragm creates a negative intrathoracic pressure, which initiates inspiration. For effective airflow to occur, however, the airway must be patent and this requires the participation of other muscle groups.

### ■ Question:

Where are these muscles located, and how is the timing of their activity related to that of the diaphragm during inspiration?

### ■ Answers:

1. *Response to hypoxemia:* In the adult, lowering the inspired oxygen concentration from 0.21 (room air) to 0.15 results in an increase in minute ventilation, which is sustained during a 5-minute study period. Newborn infants respond differently to a reduction in the inspired oxygen concentration. Infants in this age group respond by increasing minute ventilation for the first minute or two, at which point minute ventilation decreases below that seen during the room air measurement. This decrease continues to the end of the 5-minute test. This pattern of response is seen in premature and newborn term infants and is not limited to those having clinical apnea. The pathophysiology of this biphasic response in neonates is presumed to be due to initial peripheral chemoreceptor stimulation followed by central depression of the respiratory center. If this study were to be repeated when the infant in Example 1 was 1 month of age, the response would be similar to that of the older child or an adult.

2. *Response to change in carbon dioxide:* Increasing the alveolar $CO_2$ concentration results in an increase in minute ventilation, presumably due to stimulation of central chemoreceptors. This response appears to be less well developed in preterm infants of less than 33 weeks' gestation. Furthermore, the response is different in infants with clinical apnea (Fig. 10-2A). In these infants the slope of the $CO_2$ response curve is less steep.

In the adult and older child, sensitivity to carbon dioxide is greater at lower arterial $pO_2$ values. In contrast, Rigatto demonstrated (Fig. 10-2B) that in premature infants the sensitivity to carbon dioxide is diminished at lower inspired oxygen concentration values. In this question, the increase in ventilation for the premature infant should be less at a diminished $PaO_2$ value (e.g., 40 mm Hg) than at a normal concentration (100 mm Hg) and for the adult greater at a $PaO_2$ of 40 mm Hg than at a normal or elevated $PaO_2$ value of 100 to 200 mm Hg.

3. *Sensory reflexes:* A change in environmental temperature can modify the respiratory pattern of the neonate. For example, the sudden exposure to a cooler temperature at birth is believed to contribute to the initiation of respiration. Similarly a rapid increase in the air temperature in the isolette of a premature infant has been associated with the development of apnea.

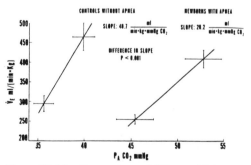

**Figure 10-2A** Comparison of $CO_2$ sensitivity obtained from ventilatory responses to changing alveolar $PCO_2$ ($PaCO_2$) in preterm infants with and without apnea. Note the less steep ventilatory response in the apneic group.

From Gerhardt T, Bancalari E: Apnea of prematurity: Lung function and regulation of breathing. *Pediatrics* 1984; 74:58. Reproduced by permission of *Pediatrics*, vol. 74, page 58, copyright 1984.

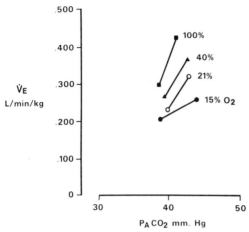

**Figure 10-2B** Carbon dioxide sensitivity measured in premature infants after achieving steady state at different concentrations of oxygen. The lower the oxygen percentage, the less response to increased inhaled carbon dioxide. This response is opposite that seen in the adult.
From Rigatto H: Apnea. *Pediatr Clin North Am* 1982; 29(5):1109. Reprinted with permission of W.B. Saunders Company.

Stimulation of chemoreceptors and taste receptors, surrounding the glottis and in the larynx, can result in a reflex decrease in ventilation or apnea in experimental animals. In a similar fashion, when saline or water is instilled in the pharynx of premature infants with apnea, a pattern of response that includes airway obstruction and central apnea can be observed. It is important to note that most apnea in premature infants occurs independently of regurgitation, but when reflux is observed in association with apnea, airway obstruction is likely to play an important role.

Stimulation of the pharynx of a newborn infant with a suction catheter can cause apnea. This is more likely to occur if the infant is already hypoxic.

4. *Mechanical receptor reflexes:* The lung is innervated with nerves that respond to both increases and decreases in lung volumes. These nerves provide afferent stimuli to the brain stem respiratory center. Similarly, the muscles of the chest wall have nerves that respond to changes in the length of the muscle spindles. These nerves return to the spinal cord and modify the activity of alpha motor nerves of the anterior horn cells. One such reflex well studied in anesthetized animals is the Hering-Breuer reflex. This reflex is mediated by the vagal afferent fibers from the lung and results in a decrease in inspiratory effort when the lung is maintained at a distended volume. When airway occlusion occurs in the adult at end expiration, the usual response is to have a longer and more forceful inspiratory effort for the inspiration immediately following the occluded breath. However, when premature infants are studied in a similar fashion, their inspiratory effort is diminished. Furthermore in premature infants with apnea the response is diminished even further (both in duration and intensity) compared to control preterm infants without apnea.

5. *Muscles controlling respiration and airway patency:* The muscles involved in generating an inspiratory effort are the diaphragm, the intercostal muscles, and the abdominal muscles. Inspiration produces a negative pressure in the airway, which causes the soft tissues of the upper airway to collapse. An opposing dilating force is provided by muscles in this region. The genioglossus is the principal muscle providing this dilating force. Contraction of the genioglossus pulls the tongue and hyoid bone toward the mandible. The geniohyoid and cervical strap muscles also produce dilating forces in the pharynx, and the posterior cricoarytenoid helps open the vocal cords. It has been shown that these muscles contract to open the airway as inspiration begins, and that reflex responses modify their activity.

Obstruction of the airway in infants can occur at the level of the pharynx. This kind of obstruction can be produced by flexing the neck of a premature infant. However, it can also occur spontaneously during episodes of apnea. Postmortem studies reported by Mathew have determined the pressures necessary to cause closure of the pharyngeal airway. Head position is a key determinant of how much pressure is needed to produce airway collapse. If the head and neck are maintained in a neutral position (at 90 degrees), collapse can occur at near atmospheric pressure. When the head and neck were in extension, negative airway pressure was needed for collapse but, in flexion, airway closure occurred with positive pressure in the airway. These postmortem pressure measurements indicate that the normal anatomy of the infant pharynx places them at risk for airway obstruction.

The information available suggests that newborn infants, particularly those born before term, exhibit considerable differences in their control of respiration. As reviewed, these differences include (1) decreased respiratory effort in response to changes in oxygen and carbon dioxide, (2) developmentally immature sensory and muscle reflexes, and (3) an upper airway anatomy that predisposes them to airway obstruction.

## CLINICAL MANAGEMENT

### Recognition of Apnea

To discuss clinical events, we must use common definitions to name the events being recognized. *Apnea* in its broadest use means cessation of breathing. When pauses in respiration occur, some combination of three clinically recognizable events becomes apparent: (1) absent respiratory effort, (2) a heart rate lower than normal, and (3) a change in color (usually cyanosis). Each of these three events can occur singly or in combination. During the past several years, it has been well established that infants exhibit interruptions in breathing either because the effort to breathe is absent (central apnea), the effort to breathe is present but the airway is temporarily blocked (obstructive apnea), or a combination of these two events occurs (mixed apnea). The following list gives the currently accepted definitions for these three types of apnea.

*Central apnea* is absence of breathing effort. The term implies that it is absence of central nervous system initiation of breathing, but should also indicate that the entire neuromuscular system of breathing has failed to initiate an inspiration.
*Obstructive apnea* is failure to breathe because of a blockage of the airway despite breathing effort.
*Mixed apnea* is a single episode of absent breathing that is due to a combination of lack of breathing effort and blocked effort.

Other terms (periodic breathing, pathological apnea, etc.) have been used to describe apnea in premature infants and to distinguish the clinical significance of certain types of respiratory pauses. The following definitions are reproduced by permission of *Pediatrics*, vol. 79, page 292, copyright 1987 [National Institutes of Health consensus development conference on infantile apnea and home monitoring: Sept. 29–Oct. 1, 1986. *Pediatrics* 1987; 79(Feb.):293].

*Periodic breathing:* "A breathing pattern in which there are three or more respiratory pauses of greater than 3 seconds duration with less than 20 seconds of respiration between pauses. Periodic breathing can be a normal event."
*Pathologic[al] apnea:* "A respiratory pause is abnormal if it is prolonged (20 seconds) or associated with cyanosis; marked pallor or hypotonia; or bradycardia."
*Apnea of prematurity (AOP):* "Periodic breathing *with* pathologic[al] apnea in a premature infant. Apnea of prematurity usually ceases by 37 weeks gestation (menstrual dating) but occasionally persists to several weeks past term."
*Symptomatic premature infants:* "Preterm infants who continue to have AOP at the time when they would otherwise be ready for discharge."

### EXERCISE 2

The following four case studies describe infants with clinically recognized episodes of acute change in clinical condition. Please read each case study and decide which *definition* or *definitions* would be applicable to these events.

***Classification of Abnormal***
***Breathing Patterns***
Central apnea
Obstructive apnea
Mixed apnea
Periodic breathing
Apnea of prematurity
Pathological apnea
Symptomatic premature Infant

You will note that in the process of defining the type of apnea, a therapeutic maneuver is frequently required. The next section discusses the management of apnea in much greater detail.

## CASE STUDY 1

A 1-day-old 1,250-g appropriate-for-gestational-age, premature female infant without respiratory distress is being examined while she is sleeping in the prone position. You note that she will breath regularly for 5 to 8 seconds, then have no respiratory effort for 3 seconds, and then resume breathing for the same period of time followed by a similar pause. This pattern repeats itself for the next minute. During this time the infant remains pink and well perfused. The heart rate remains between 130 and 140 beats per minute (BPM).

## CASE STUDY 2

The same infant from Case Study 1 later has a monitor alarm for bradycardia. When you go to the incubator, the infant has no respiratory effort. The infant is mildly cyanotic. You note the heart rate to be 80 BPM. You stimulate the infant, and she begins regular respirations and regains normal color.

## CASE STUDY 3

A 6-day-old 1540-g 33-week-gestational-age male has recovered from *respiratory distress syndrome* sufficiently to be in hood oxygen at 28%. The infant's monitor alarm sounds. When you arrive, the monitor has 60 BPM for the heart rate and 46 breaths per minute for the respirations. You look at the infant. He is making breathing efforts, but the neck is in extreme flexion, and he is cyanotic. You readjust the infant's position, and he begins to cry with a prompt increase in the heart rate to 170 BPM.

## CASE STUDY 4

The same infant from Case Study 3 has another monitor alarm. Now when you arrive the respiratory rate is 0, but the heart rate is 110 BPM. The infant has no apparent respiratory effort. As you open the doors to the incubator, the infant begins to make respiratory efforts, but you notice there are retractions. The infant is now becoming cyanotic, and the heart rate is 60 BPM. You turn the infant on his back, position his airway, suction the mouth for saliva, stimulate the infant, and give free-flow oxygen to the face. The respiratory effort becomes regular and free of retractions. The heart rate and color promptly improve.

### ■ Discussion:

All four of these case studies illustrate the difficulty associated with recognizing the three types of apnea. The diagnosis of apnea in its various forms depends on the ability to measure the features of respiratory effort and airflow. Various centers have developed the capability to study the breathing of infants in some detail. It is possible to measure and record simultaneously respiratory effort, nasal and oral airflow, the electrocardiogram, the electroencephalogram, esophageal pH, the oxygen saturation, and/or transcutaneous $pO_2/pCO_2$ while you are videotaping the infant. Such intensive study has greatly expanded our understanding of apneic events in infants. However, this type of multiple event recording is not routinely available. Therefore, the clinician must rely on observations made directly (or by available monitoring) to determine the kind of event that has occurred. Standard monitoring includes the electrocardiogram for heart rate, impedance pneumogram for respiratory effort, and pulse oximeter or transcutaneous $pO_2$ measurement to determine cyanosis. The capabilities and limitations of these common clinical monitors are discussed in the references provided.

In practical terms, the monitors of heart rate and impedance pneumography can be set to sound an alarm when the heart rate goes below a selected level (usually 80 to 100 BPM) or the chest wall ceases to move for a certain period of time (15 to 20 seconds). Monitoring for cyanosis is done by using a pulse oximeter and selecting an alarm value for the oxygen saturation ($SpO_2$). The caregiver responding to the alarm must then determine if the infant is indeed bradycardic, apneic, or cyanotic. After a very short time working in a modern neonatal intensive care unit (NICU), the newcomer understands that many times alarms sound without any apparent problem when the infant is examined. This is because either the monitor signal was wrong or the infant has already resumed breathing and appears well.

### ■ Answers:

**Case Study 1:** This infant is having *periodic breathing*. Each brief apnea is a *central apnea*. It is not apnea of prematurity because there is no pathological apnea during this episode. Here the monitoring information agrees with your observations. There are brief pauses in respiratory effort that are short and rhythmic and that do not change the infant's overall condition.

**Case Study 2:** This is an episode of *Central apnea*, which qualifies as *pathological apnea*. It is central because there is no respiratory effort. It is pathological because cyanosis and bradycardia occur during the event. This is also labeled *apnea of prematurity* because of the infant's gestational age at birth and postconceptional age. If this event had been recorded by multiple-event recording, a simultaneous cessation in airflow and respiratory effort would have been recorded followed by a slowing of the heart rate and a decrease in the $SpO_2$. With your stimulation, the airflow and respiratory effort would have returned simultaneously, followed promptly by an increase in the heart rate and then the $SpO_2$. Although multiple-event recording would have allowed greater understanding of these events, the important feature for the clinician is that cyanosis accompanied the decrease in heart rate.

**Case Study 3:** This is an apparent episode of *obstructive apnea*. The infant experienced an episode of airway obstruction because of the position of the head and neck. This event also qualifies as *apnea of prematurity* and because of the bradycardia is *pathological*. Multiple-event recording would have confirmed that airflow was blocked and documented the duration of the event and the exact decline in heart rate and $SpO_2$. In this case study, the clinician recognized that the position of the infant's neck predisposed him to airway obstruction. Furthermore, repositioning the infant's head relieved the cyanosis and bradycardia.

**Case Study 4:** This is an apparent single episode of *mixed apnea*. At first, the infant appears to have central apnea, but when respiratory effort resumes the progression to cyanosis and bradycardia suggest that the airway is obstructed. Again, this episode would qualify both as *apnea of prematurity* and *pathological apnea*. Multiple-event recording would have demonstrated that the episode began as central apnea (with cessation of effort and airflow) followed by an obstructive apneic episode (characterized by resumption of respiratory effort, but not airflow). As a result the heart rate and $SpO_2$ would decline further. Figure 10-3 illustrates an event of mixed apnea, longer in duration than described in the case study. It is important to note that the heart rate and oxygen saturation continue to fall despite chest movement. Although such recordings make interpretation of mixed apnea more certain, the significant features of this event (respiratory disturbance accompanied by bradycardia and cyanosis) are apparent to the clinician. In Case Study 4, by reasoning that airway obstruction is causing continued bradycardia and cyanosis, an appropriate intervention results in the infant's improvement.

The preceding case studies were presented as if you were observing the patient and could directly interpret the event. This is rarely the case, and your recognition of the type of apnea depends on the information provided by others. It has long been appreciated that many episodes of apnea go undocumented by nurses in a busy NICU. In a recent study by Muttitt et al., nurses clinically detected only 54% of apneic events documented by a computer. Furthermore, they were less able to recognize obstructive and mixed apnea. Interestingly, however, in the events not detected by the nurse, the patients apparently recovered without intervention.

From the previous discussion, it should be clear that it is not sufficient to simply terminate an apneic event by responding to an alarm. Everyone who works in the nursery must learn how to recognize and document the various kinds of apnea occurring in newborn infants. Only then can an appropriate management strategy be selected.

**Assessing Significance**

For the clinician a significant apnea event is one that requires determination of etiology and consideration of appropriate treatment. The definition of pathological apnea uses criteria that mark the event as abnormal for newborn infants and therefore clinically significant. The importance of such an event in terms of oxygen delivery to vital areas such as the brain is more difficult to determine. Marked bradycardia and cyanosis during pathological apnea would be expected to decrease tissue oxygenation. In fact, recent studies using Doppler ultrasound and near-infrared spectroscopy suggest that an adverse effect on cerebral blood flow does occur (Fig. 10-4).

Often the clinician is uncertain if a given episode of apnea associated with bradycardia is harmful. Bradycardia, as a cause for a monitor alarm, may be transient. Furthermore, it is

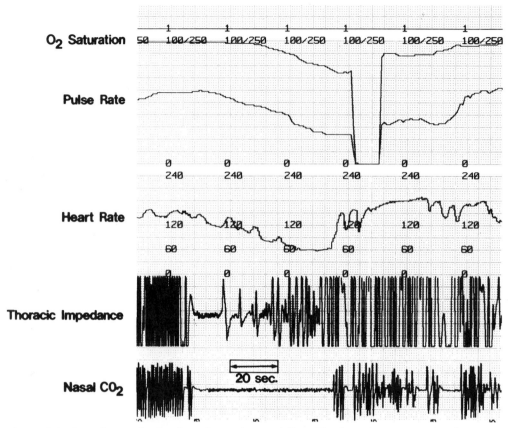

**Figure 10-3** A single episode of prolonged mixed apnea followed by three short apneas. A pulse oximeter is measuring $O_2$ saturation and pulse rate. Standard cardiopulmonary monitoring provide thoracic impedance and ECG for the heart rate. Nasal $CO_2$ is the measure of airflow. Note that the mixed apnea begins as central apnea and becomes obstructive apnea (respiratory effort by thoracic impedance fluctuation but no nasal $CO_2$ airflow) and that with resumed airflow there is immediate recovery of the heart rate although the pulse oximeter signal is lost briefly.
From Hunt CE: Cardiorespiratory monitoring. *Clin Perinatol* 1991; 18(3):481. Reprinted with permission of W.B. Saunders Company.

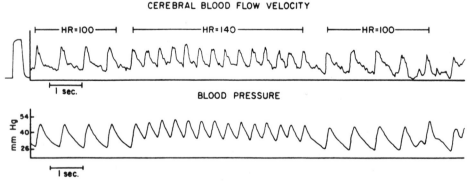

**Figure 10-4** Decrease in cerebral blood flow velocity and arterial blood pressure during apnea with bradycardia. HR is heart rate. Apnea began after single first breath. With decreasing heart rate, both systolic and diastolic flow velocity decreased. Cerebral blood flow velocity was measured by Doppler ultrasound and arterial blood pressure was from an umbilical artery catheter.
From Perlman J, Volpe J: Episodes of apnea and bradycardia in the preterm newborn: Impact on cerebral circulation. *Pediatrics* 1985; 76(3):333. Reproduced by permission of *Pediatrics*, vol. 76, page 333, copyright 1985.

common for the infant to appear normal at the time caretakers respond to the alarm. Hodgman et al. reported that in a study of premature infants monitored with electrocardiogram and impedance pneumography, more than half of the episodes of transient bradycardia were not associated with central apnea. However, of those apnea events characterized by pauses in respiration lasting 15 seconds or longer, virtually all the infants became bradycardic. Self-resolved apnea lasting between 15 and 20 seconds associated with transient bradycardia was so common that the authors suggested it was not abnormal. Other studies employing a separate channel to measure nasal airflow have demonstrated that *most* episodes of transient bradycardia in premature infants not associated with central apnea are associated with obstructive or mixed apnea. Therefore, isolated bradycardia without associated apnea is an unusual event in a preterm infant.

Measurement of oxygen saturation by pulse oximetry (SpO$_2$) is widely used to detect episodes of cyanosis. Pulse oximetry has been shown to be useful and accurate for all sizes of infants encountered in the infant intensive care unit. Upton et al. reported that there was a positive correlation with the duration of apnea and the reduction in SpO$_2$; however, some episodes of apnea less than 10 seconds in duration had a more than 15% reduction in SpO$_2$. Pulse oximetry is helpful in determining the clinical significance of a given apnea event.

Obviously, the clinician must accept some uncertainty when attempting to understand episodes of apnea in a given infant. The best you can do is use the information gained from monitoring and nursing observations to determine if the patient needs further evaluation or treatment. The definition of pathological apnea is useful for assigning clinical significance. All such events in term infants should be considered abnormal. For the premature infant brief events of self-resolving bradycardia with or without observed apnea (in the absence of other findings) may not be clinically important.

### Diagnosis of Apnea

Although brief pauses in respiration are commonly observed in newborn infants, other conditions may cause the apnea to be more severe. Apnea may be a sign of infection, tissue hypoxia, disturbances of metabolism, congenital or acquired abnormalities of the central nervous system, drugs, severe anemia, and gastroesophageal reflux. This section discusses these diagnoses in greater detail.

Infants with sepsis, pneumonia, and meningitis can all exhibit apnea as part of their disease presentations. Apnea, as part of serious bacterial infection, is usually severe and may result in ventilatory failure requiring assisted ventilation. One type of infectious agent that is particularly associated with apnea is respiratory syncytial virus (RSV). RSV often causes hypoxemia and frequently causes apnea in infants up to 44 weeks' postconceptional age.

As discussed in the previous section, low arterial oxygen levels depress respirations in newborns. Therefore, conditions that cause cyanosis can also cause apnea. This is particularly true of pulmonary diseases. Premature infants with respiratory distress syndrome (RDS) may demonstrate apnea both early on as a sign of progressive deterioration and later when the lungs improve and attempts to decrease respiratory support are made. Bronchopulmonary dysplasia will result in apnea, particularly if the infant becomes hypoxemic during sleep.

Congenital heart disease with or without associated cyanosis can cause apnea. In most instances the apnea is due to hypoxemia either secondary to the congenital heart lesion itself or to congestive heart failure. In premature infants, however, pulmonary congestion from a patent ductus arteriosus can cause apnea without apparent preceding cyanosis or overt congestive heart failure.

Structural abnormalities of the central nervous system can cause apnea. Infants with these conditions usually exhibit apnea as one sign among many indicative of an abnormal nervous system. Premature infants with intraventricular and intraparenchymal cerebral hemorrhages may also have apnea. The relationship of apnea to these hemorrhages, particularly when the hemorrhages are small in size, is uncertain. The report by Butcher-Puech et al. suggests that infants with severe hemorrhages are more likely to have obstructive apnea episodes. Seizures may present as apnea; however, it is important to note that apnea is unlikely to be the sole manifestation of a seizure disorder in a preterm infant.

Medications that depress respirations must

be considered in the differential diagnosis of apnea. Maternal narcotic analgesia in labor may cause apnea, but this is usually apparent in the delivery room. The administration of magnesium sulfate during labor may cause hypermagnesemia in the neonate, and apnea may be an early sign of magnesium toxicity, especially in infants also receiving aminoglycoside antibiotics. Maternal cocaine use can cause respiratory abnormalities in the neonate. Furthermore, there is the expected side effect of respiratory depression (including apnea) with the use of narcotics, barbiturates, and benzodiazepines in neonates. Prostaglandin $E_1$, when used to maintain patency of the ductus arteriosus will commonly have apnea as a side effect.

Anemia can be a cause of apnea. Postnatally, premature infants undergo a progressive decline in their hemoglobin concentrations (physiological anemia) that is more marked than observed in term infants. While it makes theoretical sense that reduced oxygen delivery to the central nervous system (as would occur with any progressive anemia) might be an important determinant of abnormal breathing patterns, this issue still remains controversial. DeMaio et al. showed that the frequency of periodic breathing and apnea longer than 6 seconds decreased after blood transfusion in anemic premature infants. However, in a study of transfusion therapy in premature infants, Keyes et al. could not demonstrate a relationship between hematocrit values (19% to 64%) and the infant's heart rate or respiratory rate. In this study, transfusions were given as the physicians deemed them necessary, but contrary to DeMaio's study, transfusion therapy had no effect on heart rate, respiratory rate, or the frequency of apnea (>15 seconds) and bradycardia (<80 BPM). It is difficult at present to offer clear guidelines as to when to transfuse premature infants with apnea. If, however, apnea is associated with severe anemia or increases as the hematocrit falls, or if anemia is present along with another condition causing hypoxemia, a blood transfusion is likely to be therapeutic.

Premature infants who require anesthesia for surgery may have postoperative apnea. This type of apnea occurs in premature infants who are beyond term (by postconceptional age) and in infants who have stopped having apnea preoperatively. Postoperative apnea also occurs in infants who did not have a signifi-

cant history of apnea earlier in life. When general anesthesia is used, postoperative apnea may be central, obstructive, or mixed. Former premature infants with preoperative hematocrits of less then 30% are more likely to become apneic following general anesthesia. Apnea can also occur in infants receiving spinal anesthesia, especially if ketamine is used for preoperative sedation.

Apnea has been shown to occur during episodes of gastroesophageal reflux. It is unfortunate for the clinician that regurgitation and vomiting are particularly common in neonates. Therefore, establishing the relationship of apnea with reflux in an individual patient requires monitoring for reflux (with a pH probe) and apnea simultaneously. Reflux-associated apnea can be central, mixed, or obstructive and may not be responsive to methylxanthine treatment.

Anomalies of the upper airway can lead to apnea. Choanal stenosis and atresia can cause obstructive apnea. Similarly, the micrognathia of Pierre Robin syndrome (and associated glossoptosis) can cause obstructive apnea. Infants who have anomalies of the upper airway usually exhibit feeding and breathing abnormalities other than apnea.

## EXERCISE 3

Review Case Studies 5 through 8 and answer the questions that follow each case study.

## CASE STUDY 5

You are called to see a male infant born at term gestation who has apnea at 1 hour of age. The mother was healthy during her pregnancy and received regular prenatal care. She denied alcohol, illicit drugs, and tobacco use during pregnancy. She was admitted in labor the day before her expected date of confinement. The infant was delivered by cesarean section because of cephalopelvic disproportion after 20 hours of ruptured membranes. The mother did not have signs of infection during labor. The infant needed repetitive suctioning, stimulation, and oxygen by mask in the delivery room to relieve cyanosis. In the nursery, he was noted to be tachypneic and continued to need 40% oxygen by hood. The chest x-ray was consistent with retained fetal lung fluid.

As you examine the infant at 1 hour of age, he extends his arms and legs and stops breathing. He becomes cyanotic and requires bag and mask ventilation. When another episode of apnea occurs, the infant is intubated and started on assisted ventilation.

■ **Question:**
What conditions might be contributing to the development of apnea in this case?

## CASE STUDY 5 continued
This infant is later observed to have seizures by the nurse and during an episode of electrographically confirmed seizures has apnea. He is then started on phenobarbital and is free of apnea without assisted ventilation. After 1 week of phenobarbital treatment, he again has several episodes of apnea.

■ **Question:**
What causes of apnea should now be investigated?

## CASE STUDY 6
A female infant born at 28 weeks' gestation was treated with assisted ventilation and surfactant replacement for respiratory distress syndrome. She is now 14 days old and continues to need 28% oxygen by hood to maintain a normal oxygen saturation value. Orogastric gavage feedings have been in use for the last 3 days, and several feedings have been associated with regurgitation. Six episodes of apnea have been noted by the nurses since discontinuing assisted ventilation 5 days ago. In the last hour, there have been three additional episodes of apnea associated with cyanosis requiring treatment with bag and mask ventilation. You are called during the third event because the infant will not resume regular respirations. You place an endotracheal tube and continue assisted ventilation with a respirator.

■ **Question:**
What possible causes for this change in frequency and severity of apnea would you want to evaluate?

## CASE STUDY 7
A 34-week gestation, 2,100-g female infant is transferred to your NICU because she required intubation and ventilation for respiratory failure. The infant was born earlier in the day after a rapid labor that was complicated by a small placental abruption. In the delivery room the infant cried and was assigned Apgar scores of 7 and 9. The infant went to the newborn nursery where the nurse described her as being intermittently cyanotic. The infant's breathing pattern was thought to be normal; however, when she was stimulated to cry, her color improved. When the infant's temperature had stabilized, she was placed in a bassinet. The infant was found a short time later to be cyanotic and apneic. The nurse detected a heart rate of 40 BPM and began resuscitation. The infant was intubated and was given assisted ventilation during transfer. In your nursery, the chest x-ray is normal, and the infant has a normal arterial blood gas while intubated with a ventilator rate of 6 and $FiO_2$ of 0.25.

■ **Questions:**
What diagnoses do you suspect? What would you do to evaluate this infant?

## CASE STUDY 8
A 3-month-old male infant with bronchopulmonary dysplasia has an incarcerated left inguinal hernia. He was born at 26 weeks' gestation and weighed 680 g. His bronchopulmonary dysplasia has been improving, and he has been off supplemental oxygen for the last week. The last episode of apnea was 2 weeks ago. The hernia is repaired under general anesthesia, but in the recovery room he has apnea. You are asked to assist in his management.

■ **Question:**
What conditions may be contributing to this recurrence of apnea?

■ **Answers:**

**Case Study 5:**   This term infant had severe apnea shortly after birth. The mother's history was unremarkable, and there was no indication of asphyxia during labor. Membranes were ruptured 20 hours prior to delivery by cesarean section. Respiratory distress was evident immediately after birth. Given the infant's *respiratory distress* and *ruptured membranes for 20 hours,* pneumonia and/or sepsis must be considered likely possibilities for the apnea. Hypoglycemia needs to be excluded although it is unlikely in this particular case. The pulmonary disease (presumed to be retained fetal lung fluid) could be causing hypoxemia (resulting in apnea), but noninvasive monitoring suggested that oxygenation was adequate. Abnormalities of the central nervous system must be considered. The extension movements associated with the apnea make the diagnosis of a seizure most likely. The etiology of the seizure would need to be explored and treatment given. A review of the mother's medications to exclude a possible narcotic effect is needed, but is an unlikely cause.

**Case Study 5 continued:** When the infant has been treated for a week, apnea resumes. Although again new problems such as infection and hypoglycemia should be considered, there is a greater probability that either the phenobarbital level is too high or that recurrent seizures are again causing apnea. For this particular case, the phenobarbital level was below the therapeutic range. When watched closely during the apnea episode, the infant was noted to have eye and tongue movements followed by shallow breathing, then cyanosis, and finally apnea. Apnea was controlled when the seizures were controlled.

**Case Study 6:** This 30-week postconceptional age infant had been steadily improving until several feedings were not tolerated and severe apnea developed. This sudden change in the infant's condition suggests a new problem and infection would be a likely cause. Less likely possibilities would include inadequate oxygenation (monitoring had not demonstrated this), gastroesophageal reflux with aspiration, a change in cardiac condition (e.g., patent ductus arteriosus), or a change in glucose or electrolyte concentrations. This infant had rapid onset of necrotizing enterocolitis shortly after these events occurred, suggesting that sepsis was the true etiology.

**Case Study 7:** This infant must be evaluated for all the conditions that were considered for the term infant described in Case Study 5. It is important to note that this infant's course was somewhat unusual in that following respiratory arrest she did well when treated only with intubation and minimal ventilator support. This should alert you to the possibility of an airway abnormality that the endotracheal tube corrected. In this case, the episodes of cyanosis were being caused by airway obstruction. An evaluation for an airway anomaly should begin at the nose and proceed down the respiratory tract until the cause is determined. This infant had right-sided choanal atresia and choanal stenosis on the contralateral side. Assisted ventilation was not required once an adequate airway was established.

**Case Study 8:** This infant is having postoperative apnea. A hemoglobin concentration should be determined. Respirations should be monitored and treatment for apnea given (see next section) until it resolves. The possibility of infection from the incarcerated hernia, hypoxemia from the bronchopulmonary dysplasia, or disturbances of glucose, electrolytes, or calcium must be considered.

## Therapy

Treatment begins with diagnosis and any cause that might be contributing to the onset of apnea should be evaluated. In many instances, immediate respiratory support is required before treatment for the associated cause is initiated. Treatments available for apnea include physical stimulation, medications to stimulate breathing, continuous positive airway pressure, and ventilation.

Many kinds of stimulation have been used to treat apnea in newborn infants. Cutaneous stimulation by rubbing the infant's skin is one commonly used form. This can be done in response to an apnea event in progress, but it has also been used in some nurseries prophylactically to lessen the frequency of apnea. When used as part of the infant's care, intermittent cutaneous stimulation has been reported to decrease apnea frequency in premature infants. Vestibular stimulation in the form of movement (e.g., rocking waterbed) has also been reported to lessen the frequency of apnea, but results have varied with the timing and type of stimulus used. Stimulation (like that used to awaken a sleeping infant) such as voice and a gentle jostling movement is often followed by resumed respirations and is perhaps the most time-honored and universally applied first treatment in the care of premature infants with apnea.

Theophylline and caffeine are methylxanthines that are widely used to treat apnea in infants. Theophylline and caffeine differ in chemical structure by only one methyl group and share many pharmacological properties. Methylxanthines competitively inhibit phosphodiesterase, thus preventing the degradation of adenosine 3',5'-cyclic monophosphate. This compound is involved in the function of many types of cells. Therefore, it is not surprising that a wide variety of effects have been ascribed to methylxanthines or their metabolites. Although the precise mechanisms of action of methylxanthines is unknown, they may decrease the incidence of apnea by either reducing the concentration of adenosine in the brain (adenosine is a known respiratory depressant) or by improving diaphragmatic contractility (by increasing intracellular calcium). Both methylxanthines have a number of unwanted side effects including irritability, tremors, seizures, tachycardia, gastric irritation (resulting in vomiting and hematemesis), water and sodium diuresis, and glucose intolerance. Because theophylline has a much lower therapeutic index than caffeine, side effects are more common with that agent. Both drugs require metabolism by the hepatic cytochrome P-450 system for excretion. This system matures with advancing gestational and postnatal age and once developed can vary in function. Therefore, the half-life of the methylxanthines is prolonged in infants and exhibits considerable individual variation. The therapeutic index for theophylline may be lower in infants compared to older children because of decreased protein binding.

Theophylline is absorbed well in children when it is given orally, and it also appears to be easily absorbed in premature infants, although specific studies are lacking. Many available elixirs of theophylline contain 20% alcohol; however, alcohol-free preparations are available and should be used. The intravenous form of theophylline is aminophylline, a water-soluble compound that is 70% to 85% theophylline. The dose response relationship for theophylline in premature infants with apnea has been examined by Muttitt, Tierney, and Finer who used continuous monitoring capable of detecting all three types of apnea (Fig.

10-5). These data demonstrated that 15% of infants (3 in 22) responded at a serum concentration of 4.2 mg/L, while a cumulative 73% (16 in 22) responded with a serum level of 12.7 mg/L. Increasing the serum theophylline concentration to 15.3 mg/L resulted in only one additional infant responding. There were decreases in the frequencies of all three types of apnea. Side effects were more common with blood levels greater than 10 mg/L. Therefore, not all infants who are administered theophylline respond adequately before side effects are observed. Treatment with theophylline must be monitored with frequent blood levels because of the narrow therapeutic index for the drug.

The ideal drug therapy for apnea should result in a rapidly achieved drug level that reduces apnea but does not cause side effects. For theophylline, a dose of 1 mg/kg body weight will raise the serum concentration 2 mcg/mL. The Federal Food and Drug Administration Drug Bulletin has recommended a loading dose of 4 to 5 mg/kg followed by 1 mg/kg q. 12 hours. An equivalent aminophylline dose would be a 5 to 6 mg/kg loading dose and a maintenance dose of 1.2 mg/kg q. 12 hours. Although this schedule will avoid side effects, many infants will need a higher maintenance dose administered at q. 8-hour intervals to achieve an acceptable therapeutic effect.

Caffeine is commercially available in the United States both as caffeine benzoate and caffeine citrate. Caffeine benzoate should be avoided in newborns because of a possible adverse effect on bilirubin-albumin binding. Twenty milligrams of caffeine citrate contains 10 mg of caffeine and this preparation is available as a powder (from which a parenteral solution can be made) and in an enteral form. Caffeine citrate, however, is acidic and should not be given intramuscularly. Apnea in premature infants usually responds to blood levels ranging from 8 to 20 mg/L. Toxicity rarely occurs at blood concentrations of less than 50 mg/L. Note that some infants may respond to caffeine who did not have an adequate response to theophylline. Because the half-life of caffeine in premature infants during the first month of life is usually more than 100 hours, doses are given once a day. Furthermore, breast feeding has been shown to delay caffeine elimination. Therapeutic levels are achieved by administering a loading dose of 20 mg/kg *caffeine citrate* followed by 5 mg/kg every 24 hours. Because of the wider therapeu-

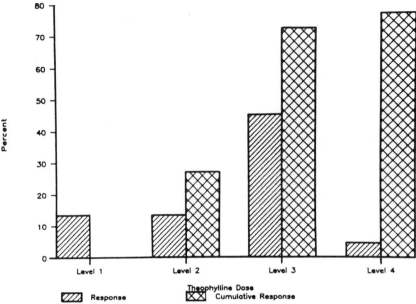

**Figure 10-5**  Percentage of premature infants who had decreased apnea with sequential increases in theophylline serum levels. Level 1 was 4.2 mg/L, level 2 was 8.5 mg/L, level 3 was 12.7 mg/L, and level 4 was 15.3 mg/L. Response means infants who did not decrease apnea until that level was reached and cumulative response means infants who had responded at that level or lower.
From Muttitt SC, Tierney AJ, Finer NN: The dose response of theophylline in treatment of apnea of prematurity. *J Pediatr* 1988; 112(1):118. Reprinted with permission of Mosby-Year Book, Inc.

tic index, blood levels can be followed less frequently when caffeine (instead of theophylline) is used, but again measurements must be available in a timely fashion to evaluate a lack of response or signs of toxicity.

Doxapram is a respiratory stimulant with mainly peripheral chemoreceptor effects. Infants receiving doxapram exhibit both a rise in minute ventilation and tidal volume. In the United States, doxapram is available only as a preparation that contains benzyl alcohol and therefore should not be used in premature infants. The drug is available without benzyl alcohol in Canada and other countries. Doxapram has been shown to be efficacious in some infants who did not respond adequately to theophylline or caffeine. Unfortunately, doxapram must be delivered by continuous intravenous infusion. Furthermore, doxapram appears to have a narrow therapeutic index and blood levels must be closely monitored. If a benzyl alcohol–free doxapram preparation is available along with drug level testing, doxapram may be a suitable alternative to methylxanthines in preterm babies. (For dosage information see Barrington et al. and Raval, Reitz, and Yeh.)

Nasal continuous positive airway pressure (NCPAP) is widely used to treat apnea in preterm infants. It is often used for the patient with apnea who also has significant pulmonary disease. For example, the infant who is recovering from RDS and is ready for a trial of extubation is commonly treated with NCPAP to maintain lung volume and prevent hypoxemia. Premature infants without pulmonary disease may also respond to NCPAP treatment. Miller, Carlo, and Martin showed that the frequency of obstructive and mixed apnea were reduced by NCPAP; however, the frequency of central apnea was not significantly affected. This suggests that the effect of NCPAP is principally on the upper airway.

Assisted ventilation is necessary for treatment of apnea when respiratory failure is present. Apnea may be so frequent and severe that immediate assistance of respiration is needed. In other infants, apnea may be viewed as one of several signs of an impending respiratory arrest. Finally, some extremely premature infants will need a low rate of ventilation (6 to 10 BPM) to prevent apnea that cannot be adequately managed by the treatments just discussed.

## EXERCISE 4

Please describe how you might respond to the following clinical situations.

### CASE STUDY 9

A male infant weighing 3.25 kg was born after a 34-week gestation to an insulin-dependent diabetic woman whose membranes ruptured 18 hours before delivery. In the delivery room the infant was stimulated and given oxygen by mask for the first 2 minutes of life. The Apgar scores were 6 and 8. At 1 hour of age, the infant was tachypneic and needed oxygen because of cyanosis. When you arrive in the nursery, the infant has been apneic for approximately 30 seconds, and the nurse is providing bag and mask ventilation. The infant becomes increasingly cyanotic and does not resume breathing with stimulation.

### CASE STUDY 10

A 5-day-old infant, born following a 32-week gestation, has recovered sufficiently from RDS to be extubated and placed in an oxygen hood with an inspired oxygen concentration ($FiO_2$) of 0.32. The hemoglobin, glucose, calcium, and electrolyte levels were normal that morning. During the next 12 hours the respiratory rate per minute increased from 44 to 60 and mild retractions were noted; however, the oxygen saturation remained normal. There have been several episodes of bradycardia associated with apnea and cyanosis. All these events have responded to stimulation.

### CASE STUDY 11

A 2-week-old premature infant (33-week postconceptional age) stopped having pathological apnea when treated with aminophylline intravenously. Four days ago he was switched to oral theophylline. Today he has begun to have pathological apnea once more. His examination is unchanged; however, there was some regurgitation after a feeding.

### CASE STUDY 12

An infant born 6 weeks ago, at 28 weeks' gestation, is now in stable condition. Since extubation 4 weeks ago, the infant has been treated with theophylline. In the last 2 weeks no monitor alarms for apnea, bradycardia, or cyanosis have been noted by the nurses.

### ■ Answers:

**Case Study 9:** If repetitive bag and mask ventilation is needed, intubation for assisted ventilation should be accomplished and cardiopulmonary monitoring should be initiated. Because of the onset of severe apnea within hours after birth, causes other than apnea of prematurity should be sought. You would proceed by treating those conditions likely to present during the first day of life (e.g., sepsis, hypoglycemia, or hypoxemia) and evaluating the response to treatment.

**Case Study 10:** This infant's changing condition is almost certainly due to an exacerbation of his underlying pulmonary disease (RDS). The increasing signs of respiratory distress and frequency of apnea suggest that additional treatment is needed. NCPAP could be used in such a case to improve lung function and prevent episodic upper airway occlusion. Furthermore, intravenous aminophylline could be used alone or in addition to NCPAP. If pathological apnea persisted, despite these treatments, a return to assisted ventilation would be indicated.

**Case Study 11:** In this case, you should first determine the serum theophylline level. If it is lower than the prior therapeutic level, the dosage should be adjusted using a loading dose of 1 mg/kg for each 2 mcg/mL increase in the plasma level desired. If the serum level is unchanged, you should strongly consider other causes for apnea, such as infection or gastroesophageal reflux. If no other cause is evident, and the serum theophylline level is in the "top normal" range, it is appropriate to use caffeine.

**Case Study 12:** The infant is now at a postconceptional age when apnea of prematurity could be expected to resolve. The theophylline should be discontinued (in the hospital); however, routine monitoring should be continued to determine the response. Many neonatologists would also make a permanent recording of the infant's breathing pattern and heart rate to prove that the apnea has resolved.

## Hospital Discharge

The decision to discharge an infant who has been hospitalized for several weeks is one that requires consideration of many factors. The clinical stability of the cardiorespiratory system is central to this decision. Is the infant ready for home care without treatment or monitoring? If the infant has ongoing apnea can discharge still occur and, if so, what monitoring or treatment must be continued at home?

## EXERCISE 5

Consider what discharge instructions you would give the family and what treatments you would use at discharge in the following situations.

1. The term infant who had apnea associated with an episode of sepsis *or* the premature infant who had mild apnea of prematurity not requiring treatment. Both infants have been free of monitor alarms for more than 2 weeks.

2. The premature infant with a postconceptional age of 37 weeks who was treated with methylxanthines for apnea after ventilation for RDS. The infant has now been off medication for 10 days and is without apnea or bradycardia by nurses' observations.

3. The premature infant with a postconceptional age of 38 weeks who continues to have monitor alarms despite methylxanthine treatment and who has had some episodes requiring stimulation. The infant is feeding orally and is otherwise doing well without incubator support.

### ■ Answers:

Your response to these three prototype examples will be greatly influenced by the local practices of the neonatologists where you trained or currently work. Needless to say, the issue of home monitoring is an extremely controversial one. On the decision to recommend home monitoring, the National Institutes of Health Consensus Development Conference Statement concluded, "Routine monitoring of asymptomatic preterm infants, as a group, is not warranted. Individual preterm infants such as those with certain residual diseases may be considered for monitoring." A recent survey by Meadow et al. concerning home monitor use for premature infants at discharge by physicians at U.S. hospitals offering neonatology training programs found variation in

practices not only between hospitals but within hospitals. This is an area of clinical practice where widely different opinions are often strongly held and there is not a current consensus. My individual response to these three situations and the basis of my opinions are described next.

Infants who may have had apnea or were at risk for apnea but who are now clinically normal when otherwise ready for discharge do not need any additional evaluation or treatment. The parents of these infants should be told that the previous apnea was a result of their prematurity (or prior illness) and has now resolved. Most parents are somewhat confused about the relationship of apnea, monitoring, and sudden infant death syndrome (SIDS). It is important to emphasize to the families that resolution of apnea as a clinical problem occurs in almost all infants by 36 weeks' postconceptional age and that apnea of prematurity is not an independent risk factor for SIDS.

In item 2 in Exercise 5, the infant had apnea that was treated with methylxanthines. The infant is now at a postconceptional age when pathological apnea due to apnea of prematurity is expected to have resolved. This infant has not had clinically detected pathological apnea off medication and is otherwise doing well. The decision to initially stop methylxanthine treatment would have been made after the infant had completed a 7- to 10-day symptom-free interval when pathological apnea did not occur. The author would discharge such an infant without further testing or treatment for apnea. Indeed, the data of Southall et al. suggest that routine home pneumograms (24-hour recordings of ECG and chest wall movement to detect respiratory effort) are not predictive of which NICU graduates are likely to experience sudden death. Therefore, many clinicians have taken the viewpoint that if episodes of apnea are not detected clinically and do not require intervention, home monitoring or treatment is not indicated when the infant is ready for discharge. Other neonatologists, because of a concern that significant apnea was not being observed or reported, would obtain a permanent recording. If significant episodes of apnea were present, they would monitor these infants at home and consider reinstituting methylxanthine treatment. Whichever approach is taken, you must understand the goals and plan of treatment when methylxanthines are used. For most infants this means a relatively brief course of treatment until the apnea has resolved. It is common for parents with infants who have had an NICU stay of several weeks to have anxiety as treatments are withdrawn. Informing parents about the natural history of apnea and describing for them your plan of management is important to lessen their view of the infant as vulnerable. Resolution of apnea should reinforce their view of the infant as increasingly competent and ready for discharge to the home.

For the infant with persistence of pathological apnea (as in item 3 in Exercise 5), an individual decision on the advisability of discharge must be made. In this case, home monitoring should be considered a diagnostic option, not a treatment. Treatment modalities include methylxanthines for prevention of apnea and cardiopulmonary resuscitation when prevention fails. Not all parents are able to provide this level of constant medical care in their home. Some infants may continue to have severe apnea or to have apnea in association with other medical problems, making discharge inadvisable. In a retrospective review (Rosen et al.) of home monitoring outcome for premature infants discharged on monitors because of persistent, clinically recognized abnormalities, 16% (13 in 89) had events requiring intervention. Furthermore, it was not possible to predict by cardiorespiratory abnormalities or clinical characteristics which infants were at risk for life-threatening events. Forming a discharge plan for infants considered to be at risk for continued pathological apnea should be done in consultation with a physician experienced in management of infants with persistent apnea requiring home medical care.

## BIBLIOGRAPHY

### Control of Respiration

1. Barrington KJ, Finer NN: Periodic breathing and apnea in preterm infants. *Pediatr Res* 1990; 27:118–121.
2. Barrington KJ, Finer NN: The natural history of the appearance of apnea of prematurity. *Pediatr Res* 1991; 29:372–375.
3. Chernick V, Warshaw JB, Kiley JP: NHLBI workshop summary: Developmental neurobiology of respiratory control. *Am Rev Resp Dis* 1989; 139:1295–1301.
4. Davies AM, Koenig JS, Thach BT: Upper airway chemoreflex responses to saline and water in preterm infants. *J Appl Physiol* 1988; 64:1412–1420.
5. Dransfield DA, Spitzer AR, Fox WW: Episodic airway obstruction in premature infants. *Am J Dis Child* 1983; 137:441–443.
6. Duara S: Structure and function of the upper airway in neonates. In Polin RA, Fox WW, eds: *Fetal and Neonatal Physiology*. Philadelphia, WB Saunders Co, 1991.
7. Durand M, Cabal LA, Gonzalez F, et al: Ventilatory control and carbon dioxide response in preterm infants with idiopathic apnea. *Am J Dis Child* 1985; 139:717–720.
8. Gauda EB, Miller MJ, Carlo WA, et al: Genioglossus and diaphragm activity during obstructive apnea and airway occlusion in infants. *Pediatr Res* 1989; 26:583–587.
9. Gerhardt T, Bancalari E: Apnea of prematurity. I. Lung function and regulation of breathing. *Pediatrics* 1984; 74:58–62.
10. Gerhardt T, Bancalari E: Apnea of prematurity. II. Respiratory reflexes. *Pediatrics* 1984; 74:63–66.
11. Henderson-Smart DJ, Pettigrew AG, Campbell DJ: Clinical apnea and brain-stem neural function in preterm infants. *N Engl J Med* 1983; 308:353–357.
12. Lee D, Caces R, Kwiakowski K, et al: A developmental study of types and frequency distribution of short apneas (3 to 15 seconds) in term and preterm infants. *Pediatr Res* 1987; 22:344–349.
13. Martin RJ, Miller MJ, Carlo WA: Pathogenesis of apnea in preterm infants. *J Pediatr* 1986; 109:733–741.
14. Mathew OP: Maintenance of upper airway patency. *J Pediatr* 1985; 106:863–869.
15. Mathew OP, Roberts JL, Thach BT: Pharyngeal airway obstruction in preterm infants during mixed and obstructive apnea. *J Pediatr* 1982; 100:964–968.
16. Miller MJ, Martin RJ: Pathophysiology of apnea of prematurity. In Polin RA, Fox WW, eds: *Fetal and Neonatal Physiology*. Philadelphia, WB Saunders Co, 1991.
17. Perlstein PH, Edwards NK, Sutherland JM: Apnea in premature infants and incubator-air-temperature changes. *N Engl J Med* 1970; 282:461–466.
18. Rigatto H: Apnea. *Pediatr Clin North Am* 1982; 29:1105–1116.

### Clinical Management: Recognition and Significance

19. Butcher-Puech MC, Henderson-Smart DJ, Holley D, et al: Relation between apnea duration and type and neurologic status of preterm infants. *Arch Dis Child* 1985; 60:953–958.
20. Dransfield DA, Philip AGS: Respiratory airflow measurements in the neonate. *Clin Perinatol* 1985; 12:21–30.
21. Hodgman JE, Gonzalez F, Hoppenbrouwers T, et al: Apnea, transient episodes of bradycardia, and periodic breathing in preterm infants. *Am J Dis Child* 1990; 144:54–57.

22. Hunt CE: Cardiorespiratory monitoring. *Clin Perinatol* 1991; 18:473–495.

23. Livera LN, Spencer SA, Thorniley MS, et al: Effects of hypoxemia and bradycardia on neonatal cerebral haemodynamics. *Arch Dis Child* 1991; 66:376–380.

24. Muttitt SC, Finer NN, Tierney AJ, et al: Neonatal apnea: Diagnosis by nurse versus computer. *Pediatrics* 1988; 82:713–720.

25. National Institutes of Health Consensus Development Conference Statement: Infantile apnea and home monitoring. *Pediatrics* 1987; 79:292–299.

26. Perlman JM, Volpe JJ: Episodes of apnea and bradycardia in the preterm newborn: Impact on cerebral circulation. *Pediatrics* 1985; 76:333–338.

27. Upton CJ, Milner AD, Stokes GM: Apnea, bradycardia, and oxygen saturation in preterm infants. *Arch Dis Child* 1991; 66:381–385.

## Clinical Management: Diagnosis

28. Brazy JE, Kinney HC, Oakes WJ: Central nervous system structural lesions causing apnea at birth. *J Pediatr* 1987; 111:163–175.

29. Chasnoff IJ, Hunt CE, Kletter R, et al: Prenatal cocaine exposure is associated with respiratory abnormalities. *Am J Dis Child* 1989; 143:583–587.

30. Church NR, Anas NG, Hall CB, et al: Respiratory syncytial virus-related apnea in infants. *Am J Dis Child* 1984; 138:247–250.

31. Cozzi F, Pierro A: Glossoptossis-apnea syndrome in infancy. *Pediatrics* 1985; 75:836–843.

32. DeMaio JG, Harris MC, Deuber C, et al: Effect of blood transfusion on apnea frequency in growing premature infants. *J Pediatr* 1989; 114:1039–1041.

33. Hay WW, Brockway BA, Eyzaguirre M: Neonatal pulse oximetry: Accuracy and reliability. *Pediatrics* 1989; 83:717–722.

34. Jennis MS, Peabody JL: Pulse oximetry: An alternative method for assessment of oxygenation in newborn infants. *Pediatrics* 1987; 79:524–528.

35. Keyes WG, Donahue PK, Spivak JL, et al: Assessing the need for transfusion of premature infants and role of hematocrit, clinical signs, and erythropoietin level. *Pediatrics* 1989; 84:412–417.

36. Kurth CD, LeBard SE: Association of postoperative apnea, airway obstruction, and hypoxemia in former premature infants. *Anesthesiology* 1991; 75:22–26.

37. Menon AP, Schefft GL, Thach BT: Apnea associated with regurgitation in infants. *J Pediatr* 1985; 106:625–629.

38. Newell SJ, Booth IW, Morgan ME, et al: Gastroesophageal reflux in preterm infants. *Arch Dis Child* 1989; 64:780–786.

39. Pickens DL, Schefft G, Thach BT: Prolonged apnea associated with upper airway protective reflexes in apnea of prematurity. *Am Rev Resp Dis* 1988; 137:113–118.

40. Sekar KC, Duke JC: Sleep apnea and hypoxemia in recently weaned premature infants with and without bronchopulmonary dysplasia. *Pediatr Pulmonol* 1991; 10:112–116.

41. Watanabe K, Harta K, Miyazaki S, et al: Apneic seizures in the newborn. *Am J Dis Child* 1982; 136:980–984.

42. Welborn LG, Hannallah RS, Luban NL, et al: Anemia and postoperative apnea in former preterm infants. *Anesthesiology* 1991; 74:1003–1006.

43. Welborn LG, Rice LJ, Hannallah RS, et al: Postoperative apnea in former preterm infants: Postoperative comparison of spinal and general anesthesia. *Anesthesiology* 1990; 72:838–842.

## Clinical Management: Treatment and Discharge

44. Barrington KJ, Finer NN, Torok-Both G, et al: Dose-response relationship of doxapram in the therapy for refractory idiopathic apnea of prematurity. *Pediatrics* 1987; 80:22–27.

45. Brouard C, Moriette G, Murat I, et al: Comparative efficacy of theophylline and caffeine treatment of idiopathic apnea of prematurity. *Am J Dis Child* 1985; 139:698–700.

46. David JM, Spitzer AR, Stefano JL, et al: Use of caffeine in infants unresponsive to theophylline in apnea of prematurity. *Pediatr Pulmonol* 1987; 3:90–93.

47. Jordan GD, Themelis NJ, Messerly SO, et al: Doxapram and potential benzyl alcohol toxicity: A moratorium on clinical investigation? *Pediatrics* 1986; 78:540–541.

48. Korner AF: What we don't know about waterbeds and preterm infants. *Pediatrics* 1981; 68:308.

49. LeGuennec JC, Billon B: Delay in caffeine elimination in breastfed infants. *Pediatrics* 1987; 79:264–268.

50. Meadow W, Lantos J, Mendez D, et al: What is the legal standard of medical care when there is no standard medical care? A survey of the use of home apnea monitoring for graduates of neonatal intensive care units. Abstract presented Oct. 26, 1991, in section on Perinatal Pediatrics at Annual Meeting of American Academy of Pediatrics.

51. Miller MJ, Carlo WA, Martin RJ: Continuous positive airway pressure selectively reduces obstructive apnea in preterm infants. *J Pediatr* 1985; 106:91–94.

52. Muttitt SC, Tierney AJ, Finer NN: The dose response of theophylline in the treatment of apnea of prematurity. *J Pediatr* 1988; 112:115–121.

53. Pelliowski A, Finer NN: A blended, randomized placebo-controlled trial to compare theophylline and doxapram for the treatment of apnea of prematurity. *J Pediatr* 1990; 116:648–653.

54. Raval DS, Reitz S, Yeh TF: Apnea. In Yeh TF, ed: *Neonatal Therapeutics*, 2nd ed. St. Louis, Mosby-Year Book, 1991.

55. Roberts JL, Mathew OP, Thach BT: The efficacy of theophylline in premature infants with mixed and obstructive apnea and apnea associated with pulmonary and neurologic disease. *J Pediatr* 1982; 100:968–970.

56. Rosen CL, Glaze DG, Frost JD: Home monitor follow-up of persistent apnea and bradycardia in preterm infants. *Am J Dis Child* 1986; 140:547–550.

57. Saigal S, Watts J, Campbell D: Randomized clinical trial of oscillating air mattress in preterm infants: Effect on apnea, growth, and development. *J Pediatr* 1986; 109:857–864.

58. Sims ME, Yau G, Rambhatla S, et al: Limitations of theophylline in the treatment of apnea of prematurity. *Am J Dis Child* 1985; 139:567–570.

59. Southall DP, Richards JM, Rhoden KJ, et al: Prolonged apnea and cardiac arrhythmias in infants discharged from neonatal intensive care units: Failure to predict an increased risk for sudden infant death syndrome. *Pediatrics* 1982; 70:844–851.

60. U.S. Department of Health and Human Services: Infantile apnea and home monitoring: Reports of a consensus development conference. NIH Publication 87-2905. 1987.

61. Use of theophylline in infants. *FDA Drug Bulletin* 1985; 15:16–17.

62. Walther FJ, Erickson R, Sims ME: Cardiovascular effects of caffeine therapy in preterm infants. *Am J Dis Child* 1990; 144:1164–1166.

# Chapter 11

# NEONATAL

# SEPTICEMIA

## Mary Catherine Harris, M.D.

Despite recent improvements in infant intensive care and the use of broad-spectrum antimicrobial agents, bacterial sepsis remains a major cause of morbidity and mortality in newborn infants. Neonatal septicemia is estimated to affect 1 to 4 infants per 1,000 live births; this incidence figure has changed little during the past 50 years. However, the mortality rate has declined by nearly 60% since 1930 and currently ranges from 15% to 45%. Unfortunately, the mortality rate in premature and very low birth weight infants has not exhibited a similar decline and remains tenfold greater than for infants with higher birth weights. Also, more than one-third of survivors ultimately develop neurological handicaps.

Most neonatal bacterial infections occur during the first week of life (i.e., early onset sepsis) following exposure to microorganisms colonizing the maternal genital tract during the intrapartum period. In the past decade, however, the improved survival of low birth weight, critically ill neonates has created a highly susceptible population of premature newborn infants who are hospitalized for extended periods of time and are at increased risk to develop nosocomial disease. As a consequence, there has been a significant increase in the number of bacterial infections that have their onset beyond the first week of life (i.e., late onset disease).

In this chapter, we follow the clinical course of two extremely low birth weight neonates who become infected. The first case describes an infant who develops early onset bacterial sepsis following premature rupture of membranes, and the second case describes an infant who becomes infected following a prolonged hospitalization. After completing the exercises, you should feel comfortable with the diagnosis and management of newborn infants with suspected and proven sepsis.

### EXERCISE 1

Listed below are four characteristics that help distinguish early onset infections from late onset (nosocomial) infections. Please insert the correct term or phrase into the appropriate location in the table.

#### *Early Onset Infection*

Time of onset

Incidence

Mortality

Morbidity

#### *Nosocomial Infection*

Time of onset

Incidence

Mortality

Morbidity

■ **Answer:**

***Early Onset Infection***

| | |
|---|---|
| Time of onset | <1 week |
| Incidence | 0.1% to 0.4% |
| Mortality | 15% to 45% |
| Morbidity | Neurological handicaps |

***Nosocomial Infection***

| | |
|---|---|
| Time of onset | Variable, beyond week 1 |
| Incidence | 5% to 25% |
| Mortality | 10% to 20% |
| Morbidity | Prolonged hospitalization |

## EARLY ONSET NEONATAL SEPTICEMIA

### Risk Factors

### EXERCISE 2

As you read the following case study, underline seven risk factors you believe contributed to this infant's early onset neonatal sepsis.

### CASE STUDY 1

AW was a 26-year-old primigravida woman who presented to the emergency room with a history of back pain, contractions, and questionable leakage of amniotic fluid for at least 1 week. Based on the dates of her last menstrual period, the pregnancy was estimated to be 24 to 25 weeks. On physical examination she had a temperature of 39°C and right costovertebral angle tenderness. Vaginal examination was consistent with rupture of amniotic membranes (positive fern test) and revealed purulent material. Urinalysis demonstrated many white blood cells and bacteria.

Amniocentesis yielded 25 cc of cloudy (foul-smelling) fluid and Gram's stain of this fluid demonstrated gram-positive cocci in chains, and many white blood cells. A cervical culture revealed a heavy growth of group B streptococcus, and she was treated with intravenous ampicillin. However, because of continued uterine irritability, intermittent abdominal tenderness, and a physical examination suggestive of chorioamnionitis, a decision was made for emergency delivery of the fetus. Antibiotics were administered just prior to delivery.

■ **Discussion:**

The neonatal period represents a time of increased susceptibility to the development of bacterial sepsis. Infants who develop early onset bacterial infections frequently demonstrate a history of one or more significant risk factors for infection associated with the peri-

partum period. Conversely, infants born after a completely uncomplicated labor and delivery have a very low risk for the acquisition of bacterial sepsis. Several factors are known to be associated with an increased risk of neonatal bacterial infection, including prematurity, premature rupture of membranes (rupture of membranes before the onset of labor), prolonged rupture of membranes (rupture of membranes ≥24 hours), signs and symptoms suggestive of chorioamnionitis (e.g., uterine tenderness, foul-smelling amniotic fluid, and fetal tachycardia), and maternal colonization with large numbers of virulent microorganisms. Furthermore, physiological abnormalities of host defense mechanisms in term and preterm infants greatly influence the risk of bacterial disease.

Many investigators have noted an increased incidence of early onset bacterial disease in premature infants. The risk of infection is greatest among the smallest infants, and may be seven- to eightfold higher than infants with birth weights greater than 2,500 g. Small-for-gestational-age (SGA) infants are also at increased risk for the development of bacterial disease. The increased susceptibility to infection in the very low birth weight population and significantly increased mortality following the onset of infection are presumably related to the functional immaturity of host defense mechanisms in those babies.

While transplacental transmission of infectious agents has been documented in infants infected with many viruses (e.g., cytomegalovirus and rubella) and some bacteria (e.g., *Listeria monocytogenes* and the *Treponema pallidum*), bacterial infection usually follows exposure of the fetus to organisms colonizing the maternal genital tract. The most obvious determinant of risk, therefore, is the presence of the *potential neonatal pathogen* in the maternal genital tract. Exposure of the fetus to the bacterial pathogen occurs either by the ascending route (following rupture of amniotic membranes) or by colonization of the neonate during passage through the birth canal. Susceptible infants either inhale bacteria (resulting in pneumonia and sepsis) or develop bacteremia following colonization of mucous membrane sites.

In Case Study 1, the mother's cervical cultures demonstrated a heavy growth of group B streptococcus (GBS). It is highly likely, therefore, that this infant became colonized in an ascending fashion following rupture of the mother's membranes. The infant in this case study had a greater chance of becoming colonized with GBS because of the *heavy* growth of that microorganism from the maternal birth canal. Similarly, the risk of sepsis is higher in those infants colonized at multiple sites. Overall, 30% to 75% of neonates born to mothers who are colonized with GBS become colonized. Approximately 1% of infants born to colonized women develop early onset sepsis. Therefore, infants born to colonized women constitute a high-risk group for the development of bacterial disease.

Another important risk factor for the development of invasive streptococcal disease is the lack of circulating fetal concentrations of type-specific antibody to the colonizing strain of GBS. This deficiency of antibody can result either from a low concentration of type-specific IgG in maternal serum or from failure to transmit sufficient antibody concentrations transplacentally because of premature delivery (nearly 60% of maternally derived immunoglobulin-G is transported to the fetus during the last 10 weeks of gestation). Immunologic defenses against *Escherichia coli* and other gram-negative organisms are mediated by IgM antibodies, which are of sufficient size (900 kilodaltons) and configuration to prevent effective transplacental passage. Therefore, during the immediate newborn period, and in early infancy, the infant has an increased probability of developing gram-negative bacterial sepsis. In that regard, it has been recently demonstrated that infants exhibit deficient opsonic activity against *E. coli* at birth and for the first several months of life.

Prior to the time of birth, the fetus lives in a highly protected, sterile environment, free from contaminating bacterial pathogens. Following delivery, the newborn infant must make the transition to an extrauterine existence in which there is a delicate balance between hostile microorganisms in the environment and the infant's intrinsic host defense mechanisms. Although development of the immune system begins early in gestation, these mechanisms do not function as efficiently as those in older children or adults. It is especially important to note that newborn infants are susceptible to infections caused by microorganisms found in their immediate environment, which are relatively avirulent. Not surprisingly, the types of bacteria causing neonatal infections are very similar to those opportunistic organisms that infect patients with compromised immune systems.

Protection against infection is provided by both nonspecific and specific immune mechanisms. Nonspecific mechanisms function effectively without prior exposure to a microorganism or its antigens, and include physical barriers (skin and mucous membranes), chemical barriers (digestive enzymes, bacteriostatic fatty acids on the skin), and phagocytic cells and complement. Specific host defenses, such as preformed antibody and T lymphocytes, provide a fast and aggressive response to "familiar" antigens, enabling the host to eliminate the organisms efficiently on repeated challenge.

Recent investigations have identified abnormalities in nearly every aspect of newborn host defense and, as such, the neonatal immune system can be described as anatomically competent yet antigenically inexperienced and functionally deficient. With regard to nonspecific immune mechanisms, the skin and mucous membrane barriers in the neonate are frequently compromised by routine procedures, allowing the penetration of bacteria into the underlying subepithelial tissues. Bacteremia is then followed by tissue invasion and necrosis. Ultimately, bacterial products are formed (endotoxin, teichoic acids, etc.) that activate phagocytic cells and complement and initiate the inflammatory response.

Investigations of phagocyte functions have uncovered several partial defects that predispose newborn infants to infection. Although studies of mononuclear cell function have been somewhat contradictory, *defective neutrophil chemotactic responses* have been consistently observed. In contrast, the phagocytic and bactericidal capacity of newborn neutrophils appears intact. Granulocytes obtained from stressed newborn infants exhibit a depressed ability to phagocytose and kill bacteria *in vitro*.

Infection in the newborn infant commonly results in a fall in the peripheral blood neutrophil count, which is accompanied by a depletion of bone marrow reserves and abnormalities of neutrophil kinetics. Numerous studies in infected neonatal animals and humans have documented both neutrophil storage pool and neutrophil proliferative pool depletion. Furthermore, because the stem cell proliferative rate is already maximal during the neonatal period, the infected neonate is unable to replenish neutrophil reserves in response to stress. Compounding those abnormalities is disturbed regulation of marrow neutrophil release in the newborn, which results in the release of nearly all the marrow's reserves at the initiation of an infectious stimulus.

Additional deficiencies have been noted in various other parts of the immune system including T and B cell functions, circulating serum antibody, and complement concentrations. Although B cells are present in adequate numbers, antibody responses to an infectious stimulus are frequently poor. Complement levels are significantly lower in term and preterm neonates, and deficient activities of both the classic and alternative pathways have been demonstrated. Furthermore, both lymphokine and cytokine generation by mononuclear cells may be diminished in newborn infants.

■ **Answers:**

1. Prematurity

2. Premature and prolonged rupture of membranes

3. Maternal fever

4. Maternal urinary tract infection

5. Maternal chorioamnionitis

6. Maternal colonization with group B streptococcus

7. Functional deficiencies of neonatal host defense mechanisms

## Predominant Organisms

### EXERCISE 3

■ **Questions:**
What is the most likely bacterial pathogen responsible for the Case Study 1 infant's sepsis? What other organisms are potential causes of early onset sepsis in this infant?

■ **Discussion:**
During the past four decades, there have been several changes in the predominant organisms responsible for early onset neonatal sepsis and meningitis (Table 11-1). Prior to the development of the sulfonamides in the 1930s, grampositive cocci, particularly group A streptococci, were responsible for most cases of neonatal sepsis. With the introduction of antibiotics in the 1940s, group A streptococcal infections declined in frequency, and gram-negative bacilli, particularly *E. coli,* became recognized as important pathogens. In the 1950s, *Staphylococcus aureus* was a major cause of bacterial sepsis. However, since the

early 1970s, group B streptococci and gram-negative enteric bacteria (e.g., *E. coli*) have emerged as the most frequent bacterial isolates from infants with early onset sepsis and meningitis. A recent updated survey of the microbiology of neonatal sepsis at Yale–New Haven Hospital from 1979 to 1988 demonstrated that these two neonatal pathogens [GBS (55%) and *E. coli* (14%)] still account for the majority of cases of early onset neonatal disease. Remember, however, that causative agents can vary significantly among differing institutions and geographic areas. The mechanism(s) responsible for the changing bacteriology of neonatal sepsis is unknown, although patterns of antibiotic usage and natural fluctuations in prevalent bacteria are likely to be involved.

■ **Answers:**
Given the recovery of a heavy growth of GBS from the maternal birth canal, this organism is most likely responsible for this infant's early onset sepsis. The amniotic fluid is likely to ultimately grow the same organism as well. However, because this mother's laboratory workup also demonstrated evidence of a urinary tract infection, a gram-negative enteric organism (e.g., *E. coli*) could be responsible for this infant's infection.

## Signs and Symptoms of Early Onset Infection

### EXERCISE 4

In the following case study, underline four signs and/or symptoms suggestive of infection.

**CASE STUDY 1 continued**
A female infant (BGW) weighing 834 g is born by emergency cesarean section and assigned Apgar scores of 7 and 8 at 1 and 5 minutes, respectively. She initially requires only oral suctioning and nasopharyngeal continuous positive airway pressure, but then develops increased work of breathing, which necessitates endotracheal intubation and mechanical ventilation with 100% oxygen.

Physical examination in the nursery reveals a lethargic, extremely premature infant with occasional spontaneous breaths, a tachycardia to 190 beats per minute (BPM), a peripheral blood pressure of 30/20, and a rectal tempera-

**Table 11-1** Predominant Pathogens in Early Onset Disease

| DECADE | PREDOMINANT BACTERIA | OTHER IMPORTANT PATHOGENS |
|---|---|---|
| 1930s | Group A streptococci | *Escherichia coli*<br>*Staphylococcus aureus* |
| 1940s | *Escherichia coli* | Streptococci |
| 1950s | *Staphylococcus aureus* | *Escherichia coli*<br>*Pseudomonas aeruginosa* |
| 1960s | *Escherichia coli* | *Pseudomonas aeruginosa*<br>*Klebsiella-Enterobacter* |
| 1970s | Group B streptococci | *Escherichia coli*<br>*Listeria monocytogenes* |
| 1980s | Group B streptococci<br>*Escherichia coli* | |

*Source:* Adapted from Philip AGS: *Neonatal Sepsis and Meningitis.* Boston, GK Hall Medical Publishers, 1985, p. 8.

ture of 36°C. The infant's color is cyanotic, and her peripheral perfusion is poor. Central umbilical arterial and venous lines are placed for the monitoring of blood pressure, the administration of fluid, and the measurement of arterial blood gases. She is begun on intravenous ampicillin and gentamicin after a blood culture is obtained. A low Dextrostix value (20 mg/dL) is appropriately treated with intravenous dextrose.

■ **Discussion:**

Most infants who develop bacterial sepsis demonstrate signs or symptoms of infection within a short time after delivery. The occurrence of infection *in utero* is suggested by the presence of fetal distress (including fetal tachycardia). However, infected infants frequently display signs that are common to a variety of newborn disorders, thus making the specific diagnosis of neonatal sepsis extremely difficult. The most prominent of these signs include respiratory distress, low Apgar scores, lethargy, fever or hypothermia, apnea, cyanosis, poor feeding, vomiting, diarrhea, jaundice, and skin rashes including petechiae, abscesses, and sclerema (hardening of the skin). Late (and frequently ominous) signs are those indicative of cardiovascular dysfunction such as tachycardia, pallor, poor perfusion, oliguria, and systemic hypotension.

■ **Answers:**

1. Respiratory distress, apnea, cyanosis

2. Lethargy, hypotonia

3. Hypothermia

4. Evidence of cardiovascular dysfunction and shock, including tachycardia, poor peripheral perfusion, and systemic hypotension

---

**Diagnosis of Early Onset Infection**

**EXERCISE 5**

---

■ **Questions:**

Review the information generated by Case Study 1 to this point. To help organize your thoughts, list the relevant *historical* information obtained from the mother and the *clinical* information obtained from the examination of the infant in the spaces provided.

1. Historical information:

2. Clinical information:

3. What *laboratory* information do you want to order at this time to help support your diagnosis of suspected neonatal sepsis?

Laboratory information:

### ■ Answers:

1. *Historical information:* Risk factors for infection in this case include fever, cloudy foul-smelling amniotic fluid, uterine tenderness, premature rupture of membranes, maternal urinary tract infection, and maternal genital colonization with pathogenic bacteria.

2. *Clinical information:* Signs compatible with sepsis include respiratory distress, apnea, cyanosis, hypothermia, lethargy, and those compatible with shock.

3. *Laboratory information:* The following laboratory tests should be obtained: blood and CSF cultures, a complete blood count with differential and platelet count, and a chest film. Ancillary tests that may be useful in the diagnosis of early onset bacterial infection include the urine latex particle agglutination test for GBS, C-reactive protein determinations, and erythrocyte sedimentation rate. These ancillary laboratory tests may have their greatest value when used as part of a sepsis screen.

---

### CASE STUDY 1 continued

The infant's initial laboratory tests (age 1 hour) revealed the following information.

  Hemoglobin = 15.3 g/dL
  Hematocrit = 46%
  White blood cells (WBCs) = 5,000/mm$^3$
  Neutrophils = 26%
  Bands = 22%
  Metamyelocytes = 1%
  Myelocytes = 1%
  Lymphocytes = 40%
  Monocytes = 10%
  Nucleated red blood cells (NRBCs) = 20
    NRBCs/100 WBCs
  Platelet count = 149,000/mm$^3$

A urine latex test was positive for GBS. Subsequently, both umbilical and peripheral blood cultures grew GBS (even though her mother was treated with antibiotics before delivery). A lumbar puncture (performed when the infant appeared clinically stable) demonstrated 3

WBC/mm$^3$, normal cerebrospinal fluid (CSF) chemistries, a negative gram stain, and no growth of organisms by 48 hours. A chest film revealed a white-out with small lung volumes and the presence of air bronchograms.

## EXERCISE 6

---

### ■ Questions:

1. Calculate this infant's (a) absolute neutrophil count, (b) absolute immature neutrophil count, and (c) immature to total neutrophil ratio (I : T ratio). What is the significance of these values?

   (a)

   (b)

   (c)

   (d)

2. How would you interpret this infant's positive urine latex test?

3. What are the etiology and clinical significance of this infant's white-out on the chest film?

4. How would you interpret this infant's spinal fluid results?

### ■ Discussion:

The primary objective for the clinician is the prompt and accurate identification and early treatment of the infected infant. Failure to consider the diagnosis of infection at the earliest possible time is likely to result in an increased morbidity and mortality. However, in the final analysis, many infants with these symptoms and signs do not prove to have bacterial infection. Therefore, many are treated in an effort to protect the one truly infected neonate. While a hazard is associated with postponing treatment for the truly infected infant, there are also risks (medical, psychological, and economical) in treating uninfected infants unnecessarily. Therefore, a secondary objective should be to rule out infection in the majority of infants and discontinue antimicrobial therapy as soon as possible.

The diagnosis of infection is most frequently made using a combination of *historical* information obtained from the mother's physician, *clinical* information obtained by examination of the infant, and *laboratory* information obtained from a variety of diagnostic tests.

Isolation of microorganisms from the blood, urine, or cerebrospinal fluid has traditionally been considered the "gold standard" for the diagnosis of sepsis or meningitis in the newborn infant. However, systemic cultures of normally sterile body fluids are not always reliable. For example, in one study of infants who died with unequivocal evidence of infection, only 82% of blood or CSF cultures were positive. Therefore, blood cultures, on occasion, may be falsely negative in the presence of true infection. The lumbar puncture is also an important part of the workup for sepsis because nearly one-third of infected infants will have concomitant meningitis. *Recent studies, however, have suggested that the chance of recovering an organism from the cerebrospinal fluid of an asymptomatic infant who is born out of a high-risk environment is extremely low.* Therefore, the wisdom of performing lumbar punctures in that particular group of infants has recently been called into question. A small, but significant, number of infants with meningitis have negative blood cultures. Therefore, when the suspicion of sepsis is high, a lumbar puncture should always be performed if the infant is clinically stable. When sepsis presents after day 3, a urine culture should be included as part of the workup. Urine cultures are infrequently positive in infants less than 72 hours of age except when there are associated renal anomalies.

The peripheral WBC count and differential count can be very useful in identifying infants at risk for acute, early onset bacterial disease. The least helpful value is the total leukocyte count; counts may be normal in more than one-third of infants subsequently proven to have bacterial sepsis (particularly early in their disease). Conversely, among infants whose total WBC counts are abnormal ($<5,000/mm^3$ or $>20,000/mm^3$), fewer than 50% are subsequently proven to be infected.

In contrast, several studies have documented the usefulness of neutrophil indices, including the absolute neutrophil count, the absolute immature neutrophil count, and the I : T ratio as indicators of early onset bacterial infection (Table 11-2). In a very large study of neonates, mostly at term, Manroe determined

**Table 11-2**  Neutrophil Indices Predictive of Bacterial Infection

| INDEX | PREDICTIVE VALUE $(mm^3)$ | POSTNATAL AGE |
|---|---|---|
| Neutropenia | <1,800 | Birth |
| | <7,800 | 12 hr |
| | <7,200 | 24 hr |
| | <4,200 | 48 hr |
| | <1,800 | 72 hr and beyond |
| Increase in the ratio of immature to total neutrophils | >0.16 | Birth |
| | >0.13 | 60 hr |
| | >0.12 | 5 days and beyond |
| Increased number of total neutrophils | >5,400 | Birth |
| | >14,400 | 12 hr |
| | >12,600 | 24 hr |
| | >9,000 | 48 hr |
| | >5,400 | 72 hr and beyond |
| Increased number of immature neutrophils | >1,120 | Birth |
| | >1,440 | 12 hr |
| | >1,280 | 24 hr |
| | >800 | 48 hr |
| | >500 | 5 days and beyond |

*Source:* Adapted from Mauroe BL, Weinberg AG, Rosenfeld CR, et al.: *J Pediatr* 1979; 95:89.

reference ranges for these three indices during the first 28 days of life. When associated with the presence of respiratory distress, the absolute neutrophil count (both neutropenia and neutrophilia) proved to be the most useful index for predicting the presence of bacterial infection. The absolute immature neutrophil count was relatively insensitive for the diagnosis of early bacterial disease, however, it had high negative predictive accuracy (elevated values were unusual in uninfected infants). The single most sensitive index for the diagnosis of infection was the I : T ratio, which identified more than 90% of infants with infection. Conversely, an infant with bacterial sepsis may have a totally normal WBC count and differential count particularly early in the illness. *Therefore, in the infant suspected of sepsis, a single WBC count and differential count should be interpreted with caution.*

The premature infant is at significantly higher risk to develop bacterial infection. Moreover, the mortality from infection is also increased in this weight group. Manroe's study principally examined term neonates. However, studies by other investigators have shown significant differences in the size of neutrophil proliferative and storage pools in the premature infant population. Therefore, we might also expect to see differences in the differential count in preterm infants. In fact, preliminary studies have suggested that previously published white cell indices may not be reliable for infants with birth weights of less than 1,500 g. Furthermore, uninfected preterm infants demonstrate increased numbers of immature neutrophils when compared to term neonates and, consequently, exhibit increased I : T ratios.

Because of the difficulty in differentiating infected from uninfected neonates, interest has been renewed in the use of auxiliary tests to aid with the diagnosis of neonatal infection. Immunoassays to demonstrate bacterial capsular polysaccharide antigens have been used to provide a specific, rapid, etiologic diagnosis long before culture results are available. Commercially available methods have been developed to detect the bacterial capsular polysaccharide antigens of GBS, pneumococcus, and *Haemophilus influenzae* by means of a variety of techniques. The greatest experience in diagnosing neonatal infections has been gained using the urine latex particle agglutination (LPA) test for the detection of GBS. Most investiga-

tors have found the urine LPA to be very sensitive (92% to 100%) and specific (84% to 100%) for the diagnosis of GBS infection in newborn infants. Recently, however, we and others have noted a high incidence of false-positive reactions for GBS antigen in urine specimens from uninfected, high-risk infants. Sanchez et al. have also reported a similar phenomenon. These positive reactions may represent (1) local contamination of the perirectal skin or urinary tract with GBS or other cross-reacting bacteria, (2) antigenuria secondary to absorption of antigen from the gastrointestinal tract, or (3) problems inherent with the latex test. At the current time, we recommend that a second (sterile) urine specimen be obtained from an infant with a negative blood culture and a positive urine LPA test. This second LPA test should be negative in infants who are free of disease. Infants with invasive GBS disease manifest prolonged antigen excretion. Therefore, the LPA test usually remains positive for several days following the initiation of antibiotics. However, the results of the LPA should always be interpreted with caution and along with other available diagnostic and laboratory information. Recently, a number of newer tests have been released that employ an enzyme immunoassay to detect streptococcal antigen in urine specimens. These tests appear to be more sensitive, specific, and easier to interpret than the LPA test and should eventually replace it as the standard test in most laboratories.

Various acute phase reactants have also been suggested as useful tests in the rapid diagnosis of acute bacterial infection. C-reactive protein is known to be elevated in most infants (85%) with severe bacterial disease, while normal values are present in the majority (85%) of uninfected patients. This protein has also been used to monitor the response to antimicrobial therapy, and to assess the possibility of recurrent infection following the cessation of antibiotics. The erythrocyte sedimentation rate (ESR) has also been shown to increase during acute bacterial infection. However, elevations of the ESR have been noted in infants with ABO incompatibility and other Coombs positive hemolytic anemias. Furthermore, the ESR neither rises quickly with the onset of sepsis, nor falls appropriately as the infant is successfully treated. Therefore, both C-reactive protein determinations and the ESR are best used as part

**Table 11-3** Components of the Sepsis
Screen in Neonates

For a sepsis screen to be positive, two or more
components must be abnormal.

Immature to total neutrophil (I : T) ratio. Abnormal value defined as I : T > 0.2.

Leukocyte count. Abnormal value defined as
total WBC <5,000 or absolute neutrophil count
<1,750.

C-reactive protein. Positive result defined as
agglutination of latex beads using undiluted
serum.

Mini-ESR. Abnormal result defined as ≥10 mm/
hr (days 0–3) or ≥15 mm/hr (≥day 4).

of a group of laboratory tests (the so-called *sepsis screen*) in neonates with suspected infections.

In the early 1980s, Philip and Hewitt evaluated the usefulness of a sepsis screen to differentiate infected from uninfected newborn infants. Their sepsis screen included the following five tests: band to neutrophil ratio >0.2, leukocyte count <5,000/mm³, C-reactive protein >0.8 mg/dL, mini-ESR >15 mm/hr, and haptoglobin >25 mg/dL. Any two or more abnormal tests constituted a positive sepsis screen. In this study the authors correctly identified 28 of 30 cases (93%) of acute bacterial infection. While the positive predictive accuracy of this screen was only 40%, the negative predictive accuracy approached 100%. Gerdes and Polin used a similar screen (Table 11-3) and obtained nearly identical results for the diagnosis of infants with early onset bacterial disease. Because the sepsis screen has such high negative predictive accuracy, its greatest usefulness is to exclude infection in uninfected babies during the first week of life. It is not particularly helpful in identifying the truly infected infant (positive predictive accuracy = 40%). Furthermore, it is somewhat surprising that the predictive accuracy from the sepsis screen is little better than that obtained from the I : T ratio alone.

### ■ Answers:

1. (a) Absolute neutrophil count = 2,500/
   mm³.
   5,000/mm³ (the total WBC) × (26%
   neutrophils, 22% bands, 1% metamyelocytes, 1% myelocytes).

(b) Absolute immature neutrophil count
   = 1,200/mm³.
   5,000/mm³ (the total WBC) × (22%
   bands, 1% metamyelocytes, 1% myelocytes).

(c) Immature to total neutrophil ratio =
   0.48 (absolute immature neutrophil
   count/absolute neutrophil count).

(d) The infant in this case demonstrated a
   low absolute neutrophil count, an elevated absolute immature neutrophil count, and an elevated immature to total neutrophil ratio, all of which are suggestive (though not specific) for the diagnosis of bacterial infection. Note, however, that previously published white cell indices may not be reliable for the diagnosis of infection in premature infants. Therefore, this information must be interpreted cautiously and in combination with other clinical and laboratory studies.

2. In this particular case, there is strong clinical suspicion that this infant has evolving GBS sepsis. The positive urine latex test provides additional confirmatory evidence of this diagnosis, which is subsequently verified when the infant's cultures become positive.

3. The etiology of this infant's respiratory distress cannot be determined by means of chest radiographs alone. This infant's white-out on the chest film may represent the presence of respiratory distress syndrome (secondary to prematurity), and/or pneumonitis secondary to GBS sepsis. It is likely that this infant has both GBS pneumonia, as well as a surfactant deficiency.

4. It is unlikely that this infant has bacterial meningitis, given her normal CSF cytology, chemistries, and negative cultures. However, antepartum administration of antibiotics may have inhibited the growth of bacteria from the CSF cultures. Therefore, any signs or symptoms attributable to the central nervous system should warrant a second evaluation of the CSF. This second evaluation should include a latex test for GBS antigen. *A word of caution:* An infant with meningitis may present with normal CSF cytology and chemistries, particularly early in the evolution of meningitis.

## Treatment of Early Onset Infection

### CASE STUDY 1 continued

After her arrival in the nursery, BGW is initially unstable. She requires very high levels of ventilatory support for the treatment of respiratory distress syndrome/pneumonia, and saline infusions to maintain systemic blood pressure and peripheral perfusion. She is initially treated with intravenous ampicillin and gentamicin; however, after culture results are known, she is treated only with penicillin. By 24 hours of life, her condition gradually begins to improve.

### EXERCISE 7

#### ■ Questions:

1. Which antibiotics would you initially have prescribed for this infant?

2. Would you have changed therapy after culture results were known?

3. How long would you continue antibiotic therapy?

4. Should this infant have been treated with an adjunctive immunotherapeutic agent such as granulocytes or intravenous immunoglobulin?

5. What other supportive therapy should this infant receive?

#### ■ Discussion:

The treatment of neonatal sepsis should begin immediately after cultures of blood, cerebrospinal fluid, and urine are obtained. Lumbar puncture should be postponed in the infant with thrombocytopenia or cardiovascular instability; however, this should not delay the initiation of antimicrobial therapy. During the first week of life infants should receive empiric therapy, which will provide broad-spectrum coverage for gram-positive organisms (particularly group B streptococcus) and gram-negative (enteric) bacteria. We recommend a combination of ampicillin and gentamicin, although ampicillin plus cefotaxime is an acceptable alternative regimen. Recommended dosages for commonly used antibiotics are shown in Table 11-4.

The GBS are very susceptible to penicillin, ampicillin, and the third-generation cephalosporins. The aminoglycoside antibiotics are relatively ineffective against GBS when used alone, although *in vitro* data suggest that the bactericidal capacity of ampicillin may be enhanced by using a combination of ampicillin and gentamicin. The choice of therapy for the treatment of gram-negative infections depends on the pattern of antibiotic resistance currently present in the nursery. The aminoglycoside antibiotics are highly effective against most gram-negative enteric bacteria. The third-generation cephalosporins are also highly efficacious, and theoretically should be less toxic than the aminoglycosides. However, because of concerns regarding the emergence of resistant gram-negative organisms with routine use of third-generation cephalosporins, most institutions favor the use of a penicillin and an aminoglycoside antibiotic for the initial treatment of early onset sepsis. This combination of antibiotics is also suitable for infants with suspected meningitis. Alternatively, a third-generation cephalosporin may be used with ampicillin.

After culture results and sensitivities are established, treatment should be modified to provide the safest and most effective antibiotic therapy. For documented GBS sepsis, treatment should continue for 10 to 14 days, and for meningitis due to GBS, 14 days beyond a negative CSF culture. Most group B streptococci are highly sensitive to penicillin or ampicillin and can therefore be treated with either of these agents alone. In the case of gram-negative infection, therapy should be in-

**Table 11-4**  Dosages of Antibiotics Commonly Used for the Treatment of Bacterial Sepsis in Newborn Infants

| ANTIBIOTIC | AGE | DOSAGE (kg) | INTERVAL/ROUTE |
|---|---|---|---|
| Ampicillin | 0–7 days | LBW: 50 mg/day | q. 12 hr IV, IM |
|  |  | FT: 100 mg/day | q. 12 hr IV, IM |
|  | >7 days | 100–200 mg/day | q. 6–8 hr IV, IM |
| Carbenicillin | 0–7 days | LBW: 225 mg/day | q. 8 hr IV, IM |
|  |  | FT: 300 mg/day | q. 6 hr IV, IM |
|  | >7 days | 500 mg/day | q. 6 hr IV, IM |
| Cefazolin | 0–7 days | 50 mg/day | q. 12 hr IV |
|  | >7 days | 50–100 mg/day | q. 8 hr IV |
| Cefotaxime | 0–7 days | 100 mg/day | q. 12 hr IV |
|  | >7 days | 150 mg/day | q. 8 hr IV |
| Ceftazidime |  | 60 mg/day | q. 12 hr IV |
| Chloramphenicol | 0–7 days | 25 mg/day | q. 24 hr IV |
|  | 7–14 days | 50 mg/day | q. 12 hr IV |
| Clindamycin |  | LBW: 15 mg/day | q. 8 hr IV |
|  |  | FT: 20 mg/day | q. 6 hr IV |
| Erythromycin estolate | 0–7 days | 20 mg/day | q. 12 hr po |
|  | >7 days | 20 mg/day | q. 6–8 hr po |
| Gentamicin or Tobramycin | 0–7 days | <1,500 g: 2.5 mg/dose | q. 24 hr IV, IM |
|  |  | 1,500–2,000 g: 2.5 mg/dose | q. 18 hr IV, IM |
|  |  | >2,000 g: 2.5 mg/dose | q. 12 hr IV, IM |
|  | >7 days | <1,500 g: 2.5 mg/dose | q. 12 hr IV, IM |
|  |  | >1,500 g: 2.5 mg/dose | q. 8 hr IV, IM |
| Kanamycin | 0–7 days | LBW: 15 mg/day | q. 12 hr IV, IM |
|  |  | FT: 20 mg/day | q. 12 hr IV, IM |
|  | >7 days | 20–30 mg/day | q. 8–12 hr IV, IM |
| Oxacillin | 0–7 days | LBW: 50 mg/day | q. 12 hr IV |
|  |  | FT: 100 mg/day | q. 12 hr IV |
|  | >7 days | 150 mg/day | q. 6 hr IV |
| Penicillin G | 0–7 days | 50,000–100,000 units/day | q. 12 hr IV, IM |
|  |  | 240,000 units/day (meningitis) | q. 8 hr IV, IM |
|  | >7 days | 100,000–500,000 mg/day | q. 6–8 hr IV, IM |
| Ticarcillin | 0–7 days | LBW: 225 mg/day | q. 8 hr IV |
|  |  | FT: 300 mg/day | q. 6 hr IV |
| Vancomycin | 0–7 days | <1,000 g: 10 mg/dose | q. 24 hr IV |
|  |  | 1,000–2,000 g: 10 mg/dose | q. 18 hr IV |
|  |  | >2,000 g: 10 mg/dose | q. 12 hr IV |
|  | >7 days | <1,000 g: 10 mg/dose | q. 18 hr IV |
|  |  | 1,000–2,000 g: 10 mg/dose | q. 12 hr IV |
|  |  | >2,000 g: 10 mg/dose | q. 8 hr IV |

dividualized using culture results and sensitivity patterns. Meningitis due to enteric organisms should be treated for a minimum of 21 days.

Because of the inability of neonatal intensive care units to substantially decrease morbidity and mortality from sepsis (particularly in preterm infants), several investigators have suggested the use of immunotherapeutic agents as adjuncts to antimicrobial therapy.

These adjunctive immunotherapies include the use of intravenous immunoglobulin, granulocyte transfusion, and exchange transfusion. The rationale behind each of these therapies is to provide immune factors that are known to be deficient in the newborn infant.

Given the known deficiencies of antibody in the preterm neonates and in term infants born to nonimmune mothers, many investigators have advocated the use of intravenous immunoglobulins to enhance the infant's immune response to bacterial infection. Immunoglobulin-G is one of the few proteins that is actively transferred across the placenta to the fetal circulation, and levels of this immunoglobulin at term gestation are greater than those in maternal plasma. IgM and IgA antibodies do not cross the placenta and serum concentrations of these antibody classes in the neonate are very low. Preterm infants delivered before 30 weeks' gestation exhibit markedly depressed levels of IgG because time has been insufficient for transplacental passage of immunoglobulin to occur. As a consequence, several studies have evaluated the therapeutic efficacy of administering intravenous immunoglobulin (IVIG) therapy as an adjunct to antibiotics in neonatal sepsis. Sidiropoulos et al. studied the therapeutic effect of IVIG in both term and preterm infants treated with antibiotics alone, or antibiotics plus IVIG. Although the overall mortality from sepsis was not significantly different in the two groups, preterm infants who received both IVIG and antibiotics demonstrated a lower mortality than those treated with antibiotics alone. Haque et al. in Saudi Arabia treated newborn infants with proven sepsis with an IgM-enriched IVIG (plus antibiotics) or antibiotics alone, and found that the mortality was decreased in the infants receiving supplemental IVIG. However, in this study the organisms recovered from the study infants were not typical of agents causing infection in the United States. Therefore, these results may not be directly relevant to the nursery population of a developed country. Furthermore, all immunoglobulin preparations are not alike. This is an important issue because in animal studies the therapeutic efficacy of an administered immunoglobulin preparation has been directly correlated with the amount of *specific antibody* against the offending pathogen. Thus, although studies suggest that IVIG may have a demonstrable therapeutic benefit in the treatment of neonatal sepsis, the results of these studies should be interpreted with caution. At the current time, the use of IVIG should be reserved for critically ill infants in whom other therapeutic modalities have failed.

Granulocyte transfusion has also been suggested as an adjunct immunologic therapy for infected newborn infants, particularly those with neutropenia. The rationale for this therapy includes knowledge of the known defects in newborn phagocytic cell function, the frequent finding of neutropenia in infected neonates, and the decreased probability of survival when neutropenia is present. In addition, adult data suggest that transfused white cells are capable of migrating to the source of inflammation and phagocytosing infecting organisms. During neonatal sepsis, however, even adequate numbers of granulocytes may not sufficiently combat infection because of the abnormalities in phagocyte function just discussed. Studies in experimental animals have suggested an efficacy for white cell transfusions in the treatment of neonatal sepsis, although to date there have been few randomized controlled studies involving human infants. In one of the first randomized clinical trials, Christensen studied a severely ill group of infants with early onset disease, leukopenia, and neutrophil storage pool depletion. These infants were randomized to receive antibiotics plus granulocyte transfusion or supportive care alone. All of the infants, including seven neonates with GBS infection, survived following a single granulocyte transfusion, while the majority of infants treated with antibiotics alone died. The number of infants in this study sample were small, and further work by these investigators has questioned the validity of these results. Although the majority of more recent studies have supported the value of white cell therapy in neonatal sepsis, a large, multicenter, prospectively randomized controlled trial will be needed before this therapy can be recommended for the treatment of infected neonates. Furthermore, white cell transfusions are not without adverse effects. The potential risks of granulocyte therapy include pulmonary sequestration of transfused cells (resulting in transient hypoxemia and respiratory distress), graft versus host disease, and the transmission of infectious agents including hepatitis, cytomegalovirus, and human immunodeficiency virus.

During the 1970s, exchange transfusion was widely used as an adjunctive immunotherapy for the treatment of severe neonatal sepsis. The rationale for the use of this therapy included delivery of circulating opsonins (antibody and complement), administration of functional granulocytes, improvement of peripheral and pulmonary perfusion, and the removal of bacterial endotoxins and other byproducts of infection. To date, however, there are no prospective controlled studies evaluating the efficacy of exchange transfusion; however, retrospective data suggest a benefit from this therapy in the treatment of neonatal sepsis. Furthermore, in the event that white cells are unavailable on an emergency basis, an exchange transfusion can provide nearly the same number of white cells as a granulocyte transfusion if fresh blood is used. Exchange transfusion, however, has been associated with several potentially life-threatening complications including electrolyte imbalance, intestinal perforation, hypoglycemia, and infection. Therefore, this therapy should be reserved for critically ill infants in whom conventional treatments have failed.

In conclusion, the administration of immunoglobulin or granulocytes or the use of exchange transfusion are adjunctive immunotherapies whose efficacy has not been proven to date. Furthermore, these therapies have been shown to have significant adverse effects and should be reserved for the most critically ill neonates in whom all other treatments have failed.

### ■ Answers:

1. In this case, there is an antenatal suspicion that the infant is infected with the group B streptococcus. However, it is best to begin antimicrobial therapy with ampicillin or penicillin in combination with an aminoglycoside, as broad-spectrum agents. This combination will be effective for the majority of neonatal pathogens.

2. After culture results are known, specific therapy can be tailored to the infecting agent (in this case, GBS). This infant should receive a 10- to 14-day course with either intravenous ampicillin or penicillin.

3. The duration of parenteral antibiotic therapy should be 10 to 14 days after a negative blood culture has been obtained.

4. The adjunctive therapies you might consider using in this infant include intravenous immunoglobulin, granulocyte transfusion, and exchange transfusion. However, there is no proven benefit to using any of these adjunctive immunotherapies in the treatment of neonatal sepsis. Therefore, their use should be reserved for critically ill infants in whom conventional treatments have failed. Because this infant's condition gradually stabilized, additional therapies were not warranted.

5. In the newborn infant with infection and systemic signs of shock, it is important to emphasize the need for vigorous supportive therapy. This infant presented with early onset sepsis and respiratory distress, so the need for mechanical ventilation should be anticipated. Ongoing hypotension should be treated with fluid administration and vasoactive agents as needed.

### Prognosis

#### CASE STUDY 1 continued

BGW gradually recovered from her GBS sepsis and pneumonitis. She received 14 days of intravenous ampicillin, and never demonstrated any signs or symptoms consistent with meningeal involvement. Serial head ultrasound determinations performed during her hospitalization were reportedly within normal limits. Subsequently, she weaned slowly from the ventilator, doubled her birth weight in 2 months, and was ready for discharge 3 months after birth. She was discharged to the care of her local pediatrician and the neonatal follow-up program.

#### EXERCISE 8

### ■ Question:

How would you best counsel this infant's family regarding BGW's prognosis?

### ■ Discussion:

As mentioned earlier in this chapter, the mortality from neonatal sepsis has not changed substantially in the last two decades and remains in the 15% to 45% range despite numerous advancements in infant intensive care. The mortality is highest in the smallest, most premature infants, particularly when signs of infection are detected within 24 hours of delivery. It is likely that these infants are infected while *in utero* and receive antimicrobial therapy only after the infection has been well established. In this population, mortality is due to respiratory failure, disseminated intravascular coagulation, shock, and multiple end-organ system failure secondary to the release of inflammatory mediators from activated phagocytic cells.

Several studies have reported significant long-term sequelae in infants who survive neonatal meningitis secondary to GBS or gram-negative enteric bacilli. These sequellae include seizures, hearing loss, mental and motor disabilities, and microcephaly and hydrocephaly. Infants who are critically ill may demonstrate short-term neurological deficits, which improve with longer term follow-up. Similarly, disorders of higher cortical function may evolve during the first few years of life. There are, however, limited data regarding prognosis and morbidity in infants with *sepsis without accompanying meningitis*. However, in a single study of infants followed for 2 to 6 years beyond their bout of neonatal sepsis, handicaps were identified in 22% of survivors. Therefore, parents should be cautioned that there is a small but significant risk of developing neurological handicaps after a bout of sepsis.

### ■ Answer:

Several studies have reported significant long-term sequelae in infants who survive neonatal meningitis. However, this infant never demonstrated evidence of meningeal inflammation, and cranial imaging studies were reportedly negative. Few data exist that assess morbidity in infants with neonatal sepsis unaccompanied by meningitis. Long-term follow-up of this infant is warranted. Furthermore, the family should know that their infant is at moderate risk (10% to 25%) to develop neurological sequelae.

---

### Prevention of Early Onset Infection

### EXERCISE 9

---

### ■ Question:

How might this infant's disease have been prevented?

### ■ Discussion:

Because of the increased susceptibility of the newborn infant to bacterial infection and the continued high mortality from bacterial disease (particularly in the premature infant), many investigators have directed their efforts to prevention. To date these efforts have focused largely on the prevention of early onset GBS disease, using either chemoprophylaxis to prevent or limit the exposure of the neonate to pathogenic organisms, or maternal immunization to stimulate the production of maternal antibodies against the offending pathogen.

The first suggestion that postnatal administration of penicillin to newborn infants would decrease the incidence of early onset sepsis came from Steigman, who administered a single intramuscular dose of penicillin G at birth to prevent neonatal gonococcal ophthalmia. The authors reported no GBS disease in their nursery while penicillin was used. Subsequently, Siegel performed a large controlled trial confirming the efficacy of penicillin therapy at birth to prevent neonatal GBS disease. However, the infants in the penicillin-treated group in this study had a significantly higher mortality rate than control subjects. Moreover, fulminant disease was relatively rare in this study and blood cultures were not obtained prior to treatment, so some cases of GBS sepsis may have been missed. These authors also reported a transient increase in resistant gram-negative organisms during the first half of the study. In a subsequent study of low birth weight infants with more fulminant disease, penicillin therapy administered at birth had no effect on the incidence or mortality from GBS disease. In summary, penicillin prophylaxis at birth does not prevent fulminant early onset streptococcal disease but may lower the mortality rate for infants who become symptomatic somewhat later.

As an alternative to treating newborn infants, maternal chemoprophylaxis during the intrapartum period has been suggested as a method to prevent neonatal GBS colonization and disease. Despite several obstacles, this approach seems logical and has proven effective. One obvious concern with this therapeutic strategy is that during pregnancy women can gain or lose colonization with GBS. Therefore, knowledge that a mother is colonized at a single time point during pregnancy will not predict with total accuracy the presence or absence of GBS at delivery. Moreover, the ratio of colonized mothers to infected infants ranges from 50 : 1 to 100 : 1, so many mothers will need to be treated in order to prevent infection in one neonate.

During the past 10 years numerous controlled clinical trials have shown that treatment of mothers with penicillin or ampicillin during labor reduces the incidence of maternal and neonatal colonization with GBS. In the 1980s Boyer et al. investigated the effects of the administration of intrapartum ampicillin on the incidence of both GBS colonization and neonatal disease. Women with prenatal carriage of GBS and perinatal risk factors such as premature labor, prolonged rupture of membranes, or fever were randomized to receive ampicillin or serve as control subjects. Ampicillin eliminated the vertical transmission of GBS in mothers without risk factors; GBS colonization was detected only in neonates born to women with intrapartum fever or in whom the duration of maternal therapy prior to delivery was brief. In addition, and most significantly, these authors noted a decrease in the incidence of GBS disease in high-risk infants. Minkoff and Mead also suggested that women about to deliver preterm infants should receive intrapartum chemoprophylaxis if they are colonized with GBS. Thus, although specific treatment guidelines have not been developed to date, intrapartum antibiotic prophylaxis appears to be efficacious in the prevention of neonatal GBS colonization and disease.

Alternatively, maternal immunoprophylaxis has been suggested as an effective and lasting method for the prevention of neonatal GBS disease. IgG is transferred across the placenta during pregnancy, and specific immunoglobulin directed against the capsular polysaccharide of GBS will offer protection against neonatal disease. Therefore, if vaccination of the mother can elicit an effective antibody response, this method might confer protection to the fetus by way of placental transfer. However, two problems arise with this approach. First some nonimmune adults do not mount an antibody response following vaccination. Second, protection may not be conferred to the fetus born prematurely because time has been inadequate for the antibody to cross the placenta. At the current time candidate vaccines are nearly ready for clinical trials. However, this approach will not be of value for the prevention of neonatal infection with gram-negative organisms in which the major humoral immunologic defense resides in the IgM fraction of immunoglobulin.

■ **Answer:**

In this case, there is probably little that could have been done to prevent this infant's early onset disease short of educating her mother about the significance of ruptured membranes and leaking amniotic fluid. It is likely that maternal colonization and peripartum infection with GBS caused her infant to become colonized and subsequently infected. While data exist to support the efficacy of chemoprophylaxis for the prevention of neonatal GBS infection, this infant was infected *in utero*. The most important management decision in this case was emergent delivery of the infected fetus.

## LATE ONSET NEONATAL SEPTICEMIA

During the past few decades, technological improvements in neonatal intensive care have permitted the survival of a population of very low birth weight infants who in the past would not have lived. These infants require hospitalization for extended periods of time and are at increased risk for the development of nosocomial disease. Although incidence figures vary widely, nosocomial infection rates as high as 25% have been reported from neonatal intensive care units; infection rates are significantly greater in infants with birth weights of less than 1,500 g.

Nosocomial infections have been shown to exert a major effect on neonatal mortality and morbidity and to prolong the duration of hospitalization. Mortality rates vary with the pathogenicity of the infecting agent and range from 33% in the entire population developing nosocomial disease to 0% to 15% following infection with coagulase-negative staphylococci, the most common organism causing neonatal nosocomial sepsis. Neurological handicaps are observed more frequently when the central nervous system is involved.

### EXERCISE 10

In the following case study, underline six risk factors that you believe contributed to this infant's late onset neonatal septicemia.

### CASE STUDY 2

BGF was the 736-g product of a 26-week gestation born to a 25-year-old mother whose labor could not be stopped with tocolytic therapy. As delivery became inevitable, Mrs. F was treated with dexamethasone and intravenous antibiotics. The infant was born by elective cesarean section and was assigned Apgar scores of 6 and 8 at 1 and 5 minutes, respectively. Despite negative blood and cerebrospinal fluid cultures, the infant received a 7-day course of ampicillin and gentamicin for presumed sepsis. The infant initially demonstrated mild respiratory distress and was maintained on minimal ventilatory support. Umbilical arterial and venous lines were placed for blood gas sampling and the administration of parenteral alimentation. At the end of the infant's second week of life, both of these lines were discontinued. At this time she was begun on breast-milk feedings, which were advanced during a 2-week period. On this regimen, she began to demonstrate acceptable growth. Enteral feedings were supplemented with intravenous dextrose, amino acids, and lipids administered through a central venous catheter.

■ **Answer:**

1. Prematurity

2. Chronic hospitalization

3. Presence of foreign bodies, including central vascular catheters and endotracheal intubation

4. Parenteral alimentation

5. Prior use of antibiotics

6. Functional deficiencies of neonatal host defense mechanisms

### EXERCISE 11

■ **Question:**

Which bacterial pathogens are most likely to cause nosocomial sepsis?

■ **Answer:**

The coagulase-negative staphylococci are currently the most common pathogens associated with nosocomial infection in most newborn intensive care units. Other potential pathogens causing nosocomial sepsis include *Staphylococcus aureus*, gram-negative enteric bacteria, and *Candida* species. This infant should receive broad-spectrum antimicrobial therapy until culture results are known.

### Risk Factors

Nosocomial infections commonly occur in very low birth weight, chronically hospitalized neonates who require invasive procedures for monitoring and support. These infections are most frequently noted in infants receiving long-term parenteral nutrition who have foreign bodies (e.g., central vascular catheters, chest tubes, and ventriculoperitoneal shunts) placed for extended periods of time. Widespread antibiotic usage is believed to be another contributing factor. Furthermore, it is important to note that abnormalities of neonatal immune function persist beyond the first month of life, and likely play a major role in the development of nosocomial sepsis. This is particularly true in the premature neonate who is at the nadir of his or her postnatal decline in serum immunoglobulin concentrations (physiological hypogammaglobulinemia).

### Predominant Organisms

Similar to the changing pattern of bacterial isolates from neonates with early onset infections, several shifts have occurred in the predominant pathogens responsible for nosocomial disease. In the early 1970s, *S. aureus* (47%) and gram-negative enteric bacilli (45%) accounted for the majority of neonatal nosocomial infections (Table 11-5). However, during the past 10 years coagulase-negative staphylococci have emerged as the predominant neonatal pathogens, particularly among infants of very low birth weight. In that regard, the most commonly isolated pathogens from neonates with nosocomial sepsis, at Yale–New Haven Hospital between 1979 and 1988, were the coagulase-negative staphylococci, *E. coli*, *Klebsiella pneumonia*, enterococci, *S. aureus*, and *Candida* species. This fluctuating pattern of bacterial isolates may reflect changing patterns of antibiotic usage and extended survival of high-risk immunocompromised neonates.

### Coagulase-Negative Staphylococci

The coagulase-negative staphylococci, previously considered avirulent commensal bacteria, are now recognized as pathogens causing a variety of human diseases. During the past 10 years, coagulase-negative staphylococci have become the bacteria responsible for the major-

**Table 11-5** Predominant Pathogens in Late Onset Disease

| DECADE | PREDOMINANT BACTERIA | OTHER IMPORTANT PATHOGENS |
|---|---|---|
| 1970s | *Staphylococcus aureus*<br>Gram-negative enteric bacteria | Group D streptococci |
| 1980s | Coagulase-negative staphylococci<br>*Escherichia coli* | Other gram-negative enteric bacteria<br>Other streptococci<br>*Staphylococcus aureus* |

ity of hospital-acquired infections in critically ill and premature neonates. Several reasons are postulated for their emergence as neonatal nosocomial pathogens. First, the organism normally resides on the newborn infant's skin, and colonization with coagulase-negative staphylococci is widespread and dense by the end of the first week of life. In a recent study by our laboratory at The Children's Hospital of Philadelphia, D'Angio et al. noted that the percentage of infants with *S. epidermidis* as their predominant surface isolate rose to nearly 100% during the first week of life. Second, in the intensive care setting, the coagulase-negative staphylococci may be selected as resistant organisms because of the widespread use of antimicrobial agents. In the study by D'Angio et al., the percentage of strains resistant to multiple antibiotics rose from 32% (on day 2) to 82% by day 7. Third, the coagulase-negative staphylococci elaborate adherence factors, which facilitate their persistence on the surfaces of catheters, shunts, and prosthetic devices. After adherence takes place, the coagulase-negative staphylococci produce and become enmeshed in a matrix of extracellular slime, which has the ability to inhibit immune mechanisms.

Colonization of the skin or respiratory or gastrointestinal tracts with coagulase-negative staphylococci occurs prior to the development of infection. Systemic infection develops following a break in the skin or mucous membrane lining, allowing the colonizing organisms to become invasive. In the D'Angio et al. study, three infants developed coagulase-negative staphylococcal sepsis with an organism that was identical to their predominant surface isolate. However, it has not been proven whether the coagulase-negative staphylococci causing invasive infections in the neonatal population represent a subpopulation of bacteria that are more virulent than those isolated from the skin. Furthermore, debilitation of the

host may be a more important variable than the virulence of the organism. Therefore, it is probably safe to conclude that development of disease due to the coagulase-negative staphylococci results from complex interactions between host and bacterial factors.

The majority of infants who develop invasive disease due to coagulase-negative staphylococci are premature. The earliest epidemiological studies ascribed this association to the complex invasive therapies required by these infants. Similarly, a high percentage of neonates with invasive disease have centrally located intravascular catheters, thus providing a portal of entry into the bloodstream for organisms resident on the skin. More recently, investigators have examined the possibility that the increased susceptibility of premature infants for serious coagulase-negative staphylococcal infections relates to deficiencies of neonatal host defense mechanisms. Several studies have noted that serum opsonic activity for *S. epidermidis* is diminished in preterm infants and that the magnitude of this deficiency is inversely proportional to gestational age. Furthermore, even among term infants the opsonic activity of transplacentally derived IgG for *S. epidermidis* is significantly less than that of the mother.

Several studies have sought to determine phenotypic markers that correlate with increased virulence of coagulase-negative staphylococci. However, no single phenotypic character of coagulase-negative staphylococci can be equated with virulence, implying that pathogenic potential must rely on the interplay of multiple bacterial and host factors. Most studies have noted the predominance of the species *S. epidermidis* among infants with invasive disease. D'Angio et al. also noted that this organism was the predominant species colonizing neonatal skin. Therefore, *S. epidermidis* may have a selective advantage for surface colonization in neonates, but it may also be a more virulent coagulase-negative staphylococcal species. Coagulase-negative staphylococci elaborate a viscous extracellular material called *slime* and several studies have noted an association between slime production and the ability to cause invasive disease. In the pathogenesis of catheter-related infections, it is likely that the bacteria adhere to catheter surfaces, then secrete and become embedded in the extracellular slime matrix. Slime may make coagulase-negative staphylococci inaccessible to phagocytes and (perhaps) to antibiotics. Slime may also inhibit neutrophil chemotaxis and phagocytosis. In addition, the coagulase-negative staphylococci elaborate a variety of exoproteins including hemolysins, proteases, urease, lipase, esterase, fibrinolysin, and deoxyribonuclease. Delta-like toxin is a hemolysin produced by coagulase-negative staphylococci that resembles the enteropathic delta toxin of *S. aureus*. In infants with gastrointestinal symptomatology the presence of free toxin has been strongly associated with the development of necrotizing enterocolitis. Nataro recently investigated whether the exoproteins elaborated by coagulase-negative staphylococci might be used as markers to detect virulent strains. Unfortunately, in this study no significant relationship existed between secretion of exoproteins or enzymes and virulence; these characteristics were equally present in both pathogenic and "contaminant" isolates. While specific roles for these bacterial factors require further investigation, they are likely to play an important part in mediating both colonization and persistence of coagulase-negative staphylococci in the local environment of the host.

In summary, the pathogenesis of neonatal nosocomial disease, particularly infection with coagulase-negative staphylococci, is most probably related to a disturbance in the delicate balance between hostile microorganisms in the environment and the functional integrity of the infant's intrinsic host defense mechanisms.

### Signs and Symptoms of Late Onset Infection

### EXERCISE 12

In the following case study, underline four signs and/or symptoms that are suggestive of a late onset infection.

### CASE STUDY 2 continued

On day 28 of BGF's life, an abrupt onset occurred of respiratory distress, tachycardia, increased abdominal girth, poor perfusion, and hypotension. Because of the high probability of infection, blood, urine, and CSF cultures were obtained. Feedings were discontinued and intravenous fluids were restarted. Large volumes of crystalloid and colloid were administered to improve perfusion and blood pressure. Respiratory support was increased to maintain adequate oxygenation and intravenous antibiotics were begun.

■ **Answers:**

1. Respiratory distress

2. Tachycardia

3. Increased abdominal girth

4. Evidence of poor peripheral perfusion and shock

### EXERCISE 13

■ **Questions:**

1. How do the signs of systemic infection due to coagulase-negative staphylococci differ from those noted with other pathogens?

2. How should the infant in this case history be evaluated for sepsis?

(a)

(b)

(c)

■ **Discussion:**

Most infants with nosocomial infections caused by coagulase-negative staphylococci will develop a variety of nonspecific signs and symptoms, frequently indolent in nature. Common presenting signs include hypo- or hyperthermia, respiratory distress or apnea, gastrointestinal disturbances (feeding intolerance, abdominal distention, and bloody stools), central nervous system abnormalities (lethargy, hypotonia, or seizures), and decreased perfusion. On occasion, the coagulase-negative staphylococci may produce severe and life-threatening disease, similar to that induced by other more virulent organisms.

Coagulase-negative staphylococci may also produce focal infection in the neonate, particularly endocarditis, meningitis, necrotizing enterocolitis, or pneumonia. However, the occurrence of focal disease is often heralded by the presence of persistent bacteremia. Infective endocarditis in association with coagulase-negative staphylococcal bacteremia is often right-sided, and follows placement of an umbilical venous catheter in the right atrium. The coagulase-negative staphylococci are also a cause of meningitis, particularly in infants with indwelling intraventricular catheters or shunts. However, meningitis may develop as a sequelae to bacteremia in the absence of an intraventricular foreign body. Meningitis due to *S. epidermidis* frequently occurs without abnormalities in cell counts or chemistry values. A temporal association of necrotizing enterocolitis with coagulase-negative staphylococcal bacteremia and intestinal colonization has also been reported. While initial reports described a milder illness (without pneumatosis intestinalis, need for surgical intervention, strictures, or mortality), other authors have reported severe, even fatal enterocolitis associated with *S. epidermidis* bacteremia.

### ■ Answers:

1. Typically, the onset of infection caused by coagulase-negative staphylococci is indolent. However, on occasion, these organisms produce severe and life-threatening disease. Therefore, the signs and symptoms of coagulase-negative staphylococcal infection may be more subtle than those produced by other organisms, but not always—*so beware!!*
2. (a) Blood, CSF, and urine cultures (preferably multiple blood cultures)
   (b) Complete blood count with a differential and platelet count
   (c) Chest and abdominal radiographs as clinically indicated

---

### Diagnosis of Late Onset Infection

#### CASE STUDY 2 continued
Laboratory testing revealed the following values:

Hemoglobin = 13.0 g/dL
Hematocrit = 38%

WBC = 27.5/mm$^3$
Bands = 30%
Neutrophils = 13%
Eosinophils = 10%
Lymphocytes = 25%
Monocytes = 12%
Platelet count = 20,000/mm$^3$

Blood cultures obtained from this infant's central venous catheter and peripheral vein both grew coagulase-negative staphylococci. CSF and urine cultures demonstrated no growth. Abdominal films demonstrated questionable pneumatosis in the distal ileum, and generalized distention. A chest film revealed hazy infiltrates bilaterally.

### EXERCISE 14

#### ■ Questions:

1. How would you interpret this infant's laboratory data?

2. Is it likely that coagulase-negative staphylococcus was the offending pathogen in this case?

#### ■ Discussion:
In the not too distant past, the coagulase-negative staphylococci were considered harmless commensal organisms, and their presence in blood cultures was presumed to represent contamination. In recent years, however, this organism has been increasingly associated with neonatal nosocomial disease. Therefore, one of the most common dilemmas facing clinicians is whether an isolate of coagulase-negative staphylococci represents true infection or blood culture contamination.

To distinguish sepsis with coagulase-negative staphylococci from blood culture contamination, multiple blood cultures should ideally be obtained prior to the institution of antimicrobial therapy. In the critically ill neonate, however, it may not always be possible to postpone the initiation of antibiotics until two blood cultures are drawn. In this situation, the clinician must make an educated guess as to whether the infant's isolate represents infection or contamination, using a combination of clinical and laboratory parameters. St. Geme et al. recently demonstrated that colony counts may help distinguish sepsis from contamination with coagulase-negative staphylococci. In this study, colony counts greater than 50 colony forming units (cfu)/mL from a "peripheral" blood culture occurred only in infants with infection, while low colony counts were observed in infants with infection or contamination. These data suggest that blood cultures that grow low numbers of coagulase negative staphylococci should not be routinely ignored as contaminated when they occur in this high-risk population of neonates.

Several studies have used hematologic parameters to diagnose coagulase-negative staphylococcal disease. Baumgart noted an increased proportion of immature to total neutrophils in the bloodstream of infected infants with sepsis due to coagulase-negative staphylococci. However, recent studies from our laboratory suggest that hematologic parameters are generally not helpful in distinguishing infants with infection from those with blood culture contamination.

### ■ Answers:

1. The white blood count has not been found useful in the diagnosis of significant infection with coagulase-negative staphylococci. While an abnormal white blood count, differential count, and I : T ratio would support the diagnosis of sepsis, the absence of such does not eliminate infection. The abnormal chest and abdominal radiographs should be interpreted as supporting the diagnosis of pneumonia and necrotizing enterocolitis, respectively.

2. In the past the coagulase-negative staphylococci were considered harmless commensal organisms, and their isolation from blood cultures was considered to represent contamination rather than true disease. Therefore, in the ideal situation, the isolation of coagulase-negative staphylococci from multiple blood cultures is helpful in proving that the actual isolate is pathogenic in nature. In this particular situation, however, given the infant's critical and unstable clinical condition, any isolate growing coagulase-negative staphylococci should be interpreted as representing disease.

### Treatment of Late Onset Infection

### EXERCISE 15

#### ■ Questions:

1. Which antibiotics would you prescribe for this infant initially?

2. How long would you continue antibiotic therapy?

3. Should this infant have received prophylactic intravenous immunoglobulin to prevent nosocomial sepsis?

#### ■ Discussion:

Treatment of neonatal nosocomial disease should be initiated immediately when sepsis is suspected. Our institution begins therapy with a combination of vancomycin and netilmicin, which offers broad-spectrum coverage against most hospital-acquired microorganisms. This treatment regimen is then modified after culture results and antimicrobial susceptibility patterns are determined. Uncomplicated nosocomial sepsis should be treated for 10 to 14 days. Infants with coagulase-negative staphylococcal meningitis should be treated for 14 days after the CSF has been sterilized. Gram-negative meningitis is treated for at least 21 days.

As in the case of early onset infection, no immunotherapeutic agents have proven of value in the treatment of nosocomial disease. Several recent studies, however, have recommended the use of intravenous immunoglobulin therapy for the prevention of nosocomial sepsis in neonates. The administration of immunoglobulins may have particular benefit for the preterm infant, especially during physiological hypogammaglobulinemia. Several studies and two multicenter trials have investigated the potential benefit of prophylactic administration of intravenous immunoglobulin, and results are thus far inconclusive. Furthermore, most of these studies have included only small numbers of infants, in whom the definition of infection was not standardized. This is particularly problematic in the case of coagulase-negative staphylococcal isolates, where it is frequently difficult to distinguish sepsis from blood culture contamination. In addition, the use of varying immunoglobulin preparations, as well as variations of dosing and frequency of administration makes the interpretation of these data difficult. Given these limitations, IVIG cannot, at present, be recommended as a useful agent for the prevention of nosocomial sepsis in newborn infants.

## ■ Answers:

1. The principles of management of neonatal nosocomial sepsis are identical to those for the treatment of early onset disease. It is best to initiate therapy with broad-spectrum coverage (vancomycin and netilmicin) that is effective for most nosocomial pathogens.

2. When the results of cultures are known, therapy can then be targeted to the specific offending pathogen. In this case, the infant had coagulase-negative staphylococci isolated from multiple blood cultures. Therefore, she should receive a 10- to 14-day course with vancomycin. The duration of antimicrobial therapy for infants with necrotizing enterocolitis is generally 14 days. However, if the clinical response to treatment is poor, treatment may be continued for an additional 7 days.

3. No. There are no adjunctive therapies that are of proven benefit for the treatment of neonatal nosocomial disease. As detailed in the section on early onset infection, these therapies should be reserved for critically ill infants in whom conventional treatments have failed. Intravenous immunoglobulin has also been suggested as a prophylactic agent to prevent nosocomial infections. At the present time, the results of large clinical trials have proven inconclusive. Therefore, prophylactic use of IVIG is not currently recommended.

## BIBLIOGRAPHY

1. Anderson DC, Hughes BJ, Smith CW: Abnormal mobility of neonatal polymorphonuclear leukocytes: Relationship to impaired redistribution of surface adhesion sites by chemotactic factor or colchicine. *J Clin Invest* 1981; 68:863–873.
2. Baker CJ, Edwards MS: Group B streptococcal infections. In Remington JS, Klein JO, eds: *Infectious Diseases of the Fetus and Newborn Infant*, Philadelphia, WB Saunders Co, 1990, pp. 742–811.
3. Baker CJ, Rench MA: Commercial latex particle agglutination for detection of group B streptococcal antigen in body fluids. *J Pediatr* 1983; 102:393–395.
4. Baker CJ: Immunization to prevent group B streptococcal disease: Victories and vexations. *J Infect Dis* 1990; 161:917–921.
5. Baker CJ: Multicenter trial of intravenous immunoglobulin to prevent late-onset infection in preterm infants. *Pediatr Res* 1989; 25:275A.
6. Baley JE, Stork EK, Warkentin PI, et al: Buffy coat transfusions in neutropenic neonates with presumed sepsis: A prospective, randomized trial. *Pediatrics* 1987; 80:712–720.
7. Baumgart S, Hall SE, Campos JM, et al: Sepsis with coagulase-negative staphylococci in critically ill newborns. *Am J Dis Child* 1983; 137:461–463.
8. Berger M: Complement deficiency and neutrophil dysfunction as risk factors for bacterial infection in newborns and the role of granulocyte transfusion in therapy. *Rev Infect Dis* 1990; 12(suppl 4):S401–S409.
9. Blanc WA: Pathways of fetal and early neonatal infection. Viral placentitis, bacterial and fungal chorioamnionitis. *J Pediatr* 1961; 59:473–496.
10. Boyer KM, Gadzala CA, Kelly PD, et al: Selective intrapartum chemoprophylaxis of neonatal group B streptococcal early-onset disease. III: Interruption of mother-to-infant transmission. *J Infect Dis* 1983; 148:810–816.
11. Cairo MS, Worcester C, Rucker R, et al: Role of circulating complement and polymorphonuclear leukocyte transfusion in treatment and outcome in critically ill neonates with sepsis. *J Pediatr* 1987; 110:935–941.
12. Cairo MS: Neonatal neutrophil host defense. Prospects for immunologic enhancement during neonatal sepsis. *Am J Dis Child* 1989; 143:40–46.
13. Christensen RD, Anstall HB, Rothstein G: Review: Deficiencies in the neutrophilic system of newborn infants and the use of leukocyte transfusions in the treatment of neonatal sepsis. *J Clin Apheresis* 1982; 1:33–41.
14. Christensen RD, Rothstein G, Anstall HB, et al: Granulocyte transfusions in neonates with bacterial infection, neutropenia, and depletion of mature marrow neutrophils. *Pediatrics* 1982; 70:1–6.
15. Christensen RD, Rothstein G: Exhaustion of mature marrow neutrophils in neonates with sepsis. *J Pediatr* 1980; 96:316–318.
16. Clapp DW, Kleigman RM, Baley JE, et al: Use of intravenously administered immune globulin to prevent nosocomial sepsis in low birth weight infants: Report of a pilot study. *J Pediatr* 1989; 115:973–978.
17. D'Angio CT, McGowan KL, Baumgart S, et al:

Surface colonization with coagulase-negative staphylococci in premature neonates. *J Pediatr* 1989; 114:1029–1034.

18. Edwards MS: Coagulase-negative staphylococcal bacteremia in neonates: Confusion continued. *Pediatrics* 1990; 86:320–322.

19. Ferrieri P: Neonatal susceptibility and immunity to major bacterial pathogens. *Rev Infect Dis* 1990; 12(suppl 4):S394–S400.

20. Fleer A, Gerards LJ, Aerts P, et al: Opsonic defense to *Staphylococcus epidermidis* in the premature neonate. *J Infect Dis* 1985; 152:930–937.

21. Freedman RM, Ingram DL, Gross I, et al: A half century of neonatal sepsis at Yale. *Am J Dis Child* 1981; 135:140–144.

22. Freeman J, Epstein MF, Smith NE, et al: Extra hospital stay and antibiotic usage with nosocomial coagulase-negative staphylococcal bacteremia in two neonatal intensive care unit populations. *Am J Dis Child* 1990; 144:324–329.

23. Freeman J, Platt R, Sidebottom DG, et al: Coagulase-negative staphylococcal bacteremia in the changing neonatal intensive care unit population: Is there an epidemic? *JAMA* 1987; 258:2548–2552.

24. Gemmel CG, Schumacher-Perdreau F: Extracellular toxins and enzymes eleborated by coagulase-negative staphylococci. In Easmon CSF, Adlam C, eds: *Staphylococci and Staphylococcal Infections.* New York, Academic Press, 1983, pp. 809–827.

25. Gerdes JS, Polin RA: Sepsis screen in neonates with evaluation of plasma fibronectin. *Pediatr Infect Dis J* 1987; 6:443–446.

26. Gladstone IM, Ehrenkranz RA, Edberg SC, et al: A ten-year review of neonatal sepsis and comparison with the previous fifty-year experience. *Pediatr Infect Dis J* 1990; 9:819–825.

27. Gonzalez LA, Hill HR: The current status of intravenous gammaglobulin use in neonates. *Pediatr Infect Dis J* 1989; 8:315–322.

28. Gray ED, Peters G, Verstegen M, et al: Effect of extracellular slime substance from *Staphylococcus epidermidis* on the human cellular immune response. *Lancet* 1984; i:365–367.

29. Greenspoon JS, Wilcox JG, Kirschbaum TH: Group B streptococcus: The effectiveness of screening and chemoprophylaxis. *Obstet Gynecol Surv* 1991; 46:499–508.

30. Gruskay JA, Abbasi S, Anday E, et al: *Staphylococcus epidermidis*-associated enterocolitis. *J Pediatr* 1986; 109:520–524.

31. Gruskay JC, Harris MC, Costarino AT, et al: Neonatal *Staphylococcus epidermidis* meningitis with unremarkable CSF examination results. *Am J Dis Child* 1989; 143:580–582.

32. Hall SL. Coagulase-negative staphylococcal infection in neonates. *Pediatr Infect Dis J* 1991; 10:57–67.

33. Haque KN, Zaidi MH, Bahakim H: IgM-enriched intravenous immunoglobulin therapy in neonatal sepsis. *Am J Dis Child* 1988; 142:1293–1296.

34. Harris MC, Polin RA: Neonatal septicemia. *Pediatr Clin North Am* 1983; 30(2):243–258.

35. Harris MC, Deuber C, Polin RA, et al: Investiga-

tion of apparent false positive urine latex particle agglutination tests for the detection of group B streptococcal antigen. *J Clin Microbiol* 1989; 27:2214–2217.

36. Harris MC, Stroobant J, Cody CS, et al: Phagocytosis of group B streptococcus by neutrophils from newborn infants. *Pediatr Res* 1983; 17:358–361.

37. Harris MC: New methods of diagnosis and treatment of neonatal sepsis. In Rathi M, ed: *Current Perinatology,* vol. II. New York, Springer-Verlag, 1990, pp. 126–143.

38. Hemming VG, Overall JC Jr, Britt MR: Nosocomial infections in a newborn intensive care unit. Results of forty-one months of surveillance. *N Engl J Med* 1976; 294:1310–1316.

39. Hill HR: Is prophylaxis of neonates with intravenous immunoglobulin beneficial? *Am J Dis Child* 1991; 145:1229–1230.

40. Johnston RB Jr: Immunotherapy and immunoprophylaxis in the newborn infant: The need for definitive clinical trails. *Rev Infect Dis* 1990; 12(suppl 4):S392–S393.

41. Kinney J, Mundorf L, Gleason C, et al: Efficacy and pharmacokinetics of intravenous immune globulin administration to high-risk neonates. *Am J Dis Child* 1991; 145:1233–1238.

42. Klein JO, Marcy SM: Bacterial sepsis and meningitis. In Remington JS, Klein JO, eds: *Infectious Diseases of the Fetus and Newborn Infant,* 3rd ed. Philadelphia, WB Saunders Co, 1990; pp. 601–656.

43. Klein JO: Current bacterial therapy for neonatal sepsis and meningitis. *Pediatr Infect Dis J* 1990; 9:783–784.

44. Laurenti F, Ferro R, Isacchi G, et al: Polymorphonuclear leukocyte transfusion for the treatment of sepsis in the newborn infant. *Pediatrics* 1981; 98:118–122.

45. Magny JF, Bremard-Oury C, Brault D, et al: Intravenous immunoglobulin therapy for prevention of infection in high-risk premature infants: Report of a multicenter, double-blind study. *Pediatrics* 1991; 88:437–443.

46. Manroe BL, Rosenfeld CR, Weinberg AG, et al: The differential leukocyte count in the assessment and outcome of early-onset neonatal group B streptococcal disease. *J Pediatr* 1977; 91:632–637.

47. Manroe BL, Weinberg AG, Rosenfeld CR, et al: The neonatal blood count in health and disease. I. Reference values for neutrophilic cells. *J Pediatr* 1979; 95:89–98.

48. Minkoff H, Mead P: An obstetric approach to the prevention of early-onset group B beta-hemolytic streptococcal sepsis. *Am J Obstet Gynecol* 1986; 154:973–977.

49. Nataro JP, Gerdes JS, Corcoran L, et al: Virulence factors of coagulase-negative staphylococci (CONS) in neonates. *Pediatr Res* 1990; 27:274A.

50. Noel GJ, Edelson PJ: *Staphylococcus epidermidis* bacteremia in neonates: Further observations and the occurrence of focal infection. *Pediatrics* 1984; 74:832–837.

51. Patrick CC, Kaplan SI, Baker CJ, et al: Persistent bacteremia due to coagulase-negative staphylo-

cocci in low birth weight neonates. *Pediatrics* 1989; 84:977–985.

52. Philip AGS, Hewitt JR: Early diagnosis of neonatal sepsis. *Pediatrics* 1980; 65:1036–1041.

53. Philip AGS: Detection of neonatal sepsis of late onset. *JAMA* 1982; 247:489–492.

54. Philip AGS: *Neonatal Sepsis and Meningitis,* Boston, GK Hall Medical Publishers, 1985.

55. Polin RA, St. Geme JW III: Neonatal sepsis. *Adv Pediatr Infect Dis* 1992; 7:25–61.

56. Pyati SP, Pildes RS, Ramamurthy RS, et al: Decreased mortality in neonates with early-onset group B streptococcal infection: Reality or artifact. *J Pediatr* 1981; 98:625–627.

57. Saez-Llorens X, McCracken GH Jr: Bacterial meningitis in neonates and children. *Infect Dis Clin North Am* 1990; 4:623–644.

58. Sanchez PJ, Siegel JD, Cushion NB, et al: Significance of a positive urine group B streptococcal latex agglutination test in neonates. *J Pediatr* 1990; 116:601–606.

59. Schmidt BK, Kirpalani HM, Corey M, et al: Coagulase-negative staphylococci as true pathogens in newborn infants: A cohort study. *Pediatr Infect Dis J* 1987; 6:1026–1031.

60. Sidebottom DG, Freeman J, Platt R, et al: Fifteen-year experience with bloodstream isolates of coagulase-negative staphylococci in neonatal intensive care. *J Clin Microbiol* 1988; 26:713–718.

61. Sidiropoulos D, Boehme U, Von Muralt G, et al: Immunoglobulin supplementation in prevention and treatment of neonatal sepsis. *Pediatr Infect Dis* 1986; 5:192–197.

62. Siegel JD, McCracken GH Jr, Threlkeld N, et al: Single-dose penicillin prophylaxis against neonatal group B streptococcal infections: A controlled trial in 18,738 newborn infants. *N Engl J Med* 1980; 303:769–775.

63. Siegel JD, McCracken GH Jr: Sepsis neonatorum. *N Engl J Med* 1981; 304:642–647.

64. Squire E, Favara B, Todd J: Diagnosis of neonatal bacterial infection: Hematologic and pathologic findings in fatal and nonfatal cases. *Pediatrics* 1979; 64:60–64.

65. St. Geme JW III, Bell LM, Baumgart S, et al: Distinguishing sepsis from blood culture contamination in young infants with blood cultures growing coagulase-negative staphylococci. *Pediatrics* 1990; 86:157–162.

66. St. Geme JW III, Polin RA: Neonatal sepsis: Progress in diagnosis and management. *Drugs* 1988; 36:784–800.

67. Steigman AJ, Bottone EJ, Hanna BA: Control of perinatal group B streptococcal sepsis: Efficacy of single injection of aqueous penicillin at birth. *Mt Sinai J Med* 1978; 45:685–693.

68. Vain NE, Mazumian JR, Swarner OW, et al: Role of exchange transfusion in the treatment of severe septicemia. *Pediatrics* 1980; 66:693–697.

69. Yoder MC, Polin RA: Immunotherapy of neonatal septicemia. *Pediatr Clin North Am* 1986; 33:481–501.

70. Yow MD, Leeds LJ, Thompson PK, et al: The natural history of group B streptococcal colonization in the pregnant woman and her offspring. I. Colonization studies. *Am J Obstet Gynecol* 1980; 137:34–38.

# Chapter 12

# CARDIAC DISEASE IN THE NEWBORN INFANT

## Michael H. Gewitz, M.D.

The evaluation and initial management of cardiovascular problems in the newborn requires not only an appreciation of the major types of anatomic defects, but also an understanding of the principles of normal and abnormal cardiopulmonary physiology and the unique factors of early postnatal life that affect them. This chapter reviews the basic factors that regulate cardiac function in the newborn and elucidates how anatomic abnormalities result in physiological aberrations; provides an overview of the evaluation processes that can lead to a diagnosis; and reviews guidelines for initial management. In this chapter, several exemplary case studies are reviewed to demonstrate the issues confronted by the practitioner in dealing with infants with possible cardiac disease.

## PHYSIOLOGICAL MANIFESTATIONS OF CARDIAC DISEASE IN THE NEWBORN INFANT

Four basic factors regulate cardiac output:

1. *Preload,* defined as the volume at end diastole that must be ejected by the ventricle, reflects systemic venous return and intravascular fluid volume.
2. *Afterload,* defined as the force opposing ventricular ejection, is related to the wall tension that must be developed by the myocardium in order to generate the intracardiac pressure required to eject a given preload. Impedance factors such as systemic or pulmonary vascular resistance are major determinants of afterload.

3. *Contractility* refers to the intrinsic properties of cardiac muscle, which provide the geometric alterations necessary for ejection. These properties are determined by the basic configuration of the cardiac ultrastructure.
4. *Heart rate* is determined by both supervening neurological and humoral input as well as by the intrinsic automaticity of the specialized cardiac conduction system.

Alterations in any of these four determinants can influence cardiac output. They are closely interrelated, however, and thus factors affecting one of these variables will affect the others. Nearly every clinical presentation involving cardiac dysfunction can be traced to alterations in one or more of these underlying physiological factors.

The classic relationship, cardiac output (CO) = heart rate (HR) × stroke volume (SV), encompasses these four basic determinants because stroke volume, the amount of blood ejected in each beat, is related to afterload, preload, and contractility. The other fundamental cardiac physiological principle, the Frank-Starling relationship, expresses the relationship between the volume of blood within the heart at the end of diastole and the pressure developed during contraction (Fig. 12-1). In essence, this law states that the cardiac output will be preserved in the face of a failing myocardium by the inherent capability of myocardial fibers to stretch, enabling cardiac volume to increase. This capability is active only to a certain point, beyond which the systolic pressure actually declines with increasing volume and heart failure results.

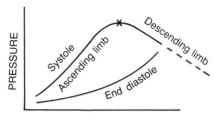

**Figure 12-1** Diagrammatic representation of Starling's Law, which relates pressure development during contraction to volume at end diastole. In general, as the volume in the heart at the end of diastole increases, the pressure developed during a systolic contraction also increases. This relationship is maintained until very large end-diastolic volumes are achieved, as exemplified by *x*, when systolic pressures start to decline with further increases in diastolic volume. The heart normally functions on the "ascending limb" of the curve, permitting it to increase stroke volume, ejection pressure, or both as diastolic volume is increased.

## ALTERATIONS IN CARDIAC OUTPUT

Conditions of early postnatal life influence each of the four physiological factors outlined earlier. In the newborn infant, heart rate assumes a preeminent role in influencing cardiac output compared to the older child or adult. Contractility is also influenced by developmental factors. Fetal research has shown that in the developing heart, compliance of the myocardium is reduced in comparison to the adult, and that for any given change in volume, greater pressure will be developed. Systemic vasomotor tone in early postnatal life is characterized by marked lability, which can result in rather dramatic shifts in left ventricular afterload by imposing great variations in resistance to ventricular ejection. Pulmonary vascular tone is well known to be significantly increased in the newborn period, and thus right ventricular afterload is normally elevated. Finally, the fluid volume status of the newborn infant undergoes great changes in the first hours and days of extrauterine life. Therefore, ventricular preload may be significantly altered in the immediate newborn period because systemic volume is a primary determinant of preload.

## TRANSITIONAL CIRCULATION

A unique aspect of early postnatal development, which is directly related to cardiac function, is the switch that must occur from the fetal cardiopulmonary circulation to a mature extrauterine system. The so-called "transitional circulation," which normally exists for only a few moments to hours after birth, may cause severe difficulties if it is not truly transient. Figure 12-2 summarizes the details of these sequential changes. Associated with anatomic changes, such as obliteration of the ductus arteriosus and closure of the foramen ovale, is the fall in pulmonary vascular resistance that must occur for satisfactory ventilation-perfusion relationships to become established within the lung and for normal oxygenation to occur.

The relaxation in pulmonary vasomotor tone should occur rapidly. At birth, systemic and pulmonary pressures are equal, but significant separation can be noted by 3 hours of life.

**Table 12-1** Factors Influencing Pulmonary Vascular Tone in the Newborn Infant

*Anatomic factors*

1. Developmental status of pulmonary vascular smooth muscle

2. Presence of congenital heart lesion affecting pulmonary blood flow and pulmonary venous pressure

*Hormonal factors*

1. Eicosanoids—prostaglandins, thromboxane, leukotrienes

2. Angiotensin system

3. Neuromediatros—acetylcholine, bradykinin, catecholamines

4. Endothelium derived agents—nitric oxide, endothelin

*Environmental factors*

1. Arterial oxygenation ($pO_2$) and carbon dioxide ($pCO_2$) status

2. Acidosis (pH)

3. Hematocrit level

4. Altitude (probably via effect of hypoxia)

*Neurological factors*

1. Hypothalamic and brain stem function

2. Reflexes—chemoreceptors, baroreceptors

3. Autonomic tone (somewhat controversial)

Failure of the elevated pulmonary artery pressures to regress can result in persistence of both intracardiac (foramen ovale) and ductal level right-to-left shunting, yielding net systemic cyanosis. Several factors are known to influence the regression of pulmonary hypertension (Table 12-1). Ventilation is of paramount importance because oxygen is a potent pulmonary artery vasodilator and carbon dioxide a vasoconstrictor. The magnitude of placental transfusion, reflected in intravascular fluid volume and left atrial pressure, is also closely related to the rate of pulmonary artery pressure decline. Delayed clamping of the cord

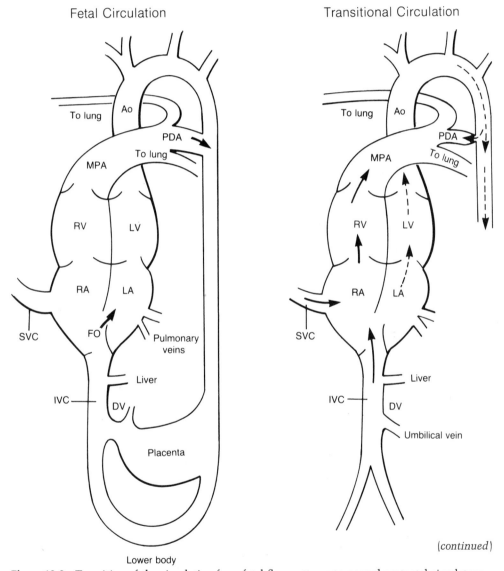

Fetal Circulation

Transitional Circulation

*(continued)*

**Figure 12-2**   Transition of the circulation from fetal flow patterns to normal postnatal circulatory scheme. The so-called "transitional circulation" is normally a short-lived situation in which the patent ductus arteriosus (PDA) and foramen ovale (FO) may be significant conduits. RV = right ventricle, RA = right atrium, DV = ductus venosus, LV = left ventricle, LA = left atrium, Ao = aorta, MPA = main pulmonary artery, SVC and IVC = superior and inferior vena cava, respectively. Solid arrows represent desaturated blood; broken arrows depict flow of oxygenated blood.
Adapted from Rudolph AM: *Congenital Diseases of the Heart*. Chicago, Year Book Medical Publishers, 1974, pp. 18–19. Adapted with permission of Mosby-Year Book, Inc.

## Neonatal Circulation

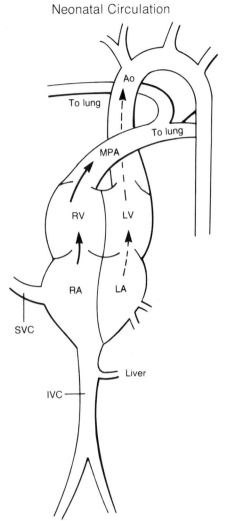

**Figure 12-2** *Continued*

has been associated with a slower decline in mean pulmonary artery pressure, which is probably related to an increased blood hematocrit and hyperviscosity. A more long-term factor is the nature of the pulmonary vascular bed itself. The process of anatomic change in pulmonary vascular smooth muscle, with regression of the medial muscle and its ultimate disappearance from vessels smaller than 50 $\mu$m in diameter, is a developmental process that occurs during a relatively long period of time. It is not fully completed until the second year of life. Thus, although pulmonary artery pressure falls and flow increases rapidly after birth, the decline in pulmonary vascular resistance proceeds at a slower pace.

Intense scrutiny has recently been devoted to defining the local pulmonary vasomotor influences of circulating hormones such as the derivatives of arachidonic acid that make up the prostaglandin cascade. In particular, $PGI_2$ (prostacyclin) is known to be a potent pulmonary vasodilator and thromboxane a vasoconstrictor. Even more recent data have demonstrated the influence of endothelial cell secretory products on pulmonary vasomotor tone. Endothelin, a compound produced locally by the endothelium, may be the most potent vasoconstrictor of all, and nitric oxide, also produced by the endothelium, is an important agent for the maintenance of vasorelaxation. These and other regulators of pulmonary vasoreactivity are under intense investigation because the status of the pulmonary vascular bed is central to the clinical impact of many neonatal circulatory disorders.

### EXERCISE 1

A. Relate each physiological principle to the phrase that best defines it.

_____1. Afterload
_____2. Preload
_____3. Contractility
_____4. Cardiac output

a. The volume of blood that must be ejected by the ventricle.
b. The intrinsic ability of cardiac muscle to shorten with an appropriate stimulus.
c. The product of stroke volume and heart rate.
d. The tension that must be generated by the heart muscle in order to eject.

B. List five of the factors that influence pulmonary vascular tone in the newborn infant.

1.

2.

3.

4.

5.

Answers for this and all exercises are provided at the end of the chapter.

## CYANOSIS

Aside from alterations in cardiac output, the other principal manifestation of cardiac disease in the newborn infant is altered oxygen saturation as represented by cyanosis. Cyanosis is classically defined as a bluish discoloration of skin or mucous membranes reflecting the presence of a minimum of 5 g/dL of reduced hemoglobin in systemic capillaries. It is clinically important to distinguish between *central* cyanosis and *peripheral* cyanosis because each has its own relevance. While peripheral cyanosis is a frequent manifestation of cutaneous vessel constriction in response to cold injury, it may also reflect severely impaired cardiac output resulting in slow transcapillary blood flow and reduction of hemoglobin at a local level. Central cyanosis can arise from a number of conditions other than congenital heart disease, and it is important for the pediatrician to be knowledgeable about the range of possible causes, since early, or no, intervention may be required. Table 12-2 lists the causes of cyanosis commonly encountered in the newborn infant.

It is frequently difficult to establish the specific causes of central cyanosis based on clinical findings alone. Nevertheless, the physiological underpinnings of the cardiac origin of cyanosis are relatively simple to understand and include at least one of the following: (1) the presence of an anatomic right-to-left intracardiac shunt associated with decreased pulmonary blood flow, (2) the association of an intracardiac right-to-left shunt with increased pulmonary blood flow, or (3) the presence of severely impaired cardiac performance resulting in pulmonary congestion with a ventilation-perfusion mismatch without an associated intracardiac shunt.

To understand these physiological concepts, several other terms must be appreciated. *Oxygen saturation* refers to the amount of oxygen actually combined with hemoglobin relative to the total amount of oxygen that could possibly be carried by the hemoglobin in any particular blood sample. This is most easily measured by spectrophotometric methods and expressed as a percentage. It can also be derived from a knowledge of pH, $PCO_2$ (carbon dioxide tension), and $PO_2$ (oxygen tension), and the application of the oxygen-hemoglobin equilibrium curve (Fig. 12-3). The normal arterial blood oxygen saturation is approximately

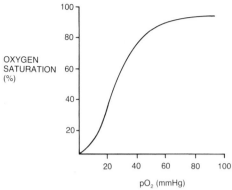

**Figure 12-3** *Oxygen-hemoglobin dissociation curve* for normal adult human blood. The sigmoidal relationship provides for nearly full saturation of hemoglobin at reduced $pO_2$. A leftward shift in the curve allows increased saturation at a given $pO_2$ level representing increased oxygen uptake by the blood.

95%. *Oxygen content* refers to the amount (mL) of oxygen in a given volume of blood (mL/dL). *Oxygen capacity* indicates the total amount (mL) of oxygen that can possibly be taken up by hemoglobin in the blood. Finally, *oxygen tension* ($PO_2$) refers to the partial pressure of oxygen in the blood (mm Hg). It can be seen from Figure 12-3 that a wide range of $PO_2$ values can result in oxygen saturation levels of greater than 90% because of the sigmoidal shape of the dissociation curve. This is an important property of hemoglobin because it enables nearly full saturation of the blood with oxygen even when there is some reduction in ventilation. A number of factors influence the oxygen-hemoglobin equilibrium curve and thus can affect the relationship between $PO_2$ and saturation. In general, factors that produce a leftward shift in the curve (alkalosis, fetal hemoglobin) result in an increase in saturation at any $PO_2$ level, thus favoring uptake of oxygen by the blood. Conversely, a rightward shift of the curve (acidosis, hypercarbia, hyperthermia) favors release of oxygen because a higher $PO_2$ is required to yield the same degree of oxygen saturation. An understanding of this relationship can be extremely important for dealing successfully with the problems posed by the cyanotic newborn infant.

On occasion, heart failure and an intracardiac right-to-left shunt coexist. The intracardiac lesion may result in mixing of desaturated blood with the systemic circulation while congestive heart failure results in pulmonary edema and alveolar hypoventilation.

**Table 12-2** Causes of Neonatal Cyanosis*

| CATEGORY | EXAMPLES | SIGNS | RESPONSE TO HYPEROXIA TEST | CHEST X-RAY | ARTERIAL BLOOD GASES |
|---|---|---|---|---|---|
| Heart disease with right-to-left shunt; *decreased* pulmonary blood flow | Tetralogy of Fallot<br>Pulmonary atresia<br>Tricuspid insufficiency | Hyperpnea<br>Heart murmur<br>Soft $S_2$ | Minimal to nil | Variable heart size<br>Diminished PVMs | pH normal or high<br>$pCO_2$ low |
| Heart disease with right-to-left shunt; *increased* pulmonary blood flow | d-Transposition<br>Anomalous pulmonary venous return | Tachypnea<br>Loud $S_2$<br>Variable heart murmur | Minimal | Large heart (unless obstructed TAPVD)<br>Increased PVMs | pH normal or low<br>$pCO_2$ normal or high |
| Heart disease with heart failure; ventilation-perfusion mismatch | Coarctation syndrome<br>Large left-to-right shunt<br>Supraventricular tachycardia | Tachypnea<br>Shock<br>Heart murmur | Good response ($PaO_2 > 150$) | Large heart<br>Pulmonary edema<br>R/O pneumonia | pH low<br>$pCO_2$ high |
| Primary pulmonary disease | RDS<br>Group B streptococcus<br>Meconium aspiration<br>Pneumothorax | Tachypnea<br>Retractions<br>Grunting, etc. | Good response (may need CPAP to prove) | Diagnostic appearance | pH low<br>$pCO_2$ high |

| Condition | Associated conditions | Clinical signs | Response to O₂ | Heart size / PVMs | Blood gas |
|---|---|---|---|---|---|
| Metabolic disease | Hypoglycemia, Methemoglobinemia | Variable: Tachypnea, Flaccid, Jittery, etc. | Minimal | Normal or large heart | pH normal or low, $pCO_2$ normal |
| Polycythemia | Twin-twin transfusion, Intrauterine growth retardation | Plethora, Signs of congestive heart failure | Minimal | Large heart, Normal PVMs | Normal or low pH, $pCO_2$ normal |
| Infection | Sepsis, Myocarditis | Shock, Marked peripheral cyanosis | Good | Large heart (unless hypo-adrenal), Pulmonary edema | pH low, $pCO_2$ high |
| Persistent fetal circulation | Meconium aspiration, LGA baby, Maternal salicylates | Hyperpnea, Differential cyanosis | Variable—transiently good (with CPAP) | Normal heart size, Decreased PVMs | pH low, $pCO_2$ may be elevated |
| Neurological disease | Intracranial bleed, Seizure disorder | Tachypnea, Focal signs, Apnea | Good | Normal | pH low, $pCO_2$ elevated |

* PVMs = pulmonary vascular markings, CPAP = continuous positive airway pressure, TAPVD = total anomalous pulmonary venous drainage. Source: Modified from Lees MH: Cyanosis of the newborn infant. *J Pediatr* 1970; 77:484. Modified with permission of Mosby-Year Book, Inc.

This child may exhibit the findings of both derangements and thus be very difficult to manage.

## EXERCISE 2

A. Place a check mark next to each of the following statements that is true.

_____1. Systemic arterial desaturation always results in visible cyanosis.

_____2. Cyanosis is possible if pulmonary blood flow is increased.

_____3. Cyanosis can be present in the absence of anatomic heart or lung disease.

_____4. Ventilation-perfusion mismatch in the lung can cause cyanosis.

_____5. Peripheral cyanosis can reflect a cardiac problem.

_____6. Central cyanosis usually reflects a cardiac problem.

_____7. Anemia may mask cyanosis.

_____8. Polycythemia may cause cyanosis in the absence of structural heart disease.

B. List four factors that produce the leftward shift in the oxygen-hemoglobin equilibrium curve depicted below.

1.

2.

3.

4.

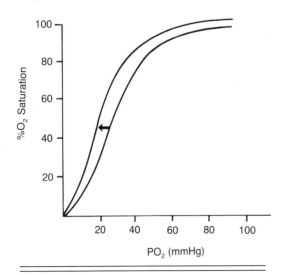

## ANATOMIC LESIONS

When you attempt to identify the specific lesion in an infant with suspected cardiac disease, it is helpful first to decide whether cyanosis or congestive heart failure is the pre-eminent problem, and then to proceed in an organized anatomic approach. For example, if you are faced with a cyanotic newborn infant with adequate ventilation and no evidence of congestive heart failure, diagnostic considerations can be limited to those anatomic lesions that result in right-to-left intracardiac shunting and normal pump function. Conversely, if congestive heart failure without cyanosis is the principal problem, an entirely different group of anatomic possibilities exists.

## LESIONS PRODUCING CYANOSIS

While direct systemic venous connection to the left heart can result in systemic desaturation, this problem usually does not present as an isolated anomaly in the newborn infant. Right-to-left atrial level shunting, however, is a common cause of neonatal cyanosis. Congenital heart lesions involving abnormalities of right ventricular inflow (tricuspid atresia, Ebstein's anomaly) or right ventricular outflow obstruction (pulmonary stenosis/atresia with intact ventricular septum) are prominent causes of shunting at the atrial level. At the ventricular level, a ventricular septal defect associated with right ventricular hypertension, such as tetralogy of Fallot or pulmonary atresia with ventricular septal defect, are the principal entities that should be considered.

Tetralogy of Fallot, the hallmark lesion of this group, actually involves three specific anatomic problems: (1) ventricular septal defect, (2) alignment of the aorta over the ventricular septal defect so that both right and left ventricular blood can egress directly into the aorta, and (3) obstruction to outflow from the right ventricle. The fourth component of the "tetrad" is right ventricular hypertrophy (Fig. 12-4). Note that the cause of cyanosis is not the reduced pulmonary blood flow itself, but rather the intracardiac right-to-left shunting, which occurs through the ventricular septal defect and *aortic override* in this lesion. The principal determinant of the degree of cyanosis in this lesion is the ratio of outflow resistance from the left ventricle to outflow resistance from the right ventricle. The lower this ratio is, the more likely that right-to-left

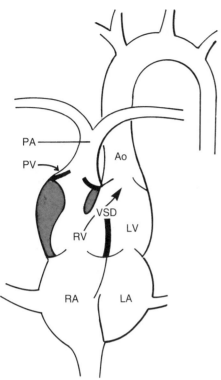

**Figure 12-4** Anatomic configuration in tetralogy of Fallot. Displacement of part of the ventricular septum results in development of a ventricular septal defect (VSD) through which desaturated blood can pass from the right ventricle (RV) out the aorta (Ao). Underdevelopment of the pulmonary artery (PA), in association with an abnormal pulmonary valve (PV) and outflow tract contributes to thickening of the right ventricle muscle. Other abbreviations as in Figure 12-2.

great vessel) and should be considered in the presence of cyanosis and decreased pulmonary blood flow. The remaining anatomic lesions that should also be considered in the child with cyanosis and decreased pulmonary blood flow are complicated anatomic derangements with multiple associated abnormalities as exemplified by transposition of the great arteries with pulmonic stenosis, double outlet right ventricle with pulmonic stenosis, endocardial cushion defect with pulmonary stenosis, or single ventricle malformations with pulmonary outflow obstruction.

The syndrome of elevated pulmonary vascular resistance, the so-called "persistent fetal circulation syndrome," deserves special mention. In this situation, massive intracardiac right-to-left shunting occurs through the foramen ovale (and often also the ductus arteriosus) because of abnormally elevated resistance at the level of the pulmonary arterioles. The consequence is severe cyanosis. This syndrome is characterized by normal cardiac anatomy and right-to-left shunting through otherwise normal fetal channels. Thus, the "lesion" is at the level of the pulmonary vascular bed and not in the heart. Two clinically important variants of persistent fetal circulation are recognized.

In the more frequent presentation, elevated pulmonary vascular resistance occurs as a reactive phenomenon to an intrapulmonary insult during the perinatal period. Frequently, meconium aspiration is part of the clinical picture. These babies are typically post-mature, large infants who have had a difficult obstetric course. Vigorous ventilatory management sometimes combined with vasodilators and blood pressure support has been successfully used to treat these infants, since achievement of respiratory alkalosis and hypocarbia may result in pulmonary arteriolar vasodilation. The recent innovation of extracorporeal membrane oxygenation (ECMO), a form of prolonged right heart bypass, appears to be a promising therapeutic modality for this problem (see Chapter 13). The second recognized form of persistent fetal circulation involves a more intractable situation in which there is a relatively fixed increase in the extent of pulmonary vascular smooth muscle. This may represent a true developmental anomaly and has been associated with other congenital anomalies such as a diaphragmatic hernia. Maternal ingestion of prostaglandin synthetase inhibitors such as aspirin has also been

shunting will occur and cyanosis will be manifest. Cyanosis from this lesion is often not apparent in the early newborn period because the right ventricular outflow obstruction may take some time to develop. It is the extreme variant, pulmonary atresia with ventricular septal defect, in which there is no direct outlet from the right ventricle to the pulmonary bed, that more commonly presents with cyanosis during the neonatal period.

Lesions at the level of the great vessels, such as patent ductus arteriosus or aortopulmonary fenestration (window), do not cause cyanosis unless complicated by pulmonary hypertension. Severe elevations of pulmonary artery pressure and pulmonary vascular resistance can result in right-to-left shunting at any level (atrial, ventricular, or related to the development of this form of persistent fetal circulation.

## LESIONS PRODUCING CONGESTIVE HEART FAILURE

A different set of anatomic possibilities must be considered when evaluating the neonate who presents with congestive heart failure as the major problem. Although these infants can manifest systemic desaturation because of alveolar hypoventilation, the principal problem is one of decreased cardiac output. Table 12-3 reviews the basic groupings you must consider in order to determine the etiology of congestive heart failure in the newborn infant. The primary anatomic lesions in this category are those that produce excessive left ventricular afterload with resultant pump failure, such as coarctation of the aorta, severe aortic stenosis, and aortic-mitral hypoplasia. These congested infants require urgent medical, and usually surgical, therapy aimed at reducing left ventricular obstruction and improving systemic blood flow. In infants with left heart hypopla-

sias, in which there is underdevelopment or even an absence of the left ventricle, mitral valve, or ascending aorta, the previously universal fatal outcomes have begun to improve with advancing surgical techniques including neonatal heart transplantation and/or surgical palliation for the univentricular heart ("Norwood" operation). These lesions are frequently associated with some degree of hypoxemia as a consequence of massive intrapulmonary shunting associated with elevated pulmonary venous pressures and pulmonary edema. If infants with such extreme congenital cardiac anomalies are to survive, early diagnosis and appropriate medical therapy are crucial. In particular, assiduous care in the control of pulmonary vascular resistance can be critical for survival until surgical therapy is accomplished.

Large left-to-right shunt lesions can also result in congestive heart failure in the newborn infant; however, in most cases failure usually develops after the immediate neonatal period. Ventricular septal defect, for example, will produce increased pulmonary blood flow if the defect is sufficiently large. The degree of

**Table 12-3**   Etiologic Considerations for Congestive Heart Failure in the Newborn Infant

| CONGENITAL HEART DISEASE | ACQUIRED HEART DISEASE | ENDOCRINE-METABOLIC | OTHER |
|---|---|---|---|
| 1. Pressure overload: Left ventricular outflow obstruction (e.g., aortic stenosis, coarctation of aorta) | 1. Myocarditis 2. Cardiomyopathy | 1. Hypoglycemia (e.g., infant of a diabetic mother) | 1. Post-asphyxial syndrome |
| 2. Volume overload: Left-to-right shunts (e.g., patent ductus arteriosus) Valvar regurgitation (atrioventricular valves) Arteriovenous fistulae Intracardiac mixing lesions (e.g., truncus arteriosus, anomalous pulmonary venous return without obstruction) | 3. Pericardial disease 4. Cor pulmonale (associated with bronchopulmonary dysplasia) | 2. Anemia or acute blood loss 3. Polycythemia 4. Calcium or magnesium disturbance 5. Electrolyte disturbance (e.g., adrenal insufficiency) | 2. Central nervous system disease (hypoventilation) 3. Sepsis |
| 3. Other structural disease Anomalous coronary artery Traumatic injury | | | |
| 4. Rhythm disturbances Supraventricular tachycardia Complete heart block | | | |

left-to-right shunting is determined by both the relative differences between pulmonary and systemic vascular resistance, and the relative compliance of the left and right ventricles. Thus, in the term infant, a delayed fall in pulmonary vascular resistance retards the development of significant left-to-right shunting. When the infant is about 1 month of age, pulmonary vascular resistance is consistently lower than systemic resistance, and large-volume left-to-right shunting can occur. Frequently, however, this situation is not clearly manifest in the otherwise normal term infant until the second month of life. The presence of a ventricular septal defect may itself be associated with elevated pulmonary pressures, thus further delaying the regression of pulmonary vascular resistance from fetal levels. An additional reason for the delayed manifestation of left-to-right shunting until the second month of life may be the change in hematocrit that "physiologically" occurs at that time. The physiological anemia of infancy noted at 6 to 9 weeks of age may result in lowered blood viscosity as well as altered systemic oxygen transport, favoring an increase in pulmonary blood and a more significant left-to-right shunt.

In certain complex situations, such as ventricular septal defect associated with left ventricular outflow obstruction (for example, coarctation of the aorta), heart failure may be present very early in postnatal life because the combined effects of an increased left ventricular afterload and the large shunt are mutually magnified. Thus, in a term infant with an apparent ventricular septal defect and heart failure in the early newborn period, the presence of an associated lesion must be seriously suspected. In contrast, the premature infant may exhibit large-volume shunting even in the first few days of life with an otherwise uncomplicated ventricular septal defect. The earlier appearance of congestive heart failure in the premature infant is presumably due to a more rapid rate of regression of pulmonary vascular resistance as a consequence of interrupted development of pulmonary vascular smooth muscle.

Other causes of heart failure without cyanosis in the newborn infant include a variety of nonstructural problems. Preeminent among these are arrhythmias, particularly supraventricular tachycardia and congenital heart block, mechanical myocardial muscle problems such as myocarditis and cardiomyopathy, and perinatal asphyxia. This latter entity may be a more common cause of heart failure than commonly recognized. The cardiac findings result from myocardial ischemia during an asphyxial insult. When the left ventricle is primarily affected, mitral regurgitation and left-to-right shunting can occur. It is not infrequent, however, for the right ventricle to be primarily involved because this chamber is more vulnerable to insult in the newborn period than at other times. With right ventricular dysfunction, tricuspid regurgitation is common, and if right ventricular pressures are sufficiently elevated, right-to-left shunting can occur.

Metabolic problems can also be important causes of congestive heart failure in the neonate. Hypoglycemia is the most frequently encountered metabolic disturbance, and regardless of the cause of low blood sugar, impaired cardiac function and gross cardiac dilatation can result. Hypocalcemia, other electrolyte disturbances, and generalized infection (sepsis) must also be considered because they can be primary causes of heart failure. Remember, however, that these problems can also be a precipitating cause of heart failure in a child with underlying anatomic heart disease. In the neonate who presents with circulatory collapse, it is not reasonable to conclude that the cause is sepsis without careful clinical evaluation for an underlying cardiac disorder.

## PATENT DUCTUS ARTERIOSUS

Of particular interest for the physician caring for the neonate is the left-to-right shunt associated with the ductus arteriosus. In the term baby, patent ductus arteriosus (PDA) may be an isolated lesion or may be associated with other significant heart disease. In some infants with a PDA and congenital heart disease, the presence of the ductus may be life-saving because of ductal-dependent systemic or pulmonary blood flow. That issue is discussed in this chapter under the "Ductal Manipulation" heading. As noted earlier, the ductus arteriosus is a critical feature of the fetal circulation. Experimental work has shown that a major percentage of ventricular output traverses the ductus in fetal life. In the fetus, the ductus is a principal conduit for the diversion of blood from the nonrespiratory lungs to the systemic circulation. During successful adaptation to extrauterine life, the ductus arteriosus undergoes closure, usually constricting nearly completely by 18 hours of life and closing permanently by 5 to 7 days. Studies of the anatomic stages of ductal closure have shown this process to be multifaceted. Functional closure precedes full anatomic closure by a considerable period (up to several months) and during the early part of this interval the ductus may be subject to reopening and to resumption of blood flow. The ductus is more likely to remain patent in the preterm infant.

The precise details of the mechanisms involved in closure of the ductus are yet to be elucidated, but recent investigations have offered several important insights. We have known for some time that oxygen tension in the blood, either perfusing the ductus or traversing through it, is an important factor in controlling ductal patency. Increasing the oxygen concentration of blood to which the ductus is exposed can result in its constriction. Although the exact mechanism of oxygen action is not certain, interaction of oxygen with cytochrome-based enzymatic systems and with vasoactive substances has been suggested as a possible mechanism. Recent work has also documented the independent importance of vasoactive agents, such as prostaglandins. Endogenous prostaglandins, $PGE_1$, $PGE_2$, and $PGI_2$ (prostacyclin) dilate the ductus. The ductus appears to be very sensitive to $PGE_2$ in particular. Other prostaglandins, specifically those of type F, may constrict the ductus, and inhibition of synthesis of the dilating prostaglandins results in ductal constriction. Acetylcholine and bradykinin are also known to reduce the caliber of the ductus arteriosus. Finally, direct neural involvement has been noted to play a possible role in ductal closure because the ductus is innervated from both vagal and sympathetic nerve fibers.

Our current understanding of the mechanism of closure of the ductus arteriosus in the term infant centers on the following schema. Following birth, the placental circulation is disrupted and pulmonary circulation is enhanced. Because the placenta is presumed to be a source for the *dilating type* prostaglandins and the lungs are a site of their metabolism, these normal postnatal events lead to a fall in circulating, dilating prostaglandins. As alveolar ventilation improves, oxygenation is increased and the relative ratio of systemic vascular resistance to pulmonary vascular re-

sistance is increased, favoring left-to-right ductal shunting. Thus, the increase in oxygen tension that occurs postnatally facilitates ductal constriction. As other circulating vasoactive agents such as bradykinin perfuse the ductus, muscular contraction of ductal smooth muscle occurs, thereby further reducing ductal flow (Fig. 12-5). These developments set in motion the anatomic processes leading to permanent ductal closure.

## EXERCISE 3

Place a check mark next to each factor that can influence the hemodynamic significance of the patent ductus arteriosus.

_____1. Arterial oxygenation

_____2. Hematocrit

_____3. Fluid volume status

_____4. Gestational age

_____5. The relative activities of E- and F-type prostaglandins

_____6. Hyperglycemia

_____7. Hydrogen ion concentration (pH)

### Patent Ductus Arteriosus in the Premature Infant

One of the well-known complications of premature birth is the development of a hemodynamically significant PDA either causing heart failure or interfering with ventilatory improvement without overt heart failure. While patent ductus arteriosus may certainly become an important cause of left-to-right shunting in the premature newborn infant without significant lung disease, the far greater clinical problem involves the association of PDA with respiratory distress syndrome (RDS). Two scenarios can develop within this clinical context. First, hypoxia and acidosis, stemming from impaired alveolar ventilation, can result in elevated pulmonary vascular resistance and right-to-left shunting through the PDA. This probably occurs at some point in nearly all babies with RDS but is clinically undetected because the right-to-left ductal shunt has no associated murmur and the hypoxemia is attributable to lung disease. Second, later in the course of RDS, usu-

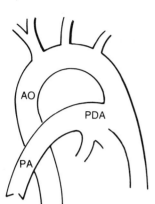

Dilators

1) PGE₁
2) PGI₂
3) Hypoxia
4) Acidosis

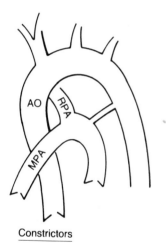

Constrictors

1) PGF$_{2\alpha}$
2) Prostaglandin synthetase
3) Increased oxygen concentration
4) Acetylcholine
5) Bradykinin

**Figure 12-5** Factors influencing the caliber of the ductus arteriosus. PGE₁ = prostaglandin E₁, PGI = prostacyclin.

ally during a time of improving pulmonary function, a left-to-right shunt through the ductus may become clinically important. This shunt can result in excessive pulmonary blood flow, left heart failure with pulmonary edema, and in some infants the need for prolonged mechanical ventilation. The multicenter national collaborative study concerning PDA in premature infants weighing less than 1,750 g found that this second scenario occurred in approximately 20% of infants enrolled in the study. Many of these preterm infants do not respond well to traditional forms of therapy aimed at improving contractility (such as digoxin) because there is usually a hyperdynamic situation with maximal cardiac performance compensating for the increased left ventricular preload (secondary to increased left atrial return) and the reduced afterload brought about by the PDA. As a direct result of the studies on the mechanism of ductal closure just noted, prostaglandin synthetase inhibitors (such as indomethacin) are now widely used to medically obliterate the unwanted PDA left-to-right shunt and to relieve the associated pulmonary circulatory overload. Surgery still has a role in selected infants that are not suitable candidates for indomethacin.

Other complications can arise from patency of the ductus in a premature infant. These include an increased frequency of intracranial hemorrhage and an increased predisposition for necrotizing enterocolitis. These problems are found in the presence of large left-to-right ductal shunts and may be related to alterations in the distribution of cardiac output to the cerebral and splanchnic vascular beds.

Much investigation is still centered on the physiological impact of a PDA in the preterm baby. This work will hopefully help to define the role of direct prophylactic treatment of the ductus and the role of early surfactant replacement therapy on ductal physiology in these babies.

## LESIONS ASSOCIATED WITH COMBINED CYANOSIS AND HEART FAILURE

Several important structural anomalies fall into this category. Transposition of the great arteries is the hallmark lesion of this group. These infants usually have increased pulmonary blood flow but are deeply cyanotic because oxygenated blood has only limited access to the systemic circulation. In simple transposition of the arteries, the pulmonary artery arises from the left ventricle while the aorta originates from the right ventricle. Venous inflow into each chamber is normal. Thus, there is arterial-venous *discordance.* The only route for oxygenated blood to reach the aorta is by shunting at the atrial level or through a patent ductus arteriosus. In addition to the anatomic abnormality, physiological differences in ventricular function may be present. In particular, the pulmonary (left) ventricle may not be able to adapt to the increased pulmonary blood flow. As a consequence, pulmonary venous congestion may result, adding to the congested picture. The degree of cyanosis in transposition of the great arteries is thus dependent on several factors. If mixing through the foramen ovale or ductus arteriosus is negligible, intense cyanosis can result with signs of cerebral hypoxia. With larger degrees of mixing at these sites or in infants with transposition of the great arteries and an associated shunt lesion, such as a ventricular septal defect, cyanosis may be less significant but congestive heart failure is likely to be a major problem. Arterial blood gas analysis will still reveal arterial desaturation, but the infant will not appear as clinically cyanotic as the newborn infant with transposition of the great arteries and no associated shunt. A further, less frequent complication of transposition of the great arteries, which commonly results in congestive heart failure, is obstruction to right ventricular outflow because of coarctation of the aorta, aortic arch interruption, or subaortic stenosis. The association of transposition of the great arteries, ventricular septal defect, and aortic obstruction should be carefully sought in any child with cyanosis and severe heart failure.

In this context, a brief review of terminology is important. In the normal heart, the aorta receives fully saturated left ventricular blood by virtue of its direct communication with the left ventricle. Normal development results in the aortic valve being positioned posterior, inferior, and to the right of the pulmonary valve (Fig. 12-6). Additionally, the venous (right) atrium is directly connected with the venous (right) ventricle and the pulmonary artery is directly linked to the right ventricle. The normal heart, then, exhibits atrioventricular *concordance* and normal great vessel relationships. In d-transposition of the great arteries (d-TGA), the atria and ventricles are still concordant because the venous atrium still empties directly into the venous ventricle.

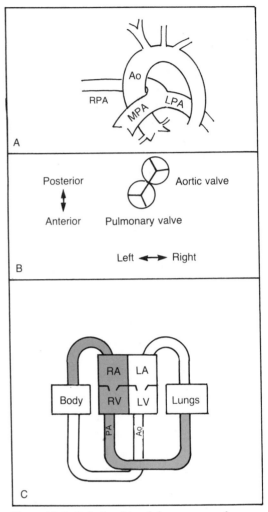

**Figure 12-6** Relationship of the great vessels (A), semilunar valves (B), and course of the circulation (C) in the normal heart. RPA = right pulmonary artery, LPA = left pulmonary artery. Other abbreviations as previously noted. Shaded areas represent desaturated blood.

However, the great vessels are now abnormally related. The term *d-TGA* refers to the position of the aortic valve: rightward ("d" or "dextro"), inferior, but now anterior to the pulmonary valve. This altered relationship leads to the aorta communicating with the right ventricle, which is in its usual anterior position, and the pulmonary artery communicating directly with the posterior left ventricle. Thus, fully saturated arterial blood returns from the lungs to the heart but is quickly pumped back again to the lungs. In a parallel fashion, venous blood returning from the body is returned to the systemic circulation without oxygenation in the lungs (Fig. 12-7).

The term *l-transposition* (l-TGA) refers to a different set of anatomic arrangements. In this lesion the great vessels are transposed with the aorta in direct communication with the right ventricle; however, the aortic valve now lies to the left of the pulmonary valve ("l" or "levo" position). This great vessel relationship is frequently seen in association with single ventricle conditions, in which there is often cyanosis and heart failure, but it is also present in so-called "corrected" transposition in which the child may be clinically normal.

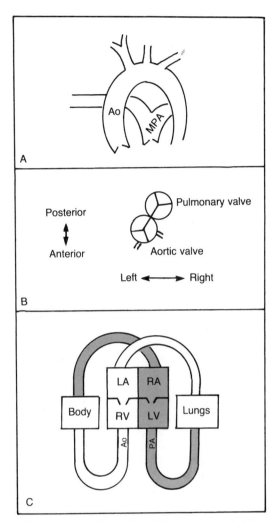

**Figure 12-8** Relationship of the great vessels (A), semilunar valves (B), and course of the circulation (C) in l-transposition of the great arteries (l-TGA) with ventricular inversion—"corrected transposition."

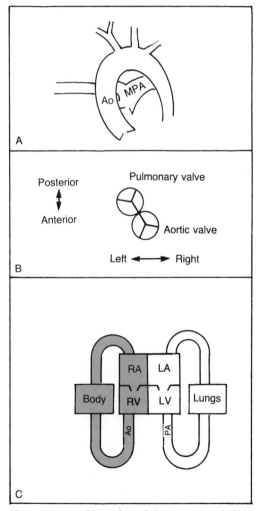

**Figure 12-7** Relationship of the great vessels (A), semilunar valves (B), and course of the circulation (C) in d-transposition of the great arteries (d-TGA). Abbreviations as in Figure 12-6.

In this lesion not only are the great vessels transposed, but atrioventricular *discordance* (Fig. 12-8) is also present. Venous inflow patterns are reversed and the right ventricle now receives fully saturated pulmonary venous blood. The aorta, arising from this malpositioned right ventricle, carries fully saturated blood to the systemic circulation and the patient is not cyanotic. Physiological correction has taken place. This is a case in which two wrongs make a right.

Other anatomic entities that may result in heart failure and arterial desaturation are double-outlet right ventricle, varieties of single ventricle, and truncus arteriosus. When these lesions are not associated with pulmonic stenosis, a large increase in pulmonary blood flow occurs in association with massive intracardiac mixing. Complete atrioventricular canal (endocardial cushion defect) is an important, relatively common lesion that produces cyanosis and heart failure. This entity is frequently associated with Down's syndrome (Trisomy 21). The etiology of congestive heart failure in this situation is usually atrioventricular valve regurgitation or subaortic obstruction. Cyanosis results from intracardiac mixing at both the atrial and ventricular levels. By definition, this lesion, in the complete form, involves defects in the posterosuperior portion of the ventricular septum and in the lower part of the atrial septum. Associated with these septal defects are fundamental abnormalities in the architecture of the atrioventricular valves (mitral and tricuspid). Frequently, portions of these valves are joined, making a common leaflet, which bridges across the crest of the ventricular septum. This leaflet may be divided or undivided and attached or unattached directly to the crest of the septum. The result of these anatomic derangements is that a common atrioventricular orifice empties both atria into both ventricles (Fig. 12-9). Thus, large degrees of bidirectional shunting can occur, depending on relative ventricular afterloads. Additionally, clefts usually exist in the atrioventricular valve tissues; thus varying degrees of atrioventricular regurgitation coexist with the intracardiac shunting patterns. As a point of reference, the term *partial atrioventricular canal* refers to a situation in which the deficiency of septal tissue involves only the lowest part of the interatrial septum. The mitral valve frequently has an associated cleft, but the tricuspid valve may be normal.

Finally, in the context of lesions causing both cyanosis and congestive heart failure, anomalous pulmonary venous return should be mentioned. In this situation, pulmonary venous drainage (containing fully saturated blood) follows an abnormal route from the lungs and returns to some point along the systemic venous pathway instead of returning to the left atrium. The entry point may be at the level of either the superior or inferior vena cava, the right atrium, or even the coronary sinus. Systemic output requires a right-to-left shunt because there is no other way for blood

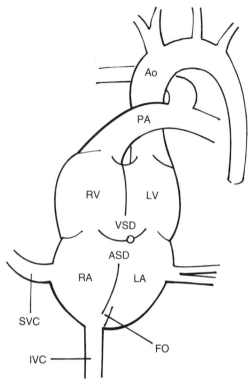

**Figure 12-9**   Anatomic configuration in complete atrioventricular canal defect (endocardial cushion defect). The common atrioventricular valve overrides the ventricular septal defect (VSD), and the atrial septal defect (ASD) is not in the same area as the foramen ovale (FO).

to fill the left ventricle (Fig. 12-10, page 270). Pulmonary hypertension is an invariable physiological component of this lesion. The presence or absence of obstruction along the venous return pathway determines whether the child manifests primarily cyanosis or heart failure, or some combination of both. In the very early postnatal period, massive right-to-left shunting will produce significant cyanosis even without obstruction. In contrast, lesser degrees of cyanosis but more severe evidence of heart failure will be present if obstruction occurs along the pulmonary venous pathway.

## EXERCISE 4

Refer to the Exercise 4 table on page 267, and by placing a check mark in the appropriate space, select one or more physiological statement(s) that relate to the cardiac lesions listed in the table.

**Exercise 4**

| LESION | 1. ASSOCIATED WITH LEFT VENTRICULAR AFTERLOAD | 2. CAN RESULT IN CYANOSIS WITH NORMAL VENTILATION | 3. ASSOCIATED WITH INCREASED PULMONARY ARTERY PRESSURE | 4. CAN RESULT IN CONGESTIVE HEART FAILURE | 5. RIGHT-TO-LEFT ATRIAL SHUNT IS PRINCIPAL FEATURE | 6. PULMONARY BLOOD FLOW INCREASED | 7. A LEFT-TO-RIGHT SHUNT IS A PRINCIPAL FEATURE |
|---|---|---|---|---|---|---|---|
| A. d-Transposition of the great vessels | | | | | | | |
| B. Coarctation of the aorta | | | | | | | |
| C. Tetralogy of Fallot | | | | | | | |
| D. Tricuspid atresia (intact ventricular septum) | | | | | | | |
| E. Myocarditis | | | | | | | |
| F. Truncus arteriosus | | | | | | | |
| G. Patent ductus arteriosus | | | | | | | |
| H. Post-asphyxial syndrome | | | | | | | |
| I. Total anomalous pulmonary venous return | | | | | | | |
| J. Aortic-mitral atresia | | | | | | | |

## EXERCISE 5

Relate each of the following statements with one of the figures shown below and on page 269 and write the figure number on the line provided. Abbreviations are as in Fig. 12-2. (Figures are adapted from Rudolph AM: *Congenital Diseases of the Heart.* Chicago, Year-Book Medical Publishers, 1974. Adapted with permission of Mosby-Year Book, Inc.)

_____A. These are parallel circulations. The magnitude of aortic saturation depends on the ductal or atrial shunt.

_____B. There is common mixing at the ventricular level. The aortic saturation reflects venous and arterial contributions.

_____C. The shunt through the PDA is right to left as is the blood flow across the atrial septum. Only 10% of the total cardiac output traverses the pulmonary circulation.

_____D. There is common mixing at atrial and ventricular levels. The height of arterial saturation reflects the relative resistances of the pulmonary and systemic vasculature.

_____E. The coronary arteries are perfused retrograde. Systemic blood flow is ductal dependent. Atrial shunting is left to right.

_____F. There is right-to-left atrial shunting. Pulmonary blood flow is dependent on left-to-right ductal shunting.

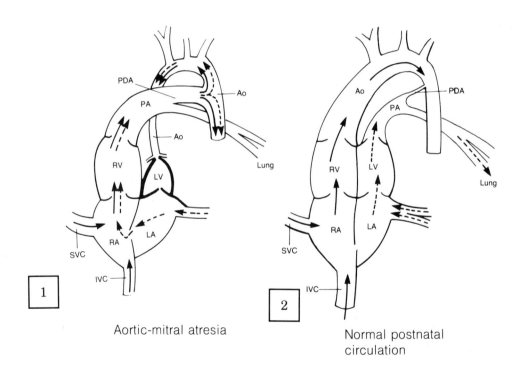

1. Aortic-mitral atresia

2. Normal postnatal circulation

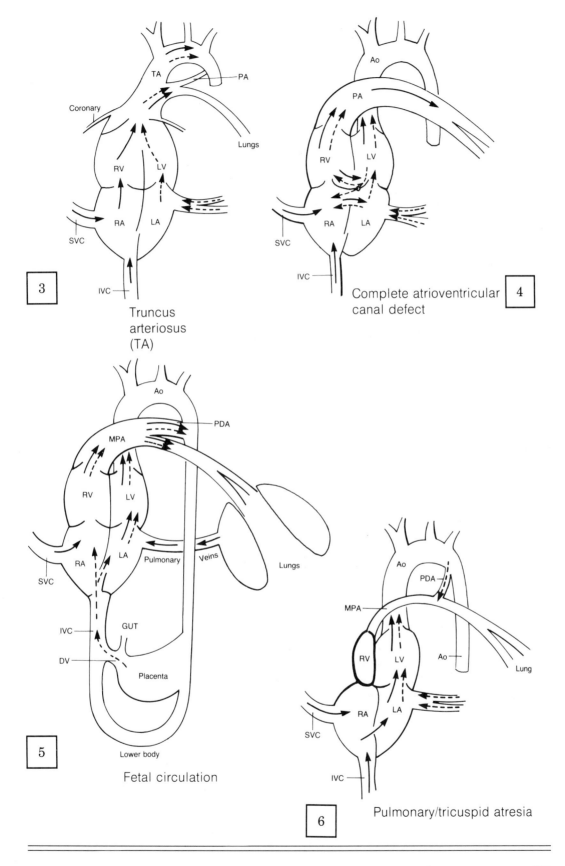

3

Truncus
arteriosus
(TA)

Complete atrioventricular
canal defect

4

5

Fetal circulation

Pulmonary/tricuspid atresia

6

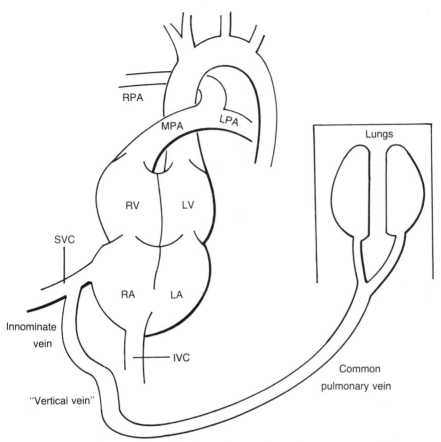

**Figure 12-10** Anatomic configuration in total anomalous pulmonary venous drainage (TAPVD). In this example, the common pulmonary vein drains eventually into the superior vena cava. In other forms, the pulmonary venous drainage may be directly to the right atrium, to the coronary sinus, or to the hepatic-inferior vena cava system.

## DIAGNOSIS

It is not vitally important to have a precise diagnosis established in the first few minutes of evaluation if the examiner can appropriately decide if heart disease is present and which general category of disturbed physiology is present. Based on appropriate knowledge of the pathophysiology and the anatomy of congenital heart disease, the clinician can interpret presenting clinical signs and supplementary laboratory studies with accuracy.

## HISTORY

A history of serious congenital heart disease in first-degree relatives of the infant under consideration is an important clue to the etiology of the infant's problems. Congenital heart disease does occur with increased frequency within certain familial contexts, and from a genetic point of view many consider polygenic multifactorial inheritance to be operative. According to this conceptualization, a hereditary predisposition to cardiac abnormality interacts with an environmental situation (such as a drug or viral teratogen) to create the appropriate milieu for the development of a specific lesion. Geneticists have assessed relative situations of risk and have determined that, in general, when a first-degree relative (mother, father, sister, or brother) has congenital heart disease, the risk of occurrence of the defect is 1% to 5%. Within this range, the rule that more common defects occur more commonly is also operative. Thus, the recurrence risk for ventricular septal defect in a family with a positive history of an affected child with that lesion would be approximately 5%, while the risk of developing a double-outlet right ventri-

**Table 12-4** Representative Prenatal Factors Associated with Congenital Heart Disease

| PRENATAL HISTORICAL FACTOR | ASSOCIATED CARDIAC DEFECT |
|---|---|
| 1. Diabetes mellitus | 1. Left ventricular out-flow obstruction: asymmetric septal hypertrophy, aortic stenosis d-transposition of the great arteries Ventricular septal defect |
| 2. Lupus erythema-tosus | 2. Congenital septal defect |
| 3. Rubella | 3. Patent ductus arte-riosus Pulmonic stenosis (peripheral) |
| 4. Alcohol abuse | 4. Pulmonic stenosis Ventricular septal defect |
| 5. Trimethadione usage | 5. Ventricular septal defect; tetralogy of Fallot |
| 6. Lithium usage | 6. Ebstein's anomaly |
| 7. Aspirin abuse | 7. Persistent pulmonary hypertension syndrome |
| 8. Coxsackie B infection | 8. Myocarditis |

cle in a baby with a positive close-family history for that lesion would be closer to 1%. These numbers, or course, need to be compared with the overall incidence of congenital heart disease in the population at large, which is 0.7% to 0.9%.

Other specific factors should also be sought in the history. Maternal rubella is well known to be a cause of congenital heart disease, specifically patent ductus arteriosus and pulmonic stenosis, but other viral agents have been associated with cardiac problems in the newborn infant. Coxsackie B infection can cause a serious, even lethal, myocarditis with severe congestive heart failure. Chronic maternal medical problems should also be elucidated. For example, maternal systemic lupus erythematosus has been associated with congenital complete heart block in the newborn infant. Similarly, maternal diabetes has been associated with a variety of neonatal cardiovascular abnormalities. A history of maternal

drug consumption, alcohol abuse, or exposure to possible teratogens such as x-rays can provide important clues as to the specific lesion. Table 12-4 lists some of the well-documented associations you should recall when you review the family and prenatal history of an infant with congenital heart disease. Of course, Mendellian syndromes and chromosomal anomalies have varying, sometimes high, de-

**Table 12-5** Representative Chromosomal and Syndrome Association with Congenital Heart Disease

| | MORE COMMON CARDIAC DEFECT(S) |
|---|---|
| ***Chromosomal disorder**** | |
| Trisomy 21 (40%) (Down's syndrome) | Ventricular septal defect Endocardial cushion defect |
| | Tetralogy of Fallot |
| | Transposition of great vessels |
| | Left ventricular outflow obstruction |
| Trisomy 18 (85%) | Ventricular septal defect |
| | Coarctation of the aorta |
| | Polyvalvular disease |
| Turner syndrome (xo) (35%) | Coarctation of the aorta |
| | Aortic valve abnormality |
| ***Syndrome (nonchromosomal)**** | |
| Noonan syndrome (50%) | Pulmonic stenosis (valvar dysplasia) |
| | Cardiomyopathy |
| | Atrial septal defect |
| CHARGE Association (80%) | PDA |
| | Ventricular septal defect |
| | Atrial septal defect |
| Vater (Vacterl) association (70%) | Ventricular septal defect |
| | Tetralogy of Fallot |
| Williams syndrome (75%) | Supravalvar arterial stenosis (aortic and/or pulmonary) |
| DiGeorge anomaly (85%) | Truncus arteriosus |
| | Interrupted aortic arch |

* (%) Refers to percentage of cases with congenital heart disease. In DiGeorge syndrome, "partial" cases have been described; otherwise the incidence is 100%. Defects listed are among more common ones and not all inclusive. In DiGeorge syndrome, chromosome 22 deletions may be involved.

grees of association with congenital cardiac defects. In Trisomy 21, for example, the incidence of cardiac defects is generally considered to be as high as 40%. In the majority of these cases, some form of ventricular septal defect is part of the problem, but a spectrum of anomalies has been described (Table 12-5).

## GENERAL CLINICAL EXAMINATION

The cardinal rules of diagnosis should apply to the evaluation of the newborn infant with suspected congenital heart disease, just as they apply to other clinical situations. *Inspection*, then, is the first step in the evaluation process. Is the infant active or does he show little spontaneous movement? Generally, with severely decreased oxygen delivery to the tissues, the newborn infant will exhibit reduced activity. Is the baby cyanotic? A gross degree of arterial desaturation will be readily apparent, but you must remember that significant hypoxemia may be present without cyanosis detectable by the naked eye. Observation of the infant's breathing pattern is of critical importance. The medical observer should differentiate between hyperpnea and tachypnea, because each entity has different implications for the underlying derangement. Hyperpnea refers to the deep, unlabored breathing at mildly elevated rates that is typical of situations in which there is decreased pulmonary blood flow. The infant exhibits an increased tidal volume in this situation, but there is a considerable degree of wasted ventilation with many well-ventilated but underperfused alveoli. Tachypnea refers to the shallow, rapid, somewhat labored breathing associated with decreased lung compliance. As such, it is a nonspecific sign and is the significant feature of primary parenchymal lung disease. From a cardiac viewpoint, tachypnea is notable in situations of pulmonary venous congestion associated with left ventricular failure, and/or pulmonary edema associated with excessive pulmonary blood flow. Other nonspecific respiratory signs that may be present in the newborn infant with heart disease include wheezing, intercostal retractions, nasal flaring, expiratory grunting, and apnea. These again reflect principally the secondary pulmonary changes associated with heart failure from any cause and are not specific signs diagnostic of heart disease. Stridor, a relatively uncommon sign in the neonate, may also represent cardiovascular disease, primarily upper airway compression from a vascular ring. While other causes of stridor in a newborn infant must be considered, the presence of a vascular ring needs to be carefully excluded in the infant with stridor because stridor is a readily remediable situation that can result in permanent tracheal damage if it is allowed to persist.

*Palpation*, the second pillar of physical diagnosis, is also required in the evaluation of the newborn infant with suspected heart disease. Pulses in all extremities should be palpated carefully. The *sine qua non* of aortic coarctation is the presence of palpable arterial pulses in the upper extremities and diminished or absent femoral pulses. Although it may be possible to exclude coarctation with the finding of one normal lower extremity pulse, you might not be able to identify symmetric pulses in the upper extremities because certain forms of coarctation, supravalvar aortic stenosis, or aortic arch hypoplasias can result in asymmetric arterial pulsation in the arms. At times the neonate with coarctation of the aorta will exhibit normal lower extremity pulses if the coarctation is the juxtaductal or preductal type and the descending aorta is perfused by right-to-left shunting through the ductus arteriosus. If this is the case, however, cyanosis of the feet as compared to the hands (*differential* cyanosis) may sometimes be observable and provide a clue to the diagnosis. Palpation will also reveal hyperactive pulses typically present in PDA or other large arteriovenous communications. Careful palpation of the precordium may also be helpful at times, particularly in hyperdynamic situations. Thrills are not commonly found in the newborn infant but may be present along the left sternal border in infants with large shunts at the ventricular level or at the suprasternal notch in neonates with significant semilunar valve obstruction. Palpation should also provide information about liver size, which is frequently though not invariably enlarged in the newborn infant with heart failure. Furthermore, liver pulsations may be observed in association with tricuspid valve disease. The newborn infant will rarely have significant peripheral edema as a sign of heart failure, but occasionally (e.g., the hydropic infant with complete heart block) this may be a striking finding. Finally, the temperature and surface characteristics of the skin may provide meaningful information as to overall peripheral perfusion.

## EXERCISE 6

Refer to the Exercise 6 table on page 274, and by placing a check mark in the appropriate space, match each of the physiological disturbances in the table with one or more of the clinical signs.

*Auscultation* in the newborn infant may be less helpful than in later life but can be important in evaluating the neonate with possible heart disease. As elsewhere in pediatrics, particular emphasis should be placed on evaluating the second heart sound. To the inexperienced ear, the fast neonatal heart rate challenges precise evaluation of the components of the second heart sound and thus extra attention may be necessary. Absence of the normal physiological splitting of the second heart sound is a significant finding and should be one of the "red flags" signaling congenital heart disease. Atresia of either great vessel will be associated with a single second heart sound, as will d-transposition of the great arteries in which the great vessels have an abnormal anterior-posterior relationship. Pulmonary hypertension associated with large right-to-left shunts will increase the intensity of the second heart sound (pulmonic component) and tend to narrow the split. Conversely, it is important to note excessive splitting of the second heart sound. Wide, *fixed* splitting (which does not vary with respiration) is associated with atrial level communications (large atrial septal defect, common atrium) or with right heart lesions such as Ebstein's anomaly. Anomalous pulmonary venous return in which the pulmonary veins drain into the systemic venous circulation or right heart may also be associated with the presence of a widely split second heart sound.

While all murmurs must be noted and described, a loud murmur may be indicative of a relatively benign situation, whereas some potentially lethal lesions may not be associated with any murmur. The most common murmurs detected in the newborn period involve the ductus arteriosus and, thus, may be transient in nature. It is also important to remember that right-to-left shunts are not associated with murmurs, and thus the intensely cyanotic infant with idiopathic persistent pulmonary hypertension (persistent fetal circulation syndrome) may not have a murmur even though massive right-to-left ductal or atrial shunting is present. In these babies, tricuspid insufficiency is often the cause of a systolic murmur. Finally, in some infants who have been asphyxiated, diminished cardiac output and heart failure may occur in the absence of a murmur.

The loudest murmurs in neonates are often those caused by atrioventricular valve regurgitation. Thus, in the postasphyxial infant, a holosystolic murmur along the right sternal border radiating toward the left should prompt you to consider tricuspid insufficiency as the cause. Similarly, in the cyanotic baby with diminished pulmonary blood flow and cardiomegaly, you should consider the possibility of pulmonic valve obstruction and associated tricuspid insufficiency if you hear a long systolic murmur over the right precordium. As a general rule, stenotic murmurs at the level of the semilunar valve are harsh, ejection-type murmurs, which are loudest in midsystole. These murmurs are frequently associated with a sharp single midsystolic sound termed a *click.* Insufficiency murmurs at the level of the atrioventricular valve level are long, nearly holosystolic, and "blowing" in quality.

Continuous murmurs are of particular interest in infancy because they represent one of the classic findings of PDA. However, the multicenter collaborative study evaluating the ductus in prematurity found that in 10% of the cases of PDA documented by other methods, a murmur was not present, and that in 60% only a systolic murmur could be heard. Thus, a continuous murmur was present in only 30% of a large number of premature babies (more than 400) with PDA. In evaluating the premature or term newborn infant with a continuous murmur, the examiner must be aware of other diagnostic possibilities because a variety of malformations can be associated with a continuous murmur (Table 12-6). The evaluation of the newborn infant with suspected cardiac disease should also include auscultation over noncardiac areas. This is particularly true in the child with congestive heart failure because bruits or murmurs may be au-

**Exercise 6**

CLINICAL SIGNS

| PHYSIOLOGICAL DISTURBANCES | 1. CYANOSIS | 2. HYPERACTIVE PULSES | 3. WHEEZING | 4. INCREASED BP IN UPPER EXTREMITIES | 5. HYPERPNEA | 6. TACHYPNEA | 7. CARDIOMEGALY | 8. DIMINISHED PERIPHERAL PULSES |
|---|---|---|---|---|---|---|---|---|
| A. Decreased myocardial contractility | | | | | | | | |
| B. Elevated pulmonary vascular resistance | | | | | | | | |
| C. Increased right ventricular afterload | | | | | | | | |
| D. Increased left ventricular afterload | | | | | | | | |
| E. Increased left ventricular preload | | | | | | | | |
| F. Large left-to-right shunt | | | | | | | | |

**Table 12-6** Causes of Continuous Murmurs in the Newborn Infant

*Acyanotic*‑‑‑‑‑‑‑‑‑‑‑‑‑‑‑‑‑‑‑‑‑‑‑‑‑‑‑‑‑‑‑‑‑‑‑‑‑‑‑‑‑‑‑‑‑‑‑‑‑‑‑‑‑

Patent ductus arteriosus

Coronary arteriovenous fistula

Other arteriovenous fistulas (pulmonary; intercostal)

Aorticopulmonary window

Peripheral pulmonic stenosis

*Cyanotic*‑‑‑‑‑‑‑‑‑‑‑‑‑‑‑‑‑‑‑‑‑‑‑‑‑‑‑‑‑‑‑‑‑‑‑‑‑‑‑‑‑‑‑‑‑‑‑‑‑‑‑‑‑‑‑

Truncus arteriosus

Total anomalous pulmonary venous drainage (to right atrium or superior vena cava)

Absent pulmonary valve leaflet syndrome (actually a "to-and-fro" murmur)

dible over the cranium or liver, indicating the presence of an arteriovenous fistula.

## EXERCISE 7

Refer to the Exercise 7 table on page 276, and by placing a check mark in the appropriate space, relate each auscultatory finding in the table with one or more of the cardiac lesions listed across the top of the table.

## EXERCISE 8

Refer to the Exercise 8 table on page 277, and by placing a check mark in the appropriate space, match each of the cardiac lesions in the table with one or more of the clinical findings.

Complementing a detailed physical examination, appropriate laboratory studies should be carried out in the newborn infant with suspected heart disease both to clarify diagnostic possibilities and to initiate a therapeutic plan. Although it is beyond the scope of this discussion to describe in detail special procedures such as cardiac catheterization, the generalist who is initially called on to see the sick newborn infant should be well versed in a number of laboratory tools.

## ARTERIAL BLOOD GAS

In nearly every situation in which heart disease is suspected, arterial blood gases should be obtained early in the evaluation. Certainly, if cyanotic heart disease is questioned, determination of arterial $PO_2$ ($PaO_2$) can be helpful. In particular, a comparison of the $PaO_2$ obtained in room air with one measured while the child is breathing 100% oxygen will help establish the presence of a fixed intracardiac right-to-left shunt. In certain situations, meaningful information can be obtained by obtaining paired blood gas samples from preductal and postductal sites. In the presence of a right-to-left ductal level shunt, as seen in the persistent fetal circulation syndrome, for example, a right radial blood gas may have a considerably higher $PaO_2$ (>20 mm Hg) than that measured from the umbilical artery. Thus, umbilical artery (descending aorta) desaturation may not in itself be sufficient to establish the presence of an anatomic intracardiac defect.

Attention should also be paid to pH and $PaCO_2$ as well. In the newborn infant with congestive heart failure, significant alveolar hypoventilation can occur, leading to retention of carbon dioxide. Cyanosis in this case is related to right-to-left shunting within the lung and signifies perfusion of poorly ventilated alveoli. Elevation of the $PaCO_2$ will also frequently be a part of this picture. In contrast, the child with cyanotic heart disease and reduced pulmonary blood flow will often exhibit increased alveolar ventilation, and thus hypocarbia, respiratory alkalosis, and an elevated pH. The presence of acidemia in a cyanotic infant, therefore, is a grave sign and indicates an urgent need for improvement in pulmonary perfusion. Similarly, in a child with impaired systemic perfusion, as in various forms of left ventricular outflow obstruction, systemic acidemia should be viewed as an indication for in-depth evaluation and therapy on an urgent basis. Transcutaneous oximetry has also been used extensively in neonates to evaluate the oxygenation status. While this tool is helpful, important caveats must be remembered when you interpret information derived from transcutaneous monitors. First, these monitors reflect oxygen saturation only; thus the results are affected by more than intracardiac shunting conditions. In particular, peripheral vaso-

CARDIAC LESION

| AUSCULTATORY FINDING | 1. d-TRANS-POSITION OF THE GREAT ARTERIES | 2. TRICUSPID REGURGI-TATION | 3. TOTAL ANOMAL-OUS PUL-MONARY VENOUS DRAINAGE | 4. PERSIS-TENT FETAL CIRCU-LATION | 5. PULMON-ARY ATRE-SIA | 6. VENTRI-CULAR SEP-TAL DEFECT | 7. AORTIC STEN-OSIS | 8. PATENT DUCTUS ARTERIO-SUS | 9. EBSTEIN'S ANOMALY |
|---|---|---|---|---|---|---|---|---|---|
| A. Widely split $S_2$ | | | | | | | | | |
| B. Single $S_2$ | | | | | | | | | |
| C. "Quadruple" rhythm | | | | | | | | | |
| D. Ejection click | | | | | | | | | |
| E. Holosystolic murmur | | | | | | | | | |
| F. Continuous murmur | | | | | | | | | |
| G. No mur-mur | | | | | | | | | |

# Exercise 8

PHYSICAL FINDINGS

| CARDIAC LESIONS | 1. DECREASED PULSES IN ALL EXTREMITIES | 2. HYPERPNEA | 3. HEART FAILURE WITHOUT HEART MURMUR | 4. RIGHT ARM BLOOD PRESSURE LESS THAN LEFT ARM BLOOD PRESSURE | 5. DIFFERENTIAL CYANOSIS | 6. CRANIAL BRUIT |
|---|---|---|---|---|---|---|
| A. Supraventricular tachycardia | | | | | | |
| B. d-TGA with PDA | | | | | | |
| C. Arteriovenous malformation | | | | | | |
| D. Postasphyxial syndrome | | | | | | |
| E. Pulmonary atresia | | | | | | |
| F. Aberrant right subclavian artery with coarctation of the aorta | | | | | | |

construction may affect the data. Furthermore, the sensitivity of these instruments is limited at extreme PaO$_2$ values. In general, transcutaneous oxygen saturation meters are most useful for trend analysis in following responses to therapy.

## OTHER BLOOD STUDIES

A complete blood count including a white cell differential count should be obtained early in the evaluation of an infant with suspected cardiac disease to rule out bacterial sepsis or viral infection. However, no single white cell parameter is diagnostic for these possibilities. It is also important to note the hemoglobin concentration because polycythemia itself can influence cardiovascular performance. Pulmonary vascular resistance may be markedly increased in the presence of the increased viscosity, and both heart failure and cyanosis can occur with normal cardiac anatomy if the red cell mass is excessive. Detailed analysis of hemoglobin may be necessary at times. For example, the infant with methemoglobinemia can manifest severe cyanosis and resemble the infant with cyanotic heart disease quite closely. Electrolytes (sodium, potassium, chloride) can also be of value in assessing the child with possible cardiovascular disease and can aid in the detection of adrenal insufficiency, a rare cause of cardiovascular instability in the newborn infant. Biochemical evaluation of renal function, as reflected in the blood urea nitrogen and creatinine, and monitoring of urine output can be helpful as clues to overall systemic perfusion and can serve as a guide to therapeutic decisions in the child with congestive heart failure. It is particularly important for the patient with PDA when you are considering the possible use of indomethacin. Glucose and calcium should also be assayed. Hypoglycemia is a well-known cause of cardiomegaly and congestive heart failure, which mimics structural heart disease. Disorders of calcium metabolism, in particular DiGeorge syndrome, are associated with specific cardiac anomalies (Table 12-5). Additionally, hypocalcemia from any etiology may have a significant negative inotropic effect. These hematologic and biochemical tests can be carried out in nearly all routine nurseries and should provide the physician with information that may significantly influence subsequent decisions.

## EXERCISE 9

From the following list of structures usually identifiable on the routine chest x-ray, label the area on the x-ray that represents the structure by placing the abbreviation in the appropriate area on the x-rays shown.

| Superior vena cava | (SVC) |
| Right atrium | (RA) |
| Right ventricle | (RV) |
| Left atrium | (LA) |
| Left ventricle | (LV) |
| Ascending aorta | (AA) |
| Pulmonary artery | (PA) |

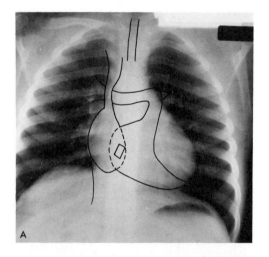

A

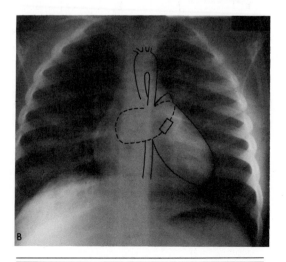

B

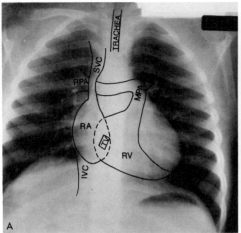
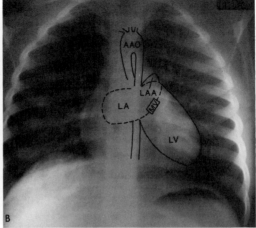

**Figure 12-11** (A) Normal anteroposterior chest x-ray film of the heart. Superimposed are the major venous structures. (B) Same x-ray film with superimposed major arterial structures. RA = right atrium, RV = right ventricle, IVC and SVC = inferior and superior vena cava, MPA = main pulmonary artery, TV = tricuspid valve, LA = left atrium, LV = left ventricle, MV = mitral valve, LAA = left atrial appendage.

## CHEST X-RAY

The chest x-ray is a widely available, easily performed test that should be part of the initial examination in every infant with suspected cardiovascular disease. The importance of the chest x-ray is evident if you consider the diagnostic possibilities according to the concepts outlined in the preceding sections. While in most situations involving the newborn infant a full four-view x-ray series is not mandatory, care should be taken to scrutinize carefully the cardiothoracic information available on the routine anterior-posterior and lateral studies. The physician should attempt to answer the following questions from the chest x-ray:

1. Is the heart enlarged?
2. Is the pulmonary blood flow increased or decreased?
3. What is the location of the aortic arch?
4. What is the position of the heart in the chest?
5. Is there primary pulmonary pathology?
6. Are the abdominal viscera normally located?
7. What is the pulmonary venous pattern?

Figure 12-11 details the cardiac structures as visualized on the normal chest x-ray film. Care should be taken to distinguish the normal thymic shadow from true cardiomegaly because in the normal newborn infant the thy-

mus is considerably enlarged. Despite thymus enlargement, overt cardiomegaly in the newborn infant is still recognizable. The side of the aortic arch can also be helpful in categorizing the diagnostic possibilities, especially when viewed within the context of the pulmonary vascular pattern. For example, the presence of a right-sided aortic arch and decreased pulmonary flow should bring to mind the possibility of tetralogy of Fallot, whereas a right aortic arch and increased flow in a child with arterial hypoxemia should suggest truncus arteriosus (Figs. 12-12 and 12-13). Left ventric-

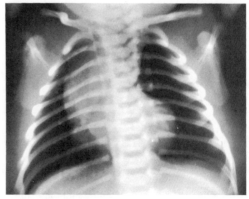

**Figure 12-12** Right-sided aortic arch and prominent apex are seen in this x-ray film from an infant with tetralogy of Fallot. The pulmonary vascular markings are reduced.

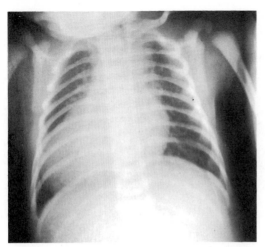

**Figure 12-13** Cardiomegaly and increased pulmonary blood flow in a child with truncus arteriosus. A right aortic arch is present.

ular obstructions are typified by extreme cardiomegaly and pulmonary venous engorgement (Fig. 12-14).

## ELECTROCARDIOGRAPHY

The electrocardiogram is another standard test that should be obtained when you evaluate the newborn infant for heart disease. Again, a systematic approach is best as you review the electrocardiogram, and it is helpful to ask several specific questions. What is the

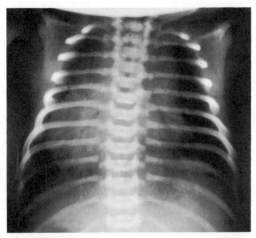

**Figure 12-14** Cardiomegaly and pulmonary congestion in a newborn infant with severe coarctation of the aorta. Despite thymic shadow, enlargement of the heart is obvious. Air bronchograms are consistent with pulmonary consolidation.

rate and rhythm? Where is the electrical axis? Are the voltages appropriate? Are the S-T and T waves normal? Assessment should also include measurement of electrocardiographic intervals (P-R, Q-T, and so forth). The electrocardiogram of the newborn infant is unique and care must be taken not to interpret neonatal data from the perspective of the electrocardiogram of an adult or older child. For example, right ventricular predominance is the norm for the newborn infant; left axis deviation is often abnormal, and a typical newborn heart rate is 120 to 140 beats per minute (BPM). Thus, the normal mean frontal axis is between 100 and 150 degrees and there should be an R wave dominance in the right precordial leads. In a patient with superiorly oriented axis (negative AVF deflection), a high suspicion of cardiac disease should exist. Similarly the T waves in the right chest leads ($V_1$, $V_{4R}$) may be upright on the first day of life, but after 72 hours T wave deflections should be negative (Fig. 12-15). Failure to proceed through this change should raise the suspicion of abnormal right ventricular hypertrophy.

Probably the most important acute feature the general physician should assess on the neonatal electrocardiogram is the rhythm. Both abnormally slow and abnormally fast rhythms can be associated with significant neonatal cardiovascular disease. Supraventricular tachycardia (Fig. 12-16) can be a cause of neonatal heart failure despite a completely normal structural cardiac anatomy. This rhythm disturbance is characterized by a heart rate of 240 to 300 BPM. Although not always the case, P waves are frequently absent on the electrocardiogram. Supraventricular tachycardia may arise *in utero* and be a cause of neonatal hydrops. More commonly, the disturbance occurs after the first week of life, although about 20% of the cases are discovered during the first week. If supraventricular tachycardia persists untreated for more than a few hours, clinical disturbances frequently appear. Hypothermia and feeding intolerance are early signs of abnormally fast rhythms, and by 24 hours congestive heart failure is usually obvious. Thus, treatment is necessary on discovery of the disorder.

In infants with supraventricular tachycardias, it is important to closely examine the post-tachycardia electrocardiogram (as well as that done during the fast heart rate episode) because the Wolff-Parkinson-White syndrome

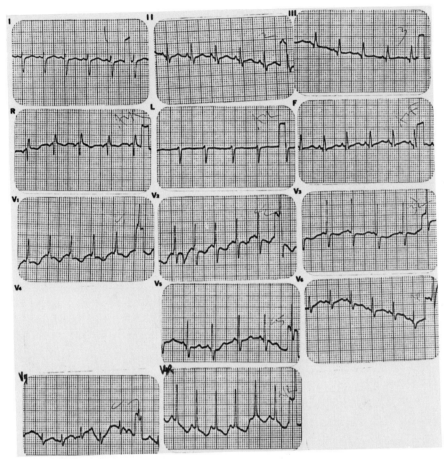

**Figure 12-15** Normal electrocardiogram in a 2-day-old, full-term infant. The predominantly negative forces in lead I indicate a right axis deviation. The rate is 165 per minute calculated by dividing the number of boxes between complexes into 1,500. Since a P wave precedes each QRS complex regularly, there is sinus rhythm. Tall R waves in the right chest leads (V$_1$, V$_2$, V$_4$R) and relatively less voltage in the left chest leads (V$_6$, V$_7$) are typical. The inverted T waves in the right chest leads are normal after the infant is 24 to 72 hours of age.

will often be evident on the postsupraventricular tachycardia tracing when it is not noticeable during the tachycardia. Wolff-Parkinson-White syndrome is characterized by a short P-R interval, a widened QRS, and a slurred upstroke of the R wave ("delta wave") as noted in Figure 12-17. It is important to recognize the Wolff-Parkinson-White syndrome because it may be more refractory to medical management than other forms of supraventricular tachycardia, and it implies a different mechanism of action, namely, the existence of an accessory electrical pathway that can bypass the normal conduction route under appropriate circumstances. Addition-

ally, Wolff-Parkinson-White syndrome is a frequent finding in congenital heart lesions such as Ebstein's anomaly of the tricuspid valve. Supraventricular tachycardia of any cause must be differentiated from sinus tachycardia. Observation of the complexes on an oscilloscopic monitor is not sufficient for this purpose, and, at minimum, an electrocardiogram rhythm strip of lead II should be done in suspect cases. A full electrocardiogram is optimal. Other atrial rhythm disturbances, such as atrial flutter and atrial fibrillation, can also occur in the neonatal period and must be promptly recognized.

At the other end of the rhythm spectrum,

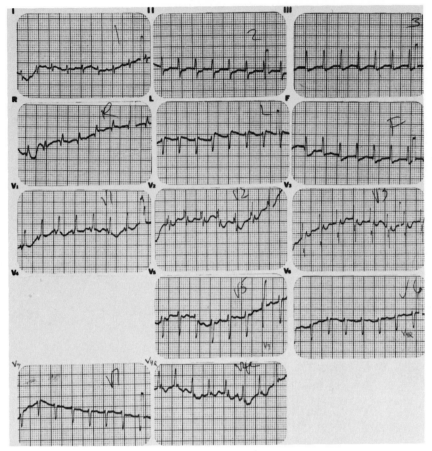

**Figure 12-16**   Electrocardiogram of an infant with supraventricular tachycardia (SVT). The rate is 185. Note the very regular rhythm and the absence of visible P waves.

congenital complete heart block can also be a cause of congestive heart failure in the newborn infant. It, too, may be initiated *in utero* and result in neonatal hydrops and fetal distress. The association of congenital complete heart block with maternal systemic lupus erythematosus has been well documented. In about one-third of the cases, congenital complete heart block is associated with complex heart disease including corrected transposition of the great arteries, endocardial cushion defects, and single ventricle. Cardiomyopathies also have been associated with congenital complete heart block. By definition, congenital heart block represents a failure of the propagation of the electrical impulse with independent activation of the chamber distal to the site of the block. Thus, the atria and ventricles are dissociated, with the atria beat-

ing at a faster rate than the ventricles (Fig. 12-18). A critical factor in the determination of symptom development is the ventricular rate. Distress is usually evident with ventricular rates below 40 to 45 BPM and rarely evident with rates greater than 60 to 70 BPM. However, the presence of anatomic cardiac disease or other extra cardiac disease may modify this picture and result in significant symptoms even at higher ventricular rates. Congenital complete heart block should be differentiated from sinus bradycardia, and, as with supraventricular tachycardia, an electrocardiogram is preferable for this purpose.

Other arrhythmias exist in the neonatal period and require evaluation, which is best accomplished by electrocardiography. These include less severe degrees of heart block, which are frequently related to digoxin therapy, and

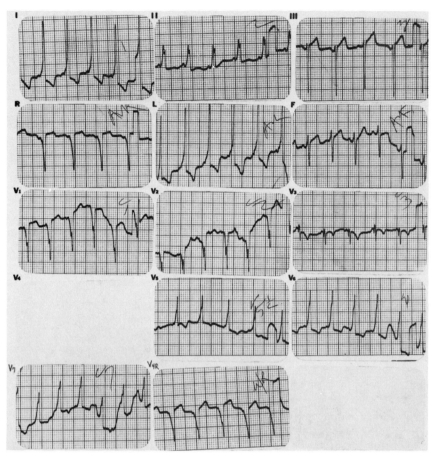

**Figure 12-17** Electrocardiogram in Wolff-Parkinson-White (WPW) syndrome. Slurring of the upstroke of the QRS ("delta" wave) is readily visible in leads I, AVL, V$_5$, V$_6$, and V$_7$. Widening of the QRS with a bundle branch block pattern is also present. The P-R interval is 0.06, which is short. The rate is 136 per minute.

other forms of tachycardia. Ventricular tachycardia in a neonate is frequently noted in association with other significant problems such as anatomic congenital heart disease, electrolyte imbalance, or myocardial disease and may at times be difficult to manage. As a general rule, in an infant with wide complex tachycardia, you should assume that ventricular tachycardia is present even though subsequent evaluation may prove otherwise.

Thus, the standard laboratory investigations generally available for evaluating the newborn infant with possible heart disease include (1) arterial blood gas analyses (in room air and in increased inspired oxygen), (2) hematologic and biochemical profiles, (3) chest x-ray, and (4) electrocardiogram. In most instances, enough information can be obtained

from these basic procedures to determine whether a cardiac problem exists and what the general nature of the problem is likely to be. In

## EXERCISE 10

Using the Exercise 10 figure at the top of page 284, identify each of the following ECG strips:

| | A B C D E |
|---|---|
| 1. Basic rhythm | _____ |
| 2. Ventricular rate | _____ |
| 3. Atrial rate | _____ |
| 4. Need for therapy (yes/no) | _____ |

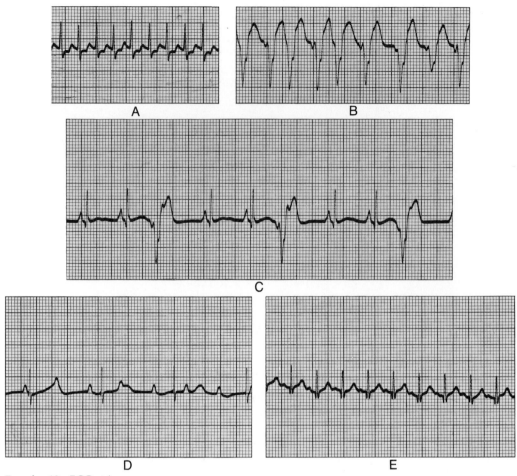

**Exercise 10**   ECG strips.

certain instances, a rather specific diagnosis can be derived when these tests are interpreted in the perspective of the clinical findings.

## ECHOCARDIOGRAPHY

Echocardiography has become a relatively first line tool in the evaluation of the child with heart disease, particularly the newborn infant. While it is beyond the scope of this discussion to discuss in detail echocardiography in the evaluation of congenital heart disease, the general physician caring for newborn infants should be aware of its availability and utility. The echocardiogram offers the cardiologist a relatively reliable means of pinpointing the cardiac anatomy for most structural lesions

and frequently obviates the need for more invasive procedures. In ambiguous situations, the echocardiogram is useful for deciding whether a more invasive procedure is indicated at all. The echocardiogram is also useful for serially following changes in cardiac performance and thus provides a more direct view of the efficacy of therapy than may otherwise be available. For anatomic delineation, two-dimensional (real-time) echocardiography offers the best noninvasive information (Fig. 12-19). The addition of color flow Doppler mapping of blood flow patterns is an important adjunct, which helps to further define not only anatomy but also the physiological impact of anatomic defects.

The echocardiogram has become the principal tool for diagnosis and assessment of ther-

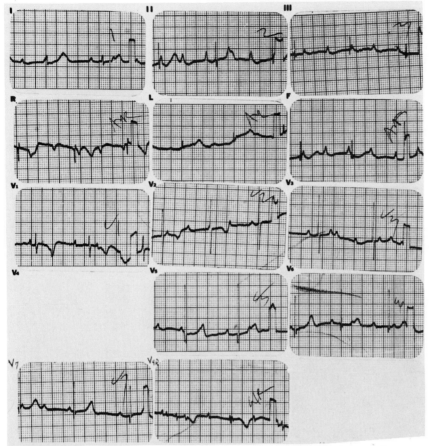

**Figure 12-18** Electrocardiogram in complete heart block. Note the absence of any regular relationship of P waves and QRS complexes. The atrial rate (p-p) is approximately 140 and the ventricular rate (R-R) is approximately 65.

apy in patent ductus arteriosus of prematurity. Doppler flow mapping, enhanced by color encoding, has made this definitive for PDA assessment (Fig. 12-20) and echocardiography is considered a precise indicator of ductal shunting. The hemodynamic effects of the ductus can thus easily be discerned and lesions that might become apparent without compensatory ductal flow (see next section) can be unmasked before pharmacological therapy is instituted.

**TREATMENT ISSUES**

While most infants with significant cardiac disease will be cared for by a pediatric cardiologist trained to handle the complex management issues of congenital heart disease, many situations arise in which the general pediatrician caring for newborn infants can provide a critical degree of care. Additionally, important steps often need to be taken relatively early in the infant's course, even before formal cardiologic assessment may be available, which may significantly affect the overall outcome for the infant.

Certainly, for the critically ill newborn infant with any form of cardiovascular disease, the general measures that are cardinal features of newborn care must also be applied. Thus, hypoglycemia and hypocalcemia must be corrected, temperature control maintained, acidosis managed, and infection treated. Artificial airway support and mechanical ventilation may also be necessary to improve any ventilation-perfusion imbalance that may be present.

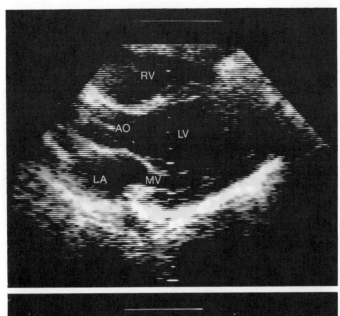

A

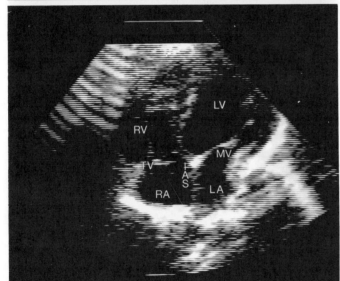

B

**Figure 12-19** (A) Two-dimensional echocardiographic cut in the long axis at the level of the left ventricular outflow tract. RV = right ventricle, LV = left ventricle, AO = aorta, LA = left atrium, MV = mitral valve. (B) Two-dimensional echocardiographic cut in the short axis at the apex showing the four cardiac chambers. TV = tricuspid valve, IAS = interatrial septum. Other abbreviations as before. (C) Standard short-axis, two-dimensional echocardiogram image of normally related great vessels. Aorta = double arrow, pulmonary artery = single arrow. (D) Standard short-axis two-dimensional echocardiogram view in d-TGA. Aorta = single arrow (arrow pointing to right coronary coming from aorta), double arrow = pulmonary artery posterior to aorta in this anomaly.

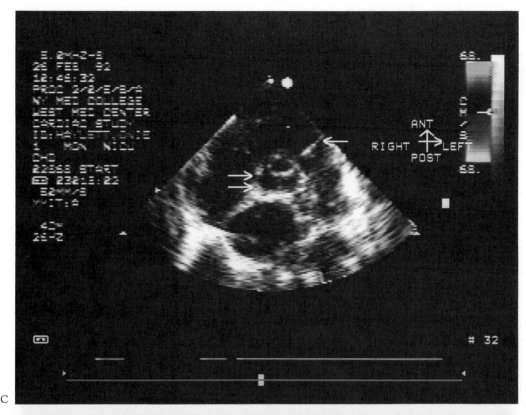

C

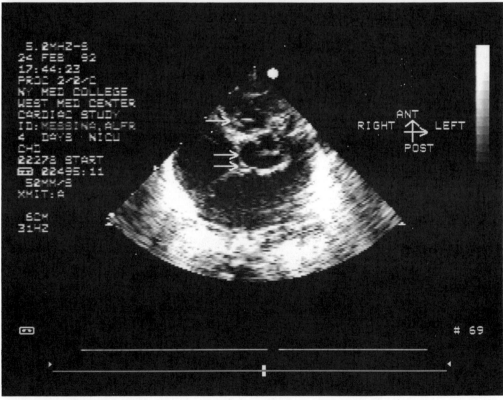

D

**Figure 12-19** *Continued*

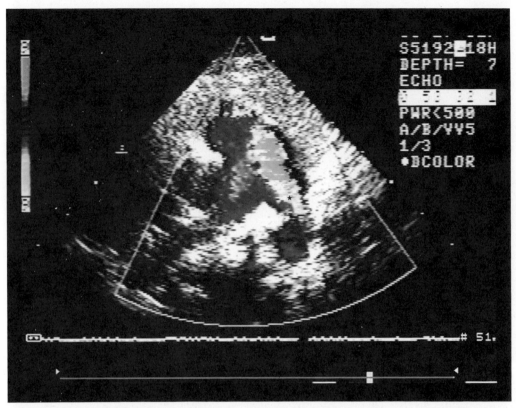

**Figure 12-20**  Two-dimensional echocardiogram with Doppler encoding showing abnormal ductal flow stream (plume*) entering into the pulmonary artery in the presence of a patent ductus arteriosus.

## DUCTAL MANIPULATION

Specific measures aimed at improving cardiac function depend on the nature of the defect. In some circumstances measures to promote ductal closure are necessary, whereas in others, methods aimed at promoting ductal patency are preferable. For the physician taking care of premature newborn infants, the more frequently encountered situation will involve procedures to close a PDA complicating the clinical course of the neonate with RDS. The nonsteroidal anti-inflammatory drug indomethacin has been extensively used to reduce the circulating concentration of dilating prostaglandins by inhibiting metabolism of the prostaglandin cascade. As noted previously, caution must be exercised to verify by echocardiography the absence of a situation in which either systemic or pulmonary blood flow is dependent on the patency of the ductus arteriosus. After this has been done and the diagnosis of patent ductus arteriosus with a significant left-to-right shunt has been established, indomethacin may be administered. At present, most clinicians employ a dosage of 0.1 to 0.2 mg/kg given intravenously and repeat it every 8 to 12 hours for three doses.

The effect of indomethacin, of course, is not limited to the patent ductus arteriosus, and prostaglandin inhibition occurs throughout the body. Because renal blood flow may be significantly affected, renal function should be assessed before the drug is administered. An abnormality in renal function, as reflected by an elevated blood urea nitrogen or creatinine (>1.8 mg/dL) or a decrease in urine output, is a contraindication to the use of indomethacin. Other contraindications to indomethacin include abnormalities in coagulation, evidence of thrombocytopenia, the presence of active central nervous system bleeding, or necrotizing enterocolitis. The efficacy of the drug should be assessed by a detailed follow-up clinical examination and laboratory evidence of decreased left-to-right shunting. A chest x-ray film showing signs of decreased pulmonary blood flow and an echocardiogram revealing decreased ductal flow are helpful to ascertain therapeutic results. The ductus may be functionally closed but not anatomically sealed. Thus, even after evidence of closure following a course of indomethacin, reemergence of the ductus arteriosus may occur and require further therapy.

Surgical closure of the PDA is certainly definitive and in most centers is carried out with exceedingly little morbidity and almost no mortality. The decision to use surgical as opposed to medical measures must be based on practical considerations. Are there contraindications to indomethacin? What are the availability and accessibility of surgical personnel? These are factors that must be determined obviously on an individual patient and center basis.

Manipulation of the PDA to maintain its patency is a maneuver of which all medical personnel caring for newborn infants should be aware. $PGE_1$ has become the agent of choice for this procedure because it is a potent ductal dilating prostaglandin and can be infused directly into the ductus through an indwelling central catheter or, more simply, into a peripheral vein. Clinical results have substantiated the efficacy of either approach, and infants can be maintained on a peripheral intravenous infusion of $PGE_1$ for several weeks until they reach a weight that permits successful surgery. Conditions in which ductal manipulation to maintain patency can be life-saving are listed in Table 12-7. While in most circumstances this drug should be administered under the supervision of a cardiologist, therapy can be initiated before a cardiovascular specialist is available for the child with cardiovascular collapse in whom a ductal-dependent

**Table 12-7** Ductal-Dependent Cardiac Lesions

---

***Ductal-dependent pulmonary blood flow***............

Pulmonary atresia with intact ventricular septum

Tricuspid atresia

Critical pulmonary stenosis

***Ductal-dependent systemic blood flow***................

Coarctation of the aorta

Aortic arch interruption

Hypoplastic left heart syndrome (aortic atresia)

---

lesion is suspected. Current recommended infusion doses are 0.05 to 0.1 $\mu$g/kg/min.

In addition to pharmacological therapy, appropriate manipulation of shunting through a PDA can be crucial for successful management of newborns with ductal-dependent systemic blood flow. These infants may be particularly sensitive to the ratio of systemic to pulmonary vascular resistance. Contrary to the usual pulmonary management of infants with cardiorespiratory disease, efforts in these circumstances should be directed at maintaining an elevated pulmonary vascular resistance in order to enhance right-to-left ductal flow. Thus, maintenance of $PCO_2$ at higher levels than usually deemed acceptable (>50 torr) may be required and iatrogenic hyperventilation should be avoided. Some centers currently administer carbon dioxide as part of the ventilatory gas mixture to achieve this goal, although this is an investigational approach at present.

## MEDICAL THERAPY FOR CONGESTIVE HEART FAILURE

The medical treatment of the infant with congestive heart failure is relatively straightforward when the problem is approached from the perspective of the physiological principles outlined earlier in this chapter under the heading "Physiological Manifestations of Cardiac Disease in the Newborn Infant." Thus, manipulations aimed at affecting the basic factors regulating cardiac output will be employed.

If congestive heart failure is found to be related to large-volume left-to-right shunting, as in ventricular septal defect or a common mixing lesion, several steps are in order. The time-tested agent of choice to improve contractility is digitalis in the form of digoxin (Lanoxin), which can be administered by intravenous, intravascular, or oral routes. Intramuscular digitalis is frequently painful, however, and absorption of digoxin from an intramuscular injection may be variable, especially in the infant with poor perfusion as a result of heart failure. Extreme caution must be used in ordering and administering parenteral digoxin to infants, since serious mistakes have frequently been committed through transcription or mathematical error. Recent data have suggested that the dose should be modified on a weight basis and have challenged the caveat that the infant may have a higher threshold to digitalis toxicity. Table 12-8 reviews dosing schedules for digoxin. Serum potassium should be monitored in a patient receiving digoxin because hypokalemia can potentiate the effects of digoxin and precipitate toxicity.

In the newborn infant, signs of digitalis toxicity principally include rhythm disturbances and feeding intolerance, specifically vomiting. Sinus bradycardia and forms of heart block are probably the most frequently observed side effects, but the development of tachyarrhythmias of either ventricular or supraventricular origin has been noted. As a general rule, the emergence of an arrhythmia in a patient on digoxin should be considered a sign of digitalis toxicity unless proven otherwise. The use of serum digitalis levels may be helpful in the evaluation of infants receiving digitalis therapy, but data regarding the specific association between a given digitalis level and toxicity in infants are not reliable. It is important to note the time of digitalis administration, since the level drawn should reflect steady-state kinetics and not peak levels. Therefore, at least 6 hours should elapse between the administration of the drug and the determination of the level. Administering digitalis will improve contractility and will also slow the heart rate by means of direct and indirect effects.

Congestive heart failure can also be treated by manipulation of intravascular volume status. In the premature newborn infant with congestive heart failure secondary to a PDA, intravenous fluid restriction and diuretic therapy alone may produce dramatic results. In most other circumstances, diuretics and digoxin should be administered concurrently. Furosemide has achieved wide acceptance as the initial diuretic and should be given parenterally in a dose of 1 to 2 mg/kg. This is usually administered at 12-hour intervals. While many centers continue furosemide as the maintenance diuretic, others prefer chlorothiazide (20 mg/kg/day) because there is an incidence of nephracalcinosis that occurs with chronic furosemide therapy. Potassium supplementation, either as potassium chloride elixir or by use of spironolactone (2 mg/kg/day), is indicated if daily diurectics are used.

The importance of maintaining the hematocrit above anemic levels is of particular merit in the newborn infant with heart failure. It is a frequent clinical observation that heart failure may be worsened in the presence of anemia, even the physiological anemia of infancy. Thus, transfusion to raise the hematocrit in the anemic infant with heart failure from any cause should be considered a primary form of therapy.

**Table 12-8**   Digitalization

**A.** *Usual doses (intramuscular or oral; intravenous doses are 75% of oral or intramuscular dose):*

| | WEIGHT (G) | TOTAL DIGITALIZING DOSE |
|---|---|---|
| Prematures | 500–1,000 | 20 μg/kg or 0.02 mg/kg |
| | 1,000–1,500 | 20–30 μg/kg or 0.02–0.03 mg/kg |
| | 1,500–2,000 | 30 μg/kg or 0.03 mg/kg |
| | 2,000–2,500 | 30–40 μg/kg or 0.03–0.04 mg/kg |
| Full term to 1 month | | 50–60 μg/kg or 0.05–0.06 mg/kg |

**B.** *Alterations in usual doses:*

1. Lower if renal function is impaired
2. Lower in presence of poor myocardial function (cardiomyopathy, myocarditis)
3. Lower in presence of metabolic imbalance, electrolyte abnormalities, hypoxia, acidosis

**C.** *Method:*

1. ½ dose immediately
2. ¼ dose 4 to 6 hours after initial dose
3. ¼ dose 4 to 6 hours following second dose
4. Maintenance dose is ⅛ of total digitalizing dose given in 2 doses per day 12 hours apart and begun 12 hours after last digitalizing dose.

Intravenous infusion of catecholamines may at times be required for cardiovascular collapse in the newborn infant. In severe forms of left ventricular outflow obstruction, such as aortic stenosis or coarctation of the aorta, this support can result in a dramatic improvement in peripheral perfusion, acid-base balance, and urine output, and help to decrease subsequent surgical mortality and morbidity. For this purpose, dopamine (2 to 10 $\mu$g/kg/min) or isoproterenol (0.05 to 0.1 $\mu$g/kg/min) are the preferable agents. In the lower dosage ranges (2 to 5 $\mu$g/kg/min), dopamine will significantly improve renal perfusion independently of its direct inotropic effect on the heart, and is currently the preferred agent. Dobutamine is also used (3 to 10 $\mu$g/kg/min) in this context but there is some controversy regarding its efficacy in premature neonates.

Finally, in certain severe situations in which surgical therapy is not an immediate option, afterload reduction has been used to treat congestive heart failure in the newborn infant. This should be done only under the direct supervision of trained personnel well versed in cardiopulmonary physiology and able to use the appropriate intravascular monitoring systems required. Hydralazine (0.2 mg/kg) has been widely used for this purpose, although nitroprusside has recently become popular because of its substantial, rapid effect. Remember, it is crucial that an infant's central fluid volume be carefully monitored if afterload reduction is used. Ideally, filling pressures such as central venous pressure should be measured whenever this modality is employed.

## ARRHYTHMIAS

As noted earlier, both tachyarrhythmias and bradyarrhythmias can result in significant cardiovascular compromise in the newborn infant, including severe congestive heart failure. In the infant with supraventricular tachycardia (SVT), maneuvers that influence vagal tone are not as successful as they are when carried out in the adult. However, a neurogenic manipulation that has demonstrated efficacy in the infant with SVT is immersion of the face in cold water or application of ice to the face. This induces bradycardia by means of parasympathetic efferents. The baby should be monitored during the procedure because asys-

tole has been reported in experimental situations using the cold water technique.

The more traditional approach to SVT (Table 12-9) has involved the use of digoxin, given parenterally, in doses similar to those given for congestive heart failure. This method is useful as a first line approach for the infant with normal peripheral perfusion and a relatively short history of the tachycardia. However, if evidence of cardiovascular collapse exists, or if the disturbance has been present for an extended period of time, cardioversion with direct current countershock is indicated. With 0.5 to 2.0 W-sec/kg, the SVT can usually be aborted. It is still necessary to commence digoxin (or propranolol) after successful countershock because recurrences are frequent. Propranolol is particularly useful in the Wolff-Parkinson-White syndrome but may be effectively used in other forms of supraventricular tachycardia as well. Verapamil, which inhibits calcium flux, and adenosine, which directly affects cardiac conduction tissue, have also been proposed for use in the newborn infant with SVT. Verapamil, however, can cause marked vasodilation, inducing hypotension and even asystole when used intravenously and thus is not recommended for emergency intravenous treatment of the young infant.

**Table 12-9**  Treatment of SVT

*Acute phase*

Asymptomatic or minimally symptomatic
    Neurogenic maneuver: ice water application to facies
    Transesophageal overdrive pacing
    Intravenous digoxin (see Table 12-8)
    Intravenous procainamide
    Intravenous adenosine

Symptomatic or unstable infant
    Direct current cardioversion (0.5 to 2 W-sec/kg)
    Intravenous adenosine

*Chronic phase*

Without Wolff-Parkinson-White (WPW) syndrome
    Oral digoxin (see Table 12-8)
    Oral propranolol
    Oral verapamil    {sequential
    Oral procainamide  {additions
    Oral amiodarone

With WPW
    Oral propranolol
    Oral verapamil and as above
    Consider electrophysiological assessment to prepare for surgical treatment if refractory to triple drug therapy

Adenosine may be a more useful agent if current investigation confirms its efficacy in the neonate. Finally, overdrive pacing through an electrical catheter placed in the midesophagus is another effective treatment for SVT, to be used by experienced personnel.

The treatment of complete heart block is also dependent on the symptoms. The critically ill newborn infant with hydrops and congenital complete heart block may require intubation, ventilatory support, treatment of acidosis, and maintenance of blood pressure with exogenous catecholamines. In general, these infants will have a ventricular rate below 50. Infusion of isoproterenol may be a helpful temporary measure in these patients until more definitive care (pacemaker therapy) can be arranged. Heart rate itself should not be the sole factor determining the need for pacing, but rather the presence of other signs of cardiac distress should be incorporated into the information needed for a therapeutic decision. It is worth emphasizing that whenever congenital heart block is suspected, experienced cardiologic consultation should be expeditiously sought.

## EXERCISE 11

For each of the conditions listed in the Exercise 11 table on page 293, select the most appropriate treatment by placing a check mark in the appropriate space. More than one treatment modality may apply for a particular condition.

## EXERCISE 12

Place a check mark next to each treatment shown below that should be part of the initial management of a cyanotic newborn infant.

_____1. Administer oxygen.

_____2. Start intravenous antibiotics.

_____3. Observe for 24 to 48 hours with monitoring of heart rate and respiration.

_____4. Administer sodium bicarbonate if ventilation is normal but pH is low.

_____5. Consider infusion of $PGE_1$.

_____6. Initiate enteral feedings to improve intestinal motility.

## SURGICAL THERAPY

Most situations that result in congestive heart failure or cyanosis of cardiac origin in the newborn period ultimately require surgical treatment. It is beyond the scope of this chapter to discuss the details of surgical therapy for congenital heart disease, but the physician caring for newborns should be aware of which situations require immediate surgical attention and which do not, and what surgical approaches are generally available.

Whenever possible, the current approach of most pediatric cardiac surgeons is to perform a complete surgical correction in the immediate newborn period, although there are still situations where surgical palliation is required. The decision to proceed with palliative therapy as opposed to total correction depends on several issues: What is the primary cardiac defect? What are the associated cardiac and extracardiac defects? What is the gestational age and weight of the patient? What is the overall condition of the baby? Can the infant physically tolerate the procedure required to correct the defect totally? These factors must be considered in each case before a decision regarding the proper surgical approach can be made.

For the child with ductal-dependent pulmonary blood flow, prostaglandin infusion as outlined earlier is only a temporary life-saving procedure. More permanent treatment is always necessary either in the newborn period or shortly thereafter. If total repair is not feasible as a newborn, palliation is accomplished through creation of an aortopulmonary communication—a *shunt*—which provides long-term satisfactory pulmonary blood flow. This communication is frequently made between the subclavian artery and the pulmonary artery on the side opposite to the aortic arch (Blalock-Taussig procedure), although under certain circumstances other sites may be used (Fig. 12-21). A proper understanding of the anatomy of the aortic arch vessels is required to create this shunt successfully. It is important to recognize that shunt procedures are used to increase pulmonary blood flow and not to decrease cyanosis *per se*. Intracardiac right-to-left shunting can cause cyanosis without decreasing pulmonary blood flow. Simple d-transposition of the great arteries is a good example of this situation, since marked cyanosis may be apparent despite increased blood flow to the lungs. In such a clinical context, a

**Exercise 11**

TREATMENT

| CONDITION | 1. CARDIOVERSION | 2. PROPRANOLOL | 3. DIGITALIS | 4. INDOMETHACIN | 5. PGE$_1$ | 6. LASIX | 7. NO TREATMENT |
|---|---|---|---|---|---|---|---|
| A. Supraventricular tachycardia | | | | | | | |
| B. Patent ductus arteriosus with congestive heart failure, term infant | | | | | | | |
| C. Coarctation of the aorta with congestive heart failure | | | | | | | |
| D. Pulmonary atresia | | | | | | | |
| E. Premature atrial contractions | | | | | | | |
| F. Patent ductus arteriosus with congestive heart failure, premature infant | | | | | | | |
| G. Congenital heart block, ventricular rate = 85, no congestive heart failure | | | | | | | |

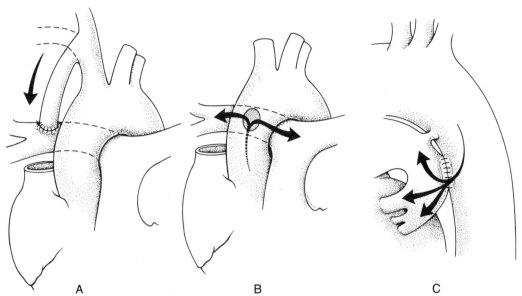

**Figure 12-21** Examples of shunt procedures employed to increase pulmonary blood flow in the newborn period. (A) Subclavian artery (right) to pulmonary anastomosis. (B) Ascending aorta to right pulmonary artery anastomosis. (C) Descending aorta to left pulmonary artery anastomosis.
From Friedman SF: Cardiac disease. In Kaye R, Oski FA, Barness LA: *Core Textbook of Pediatrics.* Philadelphia, JB Lippincott Co, 1982, p. 300. Reprinted with permission of J.B. Lippincott Company.

shunt procedure would only further increase pulmonary flow. It would certainly not be helpful, and may in fact be harmful.

As noted earlier under the heading "Lesions Producing Cyanosis," certain lesions require the establishment of intracardiac mixing in order to ensure an adequate cardiac output, acceptable oxygenation, or both. These lesions include tricuspid atresia, pulmonary valve atresia with a hypoplastic right ventricle, mitral atresia, and several more complex lesions including complex single ventricle states. Usually, this is accomplished at the time of cardiac catheterization by means of the balloon atrial septostomy (Rashkind procedure) in which a hole is iatrogenically created in the atrial septum. If this is unsuccessful, surgical septectomy is sometimes necessary for lesions in which one-stage correction is not possible.

Total intracardiac correction of congenital heart lesions in infants is carried out by open heart surgery using cardiopulmonary bypass, hypothermia, or a combination of both techniques. These procedures permit excellent visualization of the defects with adequate myocardial and visceral protection. Closed heart repairs refer to procedures carried out on extracardiac structures in which cardiopulmonary bypass is not employed. The indications

for open heart surgery in the newborn and the decision for closed heart surgery must also be critically examined in each case. No universal rules apply in either situation, aside from the general principle that total repair is always preferable to palliation if the surgical procedure is possible and safe. Recent improvements in neonatal open heart surgery have been dramatic. Currently, all forms of total anomalous pulmonary venous return are amenable to neonatal complete repair, and the arterial switch operation done within the first 10 to 14 days of life is considered the treatment of choice for simple d-transposition of the great arteries. Surgery as a newborn has become possible for defects previously considered to have uniformly fatal outcomes, such as left ventricular hypoplasia. In this circumstance, current investigations are focused on determining the relative efficacies of neonatal heart transplantation and multistage palliation (Norwood procedure) for this spectrum of defects. With these surgical advances has come increasing responsibility for early accurate diagnosis and effective perioperative medical management of the neonate with congenital heart disease. In addition, new techniques for interventional cardiac catheterization (e.g., balloon angioplasty) are likely to become more applicable to neonatal situations in the years ahead, further increasing the role of nonsurgical management for these babies.

## EXERCISE 13

Place a check mark adjacent to the lesions that may require creation of an intracardiac shunt for palliation.

_____1. d-Transposition of the great arteries

_____2. Tricuspid atresia

_____3. Aortic stenosis

_____4. Total anomalous pulmonary venous return

_____5. Mitral atresia

_____6. Pulmonary atresia

_____7. Truncus arteriosus

## EXERCISE 14

A male baby is normal at birth with Apgar scores of 8 at 1 minute and 9 at 5 minutes. On the second day, cyanosis is noted, but no heart murmur is heard and the baby's respiratory rate is 40 breaths per minute.

How would you proceed to evaluate the baby?

1.



2.



3.



4.



Based on these procedures, the following data are available: $PaO_2$ in 100% oxygen = 21 mm Hg; $PaO_2$ in room air = 18 mm Hg; $PaCO_2$ = 29 mm Hg; pH = 7.48. Chest x-ray reveals moderate cardiomegaly mildly increased pulmonary vascular markings, and a left aortic arch. The ECG shows increased right ventricular forces that are considered normal for age.

5. Can you make a diagnosis at this point?



6. What disorder is most likely?



7. How would you proceed now?



You believe that the baby has cyanotic congenital heart disease, specifically d-transposition of the great arteries. Your cardiologist has been called.

8. What step is the cardiologist likely to take?



The echocardiogram reveals findings consistent with d-transposition of the great arteries.

9. What should happen next?



## EXERCISE 15

A 2-day-old, full-term infant has become quite ill after an otherwise normal postnatal course. Feeding is a problem and the nurse has noted a fast heart rate. The baby is lethargic and "dusky" (appears cyanotic).

How would you evaluate the infant?

1.

2.

3.

4.

5.

pulses in all extremities. There is considerable hepatomegaly and the baby is noted to be tachypneic. A chest x-ray reveals cardiomegaly and pulmonary venous congestion. An ECG shows a ventricular rate of 280 with no P waves visible. Serum electrolytes are normal but the child is mildly acidotic with an arterial pH of 7.27. $PaO_2$ and $PaCO_2$ are normal. Serum glucose and calcium concentrations are normal and the complete blood count does not suggest infection.

6. What is your diagnosis?

7. What do you do?

Examination of the baby reveals decreased blood pressure with poor but equal arterial

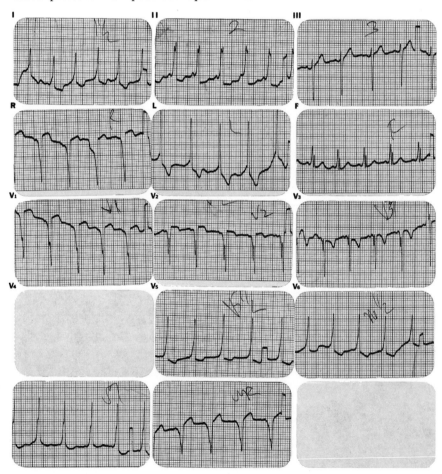

**Exercise 15**  Postconversion ECG.

The baby is quite ill with supraventricular tachycardia. Urgent therapy is required, which often may require the pediatrician to act before cardiac consultation is available. Direct current countershock is indicated for this critically ill infant. Acidosis should be corrected with bicarbonate first, if possible, and the defibrillator should be synchronized to shock on the QRS, if at all possible.

8. What other forms of therapy are possible?

Digoxin is a drug with particular efficacy to treat supraventricular tachycardia in infancy in most situations. One-half the calculated total digitalizing dose can be used initially, given intravenously in the critically ill infant. The remainder of the digitalizing dose is given during the next 16 to 24 hours in divided doses. Risk is increased with the use of cardioversion (countershock) therapy in a digitalized patient, but electrical therapy may be required if improvement has not been accomplished with digoxin.

Countershock has successfully converted the rhythm to sinus and the infant has improved clinically.

9. What should you do now?

A postconversion ECG is shown 296.

10. What does this show and what is the significance of these findings?

11. What should you do now?

While children with supraventricular tachycardia, even confirmed Wolff-Parkinson-White syndrome, can have normal anatomy, further workup to rule out congenital heart disease is indicated. Therapeutically, the child should be started on chronic anti-arrhythmic therapy for 6 to 12 months. In most situations, digoxin is used, but propranolol is an acceptable alternative and, in specific instances such as WPW, is preferable. The important points are that the child may require long-term therapy despite initial conversion, and that evaluation to rule out structural heart disease is indicated.

## ANSWERS TO EXERCISES

### ■ Exercise 1:

A.
1. d
2. a
3. b
4. d

B.
1. Pulmonary vascular smooth muscle development
2. Presence of congenital heart disease
3. Hormonal factors such as prostaglandins, angiotensin, bradykinin, and acetylcholine
4. Arterial oxygenation and acid-base balance
5. Hematocrit level

### ■ Exercise 2:

A. True statements: 2, 3, 4, 5, 6, 7, 8

B. This is a leftward shift of the curve. Responsible factors include alkalosis, hypocarbia ($pCO_2$), hypothermia, and the presence of fetal hemoglobin.

### ■ Exercise 3:

1, 2, 3, 4, 5, 7

### ■ Exercise 4:

A. 2, 4, 6

B. 1, 3, 4

C. 2

D. 2, 5

E. 4

F. 2, 3, 4, 6, 7

G. 3, 4, 6, 7

H. 3, 4, 5

I. 2, 3, 4, 5, 6

J. 1, 3, 4, 7

■ **Exercise 5:**

A. 2

B. 3

C. 5

D. 4

E. 1

F. 6

■ **Exercise 6:**

A. 1, 3, 6, 7, 8

B. 1, 7

C. 1, 5, 7

D. 3, 4, 6, 7, 8

E. 2, 3, 6, 7

F. 2, 3, 6, 7

■ **Exercise 7:**

A. 3, 9

B. 1, 4, 5

C. 9

D. 7

E. 2, 6, 8

F. 8

G. 1, 4, 9

■ **Exercise 8:**

A. 1, 3

B. 2, 5

C. 1, 3, 6

D. 1, 3

E. 2

F. 3, 4

■ **Exercise 9:**

See Figure 12-11.

■ **Exercise 10:**

A. 1. Supraventricular tachycardia
   2. 250
   3. Cannot calculate (probably 250)
   4. Yes
B. 1. Ventricular tachycardia
   2. 200 to 300

3. Probably 140
4. Yes

C. 1. Premature ventricular contractions
   2. 115
   3. 115
   4. Yes, if symptom producing, multifocal, increase with exercise, or if extrasystoles occur in multiples
D. 1. Complete heart block
   2. 65
   3. 150
   4. Yes, if symptom producing or sustained situation after open heart surgery
E. 1. Normal sinus rhythm (sinus tachycardia)
   2. 165
   3. 165
   4. No

■ **Exercise 11:**

A. 1, 2, 3

B. 3, 6

C. 3, 5, 6

D. 5

E. 7

F. 3, 4, 6

G. 7

■ **Exercise 12:**

1, 4, 5

■ **Exercise 13:**

1, 2, 4, 5, 6

■ **Exercise 14:**

1. Obtain arterial blood gases in room air and in 100% inspired oxygen.

2. Obtain chest x-ray.

3. Obtain electrocardiogram.

4. Check hematologic and biochemical profile.

5. Diagnosis of congenital heart disease is likely.

6. Cyanosis plus increased pulmonary blood flow. Suspect d-transposition of the great arteries.

7. Contact the cardiologist.

8. An echocardiogram to confirm diagnosis would be done.

9. The cardiac surgeon should be called to proceed with complete repair. Intermediary cardiac catherization may or may not be required, depending on the clinical details.

■ **Exercise 15:**

1. Full examination

2. Chest x-ray

3. Electrocardiogram

4. Hematologic profile

5. Arterial blood gas

6. Supraventricular tachycardia

7. D-C shock

8. Digoxin; application of cold water or ice to the face; transesophageal overdrive pacing; adenosine

9. Repeat electrocardiogram

10. The tracing shows a delta wave, a short P-R interval, and a widened QRS complex. This is typical of Wolff-Parkinson-White syndrome.

11. Start propranolol therapy. Arrange for a full cardiac workup. Arrange for a serial follow-up and long-term therapy.

## BIBLIOGRAPHY

1. Artman M, Graham TP: Congestive heart failure in infancy: Recognition and management. *Am Heart J* 1982; 102:1040–1055.
2. Buciarelli R, Nelson RM, Eagan EA II, et al: Transient tricuspid insufficiency of the newborn: A form of myocardial dysfunction in stressed newborns. *Pediatrics* 1977; 59:330.
3. Castaneda A: Arterial switch operation for simple and complex TGA-indication criterias and limitations relevant to surgery. *J Thorac Cardiovasc Surg* 1991; 39(supp 2):151.
4. Fox WW, Gewitz MH, Dinwiddie R, et al: Pulmonary hypertension in the perinatal aspiration syndromes. *Pediatrics* 1977; 59:205–211.
5. Gewitz MH, Phillips JB: Fetal circulation. In Polin R, Fox W, eds: *Fetal and Neonatal Physiology.* Philadelphia, WB Saunders Co, 1992.
6. Gillette PC, Garson A, eds: *Pediatric Cardiac Dysrhythmias.* New York, Gruen and Stratton, 1981.
7. Heymann MA, Rudolph AM: Neonatal manipulation: Patent ductus arteriosus. In Engle MA, ed: *Pediatric Cardiovascular Disease.* Philadelphia, FA Davis Co, 1981.
8. Hirsimaki H, Kero P, Saraste M: Grading of left-to-right shunting ductus arteriosus in neonates with bedside pulsed Doppler ultrasound. *Am J Perinatol* 1991; 8:247.
9. Katz AM: *Physiology of the Heart.* New York, Raven Press, 1977.
10. Kirklin JK, Blackstone EH, Kirklin JW, et al: Intracardiac surgery in infants under age 3 months: Incremental risk factors for hospital mortality. *Am J Cardiol* 1981; 48:500–506.
11. Lees MH: Cyanosis of the newborn infant. *J Pediatr* 1970; 77:484–498.
12. Long W: *Fetal and Neonatal Cardiology.* Philadelphia, WB Saunders Co, 1990.
13. Peckham GJ, Heymann MA, eds: Cardiovascular sequelae of asphyxia in the newborn. Report of the 83rd Ross Conference on Pediatric Research. Columbus, OH, Ross Laboratories, 1982.
14. Pigott J, Murphy J, Barber G, et al: Palliative reconstructive surgery for hypoplastic left heart syndrome. *Ann Thorac Surg* 1988; 45:122.
15. Rudolph AM: *Congenital Diseases of the Heart.* Chicago, Year Book Medical Publishers, 1974.
16. Talner NS, Sanyal SK, Halloran KH, et al: Congestive heart failure in infancy. I. Abnormalities in the blood gas and acid base equilibrium. *Pediatrics* 1965; 35:20.

# Chapter 13

□

# PERSISTENT

□

# PULMONARY

□

# HYPERTENSION

□

# OF THE NEONATE

□

*William A. Engle, M.D.*

Persistent pulmonary hypertension of the neonate, or persistent fetal circulation, is a life-threatening disorder that complicates the transition from fetal to postnatal life following delivery. This chapter reviews the physiology and pathophysiology, clinical presentation, differential diagnosis, diagnostic evaluation, treatment, and outcome of persistent pulmonary hypertension of the neonate. Following completion of this study, you should be able to do the following:

- Define persistent pulmonary hypertension of the neonate.
- Outline the fetal and postnatal circulations and list the major events that promote the normal cardiovascular transition from fetal to postnatal life.
- Discuss the factors that influence pulmonary vascular resistance during the neonatal period.
- Describe the survival rates, neurodevelopmental, and pulmonary outcomes for neonates with persistent pulmonary hypertension.
- Formulate a differential diagnosis.
- Select a diagnostic evaluation.
- Identify therapeutics and their rationale including recent advances such as high-frequency ventilation and extracorporeal membrane oxygenation.
- Describe the survival rates, neurodevelopmental, and pulmonary outcomes for

neonates with persistent pulmonary hypertension.

This chapter focuses on several case studies. Interspersed throughout the case studies will be exercises for you to consider, which are followed by discussions pertinent to each exercise. Some of the answers to the exercises may be found within the exercise discussions, while others are listed after the exercises.

## CASE STUDY 1

A 41-year-old married woman with an uncomplicated pregnancy is now entering her 43rd week of gestation. She has had weekly reactive (normal) nonstress tests and normal biophysical profiles. During the past day, fetal movements have diminished. An oxytocin challenge test reveals an invariant sinusoidal pattern and an emergency cesarean section is performed. You are asked to evaluate and treat the infant (MS) immediately following delivery. As the obstetrician incises the uterus, he informs you of the presence of thick, particulate meconium in the amniotic fluid.

## EXERCISE 1

■ **Question:**

Which of the following problems is your most immediate concern in the delivery room for this infant?

1. Hypothermia

2. Sepsis

3. Transient tachypnea of the newborn

4. Meconium aspiration

5. Hypoglycemia

■ **Answer:**

1. This is an incorrect choice. Heat loss in the delivery room is usually not a life-threatening problem although it is important to manage the infant in ways to minimize heat loss. Furthermore, hypothermia is known to increase oxygen consumption and may make resuscitation of this infant more difficult. Use of a preheated radiant warmer prepared with absorbant towels for removing wet secretions and amniotic fluid is important for all deliveries.

2. This is an incorrect choice. Although there is no maternal evidence of infection, you are correct to be concerned about infection in this infant. However, the immediate concern for this infant is prompt stabilization and resuscitation. Following stabilization, evaluation for infection and initiation of antibiotic therapy may be warranted.

3. This is an incorrect choice. Although this infant may be at risk for retained intra-alveolar and interstitial fluid (transient tachypnea of the newborn), this choice is not the most immediate concern. During stabilization of this infant, assessment of respiratory effort and liberal provision of oxygen is indicated.

4. This is the correct choice. In the presence of thick and particulate meconium, the infant is at increased risk for meconium aspiration syndrome and persistent pulmonary hypertension. Meconium staining of amniotic fluid occurs in 10% to 20% of all deliveries; meconium aspiration syndrome occurs in 1% of these cases. The immediate management of this infant during delivery should include suctioning of the oropharynx, hypopharynx, and nasopharynx by the obstetrician as the head is delivered (before the shoulders are delivered). The pediatrician's role in managing this infant includes immediate suctioning of the mouth and nares followed by visualization of the vocal cords and suctioning of the trachea until it is free of meconium. Thereafter, drying the infant, assessing respirations, heart rate, and color, and providing further resuscitation are indicated.

5. This is an incorrect choice. It is true, however, that hypoglycemia may complicate the postnatal course of this infant. Therefore, attention to glucose homeostasis is important *after* securing the airway, providing for circulatory adequacy, and assuring adequate oxygenation.

## PHYSIOLOGY AND PATHOPHYSIOLOGY OF THE TRANSITIONAL CIRCULATION

### CASE STUDY 2

A 25-year-old, gravida 2, para 1, single woman has experienced an uncomplicated pregnancy. Her previous obstetric history is noteworthy in that she delivered her first child by cesarean section because of excessive vaginal bleeding associated with placenta previa. A repeat cesarean section is performed at 39 weeks' gestation under epidural anesthesia. TT cries on delivery but is noted to be cyanotic and tachypneic (respiratory rate of 84 breaths per minute). Supplemental oxygen (the $FiO_2$, inspired oxygen fraction, is 1; i.e., 100% oxygen) at a rate of 5 L/min is immediately administered ½ inch from her mouth and nose. Cyanosis improves although her right arm, face, and head are pink whereas her left arm, trunk, and lower extremities remain cyanotic (Fig. 13-1). Transcutaneous oxygen saturations are 94% and 86% from the right hand and left foot, respectively. Perfusion of the skin and extremities is poor. There is delayed capillary refill (approximately 4 seconds) and hypotension (blood pressure = 42/31; mean BP = 31 torr). Fresh frozen plasma, 15 cc/kg, is given intravenously; this raises the systolic blood pressure to 61 torr and the mean blood pressure to 48 torr. Due to lability in oxygenation noted with stimulation, procedures are restricted and other stimuli are minimized. Transcutaneous oxygen saturations equalize and rise to 100%. Supplemental oxygen is carefully weaned as tachypnea resolves during the subsequent 15 hours. A chest radiograph demonstrates fluid in the horizontal fissure of the right lung and perihilar vascular prominence consistent with transient tachypnea of the newborn. The infant is begun on oral feedings and is discharged at 3 days of age.

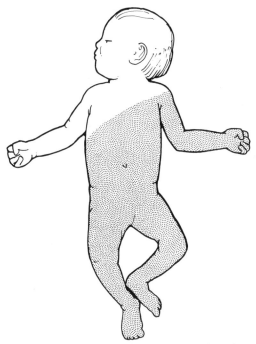

**Figure 13-1** Distribution of cyanosis in the infant in Case Study 2. The unstipled area represents a pink color, whereas the stipled area represents cyanosis. This color distribution signifies right-to-left shunting of blood across a patent ductus arteriosus.

## EXERCISE 2

1. Explain the circulatory basis for TT's skin color distribution following delivery.

2. On the three figures on pages 303 and 304, use a dotted line to represent relatively well-oxygenated blood and a solid line to represent less well-oxygenated blood, trace the expected pathways of blood flow in the fetus, the neonate described in this case study (transitional circulation) and the healthy term neonate (postnatal circulation).

### ■ Discussion:

The presence of pink color in the right arm and head (preductal blood flow distribution) and cyanosis in the left arm, trunk, and lower extremities (postductal blood flow distribution) signifies right-to-left shunting of relatively poorly oxygenated venous blood across a patent ductus arteriosus (PDA) to the systemic circulation. This shunting pattern, which is similar to the fetal circulatory pattern, is maintained because of the presence of

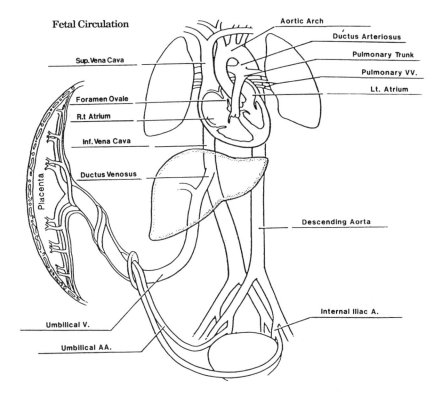

**Fetal Circulation**

Aortic Arch

Ductus Arteriosus

Pulmonary Trunk

Sup. Vena Cava

Pulmonary VV.

Lt. Atrium

Foramen Ovale

R.t Atrium

Inf. Vena Cava

Ductus Venosus

Placenta

Descending Aorta

Umbilical V.

Internal Iliac A.

Umbilical AA.

## Transitional Circulation

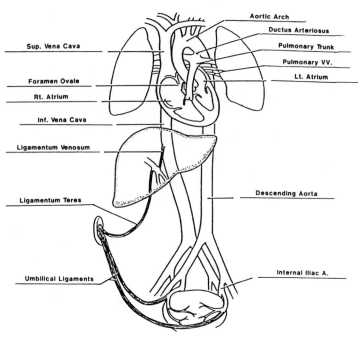

Aortic Arch
Ductus Arteriosus
Pulmonary Trunk
Pulmonary VV.
Lt. Atrium

Sup. Vena Cava
Foramen Ovale
Rt. Atrium
Inf. Vena Cava
Ligamentum Venosum
Ligamentum Teres
Umbilical Ligaments

Descending Aorta
Internal Iliac A.

## Postnatal Circulation

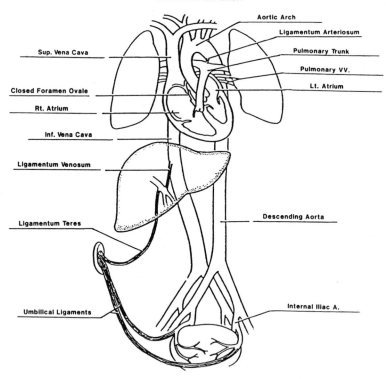

Aortic Arch
Ligamentum Arteriosum
Pulmonary Trunk
Pulmonary VV.
Lt. Atrium

Sup. Vena Cava
Closed Foramen Ovale
Rt. Atrium
Inf. Vena Cava
Ligamentum Venosum
Ligamentum Teres
Umbilical Ligaments

Descending Aorta
Internal Iliac A.

increased pulmonary vascular resistance (Fig. 13-2). The presence of this circulatory pattern after birth is termed *persistent pulmonary hypertension of the neonate* (PPHN). (Some clinicians prefer the older term *persistent fetal circulation*.) Interestingly, only about 50% of patients with PPHN will demonstrate right-to-left shunting across their ductus arteriosa. Some of these infants will have a bidirectional shunt suggestive of equal pulmonary and systemic arterial pressures. Others will have right-to-left shunting across a patent foramen ovale at the atrial level; these patients may be diffusely cyanotic due to mixing of venous and arterial blood within the atria.

The transition from a fetal circulatory pattern to a postnatal circulatory pattern is the result of several simultaneous postnatal events (Table 13-1). Prenatally, the high pulmonary vascular resistance is maintained in the fetus by a relative "hypoxemia" (partial pressure of oxygen in umbilical venous blood

is approximately 35 torr) and circulating leukotrienes, which vasoconstrict the pulmonary circulation. With the initial respiratory efforts following delivery, alveolar ventilation begins and the pulmonary vascular bed is mechanically tethered open; this causes an immediate and significant decrease in pulmonary vascular resistance. Pulmonary vascular vasodilation and increased pulmonary blood flow are further promoted by an increased oxygen tension (especially within the alveolar space), a reduction in carbon dioxide tension, and elevated concentrations of humoral vasodilators such as prostacyclin within the pulmonary circulation. Loss of umbilical venous return from the placenta and closure of the ductus venosus also contribute to a decrease in right atrial pressure. Furthermore, with loss of the low resistance placenta and increase in pulmonary venous return to the left heart, systemic vascular resistance increases. The increase in systemic vascular resistance and left atrial

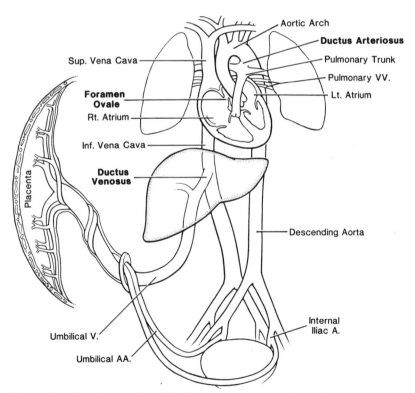

**Figure 13-2** Fetal circulation. The three major vascular shunts that maintain the fetal circulatory pattern are the ductus venosus, foramen ovale, and ductus arteriosus. Right-to-left shunting of venous blood across the foramen ovale and ductus arteriosus due to elevated pulmonary vascular resistance characterizes persistent pulmonary hypertension of the neonate.

**Table 13-1** Transition from Fetal to Neonatal Circulation*

| EVENT | PHYSIOLOGICAL CONSEQUENCE | EFFECT ON CARDIOVASCULAR SYSTEM |
|---|---|---|
| Alveolar ventilation | Decreased PVR (increased PO$_2$, prostacyclin) | Increased LA pressure |
| | Increased pulmonary blood flow | |
| | Increased pulmonary venous return | |
| Placental separation | Decreased IVC return | Decreased RA pressure |
| | Closure of ductus venosus | Increased SVR |
| Decreased RA pressure and increased LA pressure | | Closure of foramen ovale |
| Decreased PVR and increased SVR | Reversal of ductal flow | Closure of ductus arteriosus |
| | Increased PO$_2$ in ductus | |

* PVR = pulmonary vascular resistance, IVC = inferior vena cava, SVR = systemic vascular resistance, LA = left atrium, RA = right atrium.

pressure and the decrease in pulmonary vascular resistance reverses the right-to-left shunt across the ductus arteriosus and foramen ovale. The oxygen tension and pressure changes associated with reversal of right-to-left shunting then promote closure of the ductus arteriosus, foramen ovale, and ductus venosus. When these structures close, the transition from the fetal circulation to the postnatal circulation is complete (Fig. 13-3).

■ **Answers:**

1. This infant's skin color distribution represents the following:
   a. Perfusion of the face, hand, and right arm with well-oxygenated blood (derived from the left ventricle)
   b. Perfusion of the remainder of the body with poorly oxygenated blood originating in the pulmonary artery and shunting across the ductus arteriosus to the aorta
2. See the figures on pages 308 and 309.

### EXERCISE 3

Describe the physiological factors that are responsible for the following events during the transition from the fetal life to postnatal life.

1. Fall in pulmonary vascular resistance:

2. Fall in right atrial pressure:

3. Increase in left atrial pressure:

4. Increase in systemic vascular resistance:

■ **Discussion:**

**Control of Pulmonary Vascular Resistance in the Neonate:** Neonatal pulmonary vascular resistance and pulmonary blood flow are controlled by a variety of humoral, neural, physical, and mechanical influences (Table 13-2). Pulmonary vasospasm and increased pulmonary vascular resistance result when

**Table 13-2** Factors That Influence Neonatal Pulmonary Vascular Resistance

Oxygen tension
Carbon dioxide tension
Acid-base balance
Prostanoids
Alveolar distention
Physical-mechanical properties

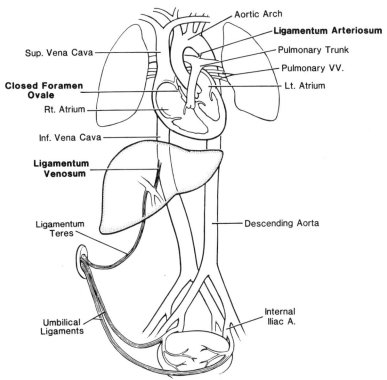

**Figure 13-3** Postnatal circulation. Transition of the postnatal circulation is characterized by closure of the foramen ovale, ductus venosus, and ductus arteriosus and formation of the ligamentum venosum, ligamentum arteriosum, ligamentum teres, and umbilical ligaments.

imbalances in these factors occur. For example, Rudolph and colleagues demonstrated that hypoxemia and acidosis are both potent initiators of increased pulmonary vascular resistance. At any given level of arterial $PO_2$, acidosis accentuates the hypoxemia-induced pulmonary vasoconstriction. Therefore, any of a number of neonatal respiratory and cardiac illnesses (Table 13-3), resulting in hypoxemia and/or acidosis, may precipitate pulmonary vasospasm, decreased pulmonary blood flow, increased right heart strain, and induce right-to-left shunting through the ductus arteriosus and/or foramen ovale. In addition ventilation-perfusion mismatching across diseased lung segments may contribute to right-to-left shunting. This shunting of relatively poorly oxygenated venous blood into the systemic circulation results in relatively low systemic oxygenation and, if uncompensated by increased cardiac output, may reduce oxygen delivery. Hypotension due to vasodilation of the systemic circulation may further exacerbate right-to-left shunting.

**Table 13-3** Illnesses Associated with Persistent Pulmonary Hypertension of the Neonate

Idiopathic persistent pulmonary hypertension of the neonate

Aspiration syndromes: meconium, blood, amniotic fluid

Sepsis/pneumonia

Hyaline membrane disease

Transient tachypnea of the newborn

Air leak phenomena: pneumothorax, pneumomediastinum, pulmonary interstitial emphysema

Pulmonary hypoplasia: congenital diaphragmatic hernia, oligohydramnios syndrome

Perinatal asphyxia

Congenital heart disease: total anomalous pulmonary venous return, transposition of great vessels, etc.

## Fetal Circulation

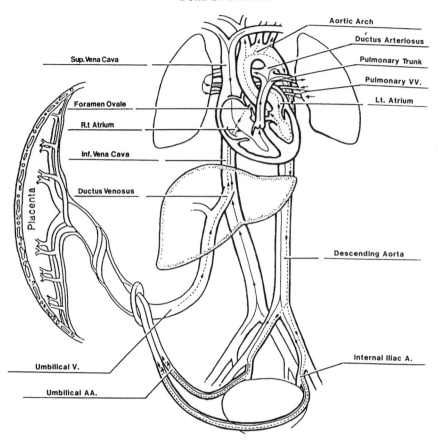

Aortic Arch
Ductus Arteriosus
Pulmonary Trunk
Pulmonary VV.
Lt. Atrium

Sup. Vena Cava

Foramen Ovale
R.t Atrium
Inf. Vena Cava
Ductus Venosus

Placenta

Descending Aorta

Umbilical V.
Umbilical AA.

Internal Iliac A.

## Transitional Circulation

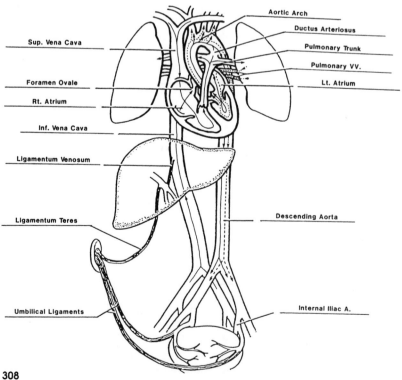

Aortic Arch
Ductus Arteriosus
Pulmonary Trunk
Pulmonary VV.
Lt. Atrium

Sup. Vena Cava

Foramen Ovale
Rt. Atrium
Inf. Vena Cava
Ligamentum Venosum

Ligamentum Teres

Descending Aorta

Umbilical Ligaments

Internal Iliac A.

## Postnatal Circulation

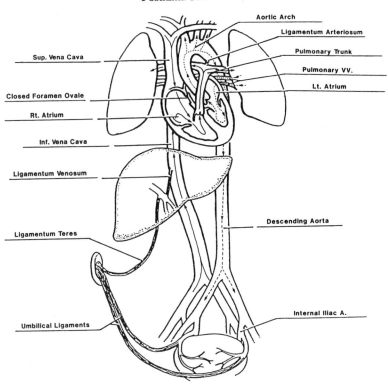

The cellular and biochemical events responsible for hypoxic vasoconstriction of the pulmonary vascular bed are uncertain. It has been demonstrated, however, that hypoxia-induced pulmonary vasospasm is a *local effect* that occurs in experimental preparations devoid of nerves. It has not been determined whether this vasoconstrictive response is a direct effect of alveolar or pulmonary arterial hypoxia, or due to vasoactive mediators induced at the tissue or circulating level. Proposed mediators of increased pulmonary vascular resistance include histamine, serotonin, leukotrienes, thromboxanes, platelet activating factor, and angiotensin II.

The effect of carbon dioxide tension on pulmonary vascular resistance is principally mediated through a direct effect on hydrogen ion concentration. In that regard, Viles and Shepherd demonstrated that alkalosis (pH > 7.5) attenuated or eliminated hypoxic pulmonary vasoconstriction in the adult cat. Further support for that concept was demonstrated by Schreiber, Heymann, and Soifer, who found that hypoxic vasoconstriction was more responsive to a metabolic alkalosis (with a normal carbon dioxide tension) than to a pure respiratory alkalosis. Note, however, that Viles and Shepherd also demonstrated that hypercarbia can act as a vasodilator in isolated lung preparations. This paradoxical effect appears to be independent of the hydrogen ion concentration.

### ■ Answers:

1. Fall in pulmonary vascular resistance:
   - Initiation of alveolar ventilation
   - Improved oxygenation
2. Fall in right atrial pressure:
   - Loss of umbilical venous return
   - Closure of the ductus venosus
3. Increase in left atrial pressure:
   - Increase in pulmonary venous return
4. Increase in systemic vascular resistance:
   - Increase in pulmonary venous return
   - Loss of the low-resistance placenta

### EXERCISE 4

List five major factors that control pulmonary vascular resistance in postnatal life.

1.

2.

3.

4.

5.

### ■ Answers:

1. Oxygen tension

2. Acid-base balance

3. Local physical mechanical properties

4. Humoral agents (prostanoids, leukotrienes, etc.)

5. Alveolar distention

---

## CASE STUDY 3

CDH, a 3,470-g male newborn infant, is delivered at 40 weeks' gestation to a 22-year-old, gravida 3, para 2 woman. The pregnancy has been complicated by polyhydramnios and a left-sided diaphragmatic hernia diagnosed by ultrasound at 6 months of gestation in the fetus. Immediately following birth, CDH is intubated and administered 100% oxygen. An orogastric tube is placed to remove swallowed air. Apgar scores are 7 and 8 at 1 and 5 minutes, respectively. Marked lability in oxygenation is noted but quickly treated by continued oxygen supplementation ($FiO_2$ = 1.0), mechanical ventilation, and volume expansion with 10 cc/kg fresh frozen plasma. Surgical repair of the left diaphragmatic hernia is performed when CDH is 3 days of age. Mechanical ventilation and oxygen supplementation are carefully weaned during the next 8 days. CDH is discharged at 11 days of age.

## EXERCISE 5

---

### ■ Question:

Which of the following factors is responsible for the elevated pulmonary vascular resistance in neonates with congenital diaphragmatic hernia?

1. Pulmonary vasoconstriction

2. Excess pulmonary blood flow

3. Pulmonary venous obstruction

4. Pulmonary vascular hypoplasia

5. Pulmonary vascular restriction

### ■ Discussion/Answer:

Although *pulmonary vasoconstriction* largely contributes to the increased pulmonary vascular resistance observed in neonates with persistent pulmonary hypertension, vascular restriction may also contribute to abnormal postnatal pulmonary vascular adaptation. *Extension of the pulmonary arterial muscle beyond the terminal bronchiolar vessels into the intraacinar vessels* (respiratory bronchiole, alveolar duct, and alveoli) results in a reduction in internal diameter of these vessels. Because resistance is inversely proportional to the fourth power of the radius, decreasing the intraluminal diameter (by increasing distal pulmonary arteriolar wall thickness) will substantially increase resistance to pulmonary blood flow. In normal neonates, vascular smooth muscle does not extend beyond the terminal bronchioles. However, in human neonates dying from persistent pulmonary hypertension, meconium aspiration syndrome, and congenital diaphragmatic hernia, distal muscular extension into intraacinar arteriolar vessels has been shown to occur. In addition to distal pulmonary arteriolar muscular extension, neonates with congenital diaphragmatic hernia are at risk for *pulmonary arterial hypoplasia* due to compression of the lung parenchyma and pulmonary vasculature by intrathoracic bowel. Table 13-4 lists other conditions associated at birth with pulmonary hypoplasia and a diminished pulmonary vascular tree. If the pulmonary vascular bed is restrictive due to vascular hypoplasia and distal pulmonary arteriole muscularization, the pulmonary arterial pressure will rise and right-to-left shunting across the foramen ovale, ductus arteriosus, or both may result.

An animal model for persistent pulmonary hypertension of the neonate has recently been developed. Ligation of the ductus arteriosus in the fetal lamb for 3 to 17 days prior to delivery results in increased wall thickness of intraacinar vessels, elevated pulmonary artery pressure, lower pulmonary blood flow, increased right-to-left ductal shunting, and abnormal pulmonary vascular reactivity. This *in utero* vascular remodeling may be the laboratory correlate for human neonates with extension of pulmonary vascular musculature into intraacinar locations. Therefore, *in utero* pul-

**Table 13-4**  Conditions Associated with Pulmonary Hypoplasia at Birth

Congenital diaphragmatic hernia or eventration

Oligohydramnios associated with renal agenesis, renal dysplasia or chronic leakage of amniotic fluid

Asphyxiating thoracic dystrophy*

Pleural effusion

Rhesus isoimmunization

Vascular anomalies

Rubella

Idiopathic (primary)

Werdnig-Hoffmann disease

Diaphragmatic amyoplasia and phrenic nerve agenesis

---

* This disease can be associated with normal lung volume at birth.
*Source:* From Geggel RL, Reid LM: The structural basis of PPHN. *Clin Perinatol* 1984; 11:538. Reprinted with permission of W.B. Saunders Company.

monary vascular remodeling may signify a preceding *in utero* stress or congenital predisposition to neonatal pulmonary vasoreactivity.

---

**CASE STUDY 4**

HIE is delivered to a 19-year-old, gravida 1, para 1 mother whose pregnancy has been complicated by the absence of prenatal care. When the woman is presented to the labor area, profound bradycardia is detected [fetal heart rate of 40 beats per minute (BPM)] and emergency cesarean section is performed. Apgar scores are 3 at 1 minute (1 for heart rate 90, 1 for gasping respiratory efforts, and 1 for reflex irritability) and 7 at 5 minutes (2 for heart rate 128, 2 for regular respirations, 1 for acrocyanosis, 1 for reflex irritability, and 1 for mild hypotonia). Although her respirations are regular, HIE has retractions and grunting respiratory efforts for which she is administered supplemental oxygen (FiO$_2$ = 1.0). Her clinical appearance is remarkable for a well-oxygenated right arm, face, and head and a cyanotic left arm, trunk, and lower extremities. The respiratory therapist places transcutaneous oxygen saturation probes on HIE's right hand and left foot to monitor oxygenation. Due to severe respiratory distress and persistent cyanosis (arterial oxygen saturation of 80% on the left foot), HIE is placed on a mechanical ventilator. The preductal transcutaneous saturation rises to 98%, whereas the postductal transcutaneous saturation remains at 81%. Umbilical arterial and venous catheters are placed under sterile conditions with the tip of the umbilical arterial line in the middle thoracic aorta (postductal). An arterial blood gas reveals a PaO$_2$ of 42 torr, a pH of 7.38, and a base deficit of 5. During placement of the umbilical lines and suctioning of the endotracheal tube, HIE's preductal oxygen saturation falls to 83%; gradual return of the preductal oxygen saturation to 97% occurs following these procedures. Lability in oxygenation persists, so minimal stimulation techniques are instituted along with administration of fentanyl and secobarbital. At this time, her physical examination is remarkable for relative pallor of the left arm, trunk, and lower body, a systolic heart murmur at the left sternal border, a loud second heart sound that splits normally, and unlabored tachypnea.

**EXERCISE 6**

---

List four clinical findings indicative of severe persistent pulmonary hypertension in this neonate.

1.

2.

3.

4.

■ **Discussion:**

Persistent pulmonary hypertension of the neonate may either be a primary disorder or occur secondary to a variety of underlying pulmonary or cardiac conditions. Most neonates with pulmonary hypertension are near-term, term, or post-term babies. The severity of clinical symptoms associated with persistent pul-

**Table 13-5**  Clinical Features of Persistent Pulmonary Hypertension of the Neonate

Near-term, term, or post-term

Onset of symptoms generally within 12 hours of age

Lability in oxygenation

Cyanosis and pallor

Heart murmur

Loud second heart sound

Tachypnea, retractions, grunting respirations

Variable chest radiograph

---

monary hypertension varies with the underlying pathology (Table 13-5).

The mildest form of persistent pulmonary hypertension of the neonate is found in infants who present immediately following delivery with cyanosis and unlabored tachypnea (see Case Study 2). In these infants, the preductal transcutaneous oxygen saturation is usually higher than the postductal reading, and this differential usually resolves quickly with aggressive administration of oxygen ($FiO_2 = 1.0$), minimal stimulation, and, in some cases, intravascular volume expansion. Chest radiographs are usually clear or may be consistent with retained intraalveolar and interstitial fluid (transient tachypnea). Right-to-left ductal shunting commonly resolves quickly, and normal physiological stability is resumed in less than 6 to 24 hours. The terms *delayed transitional circulation, transient tachypnea of the newborn,* or *transient pulmonary vascular lability* may be used to describe this mild form of persistent pulmonary hypertension of the neonate.

More severe forms of persistent pulmonary hypertension of the neonate are clinically characterized by marked lability in oxygenation, severe cyanosis, and tachypnea. A systolic heart murmur (indicative of tricuspid insufficiency) and hypotension are often seen. Chest radiographs either are normal, demonstrate mild cardiomegaly, or are consistent with an underlying pulmonary or cardiac disorder (Table 13-5). Lability in oxygenation is  the hallmark of this disorder. Because this lability may be exacerbated by minimal stresses (e.g., bathing, endotracheal tube suctioning, repositioning), caregiving techniques to mini-

mize these stresses are emphasized. In addition, sedatives (e.g., secobarbital), analgesics (e.g., morphine sulfate, fentanyl), and neuromuscular blocking agents (e.g., pancuronium, curare, vecuronium) are employed when lability in oxygenation is marked and control of ventilation is desired. When neuromuscular blocking agents are used, many clinicians begin administering anticonvulsants because of the difficulty in detecting clinical seizures in a paralyzed infant.

Cyanosis and pallor may either be generalized (if right-to-left shunting occurs principally across the foramen ovale at the level of the atria) or follow a postductal distribution if right-to-left ductal shunting is also present. Differentiating severe persistent pulmonary hypertension of the neonate from cyanotic congenital heart disease is often difficult when arterial oxygen tensions greater than 100 torr cannot be obtained and the chest x-ray is normal. Echocardiography is often helpful in making this distinction (Table 13-6). Echocardiographic features of PPHN include right-to-left shunting across the foramen ovale (and/or ductus arteriosus), elevated pulmonary artery pressure, bowing of the atrial septum into the left atrium, tricuspid insufficiency, right ventricular enlargement with septal deviation, and prolongation of the right ventricular preejection phase/right ventricular ejection time ratio.

If echocardiography is not available, several clinical maneuvers can help differentiate the cause for cyanosis (Table 13-6). These include measurement of preductal and postductal oxygen saturations or oxygen tensions (to identify right-to-left ductal shunting) and placing the infant in 100% oxygen to determine the presence of a fixed right-to-left shunt (hyperoxia test). An oxygen tension greater than 100 torr

**Table 13-6**  Diagnosis of Persistent Pulmonary Hypertension of the Neonate

Lability in oxygenation

Difference in simultaneous preductal and postductal oxygen saturations or oxygen tensions

Response to 100% oxygen

Hyperoxia-hyperventilation maneuver

Echocardiography

suggests the diagnosis of persistent pulmonary hypertension, and an oxygen tension less than 50 torr suggests a diagnosis of cyanotic congenital heart disease. If the diagnosis still remains unclear, a hyperoxia-hyperventilation maneuver may be helpful. This test entails lowering the arterial carbon dioxide tension ($PCO_2$ 20 to 25 torr) and elevating the arterial pH to at least 7.50 by overventilating the infant. Once again, if the arterial oxygen tension increases to greater than 100 torr, the patient likely has persistent pulmonary hypertension rather than cyanotic congenital heart disease.

■ **Answers:**

1. Cyanosis

2. Respiratory distress (tachypnea, retractions, and grunting)

3. Heart murmur

4. Loud second heart sound

---

## TREATMENT OF PERSISTENT PULMONARY HYPERTENSION OF THE NEONATE

### CASE STUDY 4 continued
At 6 hours of age, HIE experiences a sudden fall in oxygen saturation (preductal saturation, 72%; postductal saturation, 65%) while receiving mechanical ventilation with a peak inspiratory pressure of 32 cm $H_2O$, a positive end-expiratory pressure of 5 cm $H_2O$, a ventilator rate of 60 breaths per minute, an inspiratory time of 0.5 seconds, and a $FiO_2$ = 1.0 (100% oxygen). Bilateral pneumothoraces are diagnosed by physical examination and transillumination. Following bilateral thoracentesis and chest tube placement, oxygen saturations improve but increased ventilator support (peak inspiratory pressure = 46 cm $H_2O$) is required to increase the preductal oxygen saturation to 96% and the postductal oxygen saturation to 90%. In addition, the systemic blood pressure has fallen from a mean of 52 mm Hg [blood pressure (BP) = 64/44] to a mean of 36 mm Hg (BP = 48/28). HIE receives 10 cc/kg of fresh frozen plasma and dopamine (5 mcg/kg/min) and dobutamine (15 mcg/kg/min) are begun. Pharmacological paralysis is initiated with pancuronium bromide, and phenobarbital is begun. The postductal arterial blood gas values while be-

ing mechanically ventilated are $PaO_2$ of 33 torr, $PaCO_2$ of 45 torr, pH of 7.34, and a base deficit of 3. Preductal and postductal arterial oxygen saturations are 82% and 78%, respectively. Tolazoline (1.0 mg/kg) is administered through a catheter in the right hand; the preductal and postductal arterial oxygen saturations fall (75% and 72%, respectively) along with the systemic blood pressure (BP = 48/20, mean = 33 mm Hg). Fresh frozen plasma (20 cc/kg) is infused once more and the rates of administration of dobutamine and dopamine are increased to 20 mcg/kg/min and 15 mcg/kg/min, respectively. In response to these interventions, the systolic blood pressure increases to 72 mm Hg. Subsequent postductal arterial blood gas values are $PaO_2$ of 30 torr, $PaCO_2$ of 43 torr, pH of 7.35, and base deficit of 4. Sodium bicarbonate (2 mEq/kg) is given, the peak inspiratory pressure is increased to 50 cm $H_2O$, and the ventilator rate is raised to 80 breaths per minute. The subsequent arterial blood gas values are $PaO_2$ of 34 torr, $PaCO_2$ of 24 torr, pH of 7.53, and base deficit of 4.

### EXERCISE 7

Describe the physiological rationale for the following treatments used to treat persistent pulmonary hypertension of the neonate.

***Treatment***
1. Fresh frozen plasma infusion

2. Dopamine, dobutamine

3. Tolazoline

4. Sodium bicarbonate

5. Hyperventilation

***Rationale***
1.


2.

3.



4.



5.



## ■ Discussion:

Systemic blood pressure support with volume expanders (fresh frozen plasma, normal saline, red blood cells, albumin, etc.) and vasopressor agents (dopamine, dobutamine, isoproterenol, epinephrine, norepinephrine) have the theoretical potential to elevate systemic blood pressure to levels greater than pulmonary artery blood pressures (thereby diminishing right-to-left shunting across the foramen ovale and ductus arteriosus) (Table 13-6). Vasopressors are especially helpful in infants with myocardial ischemia and tricuspid regurgitation, which may be a sequelae of perinatal asphyxia. The current vasopressors of choice include dopamine and dobutamine. Most investigators prefer to use doses of dopamine that maintain renal perfusion and cardiac output (<5 to 15 mcg/kg/min) without causing vasoconstriction of the pulmonary and systemic vascular beds (>15 to 20 mcg/kg/min). The recommended dose for dobutamine is 5 to 20 mcg/kg/min; in this dosage range, positive inotropic effects are obtained and systemic vasodilation associated with higher doses is avoided. Isoproterenol, epinephrine, and norepinephrine are infrequently used in neonates with persistent pulmonary hypertension.

Because pulmonary vascular vasoconstriction contributes significantly to persistent pulmonary hypertension, selective pulmonary vasodilators that also augment cardiac output are constantly being tested. Tolazoline is an $\alpha$-adrenergic antagonist with histamine-like actions that produces both pulmonary and systemic vasodilation. It is the vasodilator most widely used to treat persistent pulmonary hypertension of the neonate, although responsiveness to the drug is quite variable. Tolazoline is contraindicated in infants with ongoing

hypotension. Nitroprusside; nitroglycerin; prostaglandins of the E, C, and D series; prostacyclin; acetylcholine; calcium channel blockers; thromboxane antagonists; leukotriene antagonists; chloropromazine; fentanyl; hydralazine; histamine; cromolyn sodium; and isoproterenol have all been studied as putative pulmonary vasodilators. Currently none appears to be uniformly beneficial when treating persistent pulmonary hypertension of the neonate.

Nitric oxide administered as an inhalation of 6 to 80 parts per million has recently been reported to reduce pulmonary vascular resistance in neonates with persistent pulmonary hypertension complicating meconium aspiration syndrome and sepsis. If these findings are confirmed in larger series of patients and inhaled nitric oxide is not found to be associated with significant methemoglobinemia, pulmonary inflammation, or systemic hypotension, this agent may become an important treatment for persistent pulmonary hypertension in the neonate. In addition to the potential therapeutic advantage of nitric oxide as a selective pulmonary vascular vasodilator, an understanding of the role of nitric oxide in maintaining pulmonary vascular tone may be a major advancement in our basic understanding of vascular tone regulation.

Alkalinization of the extracellular plasma with sodium bicarbonate and/or hyperventilation (to raise the arterial pH to 7.50 or greater) are currently used by many neonatologists to induce pulmonary vasodilation in neonates with persistent pulmonary hypertension (Table 13-7). Although the mechanism(s) by which these therapies effect a decrease in pulmonary vascular resistance are yet to be firmly established, an increase in arterial pH, rather than a decrease in arterial carbon dioxide tension, appears to contribute to this effect. In general, alkalinization with sodium bicarbonate is used as an adjunct therapy to further increase the arterial pH in an infant who is already being hyperventilated.

Both sodium bicarbonate infusion and hyperventilation must be used with caution because of their potential complications. Sodium bicarbonate is contraindicated in the presence of hypercarbia because of the potential to aggravate intracellular acidosis. A reduction in intracellular pH may result in a decrease in coronary perfusion pressure, diffuse myocardial ischemia, and diminished cardiac

**Table 13-7** Treatment of Persistent Pulmonary Hypertension of the Neonate

Treat underlying disorder

Monitor arterial oxygenation

Oxygen

Minimal stress

Support systemic blood pressure
    Volume expansion
    Vasopressor agents

Mechanical ventilation

Sedatives and/or pharmacological paralysis

Vasodilator agents

Alkalinization
    Sodium bicarbonate
    Hyperventilation
        Conventional ventilation at high rates (60 to 120 breaths per minute)
        High-frequency ventilation

Extracorporeal membrane oxygenation

output, thereby complicating the already compromised cardiac function, which may be a sequela of perinatal asphyxia.

Hyperventilation raises arterial pH by decreasing carbon dioxide tension to levels ranging from 10 to 35 torr. To achieve this effect with a conventional mechanical ventilator, pressures and rates must be increased to levels potentially injurious to the lung and brain; adverse effects may include pneumothoraces, pulmonary interstitial emphysemia, other air leaks, reduced cerebral blood flow, and (potentially) neurodevelopmental delay. High-frequency ventilation (using a high-frequency ventilator or oscillator) is a promising technology by which blood alkalinization can be induced at lower airway pressures than required with conventional mechanical ventilators. Clinical studies evaluating the efficacy of high-frequency ventilation for this application are currently in progress. The use of hyperventilation as a therapy for pulmonary hypertension has recently been questioned because of the potential for this therapy to do serious injury and demonstration by some investigators that persistent pulmonary hypertension of the neonate is treatable without hyperventilation. Currently many neonatologists reserve hyperventilation for neonates with severe persistent pulmonary hypertension unresponsive to conventional therapies.

■ **Answers:**

| *Treatment* | *Rationale* |
|---|---|
| 1. Fresh frozen plasma | Increase systemic blood pressure and decrease right-to-left shunting |
| 2. Dopamine, dobutamine | Increase systemic blood pressure and decrease right-to-left shunting |
| 3. Tolazoline | Decrease pulmonary vascular resistance by vasodilating the pulmonary vascular bed |
| 4. Sodium bicarbonate | Decrease pulmonary vascular resistance by making the infant alkalotic |
| 5. Hyperventilation | Decrease pulmonary vascular resistance by making the infant alkalotic |

**CASE STUDY 4 continued**

HIE is now 10 hours old. Despite maximal mechanical ventilation to induce hyperventilation (peak inspiratory pressure, 50 cm $H_2O$; rate, 80 breaths per minute) and aggressive medical support (dopamine, dobutamine, frequent volume expansion, sodium bicarbonate, pharmacological paralysis, and fentanyl), her arterial blood gases and clinical condition continue to deteriorate. The postductal arterial oxygen tension is now 29 torr. HIE's perfusion is poor and urine output has fallen to less than 1 cc/kg/hr. The family is extensively counseled regarding risks and benefits of extracorporeal membrane oxygenation (ECMO) and, after obtaining informed consent, preparations are made to initiate cardiopulmonary bypass. Blood, platelets, cryoprecipitate, thrombin, and heparin have been ordered. An emergency head ultrasound is normal. The extracorporeal circuit is primed and catheters are surgically inserted into the right internal carotid artery and right internal jugular vein. During catheter placement, systemic heparinization is instituted. ECMO is continued for 98 hours. HIE weans from mechanical ventilation and oxygen 72 hours following decannulation. At the time of discharge from the hospital, neurological and developmental assessments by pediatric neurology, occupational therapy, and physical therapy are normal. A follow-up examination at 3 years of age demonstrates HIE to be neurodevelopmentally and socially normal.

## EXERCISE 8

Answer the following questions about extracorporeal membrane oxygenation.

### ■ Questions:

1. Why was this infant an appropriate candidate for ECMO?

2. Which kinds of infants are inappropriate for ECMO?

3. Why isn't ECMO used in preterm infants (<34 weeks' gestation)?

4. How should the family be counseled regarding the neurological, respiratory, and developmental outcomes for neonates with pulmonary hypertension treated with ECMO?

### ■ Discussion:

Extracorporeal membrane oxygenation is prolonged cardiopulmonary bypass for neonates with respiratory or cardiac failure complicated by persistent pulmonary hypertension who are unlikely to survive despite maximal medical management. The mechanism by which ECMO leads to resolution of life-threatening persistent pulmonary hypertension of the neonate is unclear. During ECMO, oxygen delivery and carbon dioxide removal are maintained while pulmonary and/or cardiac dysfunction resolve; this recovery occurs without the potentially injurious effects of oxygen toxicity and barotrauma, which may complicate conventional therapeutic strategies.

A diagram of a venoarterial ECMO circuit is depicted in Figure 13-4. Several important observations about the use of prolonged extracorporeal circulation are apparent in this figure and deserve emphasis. First, an extracorporeal circuit is joined to the neonate by right internal carotid artery and right internal jugular vein catheters. During insertion of these catheters, both major vessels are ligated. Although collateral circulations usually exist to support flow to and away from the right hemisphere of the brain, an inherent risk of cerebral infarction and hemorrhage exists. Reconstruction of the internal carotid artery and use of venovenous ECMO are currently being investigated as methods to reduce these risks. Second, since the plastic extracorporeal circuit is thrombogenic, these infants require systemic heparinization to inhibit blood coagulation. In the critically ill, hypoxemic, and acidotic neonate treated with ECMO and systemic heparinization, the risks of intracranial hemorrhage and bleeding from other sites are 16% and 24.7%, respectively. Because of this risk, ECMO is limited to near-term, term, and postterm neonates who are at highest risk of dying despite maximal use of conventional therapies. Preterm infants are currently excluded from receiving ECMO because of the unacceptably high risk of severe intracranial hemorrhage and death. Recent advances in heparin bonding technology may allow performance of ECMO without systemic heparinization in the near future. Finally, the extracorporeal circuit is a series of mechanical devices, all of which may malfunction. Therefore, specially trained extracorporeal technical specialists must monitor the circuit continuously during treatment to detect and correct equipment malfunction and embolic phenomenon (air, fibrin clots).

Because of the potential complications associated with ECMO (Table 13-8), strict eligibility and exclusion requirements have evolved. To be eligible, neonates must generally be older than 34 weeks' gestation (birth

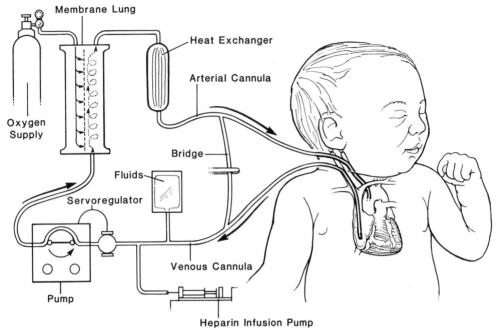

**Figure 13-4**  Diagram of the circuit used for venoarterial ECMO.
From Engle WA, Peters EA, West KW: Neonatal extracorporeal membrane oxygenation. *Indiana Med* 1989;
(May):350–357. Reprinted with permission of W.A. Engle.

weight > 2,000 g), less than 10 days old, and at high risk for dying despite receiving maximal medical supports.

To predict which infants are at highest risk for dying, two indices have been developed to quantitate the degree of respiratory failure. The first of these, the oxygenation index (OI)

is calculated as follows:

$$OI = \frac{\text{mean airway pressure} \times FiO_2 \times 100}{\text{arterial } PO_2}$$

An OI greater than 40 for greater than 2 hours or in three of five serial blood gases is predictive of an 80% mortality.

The second index, the $AaDO_2$ gradient, is calculated as follows:

$$AaDO_2 = (\text{atmospheric pressure} - \text{water vapor pressure})(FiO_2) - \text{arterial } PO_2 - (\text{arterial } PCO_2/0.8)$$

A value of 630 or greater for greater than 4 hours is predictive of an 80% mortality.

Furthermore, neonates receiving extracorporeal support *must have a reversible pulmonary or cardiac illness.* Most ECMO centers currently exclude infants with persistent pulmonary hypertension if they have a significant intracranial hemorrhage, unresponsive bleeding diatheses, irreversible major organ failure, or a chromosomal abnormality of syndrome associated with high mortality or extremely poor neurodevelopmental prognosis.

**Table 13-8**  Eligibility and Exclusion Criteria for Extracorporeal Membrane Oxygenation

---

*Eligibility*

Progressive respiratory or cardiac failure despite maximal treatment

Greater than 2-kg birth weight and/or greater than 34 weeks' gestation

Reversible lung or cardiac disease

*Exclusion*

Intracranial hemorrhage

Unresponsive bleeding diathesis

Irreversible major organ failure

Chromosomal abnormality or syndrome associated with high mortality or extremely poor neurodevelopmental prognosis

The primary diagnoses of patients most frequently requiring ECMO include meconium aspiration syndrome, overwhelming sepsis, pneumonia, respiratory distress syndrome, persistent pulmonary hypertension of the neonate, and congenital diaphragmatic hernia. As of July 1991, 5,162 near-term and term (39 ± 2.5 weeks' gestation) neonates with respiratory failure complicated by severe persistent pulmonary hypertension had been treated with ECMO; 83% of these patients have survived. There were 817 (16%) intracranial hemorrhages/infarctions, 165 (3.2%) significant gastrointestinal hemorrhages, 67 (1.3%) pulmonary hemorrhages, 416 (8.1%) cannulation site bleeding episodes, 252 (4.9%) episodes of bleeding at other surgical sites, and 370 (7.2%) other forms of hemorrhage in these patients. In addition, 2,131 mechanical complications (e.g., clot formation, tubing rupture, pump malfunction, air in circuit, and oxygenator failure) were reported; fortunately, the majority of these complications were rapidly corrected without adverse outcomes.

Historically, 40% to 80% of neonates with persistent pulmonary hypertension treated with conventional therapies alone survived. One-third of these infants suffered from chronic lung disease, 7.5% to 25% had neurosensory hearing loss, and 40% to 80% were neurodevelopmentally normal. Most recently, several investigators have demonstrated that more than 90% of near-term and term neonates with persistent pulmonary hypertension who meet criteria for ECMO (i.e., >80% risk of mortality) survive *without* the need for *extracorporeal support* or hyperventilation. The number of patients in these series is small and no neurodevelopmental and medical follow-up of these patients has yet been reported. If the patient populations reported in these series are truly similar to those populations receiving extracorporeal support and the therapeutic approaches by these investigators are proven that effective, the use of ECMO could become obsolete.

Survival rates of greater than 80% are currently being achieved in neonates treated with ECMO whose predicted survival without extracorporeal support would be less than 20%. In addition, the incidence of chronic lung disease (less than 10%), neurosensory hearing loss (4% to 21%), and neurodevelopmental outcomes (70% to 80% normal) are favorable compared to neonates receiving conventional medical support only. Although as yet unproven, most neonatologists believe that ECMO is a worthwhile therapy for selected groups of term and near-term neonates who would likely not survive if only conventional medical supports were available. Only time will tell whether this belief is true.

### ■ Answers:

1. ECMO is indicated in term and near-term neonates (>2,000 g and >34 weeks' gestation) with pulmonary hypertension who are at high risk or dying (>80%) and who are thought to have a reversible or correctable disease.

2. *Exclusion criteria:* Prematurity (<34 weeks' gestation, <2,000 g), significant intracranial hemorrhage, unresponsiveness, bleeding diathesis, major organ failure, or a chromosomal abnormality or syndrome associated with a poor neurodevelopmental prognosis.

3. Premature infants (<34 weeks' gestation) who are placed on ECMO are at high risk to sustain an intracranial hemorrhage.

4. Most survivors of ECMO are normal neurologically. The incidence of chronic lung disease is less than 10% and is somewhat dependent on the duration of mechanical ventilation and degree of lung injury prior to institution of ECMO.

### BIBLIOGRAPHY

1. Bloom RS, Cropley C: *Textbook of Neonatal Resuscitation.* American Heart Association and American Academy of Pediatrics, 1991.
2. Carson BS, Losey RW, Bowes WA, et al: Combined obstetric and pediatric approach to prevent meconium aspiration syndrome. *Am J Obstet Gynecol* 1976; 126(6):712–715.
3. Morganroth ML, Reeve JT, Murphy RC, Voelkel NF: Leukotriene synthesis and receptor blockers block hypoxic pulmonary vasoconstriction. *J Appl Physiol* 1984; 56:1340.
4. Ahmed T, Oliver W Jr: Does slow-reacting substance of anaphylaxis mediate hypoxia pulmonary vasoconstriction? *Am Rev Resp Dis* 1983; 127:566.
5. Spitzer AR, Davis J, Clarke WT, et al: Pulmonary hypertension and persistent fetal circulation in the newborn. *Clin Perinatol* 1988; 15(2):389–413.
6. Enhorning G, Adams FH, Norman A: Effect of lung expansion on the fetal lamb circulation. *Acta Paediatr Scand* 1966; 55:441.

7. Hoffman JIE, Heymann MA: Normal pulmonary circulation. In Scarpelli EM, ed: *Normal Pulmonary Physiology*, 2nd ed. Philadelphia, Lea & Febiger, 1990, pp. 233–256.

8. Heymann MA, Hoffman JIE: Pulmonary circulation in the perinatal period. In Thibeault DW, Gregory GA, eds: *Neonatal Pulmonary Care*, 2nd ed. Norwalk, CT, Appleton-Century-Crofts, 1986, pp. 149–174.

9. Galanatowicz ME, Price M, Stolar CJH: Differential effects of alveolar and arterial oxygen tension on pulmonary vasomotor tone in ECMO-perfused isolated piglet lungs. *J Pediatr Surgery* 1991; 26(3):312–316.

10. Heymann MA: Prostacyclins and leukotrienes in the perinatal period. *Clin Perinatol* 1987; 14:857–880.

11. Duke HN: The site of action of anoxia on the pulmonary blood vessels of the cat. *J Physiol* 1954; 125:373.

12. Leffler CW, Hessler JR, Green RS: Mechanism of stimulation of pulmonary prostaglandin synthesis at birth. *Prostaglandins* 1984; 28:877.

13. Leffler CW, Hessler JR, Green RS: The onset of breathing at birth stimulates pulmonary vascular prostacyclin synthesis. *Pediatr Res* 1984; 18:938.

14. Clyman RI: Ontogeny of the ductus arteriosus response to prostaglandin and inhibitors of their synthesis. *Sem Perin* 1980; 4:115–124.

15. Rudolph AM, Teitel AF, Iwamoto HS, et al: Ventilation is more important than oxygenation in reducing pulmonary vascular resistance at birth. *Pediatr Res* 1986; 20:439A.

16. Rudolph AM, Yuan S: Response of the pulmonary vasculature to hypoxia and H+ ion concentration changes. *J Clin Invest* 1966; 45:399.

17. Rudolph AM, Heymann MA: Circulatory changes in fetal lambs. *Pediatr Res* 1972; 6:341.

18. Hauge A: Role of histamine in hypoxic pulmonary hypertension in the rat. I. Blockade or potentiation of endogenous amines, kinins and ATP. *Circ Resc* 1968; 22:371.

19. Sada K, Shirai M, Ninomiya I: X-ray TV system for measuring microcirculation in small pulmonary vessels. *J Appl Physiol* 1985; 59:1013.

20. Hammerman C, Lass N, Strates E, et al: Prostanoids in neonates with persistent pulmonary hypertension. *J Pediatr* 1987; 110(3):470–472.

21. Burhop KE, Zee HVD, Bizios R, et al: Pulmonary vascular response to platelet-activating factor in awake sheep and the role of cyclooxygenase metabolites. *Am Rev Resp Dis* 1986; 134:548–554.

22. Burkov S: Hypoxic pulmonary vasoconstriction in the rat. The necessary role of Angiotensin II. *Circ Res* 1974; 35:256.

23. Viles PH, Shepherd JT: Evidence of a dilator action of carbon dioxide on the pulmonary vessels of the cat. *Circ Resc* 1968; 22:325.

24. Lyrene RK, Welch KA, Godov G, et al: Alkalosis attenuates hypoxic pulmonary vasoconstriction in neonatal lambs. *Pediatr Res* 1985; 19:1268.

25. Schreiber MD, Heymann MA, Soifer JS: Leukotriene inhibition prevents and reverses hypoxic pulmonary vasoconstriction in newborn lambs. *Pediatr Res* 1985; 19(5):437–441.

26. Reid L: Constrictive and restrictive pulmonary hypertension in the newborn and infant. *Am J Cardiovasc Pathology* 1987; 1(2):287–299.

27. Murphy JD, Rabinovitch M, Goldstein JD, et al: The structural basis of persistent pulmonary hypertension of the newborn infant. *J Pediatr* 1981; 98(6):962–967.

28. Wild LM, Nickerson PA, Morrin FC III: Ligating the ductus arteriosus before birth remodels the pulmonary vasculature of the lamb. *Pediatr Res* 1989; 25(3):251–257.

29. Abman SH, Stanley PF, Accurso FJ: Failure of postnatal adaption of the pulmonary circulation after chronic intrauterine pulmonary hypertension in fetal lambs. *J Clin Invest* 1989; 83:1849–1858.

30. Haworth SG: Pulmonary vascular remodeling in neonatal pulmonary hypertension. *Chest* 1988; 93(3):1335–1385.

31. Stenmark KR, Orton EC, Reeves JT, et al: Vascular remodeling in neonatal pulmonary hypertension. *Chest* 1988; 93(3):1275–1325.

32. Peters EA, Engle WA, Lemons JA: Persistent pulmonary hypertension of the newborn. *Indiana Med* 1989; 82(1):13–17.

33. Bonta BW: Transient pulmonary vascular lability: A form of mild pulmonary hypertension of the newborn not requiring mechanical ventilation. *J Perinatol* 1985; 8(1):19–23.

34. Riggs T, Hirschfield S, Fanaroff A, et al: Persistence of fetal circulation syndrome: An echocardiographic study. *J Pediatr* 1977; 91(4):626–631.

35. Fox WW, Duara S: Persistent pulmonary hypertension in the neonate: Diagnosis and management. *J Pediatr* 1983; 103(4):505–514.

36. Talner NS, Lister G, Fahey JT: Effect of asphyxia on the myocardium of the fetus and newborn. In Polin RA, Fox WW, eds: *Fetal and Neonatal Physiology*. Philadelphia, WB Saunders Co, 1991, pp. 759–769.

37. Weigel JT, Hageman JR: National survey of diagnosis and management of persistent pulmonary hypertension of the newborn. *J Perinatol* 1990; 10(4):369–375.

38. Fiddler GI, Chatrath R, Williams GJ, et al: Dopamine infusion for the treatment of myocardial dysfunction associated with a persistent transitional circulation. *Arch Dis Child* 1980; 55:194–198.

39. Duara S, Fox WW: Persistent pulmonary hypertension of the neonate. In Thibeault DW, Gregory GA, eds: *Neonatal Pulmonary Care*. Norwalk, CT, Appleton-Century-Crofts, 1986, pp. 461–481.

40. Drummond WH, Lock JE: Neonatal pulmonary vasodilator drugs. *Dev Pharmacol Ther* 1984; 7:1–20.

41. Stenmark KR, James SL, Voelkel NF, et al: Leukotrienes C and D in neonates with hypoxemia and pulmonary hypertension. *N Engl J Med* 1983; 309:77–80.

42. Taylor BJ, Fewell JE, Kearns GL, et al: Cromolyn sodium decreases the pulmonary vascular response to alveolar hypoxia in lambs. *Pediatr Res* 1986; 20(9):834–837.

43. Stencenko AA, Lefferts PL, Mitchell JA, et al: Vasodilatory effect of aerosol histamine during

pulmonary vasoconstriction in unanesthetized sheep. *Pediatr Pulmonol* 1987; 3:94–100.

44. Schreiber MD, Heymann MA, Soifer SJ: Increased arteriolar pH not decreased $PaCO_2$ attenuates hypoxia-induced pulmonary vasoconstriction in newborn lambs. *Pediatr Res* 1986; 20:113–117.

45. Wung JT, James LS, Kilchevsky E, et al: Management of infants with severe respiratory failure and persistence of the fetal circulation without hyperventilation. *Pediatrics* 1985; 76:488–494.

46. Cornish JD, Gertsmann DR, Clark RH, et al: Extracorporeal membrane oxygenation and high-frequency oscillatory ventilation: Potential therapeutic relationship. *Crit Care Med* 1987; 15(9):831–834.

47. Lloyd TC Jr: Influences of blood pH on hypoxic pulmonary vasoconstriction. *J Appl Physiol* 1966; 21(2):358–364.

48. Raffestin B, McMurtry IF: Effects of intracellular pH on hypoxic vasoconstriction in rat lungs. *J Appl Physiol* 1987; 63(6):2524–2531.

49. Orchard CH, Kentish JC: Effects of changes of pH on the contractile function of cardiac muscle, part I. *Am J Physiol* 1990; 258:C967–C981.

50. Weisfeldt ML, Geurci AD: Sodium bicarbonate in CPR (editorial). *JAMA* 1991; 266(15):2129–2130.

51. Kette F, Weil MH, Gazmuri RJ: Buffer solutions may comprise cardiac resuscitation by reducing coronary perfusion pressure. *JAMA* 1991; 266(15):2121–2126.

52. Hagemann JR, Adams MA, Gardner TH: Pulmonary complications of hyperventilation therapy for persistent pulmonary hypertension. *Crit Care Med* 1985; 13(12):1013–1014.

53. Cartwright D, Gregory GA, Lou H, et al: The effect of hypocarbia on the cardiovascular system of puppies. *Pediatr Res* 1984; 18(8):685–690.

54. Bifano EM, Pfannenstiel A: Duration of hyperventilation and outcome in infants with persistent pulmonary hypertension. *Pediatrics* 1988; 81(5):657–661.

55. Carter JM, Gertsmann DR, Clark RH, et al: High frequency oscillatory ventilation and extracorporeal membrane oxygenation for treatment of acute neonatal respiratory failure. *Pediatrics* 1990; 85(2):159–164.

56. Carlo WA, Beoglos A, Chatburn RL, et al: High frequency jet ventilation in neonatal pulmonary hypertension. *Am J Dis Child* 1989; 143:233–238.

57. Dworetz AR, Moya FR, Sabo B, et al: Survival of infants with persistent pulmonary hypertension without extracorporeal membrane oxygenation. Pediatrics 1989; 84(1):1–6.

58. Hirschl RB, Bartlett RH: Extracorporeal membrane oxygenation support in cardiorespiratory failure. *Adv Surg* 1987; 21:189–212.

59. Anderson HL II, OtsuT, Chapman RA, et al: Venovenous extracorporeal life support in neonates using a double lumen catheter. *ASAIO Trans* 1989; 35(3):650–653.

60. Crombleholme TM, Adzick NIS, deLorimier AA, et al: Carotid artery reconstruction following extracorporeal membrane oxygenation. *Am J Dis Child* 1990; 144:872–874.

61. Neonatal ECMO Registry of the Extracorporeal Life Support Organization (ELSO), Ann Arbor, MI, July 1991.

62. Bartlett RH, Toomasian J, Roloff D, et al: Extracorporeal membrane oxygenation in neonatal respiratory failure. *Ann Surg* 1986; 204(3):236–245.

63. VonSegesser K, Turina M: Long term cardiopulmonary bypass without systemic heparinization. *Intl J Artif Organs* 1990; 13(10):687–691.

64. Pasche B, Kodama K, Larm O, et al: Thrombin inactivation on surfaces with covalently bonded heparin. *Thrombosis Res* 1986; 44:739–748.

65. Larm O, Larson R, Olsson P: A new non-thrombogenic surface prepared by selective covalent binding of heparin via a modified reducing terminal residue. *Biomat Med Dev Artif Organs* 1983; 11:161–163.

66. Ferrara B, Johnson DE, Change P, et al: Efficacy and neurologic outcome of profound hypocapneic alkalosis for treatment of persistent pulmonary hypertension in infancy. *J Pediatr* 1984; 105(3):457–461.

67. Bernbaum JC, Russell P, Sheridan PH, et al: Long term follow up of newborns with persistent pulmonary hypertension. *Crit Care Med* 1984; 12(7):579–583.

68. Sell EJ, Gaines JA, Gluckman C, et al: Persistent fetal circulation—Neurodevelopmental outcome. *Am J Dis Child* 1985; 139:25–28.

69. Auten RL, Notter RH, Kendig JW, et al: Surfactant treatment of full term newborns with respiratory failure. *Pediatrics* 1991; 87:101–107.

70. Schumacher RE, Palmer TW, Roloff DW, et al: Follow-up of infants treated with extracorporeal membrane oxygenation for neonatal respiratory failure. *Pediatrics* 1991; 87(4):451–457.

71. Hofkosh D, Thompson AE, Nozza JR, et al: Ten years of extracorporeal membrane oxygenation: Neurodevelopmental outcome. *Pediatrics* 1991; 87(4):549–555.

72. Towne B, Lott IT, Hicks DA, et al: Long term follow up of infants and children treated with extracorporeal membrane oxygenation: A preliminary report. *J Pediatr Surg* 1985; 20(4):410–414.

73. Roberts JD, Polaner DM, Lang P, et al: Inhaled nitric oxide in persistent pulmonary hypertension of the newborn. *Lancet* 1992; 340:818–819.

74. Kinsella P, Neish SR, Shaffer E, et al: Low-dose inhalational nitric oxide in persistent pulmonary hypertension of the newborn. *Lancet* 1992; 340:819–820.

75. Engle WA, Peters EA, Gunn SK, et al: Mortality prediction in near term and term neonates with respiratory failure and interval until death. *J Perinatal* 1993; accepted for publication.

# Chapter 14

# RENAL FAILURE IN THE NEWBORN INFANT

*Joseph R. Sherbotie, M.D.*

The newborn infant, particularly the premature infant, is vulnerable to many environmental insults. Adverse events can occur during prenatal life, at any time during the birth process, or can result from the well-intentioned efforts of caregivers' actions in the nursery. Regardless of when these threatening events occur, they present a challenge to the neonate's well-being. Central to this well-being is the maintenance of an appropriate fluid and electrolyte milieu that allows the infant to function in the extrauterine environment. The kidneys and urinary tract have the primary responsibility, along with the lungs, skin, and gastrointestinal tract, for maintaining life-sustaining conditions. In caring for sick neonates, the physician is faced with decisions concerning the management of acquired or congenital renal problems and the related issue of prognosis. Is the decreased urine output an appropriate response of the kidney, or is it a manifestation of intrinsic damage? What is the cause of the renal failure? Will the kidneys heal with time and, if so, how can the caregivers avoid the life-threatening consequences of renal failure? What are realistic expectations for the infant with chronic renal insufficiency present at birth, and what kinds of decisions can be made along with the parents for treatment?

This chapter has been designed to teach the clinician how to recognize acute renal failure in the newborn infant, and provides specific recommendations for managing infants whose kidneys may not have completed their func-

tional or anatomic development. A sensible approach to the management of such patients is based on a sound understanding of how the kidney works, of differences present in the immature kidney, and understanding why chemical abnormalities may occur when renal function is limited. Case studies are presented along with exercises. Answers to all exercises are found either in or after the discussions following the exercises.

## OLIGURIA

A low urine output (<15 to 20 cc/kg/24 hr) is not a *sine qua non* of renal dysfunction. In fact, it may be a sign that the kidneys are appropriately doing their job, actively reabsorbing fluid and salt in an attempt to improve blood flow, which they sense is diminished. The following case history illustrates this concept, and provides a scheme of diagnostic criteria to evaluate renal function in the setting of oliguria.

### CASE STUDY 1

A 2,050-g male infant was born at 29 weeks' gestation to a healthy 27-year-old mother with one normal child. Through 26 weeks' gestation, the pregnancy was uncomplicated, and prenatal ultrasound and serial examinations suggested normal growth and no abnormalities. No medications or alcohol were consumed. During the last 3 weeks before delivery, persistent fetal tachycardia was noted, and maternal weight gain increased, apparently the result of a markedly enlarged uterus. The infant was delivered by cesarean section following rupture of amniotic membranes. Fetal heart tones were persistently elevated above 200 beats per minute (BPM) up until the moment of delivery. Apgar scores were 2 and 4 at 1 and 5 minutes, respectively, and the infant was intubated for respiratory distress. Physical examination was remarkable for anasarca and tachycardia. Urine output was present, but was persistently less than 0.3 mL/kg/hr. Because of the possibility of sepsis, he received intravenous ampicillin and gentamicin at the usual doses for weight.

## EXERCISE 1

### ■ Question:

Which of the abnormalities in the following table probably contributed to this infant's oliguria?

| | YES | NO |
|---|---|---|
| 1. Volume depletion | | |
| 2. Urinary tract obstruction | | |
| 3. Vascular obstruction | | |
| 4. Intrinsic renal disease | | |
| 5. Heart failure | | |
| 6. Urinary tract infection | | |
| 7. Sepsis | | |
| 8. Toxin | | |

### ■ Discussion:

*Volume depletion* (one of the most common reasons for a low urine output) is not likely in this patient, since he is edematous and well above the expected birth weight for his gestational age. Furthermore, there is no history of abnormal fluid losses, and he is not clinically dehydrated. Tachycardia is present, but for reasons other than dehydration.

*Urinary tract obstruction* is a common cause of renal insufficiency, particularly in male infants with posterior urethral valves. Oligohydramnios (decreased amount of amniotic fluid) may be observed prenatally in infants with significant urinary tract obstruction. Though these patients may present with edema at a later age, it is quite uncommon for them to present with edema in the immediate postnatal period. The possibility of obstruction, however, must not be overlooked, and a renal ultrasound study to carefully image the

kidneys, ureters, and bladder is appropriate. They were normal in this infant.

*Vascular obstruction* is more common in patients with increased blood viscosity (i.e., patients with polycythemia or depletion of effective intravascular volume) who may be at increased risk to develop renal venous thrombosis. Arterial thrombosis may be observed in infants with hypercoagulable states (e.g., protein C deficiency) or can be associated with umbilical arterial catheterization with embolization to, or thrombosis of, the renal arterial tree. In these instances, hypertension might be observed. Oliguria is not often seen unless renal arterial involvement is severe and bilateral (or when there is an affected solitary kidney). This infant's central hemoglobin concentration was high (21 g/dL) and may have been a contributing factor to the low urine output. Renal ultrasound demonstrated symmetrical kidneys and no evidence of thrombosis; however, ultrasonography is not the most sensitive way to detect vascular obstruction.

*Intrinsic renal disease* (most likely secondary to ischemia) is a definite possibility in this infant. Kidneys that are damaged by ischemia usually demonstrate both tubular and glomerular dysfunction. Tubular dysfunction is evidenced by the excretion of excessive amounts of sodium in the urine in the setting of diminished urine output. Normal kidneys reabsorb most of the salt filtered at the glomerulus when they sense diminished blood flow. Embarrassment of glomerular filtration may occur along with primary ischemic tubular damage because of obstruction of tubular lumens by cellular debris, backleak of filtered solutes across damaged tubular membranes, and decreased cortical blood flow secondary to release of vasoconstrictive hormones.

*Heart failure* is a likely etiology for the oliguria seen in this infant. The marked tachycardia and anasarca are suggestive of a markedly diminished and ineffective cardiac output. The kidneys appropriately responded in this case by increasing salt and fluid reabsorption. A cardiac evaluation would be extremely valuable in the management of this infant.

*Urinary tract infection* would not be expected to produce renal failure during the perinatal period, but may be associated with sepsis. The release of endotoxin and inflammatory mediators may increase capillary leak and result in a decreased effective circulating blood volume; this process may occasionally lead to ischemic renal failure.

*Toxin-induced* acute renal failure may be seen in the neonate. The most common causes for toxin-induced renal injury are drugs (e.g., aminoglycosides) administered after birth; however, the maternal use of medications such as angiotensin-converting enzyme inhibitors (e.g., captopril) may adversely affect renal function postnatally. This infant received an aminoglycoside antibiotic (in excessive amounts based on his wet weight), but his problems antedated their use. However, aminoglycoside antibiotics may contribute to renal insufficiency in a setting of diminished renal clearance and should be avoided or administered only with appropriate monitoring of levels in such patients. Renal damage secondary to toxic levels of aminoglycosides is most often associated with nonoliguric renal failure.

■ **Answer:**

1. no
2. no
3. no
4. yes
5. yes
6. no
7. no
8. no

## EXERCISE 2

How can we determine if this infant's oliguria is an appropriate response to intravascular volume depletion, or is secondary to intrinsic ischemic renal damage? The studies listed in the left hand column in the table below are frequently used to differentiate prerenal from ischemic acute renal failure (ARF). Please insert the expected finding in the space provided.

| | PRERENAL | ISCHEMIC ARF |
|---|---|---|
| Urine output | | |
| Urinalysis | | |

| | PRERENAL | ISCHEMIC ARF |
|---|---|---|
| Urine specific gravity | | |
| Urine (Na) | | |
| Fractional excretion of sodium (FE$_{Na}$) | | |
| BUN | | |
| Serum creatinine | | |

■ **Discussion:**

It is apparent from this exercise that the ability of the kidney to reabsorb sodium is central to distinguishing ARF from prerenal azotemia. Sodium is freely filtered at the glomerulus and is reabsorbed in the proximal tubule, thick ascending limb of the loop of Henle and the distal tubule. When the kidney (specifically the specialized portion of the distal convoluted tubule known as the *macula densa*) senses diminished tubular flow or increased tonicity of the tubular fluid, sodium reabsorption is increased. Mechanisms of increased sodium reabsorption include diminished peritubular blood flow along the proximal tubule, diminished tubular fluid flow rates, and activation of the renin/angiotensin/aldosterone axis. More sodium is absorbed isotonically at proximal tubular sites; however, increased reabsorption of sodium also occurs in more distal nephron segments. Osmotically active particles (e.g., mannitol, glucose) or anions that are filtered into the tubular fluid but are not completely reabsorbed (e.g., sulfates) may result in less reabsorption of sodium because of increased tubular fluid flow rates and a more negative luminal charge. A low urine concentration of sodium in the presence of oliguria suggests that the kidney is maximally reabsorbing salt to maintain perfusion. Normally functioning tubules will reabsorb more than 99% of the sodium filtered at the glomerulus with volume depletion.

A more critical measure of the kidney's ability to reabsorb sodium in the setting of oliguria is the fractional excretion of sodium (FE$_{Na}$). This value is calculated by comparing the amount of sodium that ends up in the urine to the amount of sodium filtered at the glomerulus. Sodium is freely filtered and appears in the glomerular ultrafiltrate in concentrations equal to that in plasma water. Creatinine is handled the same way; however, creatinine is not significantly reabsorbed or secreted by the renal tubules. Therefore, the absolute amount of creatinine found in the urine is nearly the same as that filtered at the glomerulus (though the concentration changes).

Clearance by the kidney represents the volume of blood from which a solute is totally removed in a given period of time. If sodium were not reabsorbed by the tubules, the clearance of sodium would be approximately equal to the clearance of creatinine. The renal clearance of sodium is far less than that of creatinine, the difference being the amount of sodium reabsorbed by the tubules. We can therefore calculate the fraction of sodium excreted (found in the final urine) by calculating the ratio of the clearance of sodium to the clearance of creatinine:

$$FE_{Na} = \frac{(Urine\ Na)(Urine\ Volume)}{(Serum\ Na)}$$
$$\div \frac{(Urine\ Creatinine)(Urine\ Volume)}{(Serum\ Creatinine)}$$
$$\times\ 100\%$$

Values for $FE_{Na}$ greater than 3% in association with oliguria provide strong evidence of intrinsic renal tubular damage impairing the reabsorption of salt. Caveats for more premature infants will be discussed later.

■ **Answer:**

| | PRERENAL | ISCHEMIC ARF |
|---|---|---|
| Urine output | Decreased; because of diminished circulating volume perceived by the kidney, maximal reabsorption of salt and water are expected | Decreased, though normal or even increased urine output may be seen |
| Urinalysis | Normal | Usually granular casts, renal tubular epithelial cells and debris ("muddy" urine of ATN) |

| | PRERENAL | ISCHEMIC ARF |
|---|---|---|
| Urine specific gravity | High | Usually isotonic; may be factitiously elevated in the presence of significant proteinuria |
| Urine (Na) | Low; generally below 10 to 20 mmol/L | Not depressed |
| Fractional excretion of sodium ($FE_{Na}$) | Low; usually <3% | Increased; >3%, but may be low early in ARF |
| BUN | May be elevated | May be elevated |
| Serum creatinine | Normal or minimally elevated | Usually elevated; increasing trend may be more revealing |

## HOW CAN WE TREAT RENAL FAILURE IN NEONATES?

Management of renal failure in the neonate requires a thorough understanding of fluid and electrolyte requirements and an understanding of why abnormalities occur in patients with renal failure. *Conservative management* centers around avoiding the dangerous metabolic consequences of impaired renal function. At times, this is not enough to keep the patient alive, and more *aggressive* therapeutic measures such as dialysis must be undertaken. The decision to embark on more than conservative management is closely linked to the presence of other factors contributing to the overall prognosis of the child. Measures to improve the rate of recovery of renal function and to avoid further insult (e.g., supplying substrate for renal repair, improving renal blood flow, and diminishing the adverse effects of free radicals generated during reperfusion) are currently under investigation.

### CASE STUDY 2
Baby girl AW was born prematurely to a 25-year-old, primigravida woman. The onset of

premature labor occurred at 25 weeks' gestation, and external fetal heart rate monitoring suggested fetal distress. A 750-g infant girl was born by cesarean section with Apgar scores of 1 and 3 at 1 and 5 minutes, respectively. She required mechanical ventilation soon after birth and was treated with intravenous ampicillin and gentamicin because of the possibility of sepsis. The aminoglycoside antibiotic was dosed appropriately and serum levels were followed closely. AW developed oliguria and demonstrated increasing weight over the first few days of life. Her serum creatinine concentration was 1.0 mg/dL at birth, and increased to 3.6 mg/dL by day 5 of life. At that time, serum chemistries revealed sodium = 122, chloride = 82, potassium = 8.5, and a total $CO_2$ = 14 mEq/L. Her weight had increased to 810 g, and she was edematous. Her blood pressure was persistently elevated at 110/56 mm Hg. However, there was no evidence of congestive heart failure and her perfusion was excellent.

## EXERCISE 3

### ■ Questions:

1. Based on the history, what is the most likely etiology for this infant's renal failure?

2. What features suggest that renal perfusion is normal?

### ■ Answers:

1. The history is suggestive of perinatal asphyxia, with ischemic acute renal failure the most likely possibility.

2. Clinically, the child is edematous and not volume depleted. Her blood pressure is high; however, there is no evidence of congestive heart failure, and perfusion is normal. The effective circulating volume, therefore, appears normal or excessive.

## CASE STUDY 2 continued

The following additional laboratory studies are obtained:

- *Urinalysis* reveals protein, a small amount of blood, and some granular casts, with a specific gravity of 1.008.
- *Renal ultrasound* is normal, with no evidence of hydronephrosis, obstruction, hypoplasia, or cysts.
- *Doppler* study of renal blood flow appears normal.
- *Urine, blood, and cerebrospinal fluid (CSF) cultures* are negative. (The baby is on appropriate doses of antibiotics and is not receiving any other nephrotoxic agents.)

A small amount of urine is obtained and sent for determination of sodium and creatinine concentrations:

- Urine sodium, 36 mEq/L
- Urine creatinine, 17 mg/dL

## EXERCISE 4

Calculate the fractional excretion of sodium for this patient. (Assume the serum Na = 122 mEq/L and serum creatinine = 3.6 mg/dL.)

### ■ Discussion:

The fractional excretion of sodium in the preceding case is above the commonly accepted normal value of 3%; however, premature infants (<32 weeks' gestation) typically exhibit elevated values for fractional excretion of sodium as a normal finding (even though intrinsic autoregulation keeps glomerular filtration and tubular function in relative balance). Values as high as 7% to 10% may be observed in that population. Values of 1% to 3% are normally observed in infants of >32 to 36 weeks' gestation.

In the case of AW summarized in Case Study 2, a repeat urine sodium concentration was noted to be 86 mEq/L. Therefore, the calculated fractional excretion of sodium was 15%, an abnormally elevated value in an oliguric premature infant. This suggested that this baby had intrinsic tubular damage, probably as a result of ischemia.

We now turn our attention to the management of this infant's acute renal failure. First we discuss conservative therapy.

■ **Answer:**

$$FE_{Na} = [(36 \text{ mEq/L})/(122 \text{ mEq/L})]$$
$$\div [(17 \text{ mg/dL})/3.6 \text{ mg/dL})]$$
$$\times 100\% = 6\%$$

## EXERCISE 5

■ **Questions:**

1. List the major consequences of each of the biochemical abnormalities in the following table.

| ABNORMALITY | CONSEQUENCE(S) |
| --- | --- |
| Hyperkalemia | |
| Hyponatremia | |
| Fluid overload | |
| Metabolic acidosis | |
| Hyperphosphatemia | |
| Hypocalcemia | |

2. Which of the preceding abnormalities requires immediate treatment?

■ **Discussion:**

Life-threatening biochemical abnormalities obviously need to be corrected immediately, although in practice, all serious or life-threatening abnormalities are corrected simultaneously. Any potassium concentration >6 mEq/L may have adverse consequences; however, values between 6 and 7 mEq/L are considered only moderately elevated. Patients with hyperkalemia and myocardial instability or electrocardiographic evidence of hyperkalemia (e.g., peaked T waves, widened QRS complexes, or ventricular ectopy) require immediate therapy. Seizures may be due to hyponatremia or hypocalcemia. Therefore, when these biochemical abnormalities are present in an infant with seizures, prompt treatment is also indicated. Other abnormalities may be treated as indicated by the clinical circumstance.

■ **Answers:**

1. *Hyperkalemia* may be life threatening, and it may result in life-threatening cardiac arrythmias.

   *Hyponatremia* may result in neuromuscular irritability and seizures.

   *Fluid overload* may precipitate congestive heart failure and worsen pulmonary symptoms.

*Metabolic acidosis* may interfere with the proper functioning of many enzyme systems responsible for producing energy in the body. Severe acidosis may potentiate the cardiotoxic effects of hyperkalemia.

*Hyperphosphatemia* has its major effects by resulting in a reciprocal hypocalcemia. Significant elevation of serum phosphorus and calcium (where the product of phosphorus × calcium is greater than 70 to 80 for a significant period of time) may result in soft tissue calcifications.

*Hypocalcemia,* specifically decreased free or ionized serum calcium levels, may result in neuromuscular irritability, precipitating tetany, seizures, and myocardial dysfunction.

2. *Complications requiring immediate treatment:*
   * Hyperkalemia associated with cardiac arrythmias or electrocardiographic abnormalities
   * Seizures associated with hyponatremia
   * Seizures associated with hypocalcemia
   * Severe metabolic acidosis

   *Complications requiring treatment (but not immediately):*
   * Hyperphosphatemia
   * Asymptomatic hyponatremia or hypocalcemia
   * Fluid overload
   * Asymptomatic hyperkalemia
   * Mild or moderate metabolic acidosis

## EXERCISE 6

Because of the presence of a worsening metabolic acidosis (pH = 7.19 $PCO_2$ = 40), the baby was administered sodium bicarbonate (1 mEq/kg) intravenously twice. After the second dose, the metabolic acidosis improved, but effective assisted ventilation became more difficult, requiring paralysis with a neuromuscular blocking agent.

■ **Question:**

What was overlooked?

■ **Discussion/Answer:**

Any one of several conditions could have resulted in worsening ventilation. In this particular case, the endotracheal tube was checked and was patent. The acute nature of the problem suggests that fluid overload may have been a contributing factor, but only small volumes of fluid were given. Clinically, the baby was demonstrating seizure activity prior to receiving the neuromuscular blocking agent. The serum sodium concentration was measured again and was stable (123 mEq/L); however the ionized calcium level was only 0.7 mmol/L. The administration of sodium bicarbonate almost certainly increased this infant's blood pH. As the infant's blood became more alkaline, free serum calcium would have bound to serum proteins, particularly albumin. In retrospect, the acidosis was actually maintaining this infant's ionized serum calcium levels within a reasonably safe range. The administration of sodium bicarbonate decreased the free serum calcium levels, resulting in tetany and seizures. This problem may have been avoided by measuring serum calcium levels prior to correcting the acidosis, and administering calcium if needed.

## EXERCISE 7

This baby was found to have short runs of ventricular fibrillation and widened QRS complexes on her ECG. The serum potassium concentration was 7.8 mEq/L.

### ■ Question:

Which of the following is the most appropriate therapy at this time?

1. Lidocaine drip

2. Peritoneal dialysis

3. Hemodialysis

4. Calcium chloride

5. Glucose and insulin

6. Sodium bicarbonate

### ■ Discussion/Answer:

In the presence of life-threatening hyperkalemia, *calcium chloride* or *calcium gluconate* would offer the most immediate benefit to this infant's hemodynamic status, and it should be given promptly. The other measures, designed to decrease the serum potassium concentration or remove potassium from the body, would be slower in effect. Hemodialysis might even contribute to cardiovascular instability if done prior to stabilizing the patient.

This infant's hyperkalemia may be managed in several ways (Table 14-1). Some measures are temporizing, resulting in a shift of potassium from the extracellular (ECF) to the intracellular fluid (ICF) space, while other measures actually result in the removal of potassium from the body. The temporizing measures are, in general, quicker at decreasing serum potassium levels in an emergency, but the effects may be short-lived. When hyperkalemia is present, or when it is likely to occur in the setting of acute renal failure, all potassium intake must be stopped. The newborn infant, particularly the premature infant, is less able to excrete potassium loads efficiently under normal conditions, and this may become quite problematic when renal insufficiency supervenes. Mechanisms responsible for this diminished ability to excrete potassium may include alterations in the distal tu-

**Table 14-1** Treatment of Hyperkalemia

| DRUG | ADMINISTRATION |
| --- | --- |
| Sodium polystyrene sulfonate suspension (15 g/60 mL) (Kayexalate) | 1 g/kg or 4 mL/kg of suspension q. 6 hours. Suspension may be given either po or per rectum (administered with sorbitol). |
| Calcium gluconate (10%) | 50 mg/kg intravenous for 5 to 10 minutes. Monitor with electrocardiogram. Slow infusion if heart rate slows. |
| Sodium bicarbonate | 1 to 2 mEq/kg intravenous for 5 to 10 minutes. |
| Glucose ($D_{25}W$) and insulin | 0.5 g/kg (2 mL/kg of $D_{25}W$ or 5 mL/kg of $D_{10}W$) with 0.2 units regular insulin per gram glucose (0.1 unit/kg) for 2 hours. Infuse $D_{25}W$ by way of central venous access. |

*Source:* From Karlowicz MG, Adelman RD: Acute renal failure in the neonate. *Clin Perinatol* 1992; 19(1):151. Reprinted with permission of W.B. Saunders Company.

bular concentration of Na-K-ATPase, diminished tubular flow rates, a diminished tubular fluid sodium concentration, and backleak of filtered potassium across the tubular epithelium.

---

## EXERCISE 8

### ■ Question:

What are the potential risks of each of the following therapies used to treat infants with hyperkalemia?

#### *Shift of Potassium to ICF*

| THERAPY | POTENTIAL RISK |
| --- | --- |
| Glucose, insulin | |
| Sodium bicarbonate | |

#### *Removal of Potassium*

| THERAPY | POTENTIAL RISK |
| --- | --- |
| Diuretics | |
| Sodium polystyrene sulfonate | |

### ■ Discussion:

The use of insulin and glucose may result in hypo- or hyperglycemia. Sodium bicarbonate administration may exacerbate sodium and volume overload, or precipitate tetany in the setting of hypocalcemia.

Diuretics, particularly loop diuretics, may be effective in increasing urine output in patients with oliguria. The potential side effects of diuretic therapy include volume depletion, hyponatremia, hypokalemia, metabolic alkalosis, ototoxicity (especially when loop diuretics are given along with aminoglycoside antibiotics), and idiosyncratic reactions. In addition, dosage of loop diuretics must be carefully monitored in premature infants under 31 weeks' gestation, because the potential for toxicity is greater in that population.

Sodium polystyrene sulfonate (Kayexalate) is a resin that exchanges sodium for other cations in the gut. The goal is usually the removal of potassium, but other cations including magnesium and calcium can be adsorbed. The exchange results in the absorption of sodium into the patient. Because of this, the use of cation exchange resins may result in hypomagnesemia, hypocalcemia, and exacerbation of salt and fluid overload. In addition, it may be hazardous to administer this resin when the intestinal mucosa is friable or if gastrointestinal perfusion is tenuous.

### ■ Answer:

#### *Shift of Potassium to ICF*

| THERAPY | POTENTIAL RISK |
| --- | --- |
| Glucose, insulin | Hypo- or hyperglycemia |
| Sodium bicarbonate | Salt and volume overload, alkalosis, and precipitation of tetany |

#### *Removal of Potassium*

| THERAPY | POTENTIAL RISK |
| --- | --- |
| Diuretics | Volume depletion, alkalosis, ototoxicity, electrolyte imbalance |
| Sodium polystyrene sulfonate | Hypomagnesemia, hypocalcemia, salt and fluid overload |

---

## EXERCISE 9

---

This infant's serum sodium level decreased to 112 mEq/L, and she began to have seizures. No other metabolic abnormalities were present. She was treated with diazepam when the seizures were noted.

### ■ Question:

How should the symptomatic hyponatremia be treated? Select one therapy.

1. Administer 0.9% NaCl (10 mL/kg) intravenously.

2. Change all fluids the baby is receiving to 0.9% NaCl.

3. Administer 2 to 4 mL/kg of 3% NaCl (500 mEq NaCl/L) IV slowly.

4. Begin phenobarbital.

### ■ Discussion/Answer:

Seizures caused by hyponatremia may respond poorly to the usual anticonvulsant medications. The proper treatment consists of increasing the sodium concentration in the ECF enough to ameliorate seizure activity, but avoiding rapid increases in serum sodium. Rapid correction of severe hyponatremia in adults under certain conditions may be associated with central pontine demyelinolysis, coma, and death, but this has not been well documented in children. Judicious correction of hyponatremia at any age is likely to be safest. Administering normal saline, either as a bolus or as a continuous infusion would require an inordinate amount of time to increase serum sodium levels and might result in volume overload. In contrast, administering 3 mL/kg of 3% saline would provide 15 mEq of NaCl (without significant fluid) and would increase serum sodium levels by 2 to 3 mEq/L, because the administered sodium would distribute in total body water. The goal of such therapy is to increase the serum sodium level just enough to stop the neurological symptoms. In most cases, increasing the serum sodium by a few mEq/L is often sufficient.

## EXERCISE 10

You have administered a 3% saline solution, and the seizure activity has stopped. The serum sodium concentration is now 114 mEq/L. Urine output has increased to 20 mL daily; however, her weight is 815 g (65 g above birth weight). She is still edematous, and her blood pressure is elevated. Peripheral perfusion appears normal. Urine sodium is measured again and is 70 mEq/L.

### ■ Question:

How should this infant's fluids be managed at this point? Select one therapy.

1. Begin $D_{10}$/W at an infusion rate equaling insensible water loss (1 to 2 mL/kg/hr) plus urine output (20 mL/day).

2. Begin $D_{10}$/normal saline at an infusion rate equaling insensible water loss (1 to 2 mL/kg/hr) plus urine output (20 mL/day).

3. Through a central venous catheter, administer $D_{25}$/normal saline at a rate of 1 to 2 mL/kg/hr.

### ■ Discussion/Answer:

This patient is edematous and hyponatremic. There is no evidence of intravascular volume depletion. Therefore, she is both salt and fluid overloaded. The etiology of the hyponatremia is simply too much free water. This has re-

sulted in dilution of sodium by an expanded total body water. Treatment should most appropriately be directed at administering less electrolyte free water (water without sodium and potassium) than the patient is losing. By doing this, the sodium will equilibrate in a decreasing amount of total body water, and the sodium concentration in the ECF will increase.

By administering $D_{10}$/W at a rate equaling estimated insensible water losses and urine output, the hyponatremia would worsen. The electrolyte content of the urine (70 mEq/L) reveals that 50% of it is isotonic with respect to serum sodium, and the other 50% of it represents free-water loss.

The fraction of isotonic fluid lost in the urine may be calculated as follows:

Fraction of isotonic fluid lost in urine
= (Urine Na)/(Normal Serum Na) × 100%
= [70 mEq/L]/[140 mEq/L] × 100%
= 50%

Replacing all of the urine output with electrolyte free water would result in replacing the isotonic urine losses (50% of total urine output) with free water, thereby exacerbating the hyponatremia.

Administering $D_{10}$/normal saline would result in an increase in the serum sodium concentration by 10 to 15 mEq/24 hr. Unfortunately, this patient is already volume overloaded. Therefore, increasing salt intake without reducing the fluid overload state would likely exacerbate the hypertension and might precipitate heart failure.

Increasing the serum sodium concentration by 10 to 20 mEq/24 hr is not likely to cause any neurological problems. At the same time, we would like to decrease this infant's volume overload. The most reasonable approach would be to administer fluid at a rate less than ongoing losses and to provide less free water than the infant is losing. Administering $D_{25}$/normal saline would accomplish both of these goals, and would hopefully provide enough glucose to avoid hypoglycemia. At a rate of 1 mL/hr, this regimen would provide an additional 4 mEq of NaCl daily, and would permit some weight loss because of anticipated ongoing urine output and insensible water losses. The result would be an increase in serum sodium concentration of about 10 mEq/L per 24 hours, which is a safe rate of increase.

You could attempt to increase urine output by using a loop diuretic. The enhanced urine output would permit increased fluid administration rates, and as a result would allow better nutritional support to be given. Furthermore, the response to diuretics may be a prognostic indicator, because adults with non-oliguric acute renal failure have fared better historically than those with oliguria. With very poor renal function, higher doses of loop diuretics (e.g., 3 to 4 mg/kg of furosemide) are often used. If there is no response, it should not be continued. It is important to realize that giving diuretics has little to do with improving renal function. Rather, those infants who respond may have less severe injury. Furosemide may offer some protection from further ischemic damage by decreasing the metabolic activity of the nephron segments most prone to hypoxia (e.g., the loop of Henle).

Remember that acute renal failure is often a dynamic process, and you should not rely on yesterday's data to make today's therapeutic decisions. Therefore, close attention must be paid to serum and urine chemistry values obtained on at least a twice daily basis.

## EXERCISE 11

This infant's serum phosphorus level is 12 mg/dL, and the serum calcium concentration has decreased to 5.2 mg/dL (ionized calcium 0.7 mmol/L). Because of the reciprocal relationship between serum phosphorus and serum calcium measurements, you suspect that lowering the serum phosphorus level may result in an increase in serum calcium.

### ■ Question:

What is/are the best way(s) to accomplish this goal?

1. Administer furosemide (3 mg/kg) intravenously.

2. Administer sodium polystyrene sulfonate rectally or orally.

3. Administer aluminum hydroxide orally.

4. Administer calcium carbonate orally.

5. Increase the infusion of glucose and consider administering insulin.

### ■ Discussion/Answer:

Symptomatic hypocalcemia requires immediate calcium supplementation parenterally or with dialysis. Asymptomatic hypocalcemia associated with hyperphosphatemia need not be treated as aggressively, but the potential for problems is significant. In patients with oliguric acute renal failure, furosemide will do little to increase phosphorus loss, and the cation exchange resin sodium polystyrene sulfonate is not appropriate for that purpose. Aluminum hydroxide acts as a phosphate binder in the lumen of the gut, but neonates appear to be particularly prone to the adverse effects (particularly neurological) of aluminum overload. Therefore, aluminum-containing compounds should be avoided. Calcium carbonate given orally will safely and effectively bind phosphorus in the gut, making it unavailable for absorption. This occurs to a lesser extent in patients who are not eating, presumably due to recycling of phosphorus shed into the gut. Calcium carbonate, however, may result in some constipation. Administering glucose and insulin, as is done to lower serum potassium levels, can be quite effective in quickly lowering serum phosphorus levels, because enzyme systems responsible for the cellular uptake of glucose also result in the movement of phosphorus intracellularly.

## EXERCISE 12

The infant continues to have a blood pressure of 110 to 118 over 50 to 70 mm Hg in spite of fluid restriction. Furthermore, she is developing radiographic findings consistent with pulmonary edema, and her heart is enlarged. These signs make it clear that she must have her hypertension treated. Connect the antihypertensive agents listed in the following table with their proposed mechanisms of action.

| | |
|---|---|
| Hydralazine | Blocks calcium influx through slow calcium channels |
| Nifedipine | $\beta$-blocking agent (nonselective) |
| Captopril | Direct-acting vasodilator (relaxes vascular smooth muscle) |
| Propranolol | Angiotensin-converting enzyme inhibitor |

■ **Question:**
What might be the significant side effects of each class of antihypertensive agent?

■ **Discussion/Answer:**

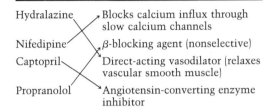

Hydralazine — Blocks calcium influx through slow calcium channels

Nifedipine — β-blocking agent (nonselective)

Captopril — Direct-acting vasodilator (relaxes vascular smooth muscle)

Propranolol — Angiotensin-converting enzyme inhibitor

*Calcium channel blocking agents* (such as nifedipine) inhibit the flux of calcium into the cell and the sarcolemma of smooth muscle and sometimes cardiac muscle. The effects are often dose dependent, and the net result is relaxation of vascular smooth muscle. Many varieties of calcium channel blocking agents are available, and they do not all have the same effects. Nifedipine acts primarily on peripheral vascular smooth muscle and has little clinically discernable effect on cardiac muscle. Other agents, such as verapamil, have greater effects on suppression of myocardial contractility, which may be clinically important. Because of this, the use of some calcium channel blocking agents with known myocardial effects may precipitate cardiac failure in patients who already have compromised myocardial function. Even nifedipine may have adverse effects on cardiac function in the setting of very severe myocardial dysfunction; however, with less severe dysfunction, cardiac output is often improved because of the decrease in afterload. Additional side effects can include mild edema and constipation. Of note, the antihypertensive effects of nifedipine may become blunted if treatment is continued for an extended period of time.

*Beta-adrenergic blocking agents* (e.g., propanolol) bind to the β-adrenergic receptor. This binding may be selective for cardiac $\beta_1$ receptors, or may be nonselective and include binding to peripheral $\beta_2$ receptors, which mediate bronchial dilation. At the doses typically used to treat hypertension, all agents have some effects on cardiac receptors. Beta-blocking agents also differ in lipid solubility, intrin-

sic sympathomimetic activity, half-life, and clearance. Each of these characteristics affects the type and frequency of side effects. Propranolol, the most common β-blocker used in newborns, is lipid soluble and is associated with central nervous system effects (e.g., sleepiness), especially early in the course of treatment. Propranolol is a nonselective blocker affecting both peripheral and cardiac β receptors. As a result of $\beta_2$ receptor blockade, bronchospasm may be precipitated. A $\beta_1$ receptor blockade on cardiac contractility and heart rate may result in congestive heart failure in patients with borderline cardiac function. Compensatory responses to hypoglycemia depend partially on stimulation of β receptors, and such responses are blunted by β-blocking drugs. The clearance of propranolol is primarily hepatic, while some other β-blocking agents are cleared to various degrees by the kidneys. The hepatic metabolism results in a *first-pass effect* when the medication is given orally, resulting in the need for a larger oral dose compared to an appropriate parenteral dose (Table 14-2). The parenteral administration of some β-blocking agents, including propranolol, may result in profound depression of cardiac output, particularly in the presence of concomitantly administered drugs that suppress cardiac output or alter cardiac rhythms.

*Direct-acting vasodilators* (e.g., hydralazine and minoxidil) act on the arterial and/or venous circulations. Hydralazine, the most

**Table 14-2** Antihypertensive Drugs in Acute Renal Failure

| DRUG | DOSAGE |
|---|---|
| Hydralazine | 0.1–0.5 mg/kg IV q. 3 hours |
| | 0.5–2 mg/kg po q. 6 hours |
| Propranolol | 0.01–0.15 mg/kg IV q. 6 hours |
| | 0.25–1.25 mg/kg po q. 6 hours |
| Captopril | 0.05–0.5 mg/kg po q. 6 hours |
| Enalapril | 0.005–0.05 mg/kg IV |
| Nifedipine | 0.25–0.5 mg/kg sublingual |
| Labetalol | 0.25–1 mg/kg IV q. 4 hours |
| Diazoxide | 1–5 mg/kg IV |
| Nitroprusside | 0.2–6 mcg/kg/min IV |

*Source:* From Karlowicz MG, Adelman RD: Acute renal failure in the neonate. *Clin Perinatol* 1992; 19(1):150. Reprinted with permission of W.B. Saunders Company.

widely used of these agents, is metabolized by the liver. Therefore, the first-pass effect mandates that higher oral doses of hydralazine be given. Side effects of hydralazine, and most direct-acting vasodilators, include tachycardia, increased cardiac output, and fluid retention. Because of this, nearly all patients require concomitant treatment with a diuretic (if they have renal function) and a $\beta$-blocking agent. On occasion, hydralazine also causes flushing, headache, and a lupus-like syndrome.

*Angiotensin-converting enzyme (ACE) inhibitors* (e.g., captopril) have undergone a remarkable growth in popularity. Most of the clinical experience with these agents in neonates and children has been with captopril, an agent that contains a sulfhydryl group incriminated in some of its undesirable side effects. These agents exert antihypertensive effects by blocking the conversion of angiotensin I to angiotensin II, a potent vasoconstrictor. In addition, these drugs also increase renin production, and modulate the kininogen system. ACE inhibitors are quite effective as antihypertensive agents and can lower blood pressure even when circulating renin levels are not elevated, suggesting that local effects in the kidney and elsewhere are of great importance in the control of blood pressure. The antihypertensive effects are exaggerated with the simultaneous use of diuretics and with volume depletion. ACE inhibitors can result in hyperkalemia and acidosis, and agents that have the potential to worsen these effects must be used with caution. Captopril in particular has been associated with the development of neutropenia; this side effect has been most commonly observed in patients with collagen vascular diseases. Doses usually effective in older children have been associated with acute renal failure in neonates. Therefore, suggested doses are much lower in the newborn (Table 14-2). These agents should be avoided in patients with bilateral renal artery stenosis or in patients with a solitary kidney and renal artery stenosis, because the maintenance of the glomerular filtration rate may be dependent on the efferent arteriolar (postglomerular) effects of angiotensin II in such cases. The metabolism of ACE inhibitors differs for different agents, so dosage adjustments may be necessary in the setting of hepatic or renal dysfunction.

The adverse effects of *diuretics* (e.g., furosemide and thiazides) typically include volume depletion and hyponatremia. This latter effect appears to be very common in newborns who often receive hypotonic fluid for nutrition. With the exception of potassium-sparing diuretics, hypokalemia is quite common as well. Furthermore, loop diuretics (e.g., furosemide) can lead to hypercalciuria, urolithiasis, and nephrocalcinosis. These latter effects are at least partially dependent on the dosage and duration of therapy. Conversely, thiazide diuretics may diminish urinary calcium excretion and may lead to hypercalcemia. Metabolic alkalosis and wasting of other minerals including phosphorus and magnesium may be seen with both major classes of diuretics. The potential for ototoxicity with the use of furosemide has already been mentioned. Only loop diuretics may be effective in patients with markedly diminished renal function.

---

## EXERCISE 13

In spite of attempts at fluid restriction, this baby's weight increases gradually. The infant has had problems with hypoglycemia and is unable to receive sufficient calories for growth. She remains mechanically ventilated and is unable to wean. Present laboratory values include arterial pH, 7.20; $PCO_2$, 36 torr; bicarbonate, 14 mEq/L; sodium, 120 mEq/L; and potassium, 7.4 mEq/L.

■ **Question:**

What are three indications for dialysis at this time?

1.

2.

3.

■ **Discussion/Answer:**

The decision to begin dialysis often depends on the presence of criteria, including the following:

1. Volume overload resistant to appropriate doses of potent diuretics.

2. Metabolic acidosis resistant to treatment with base supplementation, or when base

supplementation is contraindicated (as in the setting of hypernatremia or severe fluid overload with the potential for congestive heart failure).

3. Hyperkalemia that is symptomatic and/or cannot be effectively treated with conservative medical therapy.

4. Signs and symptoms of uremia, which might include bleeding diathesis, changes in mental status without other etiology, pericardial effusion, gastrointestinal disturbances, neurological signs (seizures, involuntary movements), and others.

In addition to these criteria, other factors important in patient care may present as relative indications to initiate dialysis in the setting of oliguric acute renal failure. These might include the need to administer significant volumes of blood products and the perceived need to supply adequate nutrition.

It is obvious from this discussion that this infant meets several of these criteria (1, 2, and 3). In addition, studies in adults have suggested that supplying adequate nutrition including sufficient protein to attain positive nitrogen balance with control of uremia improves the recovery of renal function. Therefore, it appears to be counterproductive to starve patients with protracted acute renal failure who will likely recover.

## EXERCISE 14

Since you believe dialysis is indicated, you should have some idea of the relative advantages and disadvantages of the various modalities available. Given the following statements, decide which of the modalities most closely applies to the statement. Choose between peritoneal dialysis (PD), intermittent hemodialysis (HD), and continuous arteriovenous hemofiltration (CAVH).

| | PD | HD | CAVH |
|---|---|---|---|
| 1. No need for vascular access | | | |
| 2. Continuous form of therapy | | | |
| 3. Most efficient form of dialysis | | | |
| 4. Minimizes catabolism | | | |

| | PD | HD | CAVH |
|---|---|---|---|
| 5. Most closely mimics the filtration mechanisms of the kidney | | | |
| 6. Need for a large arterial catheter | | | |
| 7. Risk of peritonitis | | | |
| 8. Hemodynamic instability | | | |

### ■ Discussion:

Peritoneal dialysis is a gentle and continuous form of dialysis, removing most solute (waste products) by diffusion across the peritoneal membrane. It involves placement of an acute or a chronic peritoneal dialysis catheter into the peritoneal cavity, and therefore is associated with the potential for contamination and the development of peritonitis. Peritoneal dialysis is technically the easiest of dialysis procedures to perform in infants and is often the first choice of many nephrologists. Fluid balance can be erratic in very sick infants. Fluid removal depends on the osmotic force generated by high concentrations of dextrose in the dialysate fluid, some of which is absorbed. While this can provide extra calories, it may lead to hyperglycemia in some patients. Protein is also lost through the peritoneal cavity where it can be removed during the course of dialysis.

Intermittent hemodialysis provides the greatest instantaneous removal rates of fluid and solute and is therefore the most efficient. The other forms of therapy, however, are equally effective in the cumulative removal of solutes because of their continuous nature. Caution must be exercised with the use of hemodialysis in neonates. For example, the use of some membrane types results in increased catabolism and sometimes leads to hypoxia. In addition, intermittent systemic anticoagulation is usually required, which may increase the likelihood of intracranial bleeding. Hemodialysis requires specialized equipment and personnel, and may be technically challenging to perform in neonates, particularly premature infants. It may result in rapid shifts of fluid and solute, leading to hemodynamic instability and serious central nervous system consequences. Because of the volume of the extracorporeal circuit, the circuit may need to be primed with blood for each treatment. Because of these limitations, intermittent hemodialysis has found its greatest place in newborns in the treatment of inborn errors of metabolism, where endogenous toxins need to be removed quickly.

CAVH most closely mimics the filtration function of the kidney. The hemofilter acts as a large glomerulus, allowing fluid and small dissolved solutes to pass freely through the membrane "pores" while not permitting protein and cellular elements to pass. Some or all of the filtered fluid (plasma water) is replaced with a sterile physiological fluid, resulting in the removal of waste products. Because the filtrate contains small solutes at the same concentration found in plasma water (the hemofilter "glomerulus" has no "tubules" to reabsorb important solutes), nonphysiological replacement fluids cannot be used. The procedure requires the placement of large-bore catheters in arteries and veins with high blood flows (preferably femoral vessels). Therefore, there are the significant risks of embolism, occlusion, or infection. Properly performed, hemodynamic stability is maintained or may be improved. Because of the continuous nature of the procedure, control of the metabolic consequences of renal failure is excellent. Variations of this technique employing a blood pump (in patients with unacceptable blood flow) and/or using sterile dialysate flowing countercurrent to blood flow (to improve solute removal) have been used in some patients. The membranes used are synthetic and biocompatible and do not appear to increase catabolic rate. Anticoagulation is required, but an attempt is usually made to only "significantly" anticoagulate the extracorporeal circuit. Circuits with small extracorporeal volumes have become available for neonates.

■ **Answer:**

1. PD

2. PD, CAVH

3. HD

4. PD, CAVH

5. CAVH

6. CAVH

7. PD

8. HD

## EXERCISE 15

The parents of this infant are concerned that they may be causing their baby to suffer. They wish to know the chances for recovery before consenting to dialysis.

■ **Question:**

What can we tell them?

■ **Discussion/Answer:**

Few studies have specifically examined the outcome of acute renal failure in the newborn infant. The results suggest outcomes similar to those seen in older children and in adults. The prognosis of acute renal failure associated with multiple organ failure is very poor in all age groups. You must decide if some or all of the extrarenal manifestations are related to the consequences of acute renal failure (e.g., respiratory failure and/or congestive heart failure secondary to volume overload) to apply this knowledge appropriately. The prognosis of isolated acute renal failure in the absence of chronic renal insufficiency in the neonate appears to be better, but generalizations are difficult to make. In small neonates with chronic renal insufficiency requiring dialysis shortly after birth, the prognosis is largely unknown. In such patients, the possibility of long-term chronic dialysis in order to reach an appropriate size for renal transplantation is a formidable (and many would contend unrealistic) undertaking. The courses of infants with chronic renal insufficiency at birth even without requiring dialysis are quite difficult to predict. The answers to the questions of these parents are very difficult, and require honesty, accuracy, and empathy from all involved in the care of the family.

## BIBLIOGRAPHY

### Physiology

1. Feld LG: Renal transport of sodium during early development. In Polin RA, Fox WW, eds: *Fetal and Neonatal Physiology.* Philadelphia, WB Saunders Co, 1992, p. 1211.
2. Siegel SR, Oh W: Renal function as a marker of human fetal maturation. *Acta Paediatr Scand* 1976; 65:481.

3. Arant BS: Postnatal development of renal function during the first year of life. *Pediatr Nephrol* 1987; 1:308.

4. Arant BS: Distal tubular sodium handling in human neonates: Clearance studies. *Contrib Nephrol* 1988; 67:130.

5. Awazu M, Kon V: Pathophysiology of acute renal failure in the neonatal period. In Polin RA, Fox WW, eds: *Fetal and Neonatal Physiology.* Philadelphia, WB Saunders Co, 1992, p. 1268.

6. Engle WD: Clinical significance of developmental renal physiology. In Polin RA, Fox WW, eds: *Fetal and Neonatal Physiology.* Philadelphia, WB Saunders Co, 1992, p. 1279.

## Diagnosis and Management

7. Feld LG, Springate JE, Fildes RD: Acute renal failure. I. Pathophysiology and diagnosis. *J Pediatr* 1986; 109(3):401.

8. Fildes RD, Springate JE, Feld LG: Acute renal failure. II. Management of suspected and established disease. *J Pediatr* 1986; 109(4):567.

9. Gaudio KM, Siegel NJ: Pathogenesis and treatment of acute renal failure. *Pediatr Clin North Am* 1987; 34(3):771.

10. Abel RM, Beck CH, Abbot WM, et al: Improved survival form acute renal failure after treatment with intravenous essential L-amino acids and glucose. *N Engl J Med* 1973; 288(14):695.

## Prognosis

11. Counahan R, Cameron JS, Ogg CS, et al: Presentation, management, complications, and outcome of acute renal failure in childhood: Five years' experience. *Br Med J* 1977; 1:599.

12. Hodson EM, Kjellstrand CM, Mauer SM: Acute renal failure in infants and children: Outcome of 53 patients requiring hemodialysis treatment. *J Pediatr* 1978; 93(5):756.

13. Niaudet P, Haj-Ibrahim M, Gagnadoux MF, et al: Outcome of children with acute renal failure. *KI* 1985; 28(suppl 17):S-148.

14. Oberkircher O, Held E, Owens E: Perintoneal dialysis as treatment for neonatal renal failure. *VIII Congress of the International Pediatric Nephrology Association* 1989; 18:021.

# Chapter 15

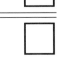

# NEONATAL SEIZURES

## *Robert Ryan Clancy, M.D.*

The behavior of healthy infants is intrinsically governed by many cyclical, neural factors that regulate the rhythms of life: respiration, sucking, feeding, wakefulness, and sleep. Sick neonates may also exhibit a variety of paroxysmal, apparently abnormal motor or autonomic behaviors that may suggest the diagnosis of *seizure* to the physician. However, not all of these events represent true epileptic seizures. By definition, epileptic seizures result from the sudden, excessive, repetitive discharging of neurons in the cerebral cortex. Only those clinical events (seizures) that simultaneously arise with the appearance of these abnormal electrical discharges, as demonstrated on the electroencephalogram, are proven epileptic seizures. The primary purpose of this chapter and first responsibility of the clinician, therefore, is to recognize the wide spectrum of clinical expression of true convulsions, and to differentiate them from other (normal or abnormal) paroxysmal activities exhibited by the sick neonate. This will allow the clinician to select those patients in need of immediate, thorough medical and neurological evaluation, to choose the most appropriate therapy, and to assign an accurate long-term neurological prognosis.

Exercises are provided throughout and the answers are given in or after the discussion following each exercise.

### SUSPECTING THE DIAGNOSIS

The following case history describes the clinical course of a very premature infant who experienced a number of potential causes of encephalopathy and seizures. As you review the history, note that the patient experienced four separate neurological events.

**CASE STUDY 1**

JM, a female infant weighing 530 g, was delivered after a 26-week gestation to a healthy 26-year-old, primigravida woman. The infant was delivered vaginally in frank breech presentation. The premature labor was attributed to an incompetent cervix. Immediately prior to delivery, the mother's temperature rose to 102°F. At birth, the recorded Apgar scores were 2 at 1 minute and 5 at 5 minutes. The infant was placed in a hood containing 100% oxygen. Her first capillary blood gases at 1 hour of age showed a $PO_2$ of 45 mm Hg, a $PCO_2$ of 53 mm Hg, and a pH of 7.24. Blood glucose was 90 mg/dL by Dextrostix measurement. A neonatal team was summoned to transport the infant to a tertiary care facility. On arrival at the referring hospital, the infant was inactive, ashen-colored, hypothermic (35°C), and intermittently apneic with periods of bradycardia to 70 beats per minute (BPM). After intubation and ventilation, the infant demonstrated improved activity and color and stabilization of vital signs. Fluids were given by an umbilical venous line. Following an uneventful transport, a blood culture was obtained and ampicillin and gentamicin were started. No lumbar puncture was performed owing to her tenuous clinical state. Because of a large insensible water loss, management of fluids and electrolytes was difficult. Serum sodium concentrations fluctuated from 125 to 157 mEq/L. The serum calcium level was 5.4 mg/dL.

**Episode 1:** On the first day of life tremors developed that were characterized by frequent rapid rhythmic oscillations of the extremities. The tremors increased when the infant was handled but could be stopped by holding or repositioning her limbs. The limb tremors were not accompanied by apnea or movements of the face, tongue, or eyes. An electroencephalogram performed during a period of tremulousness did not demonstrate seizure patterns. Following the administration of intravenous calcium gluconate, the serum calcium concentration rose from 5.4 to 8.4 mg/dL and the tremors stopped. On the third day of life, a cranial ultrasonogram was interpreted as normal. The next day motor activity diminished and a repeat cephalic ultrasound scan showed a small hemorrhage confined to the left germinal matrix. After a brief period of neurological improvement, ampicillin and gentamicin were discontinued. One day later a blood culture grew *Escherichia coli,* and tobramycin and cefamandole were started. The child again improved.

**Episode 2:**   Three days after the cessation of antibiotics, the infant began to have frequent apneic spells accompanied by bradycardia, poor color, and diminished activity. No unusual limb or eye movements accompanied these apneas. Results of an electroencephalogram were mildly abnormal. A lumbar puncture produced clear, acellular spinal fluid with a protein level of 100 mg/dL and a glucose level of 95 mg/dL.

**Episode 3:**   The next day, the house officer observed periods of irregular breathing, facial grimaces, bursts of sucking, rapid horizontal eye movements, and twitchy limb movements during sleep. Because of the difficulty of obtaining lumbar cerebrospinal fluid (CSF) for analysis, a cisternal puncture was performed that yielded 1 ml of thick purulent material containing numerous gram-negative rods. Antibiotics were changed and the infant was treated with a loading dose of intravenous phenobarbital (20 mg/kg), but the spells continued. A repeat electroencephalogram was obtained the next day to document the basis of the seizures. This electroencephalogram demonstrated that the activity in question simply represented normal rapid eye movement sleep behavior.

**Episode 4:**   The following day careful clinical observation of the patient revealed sustained periods of tonic horizontal eye deviation that had not been noticed previously. They occurred only when electrographic seizure patterns appeared in the right temporal lobe (Fig. 15-1). These minimal clinical events finally ceased after phenytoin was administered.

## EXERCISE 1

Please describe each of the four neurological events in the Exercise 1 table and decide whether or not these episodes represented seizures. Also, can you identify the causes of these events?

### ■ Discussion:

**Episode 1:**   The jitteriness was not considered to be epileptic seizures on the basis of its clinical characteristics, because the tremors were provoked by stimulation and ceased on holding or repositioning of the involved limbs.

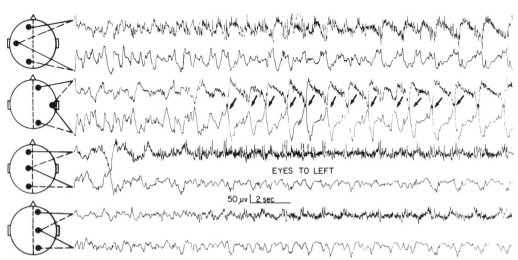

EYES TO LEFT

50 µv | 2 sec

**Figure 15-1**   JM's electroencephalogram during an epileptic seizure, clinically manifested by tonic, conjugate eye deviation to the left. The tracing reveals an electrographic seizure consisting of repetitive epileptic discharges arising in the right temporal lobe (arrows).

## Exercise 1

| NEUROLOGICAL EPISODE | EPILEPTIC SEIZURE? (YES OR NO) | EEG (NORMAL OR ABNORMAL) | POTENTIAL ETIOLOGY |
|---|---|---|---|
| Episode 1: | | | |
| Episode 2: | | | |
| Episode 3: | | | |
| Episode 4: | | | |

This was confirmed by the first electroencephalogram (EEG) in which no electrographic seizure pattern was recorded while the infant displayed the suspicious clinical behavior.

**Episode 2:** The spells of apnea and bradycardia were unaccompanied by unusual limb or eye movements. Apnea and bradycardia in the absence of other clinical signs are rarely the sole manifestations of a seizure disorder. The second EEG was mildly abnormal, but again demonstrated no seizure activity.

**Episode 3:** The normal rapid eye movement sleep behavior was initially confused with seizure activity because of the periods of rapid eye movements, sucking, and irregular breathing, but the situation was clarified by the third EEG.

**Episode 4:** The episodes of sustained tonic eye deviation were so subtle that they had originally been overlooked. They were, in fact, the only clinical expression of electrographic seizures arising in the right temporal lobe.

This case study illustrates that neurologically ill infants may exhibit a wide range of intermittent, apparently abnormal motor or autonomic behavior that does not represent true seizure activity. Conversely, true seizure activity may go unrecognized if the clinical signs are subtle. The following discussion aids you in the recognition of epileptic seizures and their differentiation from other paroxysmal clinical events that may arise in the neonate.

■ **Answer:**

See Exercise 1 answer table.

### Clinical Classification of Neonatal Seizures

In 1970, the International League Against Epilepsy proposed an extensive International Classification of Epilepsy in an attempt to standardize the existing diverse terminology describing epileptic phenomena. Unfortunately, no attempt was made to incorporate neonatal seizures into this scheme. Currently,

## Exercise 1 Answers

| NEUROLOGICAL EPISODE | EPILEPTIC SEIZURE? (YES OR NO) | EEG FINDINGS | POTENTIAL ETIOLOGY |
|---|---|---|---|
| 1. Tremulousness or jitteriness | No | Normal | Metabolic derangement: hypocalcemia; ?hyponatremia or hypernatremia |
| 2. Apnea and bradycardia | No | Mildly abnormal; no seizure patterns | Germinal matrix hemorrhage, prematurity, sepsis |
| 3. Irregular breathing, facial grimaces, sucking, rapid eye movements during sleep | No | Normal sleep EEG | Normal sleep behavior of infants |
| 4. Recurring episodes of sustained tonic eye deviation | Yes | Seizures arising in right temporal lobe | Meningitis |

no universally accepted standard classification of neonatal seizures exists that unites etiology, clinical seizure type, and electroencephalographic manifestations. Instead, a classification based solely on clinical criteria has gradually evolved. Although the clinical expression of seizures is protean, five basic seizure types are usually described: *subtle* (minimal), *tonic, focal clonic, multifocal clonic* (migratory, fragmentary), and *myoclonic.*

***Subtle Seizures:*** Subtle seizures may be difficult to recognize, even by experienced clinicians. Subtle seizures are characterized by oral, facial, or ocular activity such as repetitive, stereotyped eye deviation or jerking, eyelid blinking or fluttering, sucking, lip smacking, tongue thrusting, or drooling. Fragments of swimming or peddling limb movements may also be noted. Rarely, a cessation of spontaneous motor activity may occur. Apnea may be seen, but careful observation will usually reveal other motor activity such as tonic ocular deviation or mouthing movements. Often, the highly repetitive and stereotyped nature of the activity marks these events as convulsions rather than simply the quality of the movements. Time-synchronized video-EEG monitoring during subtle clinical seizures often shows abnormal EEG background activity but frequently fails to show coincident electrographic seizure activity. That is, subtle clinical seizures are usually not consistently based on a specific epileptic mechanism. Subtle seizures are often considered to be *nonepileptic* motor automatisms, which represent motor stereotypes released from brain stem activity centers that have been removed from the normal inhibitory braking influence of the forebrain. The clinical picture here is that acute neurological disease impairs the normal functioning of the cerebral hemispheres (and consequently the EEG background is abnormal). This results in attacks of brain stem-mediated motor automatisms termed *subtle seizures*. However, subtle clinical seizures are often not specifically triggered by epileptic spiking of the cerebral cortex. (The abnormal EEG does not show electrographic seizure patterns time-locked to the abnormal attacks of behavior.) Consequently, an EEG is usually necessary to reveal the basis of such attacks in infants who display subtle seizures.

***Tonic Seizures:*** The term *tonic* denotes an alteration in the tone of the neck, trunk, or limb musculature resulting in a change of posture. For example, the characteristic *fencer posture* produced by the asymmetric tonic neck reflex is widely regarded as manifestation of a normal alteration of tone. Abrupt, abnormal changes in the tone (and hence posture) of an infant are often loosely described as posturing, stiffening, or rigidity. Tonic seizures therefore imply episodes of increased muscle tone that alter the child's posture, resulting from a sudden excessive repetitive firing of cortical neurons. In its pure form, there is no shaking (*clonus*) of the limbs so the term *tonic-clonic seizure* would not apply. Focal tonic seizures abruptly disturb the posture of a single limb. Generalized tonic seizures are manifested by extension of both legs and flexion or extension of the arms. This may be accompanied by upward eye rolling, eyelid fluttering, or apnea. Time-synchronized video-EEG monitoring during many forms of tonic seizures often fails to display coincident ictal EEG patterns, even though the ongoing EEG background may be abnormal. Brief posturing or stiffening of one or all limbs is more often than not unassociated with electrographic seizure patterns. Sustained tonic deviation or posturing of the eyes is one example of a type of tonic seizure that has a consistent epileptic signature.

***Focal Clonic Seizures:*** The term *clonic* denotes a repetitive shaking or jerking of a group of muscles. The jerking seen in clonic seizures has two distinct components: a fast phase (usually flexion) followed by a slow phase (usually extension). In focal clonic seizures, jerking movements are confined to one limb or area of the body. Movement or repositioning of the involved limb will not affect the rate or intensity of the clonic activity as it does in the jittery infant. This type of seizure is usually easily recognized and is unlikely to be confused with nonepileptic phenomena. Clonic seizures are the most common clinical seizure type to display a reliable one-to-one correlation with ictal EEG activity, as demonstrated by video-EEG monitoring.

***Multifocal Clonic Seizures (Migratory or Fragmentary Seizures):*** These seizures are characterized by clonic limb activity in several body areas (multifocal) and may appear to migrate from one limb to another, often in a seemingly haphazard manner. Like focal clonic seizures, multifocal seizures are usually well correlated with simultaneous ictal EEG activity. Superficially, multifocal clonic seizures may resemble a state called jitteriness, tremulousness, or segmental myoclonus. The muscle activity of jitteriness or tremulousness resembles the rapid rhythmic, to-and-fro movement of tremor rather than the jerking movement of clonus. Tremors may be elicited by auditory or tactile stimulus and stopped by simply holding or repositioning the involved limb(s). Concomitant disturbances of eye movements and apnea are not usually seen. Jitteriness may occur in the same clinical setting as seizures (hypoglycemia, hypocalcemia, asphyxia, infection, drug withdrawal), so its recognition still demands a prompt, reasonable evaluation of the child. If no cause is found, the tremors do not necessarily imply an unfavorable outcome.

***Myoclonic Seizures:*** This least common of the clinical subtypes of neonatal seizures is characterized by sudden shock-like jerks of flexion of both arms and/or legs. They may occur individually or in brief series. Similar movements may be seen when eliciting the abrupt spinal-mediated withdrawal response to painful stimuli. Infrequent nonrepetitive myoclonic jerks may also appear in normal infants during periods of active (rapid eye movement) sleep. Myoclonus has an inconsistent and unpredictable correlation to coincident ictal EEG activity. Like subtle and most tonic seizures, these often appear in acutely ill or neurologically compromised infants and strongly suggest epileptic seizures. However, video-EEG monitoring frequently reveals the nonepileptic basis of these abnormal, paroxysmal movements.

## Exercise 2

| | CLINICAL SEIZURE TYPES | | | | |
| CLINICAL SEIZURE DESCRIPTION | SUBTLE | TONIC | FOCAL CLONIC | MULTIFOCAL CLONIC | MYOCLONIC |
|---|---|---|---|---|---|
| 1. Episodes of repetitive jerking or shaking confined to one limb or one-half of the body. The shaking cannot be stopped by holding or repositioning the involved body parts. | | | | | |
| 2. Episodes of sudden, brief, shock-like muscle twitches producing extension or flexion of the arms and/or legs. They may occur individually or in brief series. | | | | | |
| 3. Episodes of abrupt alteration of muscle tone resulting in disturbed body posture. They usually produce sudden stiffening of one or more limbs and may result in arching of the neck and trunk. | | | | | |
| 4. Episodes of repetitive, stereotyped eye deviation, eyelid blinking or fluttering, sucking, lip smacking, tongue thrusting, or drooling. Limb activity may accompany the ocular-facial-oral signs including swimming arm movements or peddling leg motions. | | | | | |
| 5. Episodes of repetitive jerking or shaking that involve both sides of the body and may appear to spread randomly from one limb to another. They may resemble a fragment of a generalized clonic seizure. | | | | | |

## EXERCISE 2

Using the Exercise 2 table match the descriptions of clinical seizures with the five basic seizure types by placing a check mark in the appropriate space for each seizure description below.

■ **Answers:**

1. Focal clonic

2. Myoclonic

3. Tonic

4. Subtle

5. Multifocal clonic

**Behavioral States Commonly Confused with Seizures**

*Sleep-Wake Cycle Activity:* Approximately 30 to 32 weeks following conception, four physiological states may begin to be recognized in the healthy newborn infant: wakefulness, active sleep or rapid eye movement (REM) sleep, transitional sleep, and quiet sleep [or non–rapid eye movement (non-REM) sleep]. Preterm and term infants spend the majority of their time asleep. When newborn infants fall asleep, they usually enter a period of active sleep. The infant may then exhibit facial grimaces, periods of rapid horizontal eye movements, tongue movements, sucking activity, small twitchy hand or foot movements, and large body movements (head rolling, brief posturing, squirming). Respirations are typically irregular or periodic and brief apneas may

occur. Following a period of active sleep, a transitional period of sleep ensues that is not entirely typical of either REM or non-REM sleep. When the transition is completed, a state of quiet sleep is reached in which respirations are deep and regular, no eye movements are present, and body movements are generally absent except for occasional bursts of rhythmic sucking movements. Each of these four states is accompanied by a characteristic electroencephalographic pattern.

The relative proportion of time spent in indeterminant or transitional sleep is increased in the sick neonate. REM sleep is a common state during which true convulsions may arise. The motor activities of REM sleep may sometimes be mistaken for subtle seizures. They are, however, not highly stereotyped and repetitive like epileptic seizures. When in doubt, the physician should obtain an EEG to document the true nature of the motor activity witnessed during REM sleep.

## EXERCISE 3

Using the Exercise 3 table, insert the appropriate description (wakefulness, REM sleep, transitional sleep, non-REM sleep) in the column labeled "Behavioral State."

■ **Answers:**

1. Awake

2. Active or REM sleep

3. Transitional sleep

4. Quiet or non-REM sleep

**Exercise 3**

| BEHAVIORAL STATE | EYELIDS | RESPIRATIONS | REM PERIODS | FACIAL MOVEMENTS | SMALL AND LARGE BODY MOVEMENTS |
|---|---|---|---|---|---|
| 1. | Open | Irregular, crying | − | Frequent | + |
| 2. | Closed | Periodic, irregular brief apneas | + | Frequent | + |
| 3. | Closed | Variable | − | Variable | Variable |
| 4. | Closed | Deep, regular infrequent apneas and periodic breathing | − | Sucking only | Infrequent |

***Decorticate and Decerebrate Posturing and Opisthotonos:*** Certain nonepileptic postures may be confused with genuine tonic seizures. Decorticate and decerebrate posturing may mimic the clinical appearance of a tonic seizure. Such nonepileptic posturing, however, may be stimulus sensitive; for example, triggered by painful stimulation such as endotracheal tube suctioning. In decorticate posturing, the legs are extended and the arms are flexed, adducted, and internally rotated with fisting. Typically, no change in eye position occurs. In decerebrate posturing, the legs are extended and the arms are extended, hyperpronated, and the wrists are adducted with fisting. The eyes may deviate downward with dilation of the pupils. (See Fig. 15-2.) These forms of abnormal posturing may superficially resemble epileptic seizures. The EEG is helpful in distinguishing between these nonepileptic tonic attacks and epileptic tonic seizures.

The term *opisthotonos* implies a prolonged posture of extreme arching of the neck and trunk that may be enhanced by noxious external stimuli. This sustained abnormal posture may appear in the course of a variety of encephalopathies such as meningitis, asphyxia, or cerebral hemorrhage and should not be considered a form of epileptic seizure.

Table 15-1 summarizes the clinical and laboratory features useful in distinguishing tonic epileptic seizures, decorticate posturing, decerebrate posturing, and opisthotonos.

***Jitteriness:*** This motor phenomenon has already been discussed under multifocal clonic seizures.

***Autonomic Dysfunction:*** Hiccups are characterized by powerful, repetitive contractions of inspiratory muscles and are not usually mistaken for seizure activity. Hiccups appear transiently in many healthy infants but may be prominent with brain stem dysfunction or in association with some metabolic encephalopathies. Fetal hiccups can be felt by the mother and may mimic intrauterine seizures, a rare sign of certain inborn errors of metabolism or developmental brain abnormalities.

Sick infants may exhibit other disturbed autonomic functions such as poor temperature regulation (hypothermia), respiratory irregularities (hypoventilation, hyperpnea, apnea), cardiac rate abnormalities (usually bradycardia), or fluctuations in tissue perfusion and color (episodes of flushing or ashen color). These intermittent abnormal autonomic behaviors generally are not manifestations of convulsions. Careful observation will reveal that even the apneas of the subtle seizure are usually accompanied by other peripheral phenomena such as eye deviation or sucking.

However, a small number of neonates demonstrate pure ictal apnea with no other associated clinical motor signs. Ictal apnea is often not accompanied by bradycardia, thus clini-

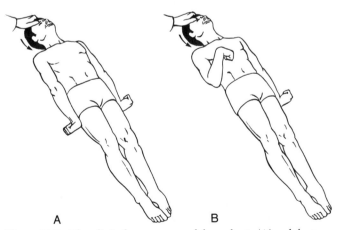

**Figure 15-2** The clinical appearance of decerebrate (A) and decorticate (B) posturing. In decerebrate posturing, the arms and legs extend and pronate, particularly on the side opposite the primary lesion.
From Plum F, Posner JB: *The Diagnosis of Stupor and Coma.* Philadelphia, FA Davis, 1980. Reprinted with permission of F.A. Davis.

**Table 15-1** Clinical and Laboratory Features Useful in Differentiation of Tonic Seizures, Decorticate Posturing, Decerebrate Posturing, and Opisthotonos

| CLINICAL EVENT | DURATION | PROVOKED BY EXTERNAL STIMULI | LEG POSTURE | ARM POSTURE | TRUNK POSTURE | CHANGE IN RESPIRATION | OCULAR POSITION | EPILEPTIC EEG CHANGES |
|---|---|---|---|---|---|---|---|---|
| Tonic seizure | Brief, intermittent | – | Extension | Flexed or extended | Usually arched (extended) | Apnea, occasionally | Blinking, upward deviation | Yes |
| Decorticate posturing | Brief, intermittent | + | Extension | Flexed, adducted, internal rotation; fisted | Extended | Typically none | Typically no change | No |
| Decerebrate posturing | Brief, intermittent | + | Extension | Extended, adducted, hyperpronated, fisted | Extended | Tachypnea, irregular breathing, apnea | Downward eye deviation, mydriasis | No |
| Opisthotonos | Prolonged, sustained posture | ± | Extension | Variable; often extended | Marked prolonged arching | Typically none | Typically no change | No |

cally distinguishing it from the familiar spells of apnea and bradycardia of prematurity. Episodic flushing of the skin may also accompany seizures in a few instances. If there is reasonable suspicion that an autonomic disturbance represents seizure activity, an EEG should be obtained.

## EXERCISE 4

Specify two special clinical circumstances in which neurologically ill neonates may be unable to display any visible clinical signs of their convulsions.

1.

2.

### ■ Discussion/Answer:

There are two special circumstances in which neurologically ill neonates may be experiencing epileptic seizures that are not apparent to the physician. Some infants with severe respiratory disease may require pharmacological paralysis (such as pancuronium) to improve the efficiency of mechanical ventilation. It is impossible to determine whether the infant in this state is awake, asleep, or even deeply comatose. All clinical neurological information is lost. If significant brain dysfunction has occurred prior to the onset of the paralysis, the possibility of seizures is real; however, clinical seizure activity will not be apparent if neuromuscular blocking agents have been administered. In this special circumstance, the physi-

cian must consider the potential benefits of periodically reversing the paralysis. This allows time to observe the infant for clinical seizures and assess the clinical neurological status, but at the risk of potential deterioration of ventilation. Alternatively, serial electroencephalographic tracings obtained during the period of therapeutic paralysis may provide some measure of neurological integrity and the presence of seizures. If the physician strongly believes that the patient is having seizures and cannot reverse the paralysis or obtain an EEG, a case may be made for empirical treatment with phenobarbital.

The second special circumstance arises in the setting of a desperately ill infant who has suffered a serious neurological insult resulting in coma. Electrographic seizures that are not accompanied by clinical seizure activity may occasionally be observed. Such infants are too compromised to manifest a clinical response to their seizures. Subclinical or occult seizures may, on occasion, be the predominant corollary of electrographic seizures in some infants (Fig. 15-3).

## Proving the Diagnosis

Although the suspicion of neonatal seizures is frequently raised, electrographic confirmation may prove a more difficult task. As noted earlier, the only absolute "proof" of seizures rests on demonstration of ongoing ictal EEG dis-

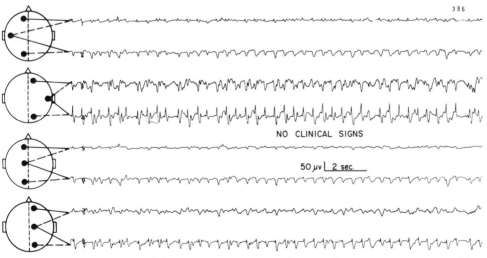

**Figure 15-3** This electroencephalogram demonstrates an electrographic seizure unaccompanied by any clinical seizure activity. This comatose term infant died of meningitis at 5 days of age.

charges concomitant with the behavior in question. Individual neonatal seizures last only a few minutes. A routine electroencephalographic tracing samples only about 40 minutes of cerebral electrical activity. The sampling error is potentially large. Consequently, the majority of routine EEGs obtained to rule out seizures are obtained between seizures (interictal) and may not prove or disprove unequivocably the occurrence of epileptic seizures. If the physician remains uncertain of the nature of the behavior and a single, routine, interictal EEG does not resolve the ambiguity, two simple maneuvers may be employed: serial EEGs or a prolonged recording (3 to 4 hours). By increasing the sampling time, the likelihood of capturing the event is improved. The medical and neurological evaluation of an infant with suspected seizures, however, should never await this absolute confirmation. The final burden of decision and diagnosis belongs to the clinician who may never know with certainty the exact nature of the neurological event expressed by the patient.

## INITIAL EVALUATION AND TREATMENT

The recognition of neonatal seizures should compel the physician to conduct an immediate investigation of their cause. The initial evaluation should proceed with these assumptions: (1) Seizures are a sign of disturbed neurological function reflecting either systemic or primary brain disease; (2) multiple factors may operate in concert in the production of seizures; and (3) the underlying cause(s) is(are) treatable and potentially injurious to the brain independent of the convulsions.

As you read the next case, you will encounter six potential etiologies that may be responsible for the generation of this infant's seizures. You will be asked to enumerate these possible etiologies and to suggest methods of treating them.

## CASE STUDY 2

AN, a male infant weighing 4,200 g, was delivered after a full-term uncomplicated gestation to a small, 21-year-old, primigravida woman. Membranes ruptured 20 hours prior to delivery. Labor was prolonged and complicated by a transverse lie and maternal fever of 101°F. Fetal heart monitoring demonstrated late decelerations, and meconium was passed by the fetus prior to delivery. A mepivacaine pudendal block was placed for maternal local anesthesia. Delivery was difficult and required midforceps extraction. The Apgar score was unrecorded at 1 minute and was 7 at 5 minutes. The infant's mouth was suctioned of meconium and he was swaddled and put to the mother's breast. Fifteen minutes later it was discovered that the umbilical cord had been torn and 60 mL of blood was found in his blanket. An initial examination revealed a pale infant with a pulse of 161 BPM and a blood pressure of 50/30 mm Hg. Breathing was noted to be periodic and was occasionally accompanied by bradycardia. The blood glucose level (Dextrostix) was below 25 mg/dL. Ten percent dextrose and water and antibiotics were administered and a neonatal transport team was summoned. During the trip, recurrent focal clonic seizures involving the left arm and leg occurred and abated after more glucose was infused.

On admission to the neonatal intensive care unit, examination revealed a pulse of 190 BPM, a blood pressure of 48/22 mm Hg, a rectal temperature of 99.6°F, and mildly labored respirations at a rate of 90 per minute. Facial bruising and a right parietal cephalohematoma were present. The child was depressed but arousable by gentle stimulation. No other frank abnormalities were noted on the remainder of the general or neurological examination. Blood was then drawn for culture and chemical analysis, and glucose was administered because the repeat blood glucose level remained below 25 mg/dL. No abnormalities of serum electrolytes, urea nitrogen, bilirubin, or calcium were present, but the low glucose by Dextrostix measurement was confirmed by a laboratory value of 18 mg/dL. A nontraumatic lumbar puncture produced slightly turbid, xanthochromic CSF with 12 white blood cells per cubic millimeter, 1665 red blood cells per cubic millimeter, a glucose level of 27 mg/dL, and a protein level of 80 mg/dL. A portable x-ray film of the skull showed a possible right parietal fracture. A subdural tap was dry. Phenobarbital was given to stop the seizures and a neurological consult was requested. At the time of the consultation the infant was noted to be depressed, but arousable. Pertinent findings included a flattened left nasolabial fold, relative paucity of activity in the left arm and leg, and an inability to fully open the left hand during the Moro reflex. Deep tendon reflexes were brisk but symmetric.

## EXERCISE 5

List six potential causes of this infant's seizures. How would you proceed to treat them?

*Etiology*
1.
2.
3.
4.
5.
6.

*Treatment*
1.
2.
3.
4.
5.
6.

### ■ Discussion:

Case Study 2 illustrates that numerous causes may be suspected in the generation of seizures but often few are identified with certainty. Furthermore, specific therapy is lacking for many of the established causes. The *initial* evaluation of the child with seizures is directed toward the discovery of significant and remediable causes. A brief general and neurological examination is performed to uncover clues regarding the possible causes of seizures. Blood and urine are analyzed for relevant metabolic or toxic disturbances. A sepsis workup is conducted including a lumbar puncture. The CSF is critically evaluated. Finally, a cranial CT scan, magnetic resonance image, or ultrasound examination is performed if a structural abnormality of the central nervous system is suspected.

### ■ Answer:

*Potential Causes*
1. Intrauterine asphyxia, abnormal fetal heart monitoring, and the long and difficult labor.
2. Central nervous system ischemia secondary to blood loss from the lacerated umbilicus.
3. Central nervous system toxicity from mepivacaine administered to the mother.
4. Sepsis and/or meningitis, in view of the maternal fever and umbilical laceration.

5. Metabolic derangement—documented hypoglycemia.
6. Trauma to the central nervous system, especially subdural hematoma. Recall that this term infant was delivered to a small primigravida woman who experienced a prolonged, difficult labor requiring forceps assistance. The x-ray film of the skull revealed a questionable fracture and the infant demonstrated a mild left hemiparesis.

*Suggested Treatment*
1. General supportive care including maintenance of cardiovascular function and ventilation, metabolic homeostasis, and treatment of seizures.
2. Blood transfusion and general medical support.
3. This possible factor can be substantiated by measuring the level of mepivacaine in the infant's blood. Forced diuresis promotes elimination of this drug from the body.
4. Isolate organisms by appropriate cultures and administration of antibiotics.
5. Administration of 10% dextrose and water.
6. MRI or CT brain scan; subdural taps.

### History and Physical Examination

The history should be reviewed with attention to possible problems encountered during *gestation* (prematurity, maternal diabetes, parity, illicit or prescribed drug use, congenital infection), *labor* (duration of ruptured membranes, maternal fever or leukocytosis, progress of labor, use of local anesthetics, abnormal fetal heart monitoring, prolongation of labor, passage of meconium), and *delivery* (use of forceps, breech presentation, difficulty of delivery, Apgar scores, type and duration of resuscitation).

The timing of the onset of the seizures is another helpful clue (Table 15-2). For example, perinatal asphyxia generally gives rise to seizures within the first day of life. On the other hand, convulsions caused by a cerebral malformation usually occur beyond the third day of life.

While completing the general physical examination, pay careful attention to vital signs,

**Table 15-2**  Peak Onset of Convulsions

24 hours
  Bacterial meningitis
  Direct effect of drugs, cocaine
  Laceration of tentorium of falx
  Perinatal asphyxia encephalopathy
  Pyridoxine dependency
  Rubella, toxoplasmosis, cytomegalovirus
  Sepsis
24 to 72 hours
  Bacterial meningitis
  Cerebral contusion with subdural hemorrhage
  Cerebral dysgenesis
  Drug withdrawal
  Intraventricular hemorrhage in the premature infant
  Nonketotic hyperglycinemia
  Sepsis
  Subarachnoid hemorrhage
  Urea cycle disturbances
72 hours
  Cerebral dysgenesis
  Kernicterus
  Ketotic hyperglycinemias
  Nutritional hypocalcemia
  Smith-Lemli-Opitz syndrome
  Urea cycle disturbances
1 week
  Cerebral dysgenesis
  Fructose dysmetabolism
  Herpes simplex
  Ketotic hyperglycinemias
  Maple syrup urine disease
  Urea cycle disturbances

*Source:* Modified from Fenichel GM: *Neonatal Neurology.* Churchill Livingstone, New York, 1980, p. 22. Modified with permission of Churchill Livingstone.

respiratory pattern, estimation of gestational age, size of the liver and spleen, and signs of somatic dysmorphism. The skin should be inspected for jaundice, rash, or neurocutaneous stigmata such as axillary freckles (observed in neurofibromatosis) or port wine nevus (which may be seen in the Sturge-Weber syndrome). The cranium should be observed for evidence of trauma (needle puncture sites on the scalp, fractures, or extreme molding).

The neurological examination is directed toward establishing the level of consciousness and estimating the intracranial pressure (fontanelle tension and degree of suture separation). The fundi must be visualized. The integrity of brain stem function is established by observing pupil equality and light reactivity, spontaneous and reflex eye movements, sucking, and swallowing. The quality and symmetry of activity, muscle tone, posture, and deep tendon reflexes should be noted.

We now review each of the major treatable causes responsible for neonatal seizures.

***Metabolic Disease:***  The whole blood glucose concentration is most conveniently measured by Dextrostix. If the estimate is low, the test is immediately repeated and confirmed. An infusion of 10% dextrose and water is administered (Table 15-3) after serum is obtained to determine levels of sodium, glucose, calcium, phosphorus, magnesium, urea nitrogen, and bilirubin. Calcium, magnesium, or both are administered if a deficiency state of either mineral is documented. The diagnosis of pyridoxine dependency rests on the family history, the presence of intractable seizures resistant to anticonvulsants and the immediate cessation of seizures following the infusion of vitamin $B_6$.

The clinical picture of irritability, poor feeding, hypotonia, hiccuping, vomiting, seizures, and progressive stupor suggests an inborn error of metabolism. In this setting, the anion gap should be calculated and blood ammonia, ketones, and pH determined. A positive urine 2,4-dinitrophenylhydrazine (DNPH) reaction suggests the presence of alpha keto acids observed in maple syrup urine disease, methylmalonicacidemia, and propionic acidemia. The specific biochemical diagnosis depends on the profile of CSF, blood and urine amino acids, or organic acids demonstrated by thin layer chromatography. General medical treatment consists of withholding further protein intake, intravenous hydration, correction of the metabolic acidosis, treatment of seizures, and occasionally peritoneal dialysis or hemodialysis. More specific treatment is available for some of the biochemical lesions that are vitamin responsive.

***Drug Effects—Drug Exposure:***  Prior to delivery, mepivacaine may inadvertently reach the infant when the obstetrician injects this local anesthetic into the mother. The drug may be delivered through an accidental fetal scalp injection or may reach the child via the placenta. The subsequent clinical course may mimic acute hypoxic-ischemic encephalopathy with depressed Apgar scores, hypotonia, apnea, bradycardia, and seizures. However, unlike the early phase of asphyxia, mepivacaine intoxication may produce total ophthalmoplegia (fixed and dilated pupils with absent doll's eye movements). The suspicion of

**Table 15-3** Recognition and Treatment of Metabolic Deficiency States

| DEFICIENCY STATE | BLOOD LEVEL | REPLACEMENT SOLUTION | DELIVER ROUTE | LOADING DOSE | MAINTENANCE DOSE | COMMENT |
|---|---|---|---|---|---|---|
| Hypoglycemia | <40 mg/dL | 10% dextrose (100 mg/mL) | IV | 2 mL/kg (200 mg/kg) | 4–6 kg/min IV, depending on blood glucose levels | Keep blood glucose in normal range if frequent, recurring seizures are present. |
| Hypocalcemia | <7.0 mg/dL | 5% calcium gluconate (50 mg/mL) | IV | 4 mL/kg (200 mg/kg) | 250 mg/kg/day po or IV, as needed | Monitor cardiac rate by EKG during loading dose. |
| Hypomagnesemia | <1.5 mg/dL | 50% $MgSO_4$ (500 mg/mL)<br>2–3% $MgSO_4$ (20–30 mg/mL | IM<br>IV | 0.2 mL/kg (100 mg/kg)<br>2–6 mL/kg | 0.2 mL/kg IM as needed<br>— | Infusion of $MgSO_4$ may produce hypotonia and weakness due to curare-like neuromuscular blockade. |
| Pyridoxine dependency | Diagnosis rests on family history and cessation of seizures after administration of vitamin $B_6$ | Pyridoxine hydrochloride | IV | 50 mg | 10–40 mg/day | Administer with EEG monitoring if possible. |

mepivacaine intoxication may be confirmed by measuring the infant's blood level of mepivacaine, and the needle puncture site on the scalp may be visible. Elimination of this drug is promoted by forced diuresis.

There are a variety of mechanisms by which cocaine can precipitate seizures in the newborn infant. Cocaine exerts a powerful stimulant effect, which can excite the immature central nervous system (CNS) to seize. This can occur just after birth by direct transplacental intoxication of the infant or later via oral consumption from breast feeding. Cocaine can also lead to cerebral infarction or a hemorrhage, which in turn may be responsible for seizures. Finally, CNS malformation due to the suspected teratogenetic effects of the drug or prenatally acquired infection are possible.

Theophylline toxicity in the neonate may be manifested by cardiovascular, gastrointestinal, or CNS disturbances. Neurological signs may include vomiting, jitteriness, and occasionally seizures. Serum levels of theophylline associated with convulsions generally exceed 75 mg/dL.

***Drug Withdrawal:*** Passive addiction of the infant to a variety of substances abused by the mother during the gestation may result in a withdrawal syndrome. Seizures accompany the withdrawal symptoms in a small percentage of these children. The most commonly involved substances include heroin, methadone, and secobarbital, but propoxyphene (Darvon) and alcohol have also been incriminated.

***Infection:*** Blood, urine, and spinal fluid should be obtained for bacterial cultures, and broad spectrum antibiotics administered before culture results are known. Serum titers for *toxoplasmosis* and *rubella*, and viral cultures for *rubella*, *cytomegalovirus*, and *herpes simplex virus* (TORCH) should also be obtained. Although the initial lumbar puncture is usually performed when meningitis is suspected, other useful information may be obtained from CSF analysis. We now review the CSF profile (appearance, cell count, and glucose and protein content) in healthy infants and those with CNS disease.

***Analysis of Cerebrospinal Fluid—Appearance:*** Normal spinal fluid is colorless and crystal clear. Yellow discoloration (xantho-

chromia) (1) may appear within 12 hours of cerebral hemorrhage owing to the liberation of red blood cell pigments, (2) may represent excessive free or conjugated bilirubin in a jaundiced child, (3) may appear without previous hemorrhage if protein content in the cerebrospinal fluid exceeds 150 mg/dL, and (4) may be an isolated finding in a normal child. The presence of cells in the fluid disturbs its crystalline clarity and imparts a turbidity or cloudiness to its appearance. Total cell counts above 400/mm$^3$ produce this effect. Visibly bloody (pink) fluid implies a red blood cell count of at least 6,000/mm$^3$.

***Red Blood Cell Count:*** Spinal fluid obtained by a nontraumatic lumbar puncture in a healthy neonate has a mean red blood cell count (RBC) of 30/mm$^3$. Many physicians are willing to accept much higher counts as within the normal range, but counts in excess of 100/mm$^3$ should probably be considered significant. The real question is whether this "significant" amount is due to a traumatic spinal tap or represents genuine brain pathology. In practice, the *three tube test* is employed to make this distinction (Table 15-4). The protein content of bloody spinal fluid is artificially elevated by serum protein in the amount of 1 mg/dL for every 1,000 RBCs present. The presence of a significant number of RBCs in a nontraumatic sample of CSF suggests cerebral contusion, infarction, primary subarachnoid hemorrhage, intraventricular hemorrhage, or a hemorrhagic infection such as herpes simplex virus meningoencephalitis.

***White Blood Cell Count, Glucose, and Protein:*** The range and mean values of these parameters have been determined for noninfected high-risk infants (Table 15-5). The white blood cell count and protein content of CSF fall precipitously toward adult levels by 3 months of age. In infants, a traumatic spinal tap should not produce a significant white blood cell pleocytosis on lumbar punctures repeated within a few days.

### EXERCISE 6 *Interpretation of the CSF Profile*

A 4-day-old term infant was evaluated for seizures. Results of general and neurological examinations were normal. No metabolic disturbance was identified. The serum glucose concentration was 150 mg/dL, the hematocrit

**Table 15-4** Differential Features of Subarachnoid Hemorrhage and Traumatic Puncture: The Three Tube Test

| CEREBROSPINAL FLUID FINDING | SUBARACHNOID HEMORRHAGE | TRAUMATIC PUNCTURE |
|---|---|---|
| Appearance | Equal blood in all tubes | First or last tube is bloodier; others are clearer |
| Supernatant fluid color | Pigment in excess of protein level | Clear |
| RBC count and hematocrit | Essentially similar in all tubes | Variable in different tubes |
| White blood cell count | Proportional to peripheral RBC count in earliest stages, relatively increased later | Proportional to peripheral RBC count |
| Clot formation | Absent | Occurs rarely |
| Repeat puncture at higher interspace | Findings similar to those at initial tap | Usually clear |

*Source:* From Fishman RA: *Cerebrospinal Fluid in Diseases of the Nervous System.* Philadelphia, WB Saunders Co, 1980, p. 172. Reprinted with permission of W.B. Saunders Company.

was 46%, RBC count $4.68 \times 10^6/mm^3$, and white blood cell count was $7.8 \times 10^3/mm^3$. Only one tube of spinal fluid could be obtained. The first three drops of cerebrospinal fluid were bloody, but subsequently cleared. The fluid was turbid and slightly xanthochromic after centrifugation. Laboratory analysis demonstrated an RBC count of $15,000/mm^3$, white blood cell count of $75/mm^3$, a glucose concentration of 45 mg/dL, and a protein concentration of 235 mg/dL. The Gram's stain was negative and cultures were obtained. How would you interpret this cerebrospinal fluid profile?

**■ Questions:**

1. What significance do you attach to the xanthochromia and turbidity?

2. Is the white blood cell count $(75/mm^3)$ compatible with a traumatic lumbar puncture or has some other event taken place?

**Table 15-5** Examination of Cerebrospinal Fluid in Noninfected High-Risk Neonates

| | TERM | PRETERM |
|---|---|---|
| White blood cell count (cells/mm³) | | |
| Range | 0–32 | 0–29 |
| Mean | 8.2 | 9.0 |
| Protein (mg/dL) | | |
| Range | 20–170 | 65–150 |
| Mean | 90 | 115 |
| Glucose (mg/dL) | | |
| Range | 34–119 | 24–63 |
| Mean | 52 | 50 |
| Ratio of cerebrospinal fluid to blood glucose | | |
| Range | 44–248 | 55–105 |
| Mean | 81 | 74 |

3. Do the protein and glucose levels fall within the normal limits for age?

4. Do you think the cerebrospinal fluid will be culture positive?

*Source:* Modified from Sarff LD, Platt LH, McCracken GH: Cerebrospinal fluid evaluation in neonates: Comparison of high risk infants with and without meningitis. *J Pediatr* 1976; 88:473. Modified with permission of Mosby-Year Book, Inc.

**■ Discussion/Answers:**

1. The xanthochromia may simply reflect the high protein level (235 mg/dL) and does not necessarily imply recent CNS hemorrhage.

Likewise the turbidity reflects the presence of an increased total cell count (15,075 cells/mm$^3$).

2. The peripheral blood ratio of white blood cells to red blood cells is $(7.8 \times 10^3/4.68 \times 10^6)$ or 1.6/1000. The 15,000 RBCs in the cerebrospinal fluid account for $(15,000) \times (1.6/1000) = 24$ white blood cells. The "corrected" white blood cell count is $(75 - 24) = 53/$mm$^3$ (too high).

3. The 15,000 RBCs are responsible for (15,000 RBCs × 1 mg of protein/1,000 RBCs) = 15 mg of protein. The "corrected" level of protein (235 − 15) = 200 mg/dL exceeds the range of 20 to 170 mg/dL, reported in noninfected newborn infants. Although the level of CSF glucose is in the normal range, the ratio of CSF glucose to blood glucose of 45/150 = 30% is low.

4. The spinal fluid cultures from this patient yielded a heavy growth of *E. coli* within 48 hours.

## STRUCTURAL ABNORMALITIES OF THE CENTRAL NERVOUS SYSTEM

A variety of structural abnormalities of the central nervous system may give rise to neonatal seizures. These disturbances may operate at microscopic or macroscopic levels. Examples of the former include the subtle disorganization of neural elements in some congenital brain malformations or the selective neuronal necrosis and edema that follow perinatal asphyxia. Macroscopic structural lesions include gross developmental brain anomalies (Fig. 15-4), frank cerebral infarction, and subarachnoid, intraventricular, or parenchymal hemorrhage. The lumbar puncture and cranial imaging examination provide invaluable assistance in establishing these diagnoses. Unfortunately, treatment for these conditions is nonspecific and directed toward the general medical support of the patient.

Subdural hematoma is one variety of structural injury responsible for neonatal seizures that requires constant consideration and early recognition. This is a treatable disease and may be fatal if uncorrected. Traumatic brain injury producing a subdural hematoma classically occurs in a large, term infant born to a small primigravida mother following a pro-

longed and difficult delivery, or often a precipitous birth in a multiparous mother. Many variations on this theme exist, so a healthy index of suspicion is mandatory. Infratentorial blood clots produce *posterior fossa* signs (early stupor or coma, irregular respirations, bradycardia, quadriparesis, and disturbed pupillary reactions and eye movements). Treatment may involve a craniotomy to remove the blood clot from the posterior fossa. Supratentorial subdural hematoma consists of blood overlying the cerebral convexity, and if associated with contusion of the underlying cortex may produce contralateral hemiparesis and focal seizures. Later, as the clot enlarges, intracranial pressure increases, mental alertness declines, and death may follow brain herniation. If the diagnosis of subdural hematoma is being seriously considered, imaging by ultrasound magnetic resonance imaging or CT scan is warranted, and the assistance of a neurosurgeon should be sought. If clinically warranted, a subdural tap should be performed to establish the presence of a convexity hemorrhage.

## EXERCISE 7

Compare the clinical features of supratentorial and infratentorial subdural hematomas by filling in the appropriate spaces in the Exercise 7 table on page 354.

■ **Answer:**
See Exercise 7 answer table on page 354.

## ANTICONVULSANTS

Why should we aggressively treat neonatal seizures with drugs? Do seizures themselves further injure an already compromised nervous system? We have just seen that epileptic seizures are a sign of neurological dysfunction and are usually not a disease *per se*. How could an innocent appearing subtle seizure be harmful to the neonatal brain if it does not interfere significantly with the child's cardiorespiratory status? These simple questions have not yet been fully answered. Several points should be borne in mind when contemplating treatment of neonatal seizures:

1. Clinical seizure activity may be subtle and go unrecognized; the clinician may substantially underestimate the true frequency of occurrence of seizures.

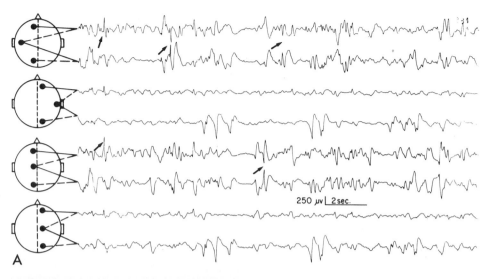

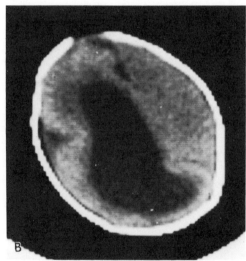

**Figure 15-4** (A) This electroencephalogram is grossly abnormal as evidenced by continuous, chaotic, high-voltage slow waves arising from the left hemisphere. Abundant epileptiform "spikes" appear in multiple locations (arrows). (B), CT scan demonstrates a developmental brain anomaly with left macrocrania and dilation of the left lateral ventricle. Fissure formation in the left hemisphere is simplified and imperfect.

2. Despite the apparently innocuous clinical appearance of some seizures, their electrographic expression may be dramatic and engage large portions of the cerebral cortex.

3. Seizures may significantly increase cerebral blood flow and exacerbate preexisting disturbances of brain perfusion.

4. A striking depletion of intracellular phosphocreatine (a major source of neuronal bioenergetics) occurs during seizures that is reversed when seizures are terminated by phenobarbital.

5. During frequent or prolonged seizures in immature animals, rapid depletion of intraneuronal glucose occurs. Lactic acidosis may also develop.

6. Neonatal rats subjected to one seizure per day subsequently demonstrated a significant reduction in brain weight and macromolecule content (DNA, RNA, protein, cholesterol).

In light of these considerations, it seems warranted to attempt prompt termination of seizures by the use of anticonvulsants. These agents act nonspecifically in the control of seizures, but do nothing to alleviate their underlying cause. Phenobarbital, for example, may control seizures caused by asphyxia, infection,

### Exercise 7

|  | SUPRATENTORIAL SUBDURAL HEMATOMA | INFRATENTORIAL SUBDURAL HEMATOMA |
|---|---|---|
| Location |  |  |
| Mental status |  |  |
| Vital signs |  |  |
| Ocular signs |  |  |
| Motor abnormalities |  |  |
| Seizures |  |  |
| Treatment |  |  |

brain malformation, or hypocalcemia. Before you select and administer any anticonvulsant, you should possess a working knowledge of their general pharmacological properties (Table 15-6).

### CASE STUDY 3

RC, a male infant weighing 3,700 g, as delivered after an uncomplicated 40-week gestation to a healthy 28-year-old, gravida 1, para 1 woman. Following the spontaneous rupture of membranes, the umbilical cord prolapsed. An emergency cesarean section was performed. The infant's Apgar scores were 1 at 1 minute and 3 at 5 minutes. The infant was immediately re-

suscitated and taken to the intensive care nursery where he required mechanical ventilation. Frequent multifocal clonic seizures began at 12 hours of age. The general physical examination was unrevealing. The neurological assessment demonstrated a depressed mental status, but intact pupillary light reactions and full reflex eye movements (doll's eyes reflex). Sucking and swallowing reflexes were diminished. A little spontaneous motor activity and generalized hypotonia was observed, but no lateralized abnormality of activity, posture, or tone. Serum glucose and electrolyte concentrations were normal. The CSF profile was normal. A cranial ultrasound examination suggested the pres-

### Exercise 7 Answers

|  | SUPRATENTORIAL SUBDURAL HEMATOMA | INFRATENTORIAL SUBDURAL HEMATOMA |
|---|---|---|
| Location | Overlying the convexity of the cerebral hemisphere; above the level of the cerebellar tentorium. | Below the cerebellar tentorium, in the posterior fossa. |
| Mental status | Initially normal or nearly normal. As the blood clot enlarges and the intracranial pressure builds, coma may result. | Early onset of stupor or coma. |
| Vital signs | Initially normal. | Early onset of bradycardia and irregular respirations or apnea. |
| Ocular signs | Initially normal. | Early onset of disturbed pupil reactions and eye movements. |
| Motor abnormalities | May demonstrate a hemiparesis contralateral to the hematoma. | Quadriparesis. |
| Seizures | May arise from an associated contusion of the cerebral cortex underneath the hematoma. | Not generally present unless other causes for seizures exist. |
| Treatment | Subdural taps through the anterior fontanelle. | Evacuation of the blood clot from the posterior fossa by a neurosurgeon. |

Table 15-6  General Pharmacological Properties of Phenobarbital, Phenytoin, Diazepam, and Lorazepam

| | PHENOBARBITAL | PHENYTOIN | DIAZEPAM | LORAZEPAM |
|---|---|---|---|---|
| Delivery route | IV, IM, po | IV | IV | IV |
| Initial loading dose | 20 mg/kg | 20 mg/kg | 0.25 mg/kg | 0.05 to 0.1 mg/kg |
| Rate of administration | Give IV dose over 20 minutes | Give IV dose no faster than 1 mg/kg/min with EKG monitoring | Give IV dose over 2 minutes | Give IV dose over 2 minutes |
| Maintenance dosage | 3–4 mg/kg/day divided every 12 hours | 3–4 mg/kg/day divided every 12 hours | 0.25 mg/kg every 15–30 minutes after load prn | 0.05 to 0.1 mg/kg prn (after loading dose) |
| Timing of first maintenance dose | 12 to 24 hours after loading | 12 to 24 hours after loading | 15 to 30 minutes after loading | Up to 12 hours |
| Therapeutic level | 20–40 µg/mL | 10–20 µg/mL | — | — |
| Serum half-life | Varies from 40 to 100 hours depending on age and duration of drug usage | Newborn: approximately 104 hours; by 1 month, 2–7 hours | 31–75 hours but seizure control may be much shorter | 12 hours |
| Possible adverse effects | Respiratory depression, hypotension, lethargy—if given in excess or too rapidly | Heart block, hypotension if given too rapidly | Respiratory depression; hypotension | Respiratory depression; hypotension |

ence of *diffuse cerebral edema*, but no focal structural disorder was identified.

You have decided to begin administering an anticonvulsant to the patient. Before you write the order to begin the drug, can you answer the questions in Exercise 8?

## EXERCISE 8

### ■ Questions:

1. Which anticonvulsant did you choose to begin therapy? Why?

2. What adverse side effects of the drug do you anticipate?

3. What serum concentration of the drug is required to stop the seizures?

4. What initial loading dose of the drug is needed to achieve the desired serum concentration?

5. Is the initial loading dose the same for term and premature infants?

6. By which route will you administer the drug initially?

7. What is the proper rate of administration of the drug?

8. How much drug is required daily to maintain the serum concentration at the desired level?

9. When will you administer the first maintenance dose?

10. By what route will you administer maintenance dosages?

11. If your first drug selection fails, which second drug will you add to the anticonvulsant regimen?

12. When will you discontinue the anticonvulsants?

### ■ Discussion/Answers:

**Phenobarbital:** Phenobarbital is currently the drug of choice for managing neonatal seizures. It may be administered intravenously, intramuscularly, or orally to produce blood levels in the therapeutic range of 20 to 40 $\mu$g/mL. The initial loading dose in the premature or term infant of 20 mg/kg (intravenously administered over 20 minutes) will achieve an average blood level of 20 $\mu$g/mL. Excessively rapid administration may lead to depression of respiration, blood pressure, and alertness. Phenobarbital is eliminated from the body slowly. The serum half-life is variable and depends on the age of the child and the duration of exposure to the drug. For example, after 14 days of treatment the half-life is about 100 hours and falls to 40 hours by 28 days. Twelve to 24 hours following the initial loading dose, the first maintenance dose (3 to 4 mg/kg/day divided every 12 hours) is given. Subsequent changes in the maintenance dose will result in a new steady-state blood level within five half-lives. For example, if the half-life of phenobarbital for a child is 50 hours, and the maintenance dose is increased from 3 to 5 mg/kg/day, the resulting higher blood level will plateau in $5 \times 50$ hours (about 10 days).

**Phenytoin:** Phenytoin (Dilantin) is another effective anticonvulsant for treatment of seizures in the newborn infant. It is not well absorbed orally or intramuscularly so that blood levels in the therapeutic range of 10 to 20 $\mu$g/mL can only be reliably achieved intravenously. In the term or preterm infant an initial loading dose of 20 mg/kg is administered at a rate of about 1 mg/kg/min to achieve an average serum level of 15 $\mu$g/mL. Excessively rapid administration may produce heart block and hypotension. Thus, electrocardiographic monitoring during the initial loading is recommended. Maintenance doses of 3 to 4 mg/kg/day divided every 12 hours are begun 12 to 24 hours following the first loading dose. The serum half-life of phenytoin is also age dependent and may fall during the immediate neonatal period from 104 hours to 2 to 7 hours. The clinical signs of phenytoin toxicity observable in older individuals (nystagmus at 20 to 30 $\mu$g/mL, ataxia at 30 to 40 $\mu$g/mL, encephalopathy at more than 40 $\mu$g/mL) are not seen in infants. Frequent blood level determinations are necessary to guide dosage adjustments.

If neonatal seizures persist despite the use of both phenobarbital and phenytoin, diazepam or lorazepam may need to be added to the regimen. These drugs may be used for short-term seizure control, especially if the child is in status epilepticus. Neither drug is indicated to treat infrequent, brief, isolated convulsions.

**Diazepam:** Diazepam (Valium) may be administered intravenously to help control status epilepticus. The average effective dose is 0.68 mg/kg. In practice, a dose of 0.25 mg/kg given for a period of 2 minutes is often used because many physicians fear respiratory depression and circulatory collapse at excessive dosages. Despite a reasonably slow elimination rate (half-life of 25 hours in premature infants, 31 hours in term babies), the clinical response may be short-lived, necessitating repeated administrations as often as every 15 to 30 minutes. The physician must be prepared to intubate and ventilate his patient if respiratory depression follows administration of diazepam. Diazepam is usually discontinued if no beneficial effects are observed after several doses are given.

**Lorazepam:** Lorazepam (Ativan) is an alternative to diazepam, which has enjoyed growing acceptance. A typical dose of 0.05 to 0.1 mg/kg/dose may be administered intravenously over 2 minutes or longer. The clinical response may be significantly prolonged (up to 12 hours) compared to the shorter duration of action of benzodiazepam. Possible side effects include hypotension and respiratory depression.

### Long-Term Treatment

After the physician has initiated a course of anticonvulsant therapy, the vexing question of timing their discontinuation must be addressed. Diazepam and lorazepam are short-term remedies for treating status epilepticus, and it is difficult to orally maintain phenytoin concentrations in a therapeutic serum range during early infancy. Therefore, the issue of long-term treatment usually involves the duration of administration or oral phenobarbital after the acute seizure disorder has subsided. Each case must be judged individually since no universal policy applies. The following information may assist your decision.

1. Although phenobarbital is generally well tolerated, it may disturb behavior, attention span, or learning abilities in some infants. The effect of chronic phenobarbital consumption on the developing nervous system is not well understood presently. Preliminary work using animal models suggests it may not be totally benign.
2. It is not true that administration of phenobarbital during infancy will prevent the later development of epilepsy.
3. The incidence of epilepsy following neonatal convulsions is quite variable. Those survivors of neonatal seizure who later appear neurologically and developmentally normal have less than a 20% chance of developing epilepsy in later life. If the child has suffered cerebral palsy and/or mental retardation following neonatal convulsions, the chance of subsequent development of epilepsy is much higher.

With this in mind, a few general guidelines may be suggested to formulate the decision of when to stop administering phenobarbital:

1. If the child continues to have seizures, despite medication, or has an ongoing cause of seizures (such as cerebral malformation or an inborn error of metabolism), medication should not be stopped.

2. It is reasonable to consider stopping anticonvulsants at discharge from the nursery or as early as 3 months of age if the child is seizure-free, appears developmentally and neurologically normal, and exhibits an EEG devoid of any frank epileptic disturbance. If seizures do recur after therapy is stopped, medication will simply have to be restarted.

3. Some physicians will continue anticonvulsant treatment for a year or longer if the child exhibits any neurological sequelae such as motor or intellectual handicaps. Still, many of these patients will not have recurring seizures and may be particularly vulnerable to the adverse behavioral side effects of phenobarbital. The predictive power of the EEG in forecasting epilepsy has not yet been determined for these children.

## ESTIMATING THE PROGNOSIS

The physician's statement of prognosis should reflect his or her perception of the probable result of the illness—a forecast of expected outcome based on certain details of the disease. Formulating a neurological prognosis for infants with neonatal seizures is often difficult. Anxious parents expect the physicians to make a reasonable estimate of the severity of their child's illness in terms of life-threatening potential or the likelihood of chronic incapacitating neurological sequelae.

Three broad prognostic categories can be defined for neonatal seizures. A *favorable prognosis* implies at least an 85% to 90% chance of survival and subsequent normal development. An *unfavorable prognosis* suggests a high likelihood (85% to 90%) of death or serious handicap in survivors. A *mixed or uncertain prognosis* is correlated with intermediate rates of mortality and morbidity. To assign an infant to one of these broad prognostic categories, the physician must weigh the following considerations: the conceptional age of the patient, the etiology of the seizures, the appearance of the EEG between the seizures, and the duration of the seizures.

## Conceptional Age

The incidence of seizures in the neonatal period far exceeds that of any comparable period during the human life span. One might conclude, therefore, that seizures arise in an immature cerebral cortex with relative ease. Studies of experimental epilepsy in newborn animals reveal, however, that it is considerably more difficult to provoke and maintain convulsions in the immature cerebral cortex than in the mature one. The high incidence of convulsions in human newborn infants probably reflects the high concentration of potential neuropathic conditions in the neonatal period. Premature infants are more refractory to convulsions than term neonates, but have a remarkably high morbidity and mortality in the wake of their seizures. It would appear that only the most severe neurological insults are capable of producing seizures in the very immature brain.

## Etiology of the Seizure

The underlying etiology of the seizure state plays a fundamental role in the determination of prognosis. For example, infants with seizures caused by *herpes simplex* encephalitis will consistently fare worse than infants whose seizures arise from late onset hypocalcemic tetany. Table 15-7 provides a general outline of expected outcome for various etiologies.

## Interictal Electroencephalogram

Much useful prognostic information may be gained by a careful analysis of the EEG obtained between seizures (interictal) in term and premature infants. The neonatal EEG is remarkably complex and should be obtained and interpreted by experienced laboratory personnel. In term neonates with seizures, a normal interictal EEG forecasts a high probability of future neurological health. Conversely, certain severely abnormal electroencephalographic patterns (for example, flat or isoelectric) are highly predictive of a fatal outcome or severe neurological sequelae in term and premature survivors. Within weeks of a serious

**Table 15-7** Influence of Etiology on Prognosis for Infants with Neonatal Seizures

| ETIOLOGY | FAVORABLE OUTCOME | MIXED OUTCOME | UNFAVORABLE OUTCOME |
|---|---|---|---|
| Toxic-metabolic | Simple late onset hypocalcemia<br>Hypomagnesemia<br>Hyponatremia<br>Mepivacaine toxicity | Hypoglycemia<br>Early onset complicated hypocalcemia<br>Pyridoxine dependency | Some aminoacidurias |
| Asphyxia | | Mild hypoxic-ischemic encephalopathy | Severe hypoxic-ischemic encephalopathy |
| Hemorrhage | Uncomplicated subarachnoid hemorrhage | Subdural hematoma<br>Intraventricular hemorrhage (Grades I and II)* | Intraventricular hemorrhage (Grades III and IV)* |
| Infection | | Aseptic meningoencephalitis; some bacterial meningitides | Herpes simplex encephalitis; some bacterial meningitides |
| Structural | | Simple traumatic contusion | Malformations of central nervous system |

\* Grade I: Hemorrhage confined to the germinal matrix.
Grade II: Hemorrhage involves the germinal matrix and the ventricle; however, the ventricle is normal in size.
Grade III: Hemorrhage involves the germinal matrix and the ventricle which is enlarged, distended with blood.
Grade IV: Hemorrhage has extended beyond the germinal matrix and the ventricle into the parenchyma of the brain.

neurological insult, substantial nonspecific normalization of the EEG may occur. Unfortunately, this does not imply a normal outcome for the child. Neurological prognostication should rely on electroencephalographic findings during the acute phase of the illness when the most abnormal EEG findings are present. If serial tracings are obtained during the course of the disease, prognosis depends on the worst tracing obtained.

## Abundance of Seizures

Currently no firm clinical data are available to indicate that isolated, infrequently recurring seizures significantly affect neurological outcome. However, status epilepticus or abundant, frequently recurring epileptic seizures that cannot be controlled with anticonvulsants may carry substantial risk of death or a lifelong neurological handicap.

## EXERCISE 9

Consider the following clinical case summaries and attempt to assign a prognosis (favorable, unfavorable, or mixed outcome) to these patients.

**Case 1:** A 980-g infant appropriate for gestational age infant demonstrated status epilepticus on the third day of life following severe asphyxia and the demonstration of a Grade IV intraventricular hemorrhage. An interictal EEG was read as grossly abnormal and virtually isoelectric.

**Prognosis:**

**Case 2:** A term infant demonstrated poor feeding, lethargy, and mild jaundice on the fourth day of life. A sepsis workup was performed and analysis of CSF revealed pleocytosis and depressed glucose. Antibiotics were promptly started. Infrequent seizures began on the fifth day of life, but were easily controlled with phenobarbital. Group B streptococcus quickly grew from the culture of CSF. An EEG was read as "mildly abnormal for age."

**Prognosis:**

**Case 3:** A term infant had a single focal seizure on the seventh day of life following an uneventful pregnancy, labor, and delivery. Results of general physical and neurological examinations appeared normal. A detailed evaluation for infection or metabolic derangement was negative. Her EEG demonstrated an unexpectedly bizarre, abnormal background. Magnetic resonance imaging of the head revealed the presence of a definite cerebral malformation.

**Prognosis:**

**Case 4:** A term infant appeared entirely well until the eighth day of life when she became remarkably jittery. Recurring focal clonic seizures appeared about 12 hours later. Evaluation disclosed a serum calcium of 5.5 mg/dL and magnesium of 1.8 mg/dL. The seizures and jitteriness resolved promptly with the infusion of intravenous calcium.

**Prognosis:**

**Case 5:** A term infant was delivered by emergency cesarean section after fetal heart rate monitoring revealed severe late decelerations. Early heavy meconium had been passed after the membranes ruptured. The Apgar scores were 4 at 1 minute and 5 at 5 minutes. The initial arterial pH was 6.98. Acute tubular necrosis of the kidneys was documented. Persistent fetal circulation developed and required the use of pancuronium and tolazoline. Despite these measures, the arterial $PO_2$ persisted below 40 mm Hg. During the period of administration of pancuronium, the child's neurological status was monitored with serial EEGs, which demonstrated grossly abnormal electrical patterns and numerous seizures. The seizures persisted electrographically despite the administration of adequate doses of both phenobarbital and phenytoin.

**Prognosis:**

■ **Answers:**

Case 1. Unfavorable outcome

Case 2. Mixed outcome

Case 3. Unfavorable outcome

Case 4. Favorable outcome

Case 5. Unfavorable outcome

---

# BIBLIOGRAPHY

## Suspecting the Diagnosis

1. Rose AL, Lombroso CT: Neonatal seizure states. *Pediatrics* 1970; 45:404.
2. Berger A, Sharf B, Winter ST: Pronounced trem-
ors in newborn infants: Their meaning and prognostic significance. *Clin Pediatr* 1975; 14:834.
3. Sarnat M: Pathogenesis of decerebrate "seizures" in the premature infant with intraventricular hemorrhage. *J Pediatr* 1975; 87:154.
4. Brown JK, Ingram TTS, Seshia SS: Patterns of decerebration in infants and children: Defects in homeostasis and sequela. *J Neurol Neurosurg Psychiatry* 1973; 36:431.
5. Feinchel GM, Olson BJ, Fitzpatrick JE: Heart rate changes in convulsive and nonconvulsive apnea. *Ann Neurol* 1979; 6:171.
6. Willis J, Gould JB: Periodic alpha seizures with apnea in a newborn. *Dev Med Child Neurol* 1980; 22:214.
7. Ariagno R: Development of respiratory control. In Korobkin R, Guilleminault C, eds: *Advances in Perinatal Neurology*. New York, Spectrum Publications, 1979, p. 249.
8. Mizrahi EM, Kellaway P: Characterization and classification of neonatal seizures. *Neurology* 1987; 37:1837–1844.
9. Clancy RR, Legido A, Lewis D: Occult neonatal seizures. *Epilepsia* 1988; 29:256–261.
10. Younkin DP, Delivoria-Papadopoulos M, Maris J, et al: Cerebral metabolic effects of neonatal seizures measured with in vivo ³¹-P NMR spectroscopy. *Ann Neurology* 1986; 20:513–519.
11. Wasterlain CG, Vert P: *Neonatal Seizures*. New York, Raven Press, 1990.

## Initial Evaluation and Treatment

12. Hillman LS, Hillman RE, Dodson WE: Diagnosis, treatment, and followup of neonatal mepivacaine intoxication secondary to paracervical and pudendal blocks during labor. *J Pediatr* 1979; 95:472.
13. Howell J, Clozer M, Aranda J: Adverse effects of caffeine and theophylline in the newborn infant. *Semin Perin* 1981; 5:359.
14. Schreiner RL, Kleinman MB: Incidence and effect of traumatic lumbar puncture in the neonate. *Dev Med Child Neurol* 1981; 21:483.
15. Escobedo M, Barton LL, Volpe J: Cerebrospinal fluid studies in an intensive care nursery. *J Perinat Med* 1975; 3:204.
16. Sarff LD, Platt LH, McCracken GH: Cerebrospinal fluid evaluation in neonates: Comparison of high risk infants with and without meningitis. *J Pediatr* 1976; 88:473.

## Anticonvulsants

17. Lou HC, Friis-Hansen B: Arterial blood pressure elevations during motor activity and epileptic seizures in the newborn. *Acta Paediatr Scand* 1979; 68:803.
18. Wasterlain CG, Duffy TE: Status epilepticus in immature rats. *Arch Neurol* 1976; 33:821.
19. Wasterlain CB, Plum F: Vulnerability of developing rat brain to electroconvulsive seizures. *Arch Neurol* 1973; 29:38.
20. Painter MJ, Pippenger C, MacDonald H, et al: Phenobarbital and diphenylhydantoin levels in neonates with seizures. *J Pediatr* 1978; 92:315.

21. Dodson WE, Prensky AL, DeVivo DC, et al: Management of seizure disorders: Selected aspects. *J Pediatr* 1976; 89:527.
22. Smith BT, Masatti RE: Intravenous diazepam in the treatment of prolonged seizure activity in neonates and infants. *Dev Med Child Neurol* 1971; 13:630.
23. McInerny TK, Schubert WK: Prognosis of neonatal seizures. *Am J Dis Child* 1969; 117:261.
24. Holden KR, Freeman JM, Melits ED: Outcome of infants with neonatal seizures. In Wada JA, Penry JK, eds: *Advances in Epileptology. Epilepsy International Symposium.* New York, Raven Press, 1980, p. 155.

**Estimating the Prognosis**

25. Sea AR, Bray PT: Significance of seizures in infants weighing less than 2500 grms. *Arch Neurol* 1977; 34:381.
26. Knauss TA, Marshall RE: Seizures in a neonatal intensive care unit. *Dev Med Child Neurol* 1977; 19:719.
27. Monod N, Pajot N, Guidasci S: The neonatal EEG: Statistical studies and prognostic value in full term and preterm babies. *Electroencephalogr Clin Neurophysiol* 1972; 32:529.
28. Tharp BR, Cukier F, Monod H: The prognostic value of the electroencephalogram in premature infants. *Electroencephalogr Clin Neurophysiol* 1981; 51:219.
29. Dreyfus-Brisac C, Monod N: Electroclinical studies of status epilepticus and convulsions in the newborn. In Kellaway P, Peterson I, eds: *Neurological and Electroencephalographic Correlative Studies in Infancy.* New York, Grune and Stratton, 1964, p. 250.
30. Ellison PH, Largent JA, Bahr JP: A scoring system to predict outcome following neonatal seizures. *J Pediatr* 1981; 99:455.
31. Clancy RR, Legido A: Postnatal epilepsy following EEG confirmed neonatal seizures. *Epilepsia* 1991; 32:69–76.

# Chapter 16

☐

# INTRAVENTRICULAR

☐

# HEMORRHAGE

☐

## *Walter C. Allan, M.D.*

Intraventricular hemorrhage (IVH) is the major acute neurological event affecting preterm infants. It is important to recognize that the meaning of the term *IVH* has evolved over the past several years to become a code word for a complex of lesions affecting the central nervous system (CNS) of the preterm infant. Each of these lesions, germinal matrix, intraventricular, and intraparenchymal hemorrhage, as well as periventricular leukomalacia, has a distinct pathophysiology and differing sequelae. Furthermore, some represent primarily hemorrhagic lesions and others, primarily ischemic CNS injury. The clinical recognition of CNS injury even in cases of extensive hemorrhage may be difficult, while the consequences of such an injury are likely to be significant. This has made screening cranial ultrasound scanning an important part of neonatal intensive care. During the last 15 years considerable natural history and research information has become available concerning the IVH complex of lesions. This information has led to subtle changes in neonatal intensive care and a resultant decline in the incidence of some forms of IVH. Controversy still surrounds some treatment issues especially involving prevention of IVH and posthemorrhagic hydrocephalus. The cases that follow attempt to highlight these controversies and review the fundamentals of pathophysiology, cranial ultrasonography, and the clinical correlates of the IVH complex of lesions.

### CASE STUDY 1

BGB, a 33-week gestation infant girl, was born to a 20-year-old, gravida 3, para 1, abortus 1 woman following an unremarkable pregnancy. Spontaneous rupture of membranes occurred on the day of delivery. The infant was born by emergency cesarean section because of prolonged bradycardia. Apgar scores were 5 and 8 at 1 and 5 minutes, respectively. Meconium was noted, but was not present below the vocal cords. Following resuscitation and stabilization, the child's arterial blood gases showed a pH of 7.45, $PaCO_2$ of 29 torr, $HCO_3$ of 19 mEq/L, and $PaO_2$ of 103 torr. From the moment of birth, the infant's course was complicated by overwhelming sepsis, respiratory distress syndrome, and severe hypotension requiring administration of dopamine. The child was stuporous and had infrequent spontaneous movements without eye opening. The cranial ultrasound scan obtained at 44 hours of age is shown in Figure 16-1.

### EXERCISE 1

The scan shown in Figure 16-1 is normal. However, the static images are not without artifact, a major problem in interpreting static images. Match the number on the artist's sketch of the coronal and sagittal scan of Figure 16-1 with the correct answer in the following list.

| STRUCTURE | NUMBER |
| --- | --- |
| Periventricular white matter obscured by artifact (coronal scan) | |
| Caudate notch | |
| Interhemispheric fissure | |
| Temporal horn of lateral ventricle | |
| Germinal matrix region | |
| Choroid plexus | |

continued

| STRUCTURE | NUMBER |
| --- | --- |
| Artifact from edge of fontanelle | |
| Artifact from edge of lateral ventricle | |
| Anterior horn of lateral ventricle | |
| Sylvian fissure | |
| Occipital horn of lateral ventricle | |
| Cavum septiae pellucidae | |

### ■ Discussion:

Familiarity with cranial ultrasound images is an essential part of the practice of neonatology, especially if the neonatologist is the person providing the family with prognostic information. However, a hearty skepticism is needed if the only images viewed by the attending physicians are static images. A review by videotape is the best way to determine if the "abnormalities" noted on scan are pathological or artifactual. If this option is not available (and often even if it is) the persistence of abnormal findings on multiple scans taken over weeks to months is the only way to prove injury has occurred.

The areas of most interest to the neonatologist are the germinal matrix region on coronal scan, the caudate notch on sagittal scan, the periventricular white matter regions on both views and, of course, the lateral ventricles. These are the areas where hemorrhagic and ischemic lesions occur.

### ■ Answer:

| STRUCTURE | NUMBER |
| --- | --- |
| Periventricular white matter obscured by artifact (coronal scan) | 6 |
| Caudate notch | 7 |
| Interhemispheric fissure | 1 |
| Temporal horn of lateral ventricle | 11 |
| Germinal matrix region | 2 |
| Choroid plexus | 9 |
| Artifact from edge of fontanelle | 12 |
| Artifact from edge of lateral ventricle | 8 |
| Anterior horn of lateral ventricle | 5 |
| Sylvian fissure | 3 |
| Occipital horn of lateral ventricle | 10 |
| Cavum septiae pellucidae | 4 |

### CASE STUDY 1 continued

BGB was able to be supported with relatively high ventilator settings until the fourth day of life. At that point, she had an episode of bradycardia and hypotension and required bolus infusions of fluid and an increase in the concentration of intravenous dopamine. She was ultimately discovered to have a plugged endotracheal tube. The arterial blood gases obtained during this episode are as follows:

| TIME | pH | $PaCO_2$ | $HCO_3$ | $PaO_2$ | REMARKS |
| --- | --- | --- | --- | --- | --- |
| 5 P.M. | 7.45 | 25 | 17 | 78 | Hypotension |
| 6 P.M. | 7.52 | 19 | 15 | 143 | Preplugged tube |
| 6:30 P.M. | 6.85 | 105 | 17 | 117 | Plugged tube |

Following this episode the infant seemed less responsive and had a slightly fuller fontanelle. The next morning a repeat cranial ultrasound scan was obtained (see Fig. 16-2).

### EXERCISE 2

### ■ Questions:

1. What do the coronal and sagittal ultrasound scans demonstrate that was not present in the scan obtained 48 hours earlier?

2. Is there any parenchymal involvement?

3. Is the left periventricular white matter region on the static image of the coronal view normal or abnormal? What could you do to clear up this uncertainty?

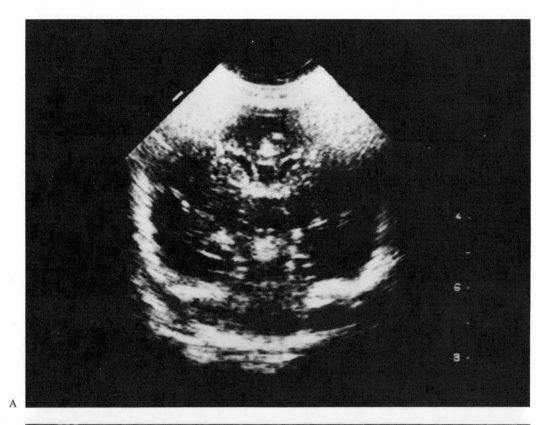

A

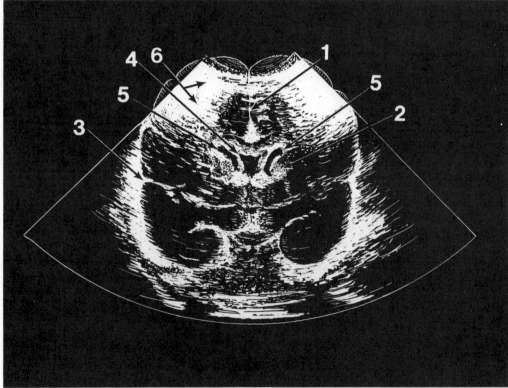

B

**Figure 16-1** (A) Coronal scan. The right side of the photograph represents the left of the infant. All coronal scans are shown in this convention. (B) Illustration of important structures and diagrammatic representation of the brain superimposed on the scan in part (A).

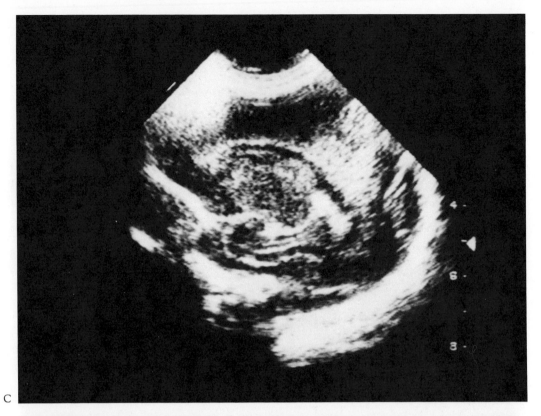

C

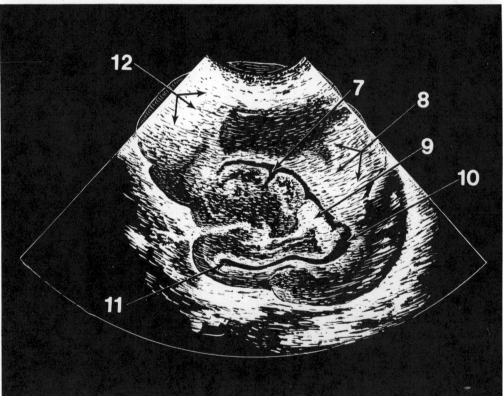

D

**Figure 16-1** *Continued* (C) Sagittal scan. The infant is looking to the left, and the occiput is on the right. All sagittal scans are shown in this convention. (D) Illustration of important structures and diagramatic representation of the brain superimposed on the scan in part (C).

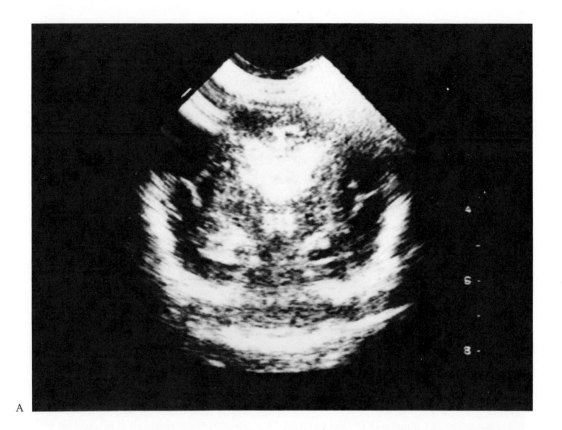

A

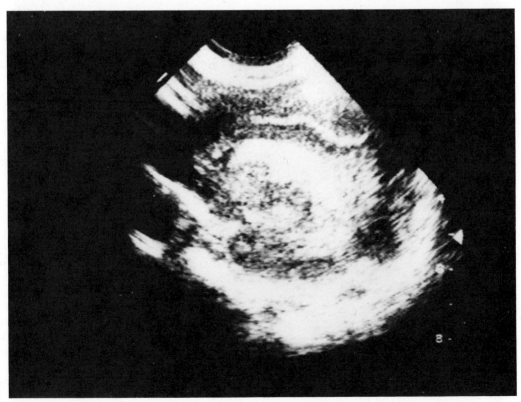

B

**Figure 16-2** (A) Coronal scan at day 5 in Case Study 1. (B) Sagittal scan at day 5 in Case Study 1.

4. What clinical signs suggest an intracranial hemorrhagic event may have occurred?

5. Based on the table of blood gases and events presented earlier, what physiological mechanisms might be evoked to explain the formation of this infant's large intraventricular hemorrhage?

6. What is the vascular site of origin of intraventricular hemorrhage? What anatomical factors make these vessels susceptible to hemorrhage?

7. What is the overall incidence of IVH in infants of less than 35 weeks' gestation?

8. What effect does extreme prematurity have on the incidence of IVH?

9. How has the incidence of IVH changed in recent years?

### ■ Answers:

1. A large germinal matrix and intraventricular hemorrhage are shown that extend into the area of the third ventricle.

2. Parenchymal involvement (either hemorrhagic or ischemic) may be present, but cannot be seen with any certainty on these static images.

3. The area of left periventricular white matter is obscured on the coronal scan by artifact from the edge of the anterior fontanelle. Review of the scan on videotape would clear up this issue as could repeating the scan.

4. This infant exhibited a change in activity and a full fontanelle. These two findings are statistically associated with the occurrence of IVH found by ultrasound scan, but have only a limited predictive value. Table 16-1 lists the clinical signs associated with autopsy-confirmed and ultrasound (US) or computerized tomography (CT)-confirmed IVH. As might be expected, more severe lesions were noted among the autopsy-confirmed cases. Therefore, it is not surprising that these infants were quite symptomatic and displayed signs compatible with the "catastrophic" and "saltatory" deterioration syndromes first described by Volpe in 1974. Those data, however, were collected prior to the availability of CT and ultrasound scans. As can be seen in Table 16-1, clinical signs are poor predictors of CT- or ultrasound-confirmed lesions. This, coupled with the ease of obtaining cranial ultrasound scans at the bedside, has made ultrasound scanning the preferred method for screening and evaluating any potential CNS cause of clinical deterioration in the neonatal intensive care unit.

5. The arterial blood gas results indicate that a sudden hypercarbic episode occurred at the time of the plugged endotracheal tube. Hypercarbia has been statistically associated with the occurrence of IVH. It is postulated that local metabolic changes produced by hypercarbia may cause vasodilation in vessels feeding the germinal matrix vascular bed and, in turn, the resultant high flow may induce hemorrhage. Although not severe enough to produce a metabolic acidosis, the episode of hypotension that occurred at 5 P.M. may have further injured this same vascular bed. Recurrent hypotension is postulated to produce underperfusion of the brain because of lack of autoregulation in preterm infants. This, in turn, results in local injury to the germinal matrix vascular bed, which increases the risk of vascular rupture and hemorrhaging when reperfusion or hyperperfusion occur (such as after hypercarbia).

**Table 16-1**  Clinical Signs and Symptoms in IVH

| ASSOCIATED WITH AUTOPSY CONFIRMATION* | ASSOCIATED WITH CT/US SCAN CONFIRMATION† | | |
|---|---|---|---|
| SYNDROME | SIGN/SYMPTOM | IVH | NO IVH |
| **Catastrophic deterioration** | | | |
| Evolves in minutes to hours | Falling hematocrit | 68% | 28% |
| Coma | Full fontanelle | 54 | 20 |
| Fixed pupils, no eye movements | Change in activity | 38 | 11 |
| Hypoventilation/apnea | Low tone | 30 | 10 |
| Tonic seizures, decerebrate rigidity, flaccidity | Abnormal eye signs | 11 | 0 |
| **Saltatory deterioration** | | | |
| Evolves in hours to days | Seizures | 11 | 0 |
| Neurological features as above that wax and wane | Tight popliteal angle | 84 | 11 |
| | No visual tracking | 79 | 21 |

* As described by Volpe.[1]
† Compiled from data in Refs. 16 and 17.
*Source:* From Allan WC: The IVH complex of lesions: Cerebrovascular injury in the preterm infant. *Neurologic Clin* 1990; 8:533. Reprinted with permission of W.B. Saunders Company.

All of these mechanisms are speculative, and physiological measurements in experimental animals as well as Doppler, near-infrared spectroscopy, and xenon washout cerebral blood flow studies in human neonates have yielded conflicting evidence. Table 16-2 organizes these multiple observations and resultant hypotheses into those factors associated with the premature infant's cerebrovasculature, those resulting from prematurity itself, and those that are the consequence of respiratory distress syndrome.

6. An *immature vascular rete* is the term used by Pape and Wigglesworth to describe the germinal matrix vessels that are the site of origin of IVH. The hemorrhage presumably begins in the germinal matrix and then ruptures into the ventricles. The vessels within the germinal matrix have a simplified structure and lack features that allow them to be identified as arterioles, venules, or capillaries. These vessels are replaced with a more mature vasculature by 36 weeks' gestation. Figure 16-3 shows a hypothetical scheme that integrates the factors listed in Table 16-2 into a model to describe the pathophysiology of IVH and the IVH complex of lesions. Further discussion of parenchymal injury is covered in later cases.

7. IVH occurs in approximately 20% of infants of less than 35 weeks' gestation.

8. In infants weighing less than 1,000 g, the incidence is approximately 30%.

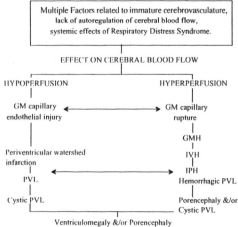

**Figure 16-3**  Interrelations of ischemic and hemorrhagic parenchymal lesions.

**Table 16-2** Pathogenesis of IVH Complex: Observations and Hypotheses

*Factors associated with preterm cerebrovasculature*

*Observation:* The incidence of IVH varies inversely with gestational age, suggesting that maturational factors are important.

*Hypothesis:* The poorly supported *vascular rete* of the germinal matrix, the increased cerebral blood flow to the area, and the unique periventricular watershed characteristics of the preterm infant are the important maturation-related factors.

*Other factors associated with prematurity*

*Observation:* Asphyxia and hypotension at birth are common in preterm infants with IVH.

*Hypothesis:* The germinal matrix and periventricular white matter are susceptible to ischemic injury, setting the stage for IVH.

*Observation:* Autoregulation of cerebral blood flow is impaired in asphyxiated newborns.

*Hypothesis:* Infants' CBF is "pressure passive" and they respond to systemic pressure changes by worsening ischemia (low blood pressure) or capillary hemorrhage (high blood pressure).

*Observation:* Coagulation factors are deficient in preterm infants with IVH.

*Hypothesis:* Preterm infants have impaired platelet/capillary interactions that contribute to hemorrhage.

*Factors associated with respiratory distress syndrome*

*Observation:* Hypoxia, hypercarbia, mechanical ventilation, pneumothorax, patent ductus arteriosus, prostaglandins, and therapies (for example, sodium bicarbonate, fluid resuscitation, pressor agents) are associated with IVH.

*Hypothesis:* Abrupt changes in systemic arterial and/or venous pressures are transmitted directly to the germinal matrix capillary bed and result in a combination of ischemia and hemorrhage. Local vasodilation is produced by metabolic factors and aggravates the ischemia and hemorrhage.

*Source:* From Allan WC: The IVH complex of lesions: Cerebrovascular injury in the preterm infant. *Neurologic Clin* 1990; 8:532. Reprinted with permission of W.B. Saunders Company.

9. The incidence of IVH has steadily declined during the past decade as shown in the data from Maine Medical Center of Table 16-3. The explanation for this steady decline is currently unknown.

**CASE STUDY 2**

BRP, a 970-g infant girl (twin A), was born following a 28-week gestation. Her mother, a healthy 33-year-old gravida 2 para 1 woman, went into spontaneous preterm labor and delivered both twins vaginally. The child's Apgar scores were 7

**Table 16-3** Declining Incidence of IVH*

| | MAINE MEDICAL CENTER INCIDENCE OF IVH BY GRADE 1980–1989† INFANTS <35 WEEKS' GESTATION | | | | | | | | | | | |
|---|---|---|---|---|---|---|---|---|---|---|---|---|
| YEAR | NO IVH | | GMH | | smIVH—% | | LgIVH—% | | IVH/IPH—% | | DIED | TOTAL |
| | (N) | (%) | (N) | (%) | (N) | (%) | (N) | (%) | (N) | (%) | (N) | (N) |
| 80–81 | 180 | 60 | 27 | 9.% | 38 | 13.% | 21 | 7.% | 6 | 2.% | 26 | 298 |
| 82–83 | 173 | 64 | 19 | 7.% | 26 | 10% | 20 | 7.% | 5 | 2.% | 27 | 270 |
| 84–85 | 211 | 71 | 22 | 7.% | 16 | 5.% | 15 | 5.% | 10 | 3.% | 24 | 298 |
| 86–87 | 277 | 77 | 30 | 8.% | 15 | 4.% | 9 | 2.% | 10 | 3.% | 21 | 362 |
| 88–89 | 313 | 81 | 11 | 3.% | 19 | 5.% | 9 | 2.% | 8 | 2.% | 25 | 385 |
| Totals | 1,154 | 72 | 109 | 7.% | 114 | 7.% | 74 | 5.% | 39 | 2.% | 123 | 1,613 |

* IVH = intraventricular hemorrhage; GMH = germinal matrix hemorrhage; smIVH = small IVH, hemorrhage occupying <50% of ventricle; LgIVH = large IVH, hemorrhage occupying >50% of ventricle with ventricular dilatation; IVH/IPH = IVH with associated intraparenchymal hemorrhage.
† Extends previously published results of ref. 3.

and 7 at 1 and 5 minutes, respectively. In the neonatal intensive care center, signs of respiratory distress developed and the infant was intubated and given artificial surfactant. On day 2 of life a cranial ultrasound scan was normal. On day 3 an unexpected deterioration occurred. This was heralded by sudden onset of pallor, a fall in oxygen saturation, and the development of metabolic acidosis. The child was given lactated Ringer's solution, packed red blood cells, and bicarbonate. She was reintubated three times before ventilation improved. Despite multiple transfusions, her hematocrit fell from the previous day's level. This suggested an intracranial hemorrhage might have occurred. The following day the presence of a hemorrhage was confirmed by ultrasound scan. The scan obtained on day 8 of life is shown in Figure 16-4.

## EXERCISE 3

### ■ Questions:

1. Compare this scan with that obtained in Case Study 1 (Fig. 16-2). What scan characteristics indicate that hemorrhage occurred acutely in Case Study 1 and subacutely in Case Study 2? When do you think hemorrhage occurred in Case Study 2?

2. What structure are the arrows pointing to on the coronal scan? Assuming that the arrows are pointing to the same structure in each hemisphere, why do they look so different?

3. What grade of IVH has occurred? What grade of IVH occurred in Case Study 1?

4. The major rationale for grading an IVH is to predict outcome. Which kind of hemorrhage is more likely to result in an adverse neurological outcome—a large intraventricular hemorrhage or an intraparenchymal hemorrhage (IPH)?

5. What are the acute sequelae of a large IVH?

### ■ Answers:

1. The ultrasound scan from Case Study 1 suggests that an acute hemorrhage has occurred; the germinal matrix and intraventricular hemorrhage have blurred together and the ventricular walls are indistinct. The hemorrhage in Case Study 2 has well-defined margins and may have contracted somewhat. In addition, ventricular dilatation is evident. This suggests that the hemorrhage is 3 to 5 days old. Ten to 14 days after an intraventricular hemorrhage has occurred, an intraventricular clot will develop and will appear on the ultrasound scan as a mass with a hypoechoic center and hyperechoic edges. The intraventricular blood will persist in this state until resorbed.

2. The anterior temporal horns are dilated and thus visible. The right temporal horn contains hemorrhage visible on the sagittal scan.

3. Both infants would be classified as having a *large IVH*. Table 16-4 describes a scheme for grading IVH and the IVH complex of lesions. Comparison with the system of Papile et al., a CT scan-based system, is listed. Many parenchymal lesions can only be recognized by their persistence and characteristic late ultrasound or CT appearance as shown in the table.

4 & 5. Parenchymal hemorrhage is statistically associated with an adverse neurological outcome. Large IVH is more likely to produce the acute sequelae of IVH, posthemorrhagic hydrocephalus (PHH).

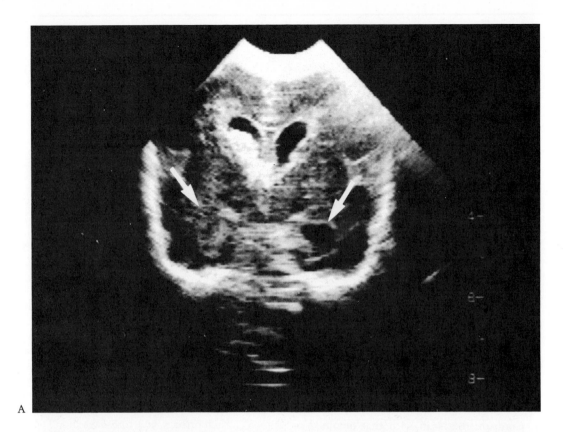

A

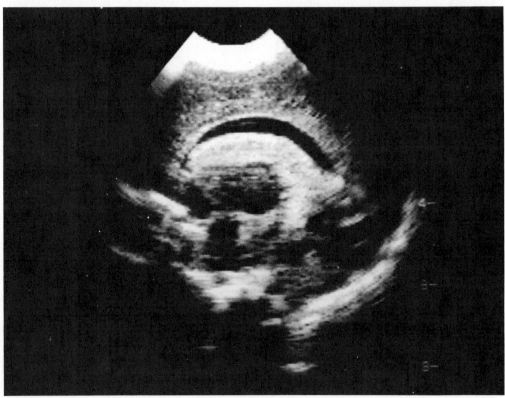

B

**Figure 16-4** (A) Coronal scan at day 8 in Case Study 2. Note the arrows. (B) Sagittal scan at day 8 in Case Study 2.

**Table 16-4**  Classification of IVH and Parenchymal Echodensities

| CLASS | EARLY SCANS* | LATE SCANS |
| --- | --- | --- |
| Germinal matrix hemorrhage (GMH) | Formerly Grade 1 (1) | Germinal matrix cyst or complete resolution |
| Small intraventricular hemorrhage (IVH) | Formerly Grade 2a (2)—GMH + IVH filling <50% of ventricle | Ventriculomegaly in 33%; rarely post-hemorrhagic hydrocephalus |
| Large intraventricular hemorrhage | Formerly Grade 2b (3)—GMH + IVH filling >50% of ventricle with ventricular dilation | Ventriculomegaly in 40%; posthemorrhagic hydrocephalus in 45% |
| Intraparenchymal | Formerly Grade 3 (4)—bright triangular echodensity in white matter with its apex superolateral to the ventricle and its base toward the cortex merging with large IVH | Porencephalic cyst |
| Periventricular leukomalacia (PVL) | Distinct triangular echodensity similar in appearance to IPH but less bright and separate from the ventricle | Cystic PVL |
| Flare | Diffuse echodensity parallel to the ventricle extending from the anterior horn to the atrium | Prolonged flare persists >2 weeks to be significant |
| Intraparenchymal echodensity | Indistinct echodensity in the periventricular white matter | Resolves <2 weeks to be nonsignificant; may develop into cystic PVL or prolonged flare |

* Grades listed are from Ref. 5; those in parentheses refer to the system of Papile et al.[4]

## CASE STUDY 2 continued

One week following the scan shown in Figure 16-4, the scan depicted in Figure 16-5 was obtained. Since head growth was proceeding normally, no intervention occurred. During the subsequent week the occipital-frontal circumference (OFC) increased from 24.5 to 26.5 cm. Lumbar punctures were performed on two successive days. However, only 4 mL of slightly xanthochromic cerebral spinal fluid (CSF) could be obtained with the second spinal tap. Therefore, the decision was made to perform external ventricular drainage by percutaneously placing an intravenous-type catheter (20-gauge insertion needle) in the right lateral ventricle through the right coronal suture at the edge of the anterior fontanelle. (A detailed description of this method is described in Ref. 5.) By means of this procedure, 40 mL of very dark, xanthochromic, ventricular fluid, containing some particulate matter, drained in the first 24 hours. During the ensuing week, the catheter was left in place, and 140 mL of CSF was drained. The scan obtained at removal of the catheter is shown in Figure 16-6. When rapid head growth (greater than 2 cm per week) and recurrent ventricular dilation occurred, a repeat external ventricular drainage was performed. This procedure was carried out on five separate occasions; each insertion and drainage lasting 3 to 7 days, over the course of 2 months as the child matured. During the last 6 weeks of hospitalization routine head growth occurred. Ventricular size was stable by cranial ultrasound scan. At discharge the scan shown in Figure 16-7 was obtained. The child went home weighing 2,525 g and appeared clinically well.

## EXERCISE 4

■ **Questions:**

1. In Figure 16-5 what is the structure marked by an arrow on the coronal scan? Why is it so prominent?

2. Why was lumbar puncture delayed for a week despite the presence of ventricular dilation apparent in Figure 16-5?

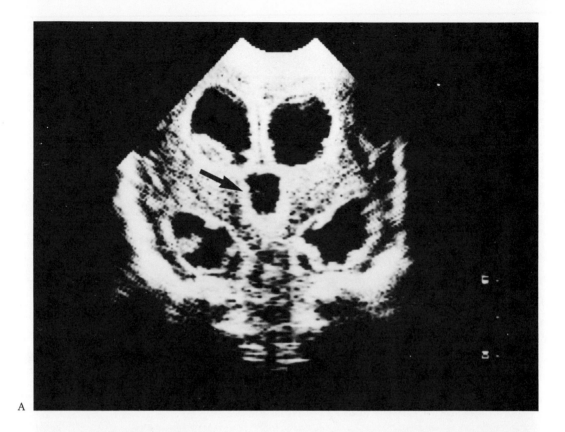

A

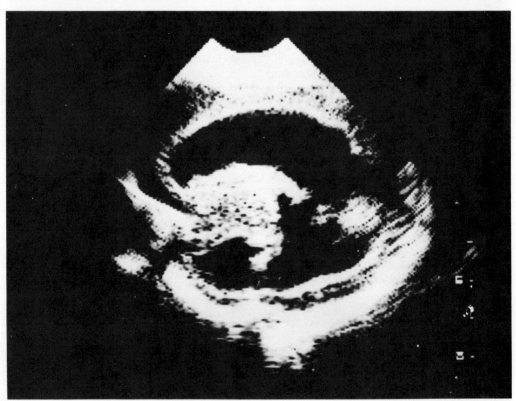

B

**Figure 16-5** (A) Coronal scan at day 15 in Case Study 2. Note the arrow. (B) Sagittal scan at day 15 in Case Study 2.

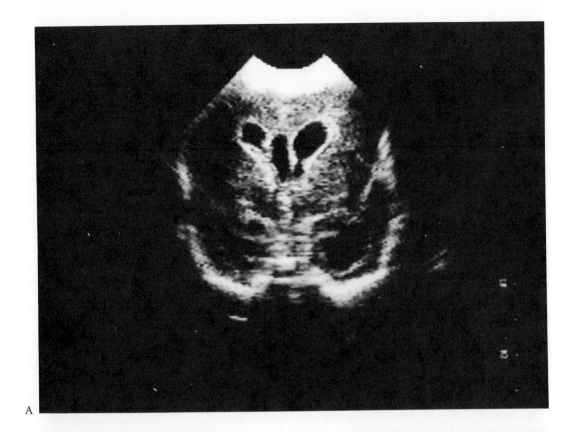

A

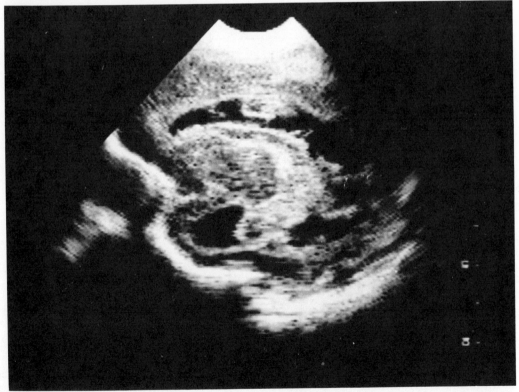

B

**Figure 16-6** (A) Coronal scan in Case Study 2 following 1 week of EVD. (B) Sagittal scan in Case Study 2 following 1 week of EVD.

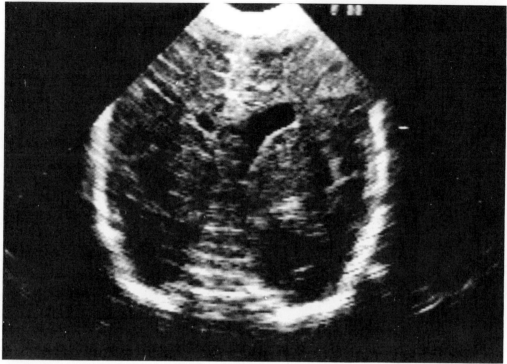

**Figure 16-7** Coronal scan in Case Study 2 at discharge.

3. What are two possible causes of PHH? What abnormalities would you expect in the CSF that might confirm one of these causes? What is the significance of the difference in color of the CSF obtained by lumbar puncture and that obtained following placement of the ventricular catheter?

4. In addition to serial lumbar punctures, what other treatments have been used in infants with PHH? What basic principle of PHH treatment is demonstrated by comparing the ultrasound scans shown in Figure 16-5 and Figure 16-6?

5. What is the overall incidence of PHH in infants with an intraventricular hemorrhage who are less than 35 weeks' gesta-

tion? How many of these infants will need permanent placement of an ventriculo-peritoneal (VP) shunt?

6. Given the ultrasound scan at discharge, do you think PHH is likely to recur? How would you know?

■ **Answers:**

1. The structure identified in Figure 16-5 is the third ventricle, which is dilated by possible obstruction of the aqueduct of Sylvius.

2. The delay in initiating serial lumbar punctures is a judgment call and somewhat controversial. In our institution we have rigorously (some might say "rigidly") stuck to a

clinical definition of PHH for the past decade. We define PHH as rapid head growth (greater than 2 cm increase in OFC per week) with associated ventricular dilatation such as that seen in Figure 16-5. We distinguish clinical PHH from simple ventriculomegaly, that is, large ventricles on cranial ultrasound scan alone. We believe that attempts to intercede in cases of ventriculomegaly will result in overtreatment and a false sense of success because ventriculomegaly is both common and spontaneously reversible.

3. PHH can result either from an inflammatory arachnoiditis in the posterior fossa resulting in communicating hydrocephalus (i.e., the ventricular CSF communicates with the lumbar space, but does not get absorbed over the convexity) or obstruction of the aqueduct of Sylvius leading to noncommunicating hydrocephalus. The ventricular fluid in this case contained 3,900 red blood cells/mm$^3$, 3300 white blood cells/mm$^3$, a protein concentration of 255 mg% and a glucose concentration of less than 10 mg%. These findings are indicative of a chemical meningitis induced by the red blood cells and blood products in the CSF. The CSF obtained by lumbar puncture differed in color from the ventricular fluid suggesting that noncommunicating hydrocephalus was present. This hypothesis was supported by the presence of a dilated third ventricle on ultrasound scan (Fig. 16-5).

4. In addition to serial lumbar punctures, acetazolamide, furosemide, glycerol, isosorbide, and early placement of a VP shunt have been used to decompress the dilated ventricles in infants with PHH. The fundamental goals of all treatments are (1) to relieve intracranial hypertension, (2) to produce a decrease in ventricular size, and (3) to reexpand the compromised cortical mantle. Our system of assessment and treatment is outlined in the flow chart of Figure 16-8.

5. Most studies report a 1% to 2% incidence of PHH. Permanent placement of a VP shunt is needed in at least 50% of these infants, regardless of the temporizing ventricular drainage methods. The four most commonly used CSF drainage methods include indwelling ventriculostomy, ventric-

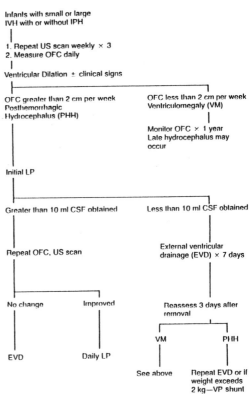

**Figure 16-8** Flow chart for the management of ventricular dilation following small or large IVH. From Allan, WC: The IVH complex of lesions: Cerebrovascular injury in the preterm infant. *Neur Clin* 1990; 8:537. Reprinted with permission of W.B. Saunders Company.

ular catheter with a reservoir, direct percutaneous ventricular taps, and intermittent external ventricular drainage. The incidence of PHH at our institution by grade of intraventricular hemorrhage is shown in Table 16-5. As indicated, PHH occurs only in cases of large IVH or IVH/IPH. At the Maine Medical Center 12 cases (0.8% of all infants of less than 35 weeks' gestation) have required VP shunt placement over an 8-year time period.

6. PHH is likely to recur if ventricular dilation persists at discharge. In rare instances PHH may recur during the first year of life in a patient in whom ventriculomegaly and rapid head growth had resolved. Weekly to monthly determinations of head circumference is a useful way to monitor the child for recurrence. Under a year of age, cranial ultrasound scans can be done through the anterior fontanelle to confirm or deny re-

**Table 16-5** Posthemorrhagic Hydrocephalus in Infants Less Than 35 Weeks' Gestation for 1981–1989 Period*

| | TOTAL NUMBER <35 WEEKS | GMH | SMALL IVH | LARGE IVH | IVH/IPH | DIED BEFORE EVALUATION |
|---|---|---|---|---|---|---|
| Total number | 1,498 | 92 | 85 | 60 | 34 | 110 |
| Number with PHH | 24 | 0 | 0 | 14 | 10 | 0 |

* GMH = germinal matrix hemorrhage, IVH = intraventricular hemorrhage, IPH = intraparenchymal hemorrhage.

turn of PHH when the OFC is crossing isobars on the head growth chart.

---

### CASE STUDY 3

MY, an 1,150-g infant boy was born following a 30-week gestation to a 15-year-old woman who did not realize she was pregnant and presented to an emergency room for "probable appendicitis." Apgar scores were 2 and 4 at 1 and 5 minutes, respectively. The child was intubated in the emergency room and transported to a tertiary care center. His initial blood gas analysis in the newborn intensive care unit revealed a pH of 7.05 and a $PaCO_2$ of 57 torr. Soon after admission, the infant required intubation and cardiovascular resuscitation with intravenous fluids. His hospital course was significant for the occurrence of severe respiratory distress and multiple pneumothoraces requiring placement of three chest tubes. On day 3 the ultrasound scan shown in Figure 16-9 was obtained. By day 16 the OFC was increasing by 2 cm per week and the ultrasound scan depicted in Figure 16-10 was obtained.

### EXERCISE 5

#### ■ Questions:

1. Where has the hemorrhaging occurred on the coronal and sagittal scans shown in Figure 16-9? What is the grade or classification of this hemorrhage?

2. Explain the pathophysiology of intraparenchymal hemorrhage (IPH).

3. Based on the initial scan, what prognostic information would you give to this family?

4. What do the images in Figure 16-10 indicate? How should this problem be managed?

5. What is abnormality is apparent in Figure 16-10B?

#### ■ Answers:

1. Figure 16-9 demonstrates a left germinal matrix hemorrhage, intraventricular hemorrhage, and IPH. The hemorrhage can be classified either as Grade IV (Papile) or a large IVH/IPH.

2. Intraparenchymal hemorrhage is believed to represent either *hemorrhage into an area of periventricular infarction* or a site of *hemorrhagic venous infarction* (or possibly both). Most recent studies suggest venous infarction is more probable. Venous infarc-

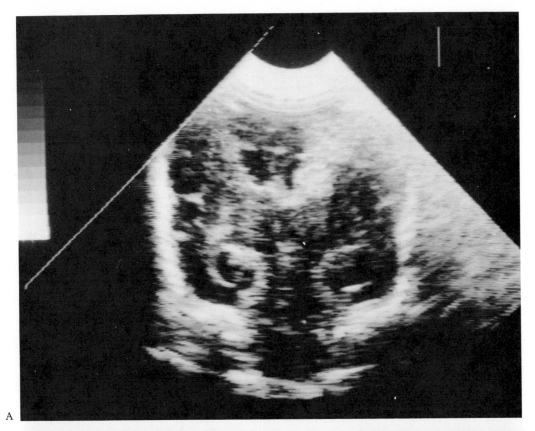

A

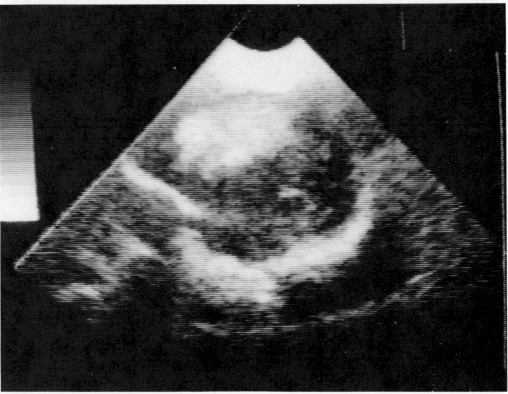

B

**Figure 16-9** (A) Coronal scan in Case Study 3 at day 3. (B) Sagittal scan, lateral to the ventricle, in Case Study 3 at day 3.
From Allan, WC: The IVH complex of lesions: Cerebrovascular injury in the preterm infant. *Neur Clin* 1990; 8:540–548.

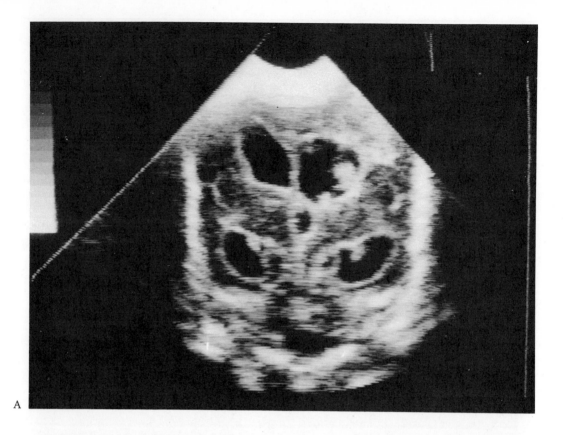

A

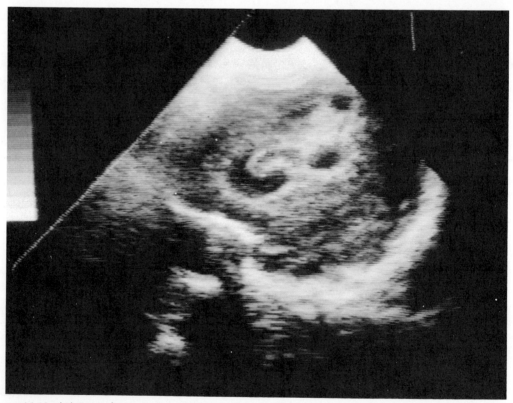

B

**Figure 16-10** (A) Coronal scan in Case Study 3 at day 16. (B) Sagittal scan, lateral to the ventricle, in Case Study 3 at day 16.
From Allan, WC: The IVH complex of lesions: Cerebrovascular injury in the preterm infant. *Neur Clin* 1990; 8:540–548.

tions are thought to result from venous stasis in the medullary and terminal veins in the deep white matter contiguous to a germinal matrix and/or intraventricular hemorrhage. In contrast, hemorrhage into areas of periventricular infarction is believed to occur at sites of reperfusion. That is, large IPHs are usually found in the anterior portion of a diffuse area of hypoperfused white matter, where a *watershed* infarction had occurred.

3. The family should be told that it is quite likely that PHH will develop during the acute phase of their child's illness. Furthermore, it is possible that as the infant develops, cerebral palsy [either spastic diplegia (R>L) or a spastic right hemiparesis] and mental impairment (usually of a mild degree) may result.

Studies examining the outcome of infants with IVH continue to emerge. Recently, Lowe and Papile followed up a group of 38 children with birth weights of less than 1,500 g with and without IVH. They were evaluated at age 5 to 6 years and compared to age-matched full-term control infants. The very low birth weight infants scored significantly lower on all test parameters. Furthermore, the 11 very low birth weight infants with germinal matrix hemorrhage (GMH) or small IVH in this group scored significantly lower than those without GMH/IVH on combined test scores. Because of these findings, the authors suggested that even small hemorrhagic injuries may have an adverse effect on overall performance of affected children at school age.

More striking neurodevelopmental deficits have been exhibited by children with parenchymal lesions. Several authors have examined the outcome of infants with parenchymal lesions on screening ultrasound scan. These studies paid particular attention to the evolution of parenchymal echodensities over time. That is, although they classified outcome by the appearance of the initial scan, they also reported the frequency of cystic changes in the areas of injury. As noted in Table 16-4, it is the evolution of parenchymal lesions to cystic periventricular leukomalacia or porencephalic cysts that allows confirmation of a definitive diagnosis of parenchymal injury. Since you would expect parenchymal injuries to be the origin of neurodevelopmental dysfunction, classification of outcome data by whether or not cystic parenchymal lesions occurs should have the highest predictive value. As evidence of this, the predictive value of "late" changes versus initial scan findings is shown in Table 16-6. It is obvious that the late cystic change of an intraparencymal lesion has the highest predictive value of adverse outcome. Thus the developing cyst seen in Figure 16-10B is an ominous sign.

4. PHH is evident. CSF drainage by lumbar puncture may be initiated and, if unsuccessful, drainage of ventricular CSF by external ventricular drainage is recommended.

5. Cystic changes in the area of parenchymal hemorrhage are apparent.

**Table 16-6**  Prediction of Outcome Based on Degree of Parenchymal Injury with US Scans

| DIAGNOSIS | EARLY SCAN RESULTS* | | | | | LATE SCAN CYSTS | |
| | NO LESION | GMH | IVH | IPH | PVL | UNILATERAL | BILATERAL |
|---|---|---|---|---|---|---|---|
| Developmental quotient <50 | 0.6† | 4.1 | 10.9 | 12.5 | 11.8 | 2.4 | 45.8 |
| Cerebral palsy | 3.6 | 8.2 | 17.8 | 62.5 | 17.6 | 30.9 | 62 |

* GMH = germinal matrix hemorrhage, IVH = intraventricular hemorrhage, IPH = intraparenchymal hemorrhage, PVL = periventricular leukomalacia.
† Numbers given are percent of incidence of diagnosis per US finding.
*Source:* Adapted from Cooke RWI: Early and late cranial ultrasonographic appearances and outcome in very low birthweight infants. *Arch Dis Child* 1987; 62:934–935. Adapted with permission of the British Medical Association.

### CASE STUDY 3 continued

External ventricular drainage was performed on three occasions between the 16th and 40th day of life, following which the OFC began to follow a normal growth curve. The child was discharged to a foster family at 90 days of age. The scan obtained at discharge is shown in Figure 16-11. Neurological examination between 6 and 9 months postconceptional age showed a subtle right hemiparesis with some fisting of the hand and decreased movement of the leg. However, with physical and occupational therapy, he progressively improved and by 16 months chronological age he was walking. His neurological examination at that time point was normal (without signs of hemiparesis). A CT scan obtained at 22 months is shown in Figure 16-12. In second grade he was thought to have a learning disability and demonstrated a 15-point difference between verbal and performance IQ testing. At 6.5 years of age he had a generalized tonic-clonic seizure in his sleep observed by his stepbrother. An electroencephalogram showed left posterior parieto-occipital spikes. He is now seizure free while receiving carbamazepine. Growth and development have otherwise been normal.

### EXERCISE 6

#### ■ Questions:

1. What is the name of the cystic structure located in the left hemisphere on Figure 16-11?

2. The CT scan in Figure 16-12 demonstrates asymmetry of the lateral ventricles. What would account for this asymmetry? What is the significance of this finding?

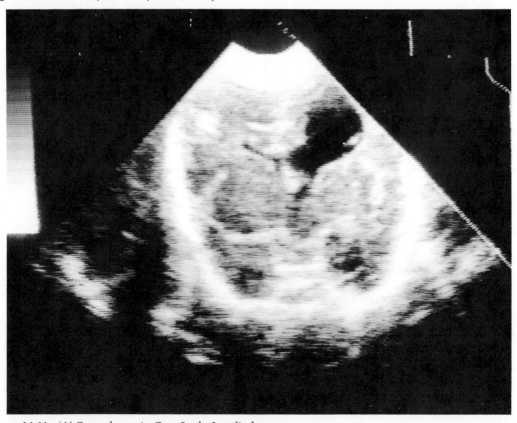

A

**Figure 16-11** (A) Coronal scan in Case Study 3 at discharge.
From Allan, WC: The IVH complex of lesions: Cerebrovascular injury in the preterm infant. *Neur Clin* 1990; 8:540–548.

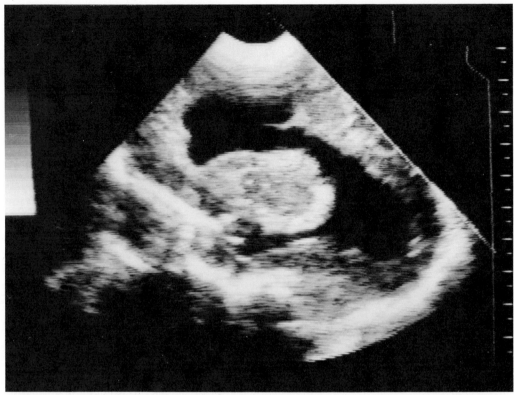

B

**Figure 16-11** *Continued* (B) Sagittal scan in Case Study 3 at discharge.

3. What are the chances of neurodevelopmental dysfunction based on the early and late ultrasound scans in this child? (Refer to Table 16-6.)

4. Is the seizure disorder that developed at age 6.5 years related to the findings on the CT scan?

■ **Answers:**

1. A porencephalic cyst is apparent in the left hemisphere. Porencephalic cysts are defined as single large space(s) communicating broadly with a lateral ventricle. The development of porencephaly is a characteristic response of the neonatal brain in which areas of chronic infarction are replaced by a sharply defined cystic cavity.

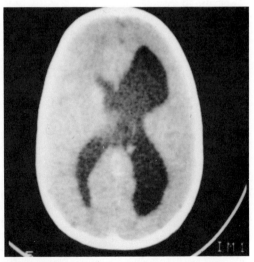

**Figure 16-12** CT scan in Case Study 3 at 22 months. The left side of the photo is the child's right.

From Allan, WC: The IVH complex of lesions: Cerebrovascular injury in the preterm infant. *Neur Clin* 1990; 8:540–548.

2. The asymmetry can be accounted for by the presence of the porencephalic cyst in association with generalized enlargement of the left lateral ventricle. This suggests that there has been more diffuse left hemisphere white matter injury. A spastic hemiparesis or learning disability may result.

3. Based on the early scan demonstrating an IPH, a developmental quotient less than 50 would be expected in 12.5% of such children and significant neurological deficit would be expected in 62.5%. Similarly, based on the later scan demonstrating unilateral porencephaly, a developmental quotient of 50 would be expected in 2.4% of affected infants and a neurological abnormality in 30.9%. Interestingly, but not surprisingly, this child fell into the group without significant developmental or neurological deficits—the most probable outcome based on the scan findings. The early scan finding of IPH alone overestimated the chance for an adverse outcome. It is obvious that waiting to see if bilateral cystic change occurs gives a better estimate of eventual performance.

4. The seizure disorder is undoubtedly related to his periventricular injury. The spikes are emanating from the left hemisphere, which contains the previously injured areas. This would suggest that, at times, cortical injury occurs in association with deep white matter injury and may produce an epileptic focus. This is an unusual outcome in our experience.

## CASE STUDY 4

An 1,170-g male infant was born following a 29-week gestation to a 29-year-old, gravida 2, para 1 mother. The mother developed toxemia and hypertension and was referred to the Perinatal Unit at Maine Medical Center. Fetal monitoring revealed spontaneous heart rate decelerations consistent with fetal distress and a cesarean section was performed. At delivery the infant was limp, cyanotic, bradycardic, and apneic, and he required immediate intubation. Apgar scores were 5 and 6 at 1 and 5 minutes, respectively, and the umbilical cord pH was 7.24. He was administered exogenous surfactant in the delivery room and then transferred to the intensive care nursery where he was placed on assisted ventilation. Initial cranial ultrasound scans at days 2, 7, and 14 were unre-

markable. On day 8 of life he had an episode of abdominal distention associated with marked tenderness. However, abdominal films failed to reveal free air and he was treated with supportive care and antibiotics (blood cultures were negative). A further episode of temperature instability and apnea occurred at 30 days of age. Treatment for sepsis was initiated for the third time, but again cultures were negative. No persistent hypotension, seizures, or further untoward events occurred. A cranial ultrasound scan was obtained at 51 days as part of discharge planning. This scan is shown in Figure 16-13.

## EXERCISE 7

### ■ Questions:

1. What lesion is apparent? Where is it located?

2. What cranial ultrasound lesion usually precedes the lesion seen in Figure 16-13? Why might the initial lesion be easily overlooked?

3. Review of the previous ultrasound scans failed to reveal any convincing abnormality. Can you speculate when the injury occurred that produced the abnormality seen on the discharge scan? What is the pathophysiology of such a lesion?

4. What neurological sequelae are likely to result from this lesion? What makes the probable neurodevelopmental outcome more bleak for this patient compared to the patient with the parenchymal lesion in Case Study 3.

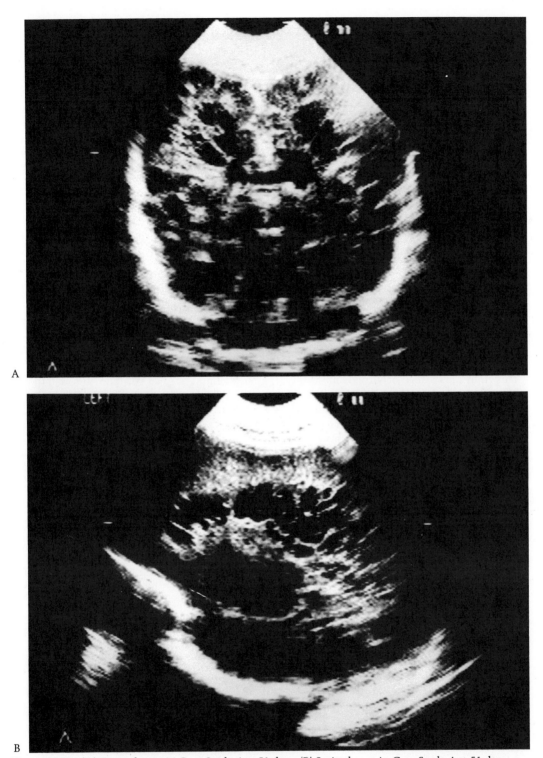

A

B

**Figure 16-13** (A) Coronal scan in Case Study 4 at 51 days. (B) Sagittal scan in Case Study 4 at 51 days.

## ■ Answers:

1. Cystic periventricular leukomalacia (PVL) is apparent on this ultrasound scan. This striking collection of cysts occupies almost the entire periventricular white matter from anterior to posterior.

2. A parenchymal echodensity, in one of its many forms [PVL, intraparenchymal echodensity (IPE), or a diffuse "flare"], usually precedes the severe cystic change seen in this case. A "flare" and IPE can often be mistaken for artifact and vice versa. Thus, parenchymal injury could have been overlooked. This case illustrates the value of obtaining a late ultrasound scan in preterm infants. At least monthly scans seem warranted in preterm infants at high risk for PVL, because cysts may develop without any prior lesion and then disappear as a gliotic scar forms. The only sign that may remain is a subtle degree of ventricular dilatation with increased sulcal markings in the area of the trigone.

3. This injury may have occurred some time between 2 and 4 weeks of life, because no scans were obtained during that time and it usually takes 2 weeks to develop the degree of cystic change noted in Figure 16-13. However, this is purely speculative, because no clinically obvious ictus occurred to the degree that would be expected given the pathophysiology of this lesion. As mentioned above, cystic PVL is thought to be the result of watershed infarction in the preterm infant's brain. The watershed area of cerebral "*irrigation*" in the preterm infant is in the periventricular white matter between the centripetal ependymal arterioles and the centrifugal cortical arterioles. This area is felt to lie 9 mm from the ventricular wall (from anterior to posterior), but is most prominent at the trigone of the lateral ventricle. The lesions in this child map to this area in a striking fashion. A watershed infarction is felt to be a largely ischemic lesion and is most highly correlated, clinically, with shock and meningitis. A schematic illustrating selective pathophysiological mechanisms is provided in Figure 16-3.

4. Spastic diplegia is the classic sequel of PVL. In this form of cerebral palsy, the legs are affected more than the arms, and because this is largely a white matter lesion, intellectual function is usually preserved. The bilateral nature of the parenchymal involvement as well as its extension anterior to posterior would make this particular child more likely to have significant neurodevelopmental impairment. From Table 16-6 the probability of poor developmental quotient and cerebral palsy for this patient are 45.8% and 62%, respectively. At corrected age 12 months, this child is sociable but does not roll over or sit and has signs of spastic diplegia.

---

## BIBLIOGRAPHY

1. Volpe JJ: Neonatal intracranial hemorrhage-iatrogenic etiology? *N Engl J Med* 1974; 291:43–45.
2. Pape KE, Wigglesworth JS: Haemorrhage, ischemia and the perinatal brain. In *Clinics in Developmental Medicine*, Numbers 69/70. London, Heinemann International Medical Publications, 1979.
3. Phillip AGS, Allan WC, Tito A, et al: Intraventricular hemorrhage in preterm infants: Declining incidence in the 1980s. *Pediatrics* 1989; 84:797–801.
4. Papile L, Burstein J, Burstein R, et al: Incidence and evolution of subependymal hemorrhage: A study of infants with birth weights less than 1500 grams. *J Pediatr* 1978; 92:529–534.
5. Marrow PJ, Dransfield DA, Mott SH, et al: Posthemorrhagic hydrocephalus: Use of an intravenous-type catheter for cerebrospinal fluid drainage. *Am J Dis Child* 1991; 145:1141–1146.
6. Allan WC, Holt PJ, Sawyer LR, et al: Ventricular dilation after neonatal periventricular-intraventricular hemorrhage. *Am J Dis Child* 1982; 136:589–593.
7. Allan WC, Dransfield DA, Tito AM: Ventricular dilation following periventricular-intraventricular hemorrhage: Outcome at age 1 year. *Pediatrics* 1984; 73:158–162.
8. Volpe JJ, Herscovitch P, Perlman JM, et al: Positron emission tomography in the newborn. Extensive impairment of regional cerebral blood flow with intraventricular hemorrhage and hemorrhagic intracerebral involvement. *Pediatrics* 1983; 72:589–601.
9. Lowe J, Papile L: Neurodevelopmental performance of very-low-birth-weight infants with mild periventricular, intraventricular hemorrhage. Outcome at 5 to 6 years of age. *Am J Dis Child* 1990; 144:1242–1245.
10. McMenamin JB, Shackelford GD, Volpe JJ: Outcome of neonatal intraventricular hemorrhage with periventricular echodense lesions. *Ann Neurol* 1984; 15:285–290.
11. Guzzetta F, Shackelford GD, Volpe S, et al: Periventricular intraparenchymal echodensities

in the premature newborn: Critical determinant of neurologic outcome. *Pediatrics* 1986; 78: 995–1006.

12. Weindling AM, Rochefort MJ, Calvert SA, et al: Development of cerebral palsy after ultrasonographic detection of periventricular cysts in the newborn. *Dev Med Child Neurol* 1985; 27:800–806.

13. deVries LS, Dubowitz LMS, Dubowitz V, et al: Predictive value of cranial ultrasound in the newborn baby: A reappraisal. *Lancet* 1985; 2: 137–140.

14. Graziani LJ, Pasto M, Stanley C, et al: Neonatal neurosonographic correlates of cerebral palsy in preterm infants. *Pediatrics* 1986; 78:88–95.

15. Cooke RWI: Early and late neurosonographic appearances and outcome in very low birthweight infants. *Arch Dis Child* 1987; 62:931–937.

16. Dubowitz LMS, Levene MI, Morante A, et al: Neurologic signs in neonatal intraventricular hemorrhage: A correlation with real-time ultrasound. *J Pediatr* 1981; 99:127–133.

17. Lazzara A, Ahmann PA, Dykes FD, et al: Clinical predictability of intraventricular hemorrhage in preterm infants. *Pediatrics* 1980; 65:30–34.

# Chapter 17

# THE INFANT WITH MULTIPLE ANOMALIES

*JoAnn Bergoffen, M.D.*

*Elaine H. Zackai, M.D.*

## DIAGNOSTIC APPROACH

The term *dysmorphology* was coined by Dr. David Smith in the 1960s to describe the study of human congenital malformations. A more exact definition is "the study of abnormal form," emphasizing a focus on structural abnormalities of development. Birth defects, in isolation or in combination as syndromes, number in the thousands. In fact, about one-third of hospitalized children have genetic conditions (Table 17-1). Each condition has its own implications for management, prognosis, and recurrence risk. Therefore, it is important to create a systematic approach to the malformed infant.

The purpose of this chapter is to take you through such a process. We present the case history of an infant born with multiple anomalies, followed by questions referring to the case. A discussion of the material needed to answer the questions and the answers (in italics) complete each section. We conclude this chapter by arriving at a diagnosis for the patient presented and provide an approach for genetic counseling for the family.

## CASE STUDY 1

JK was a 2,400-g product of a 39-week pregnancy born to a 38-year-old, gravida 3, para 1021 woman (two spontaneous abortions) and a 44-year-old father, both of Italian descent.

The mother reports having an upper respiratory infection during the first month of gestation for which she took over-the-counter cold medications. At 8 months' gestation, decreased fetal movements were noted and on examination, fundal height was less than expected. Spontaneous labor and delivery occurred at 39 weeks. Apgar scores were 7 at 1 minute (−1 tone, −2 color) and 8 at 5 minutes (−1 tone, −1 color). On initial examination, JK was found to have hypotonia, hypospadias, a small extra digit after the fifth finger on both hands, and microcephaly.

## EXERCISE 1

Identify four important pieces of information in the pregnancy history that will help you establish a diagnosis for this child's malformations.

1.

2.

3.

4.

**Table 17-1** Frequency of Genetic Disorders Among Pediatric Hospital Admission in North America

| CAUSE | SEATTLE | MONTREAL |
|---|---|---|
| Chromosomal | 0.6% | 0.4% |
| Single gene | 3.9% | 6.9% |
| Polygenic | 48.9% | 29.0% |
| Nongenetic | 46.6% | 63.7% |
| Number of admissions | 4.115 | 12.801 |

*Source:* From Gelehrter TD, Collins FC: *Principles of Medical Genetics.* © 1990, the Williams & Wilkins Co., Baltimore, p. 3. Reprinted with permission of the Williams & Wilkins Co. and T.D. Gelehrter. Data from Hall JG, Powers EK, McIlvaine RT, et al: The frequency and financial burden of genetic disease in a pediatric hospital. *Am J Med Genet* 1978; 1:417–436; and Scriver CR, Neal JL, Saginur R, et al: The frequency of genetic disease and congenital malformation among patients in a pediatric hospital. *Can Med Assoc J* 1973; 108:1111–1115.

### ■ Discussion:

In a child with congenital malformations, vital information can be learned by taking a careful pregnancy history. Remember that parents will often focus on issues they feel are most important (e.g., "I fell when I was pregnant") and inadvertently leave out clues that may ultimately prove more informative. Therefore, it is critically important to develop an organized approach to obtaining a case history, so that key information will not be inadvertently overlooked. The following issues should be addressed when the history is taken.

**Maternal and Parental Age at Conception:** Mothers older than 35 years of age are at increased risk for having children with chromosomal abnormalities secondary to nondisjunction. Nondisjunction can be defined as aberrant segregation leading to loss or gain of one or more chromosomes by a daughter cell. Nondisjunctional events occur during meiosis or mitosis and are observed more frequently during meiosis in older women. The most common chromosomal abnormalities resulting from nondisjunction are Trisomy 13, Trisomy 18, Trisomy 21, and the XXX and XXY syndromes. Note that in 90% to 95% of patients with Trisomy 21 the meiotic error is maternal in origin. Very young mothers also have a small but significantly increased risk to deliver an infant with a birth defect or chromosomal abnormality. *In the case of JK, his mother is 38 years old. This should raise some*

concern that a nondisjunctional event has occurred with this pregnancy.

Paternal age is also an important consideration. Older fathers have been shown to be at increased risk for fathering children with fresh mutations for a variety of autosomal dominant conditions (e.g., achondroplasia). *In the case of JK, his father is 44 years old. This may be an important diagnostic clue.*

**Maternal Issues:** The maternal history can be extremely valuable in pinpointing a diagnosis and/or etiology. Questions that may help lead to the diagnosis include:

• Does the mother have any chronic health issues (e.g., diabetes)?
• Did she suffer from any illnesses during this pregnancy?
• Were there signs of infection during the pregnancy, or did she experience an unexplained fever? A number of pathogens that produce a relatively mild clinical disease in adults or children have been associated with birth abnormalities and congenital defects when the infections are acquired prenatally. Such well-known infectious agents include *toxoplasma, treponema pallidum, rubella virus, cytomegalovirus, herpes simplex virus,* and *human immunodeficiency virus* (TORCH infections).
• How did this pregnancy compare to prior pregnancies? Were the mother's nutrition and weight gain appropriate and comparable to previous pregnancies?
• Did vaginal bleeding occur?
• Was there any leakage of amniotic fluid prior to delivery? Oligohydramnios (<500 mL of amniotic fluid) is caused either by chronic leakage of amniotic fluid or by any malformation that leads to impaired urine output such as renal agenesis/dysgenesis or urinary tract obstruction. Pulmonary hypoplasia, intrauterine growth deficiency, and fetal compression resulting in limb positional defects and characteristic facies are often the sequelae of oligohydramnios. This oligohydramnios sequence is known as Potter syndrome (Fig. 17-1). Polyhydramnios (>2 L of amniotic fluid) may be caused by a variety of conditions. Fetal anomalies that result in an impaired ability to swallow amniotic fluid (e.g., anencephaly or central nervous system disorders) or

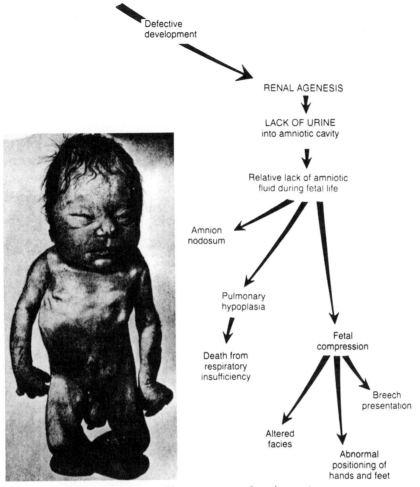

The consequences of renal agenesis.

**Figure 17-1**  The consequences of renal agenesis.
From Jones KL, ed: *Smith's Recognizable Patterns of Human Malformation*, 4th ed. Philadelphia, WB Saunders Co, 1988, p. 573. Reprinted with permission of W.B. Saunders Company.

move the amniotic fluid into the intestinal tract (e.g., structural gastrointestinal disorders such as esophageal atresia) comprise the largest categories. Excess amounts of amniotic fluid have also been observed in association with fetal circulatory disorders, multiple gestations, maternal diabetes, erythroblastosis fetalis, preeclampsia, and some dwarf syndromes.

**Teratogen Exposures:**  Many drugs are known to be teratogenic (Table 17-2) and are capable of producing physical defects in the developing embryo. Therefore you should ask if *any* drugs were taken during the pregnancy. It is important to specifically ask about vita-

mins, over-the-counter drugs, prescribed drugs, and illicit drugs. It is also important to determine when in the pregnancy the drugs were taken, the quantities of each drug taken or administered, and the duration of drug use. Fortunately, most teratogenic drugs exert a deleterious effect in only a minority of exposed fetuses. On the other hand, proving that a drug is teratogenic is difficult. For example, it has been estimated that a trial involving 35,000 subjects would be needed to prove that a drug increased the incidence of malformations by 1%. *In the case of JK, his mother took an over-the-counter cold medication, which is not believed to cause malformations.*

Be certain to question specifically about the use of alcohol. Find out when and how often

**Table 17-2**  Teratogens

| DRUG | MAJOR TERATOGENIC DEFECT |
|---|---|
| Thalidomide | Limb defects |
| Lithium | Ebstein's tricuspid valve anomaly |
| Aminopterin | Craniofacial and limb anomalies |
| Methotrexate | Craniofacial and limb anomalies |
| Phenytoin | Facial dysmorphism, dysplastic nails |
| Trimethadione | Craniofacial dysmorphism, growth retardation |
| Valproic acid | Neural tube defects |
| Androgens | Virilization |
| Tetracycline | Teeth and bone maldevelopment |
| Warfarin | Nasal hypoplasia, bone maldevelopment |
| Accutane (retinoic acid) | Craniofacial and cardiac defects |
| Propylthiouracil | Goiter |
| Radioactive iodine | Hypothyroidism |

during the pregnancy alcohol was used, and determine the amounts imbibed. Alcohol is known to be a teratogenic agent. The risk of malformations is 10% if the mother consumes 1 to 2 oz. of absolute alcohol per day, 19% if she consumes 2 oz., and 40% if she consumes more than 4 oz. per day. Unfortunately, the strongest relationship between maternal drinking and fetal outcome seems to exist in the month preceding the recognition of pregnancy. The effects of binge and social drinking are also still under current investigation. Fetal alcohol syndrome is made up of a triad of diagnostic findings: facial abnormalities (small head circumference, low nasal bridge, short palpebral fissures, midfacial hypoplasia, indistinct philtrum, and thin upper lip), growth deficiency (with little postnatal catchup), and mental retardation (in the mild to moderate range). While a dose-response relationship may exist between the amount of alcohol consumed by the mother and the severity of fetal anomalies, the pathophysiological mechanism responsible for the abnormal development remains unknown.

**Prenatal Care:** Numerous tools are now available to assess maternal and fetal well-being throughout pregnancy. Nevertheless, prenatal care is not always utilized by all pregnant women. You should determine what kind of care the mother received during her pregnancy and what evaluations were performed prior to the time of birth (glucose tolerance testing, ultrasound examinations, chorionic villus sampling, amniocentesis, biophysical profile, etc.).

**Fetal Factors:** Analyses of fetal activity are an important part of the evaluation of fetal well-being. One should routinely inquire when the mother first felt the baby move. Decreased fetal movement can be a sign of fetal distress or it may indicate that a neurological problem is present. *In the case of JK, his mother noted decreased fetal movement at 8 months' gestation, which suggests a neurological problem may have been present at that time.*

Intrauterine growth retardation (IUGR) may be caused by genetic or environmental factors. Be sure to ask if the fetus was appropriately growing throughout gestation, and if there were any differences between this infant's growth and patterns observed in previous pregnancies. Factors associated with poor fetal growth are quite heterogeneous and include chromosomal abnormalities, dysmorphic syndromes, intrauterine infections, metabolic disorders, multiple gestations, poor maternal nutrition, reduced uteroplacental blood flow (secondary to maternal vascular disease or hypertension), toxin exposure (such as maternal smoking, drinking, or drug use), and structural placental abnormalities. *In the case of JK, the fundal height was less than expected at 8 months gestation, which is indicative of a fetal, maternal, or placental problem.*

### EXERCISE 2

List two features of the family history that provide clues to the etiology of this child's malformations.

1.


2.

## ■ Discussion:

When the family history is obtained, you should ask about prior miscarriages or stillbirths. A maternal history of more than two first-trimester miscarriages increases the probability of finding a balanced translocation in one of the parents (balanced translocations are exchanges of chromosomal segments in which the diploid genetic content is maintained). Balanced translocations in either parent, in turn, increase the risk of producing an unbalanced translocation in the fetus, in which there is aneuploidy for one or more chromosomal segments. Twenty five percent of stillbirths exhibit single or multiple malformations, and at least half of these infants have a genetic etiology for their birth abnormalities. Sider et al. have recommended that couples with two or more pregnancy losses (spontaneous abortions or stillbirths) should have a routine cytogenetic analysis. *In the case of JK, the maternal history was significant for two previous spontaneous abortions.*

It is very important to determine if the parents are related. *In the case of JK, both parents are of Italian descent. On further questioning, it was revealed that the mother's grandfather and father's grandfather came from the same small town in Italy. The parents were unaware that they were second cousins prior to their marriage.*

The best way to record a family history is to construct a pedigree (Fig. 17-2). This is a schematic diagram that depicts relationships among family members. It is also a place for recording a brief summary of any conditions that may be of importance. The patient is often referred to as the index case, the proband, or the propositus. It is important to see if any family members have similar abnormalities to those in the proband. Most findings will be normal familial variants. You should also ask about abnormalities not displayed by the proband, because they may represent malformations or diseases of genetic origin that directly affect the proband's problem.

Positive findings in other family members can help determine the pattern of inheritance. In autosomal dominant conditions, the trait appears in every generation without skipping any (unless the proband represents a new mutation). Both males and females can manifest the trait and both can pass it to their offspring. On the other hand, autosomal recessive traits usually appear only in siblings and not in the parents. Both males and females are equally affected. In X-linked recessive traits, the incidence is much higher in males than females.

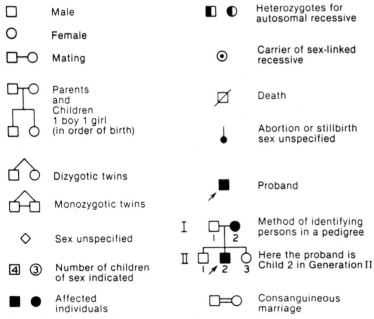

**Figure 17-2** Standard pedigree symbols.
From Thompson JS, Thompson MW: *Genetics in Medicine*, 4th ed. Philadelphia, WB Saunders Co, 1986, p. 46. Reprinted with permission of W.B. Saunders Company.

In this form of inheritance the trait is transmitted from affected fathers through carrier females (who may be variably affected) to affected sons. Therefore, these traits are never transmitted directly from father to son.

As in the case of JK, parents may be consanguineous. Consanguinity implies that two people can trace their genetic lineage back to a common ancestor, i.e., they are blood relatives. The concern is that both parents may carry a single copy of the same mutant autosomal recessive gene. If each of them contributes this mutant gene to their child, the double dose will cause a genetic disease. Clues that suggest possible consanguinity include finding the same surname on both sides of the family, tracing the origin of the families to the same limited geographic area, or establishing membership in a religious or ethnic group whose small size or established customs promote some degree of inbreeding.

=====

### CASE STUDY 1 continued

Physical examination was remarkable for a length of 46 cm, weight of 2,400 g, and head circumference of 31 cm. The anterior fontanelle was small (1 × 1 cm). Also present were micrognathia, clefting of the hard and soft palate, bilateral postaxial polydactyly, bilateral syndactyly of toes two and three, cryptorchidism, and a third-degree hypospadias. Generalized hypotonia was noted, and the cry was weak and high pitched. JK's ears appeared low set. The

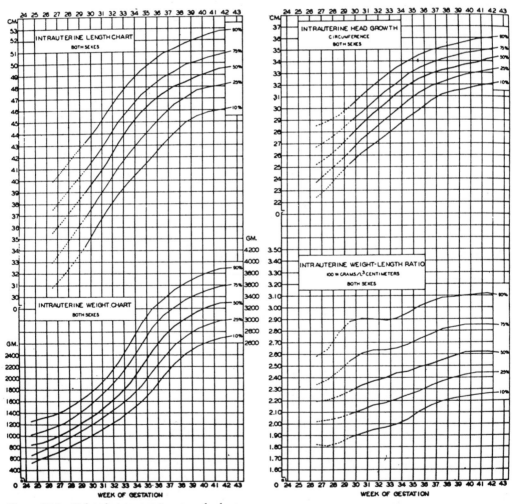

**Figure 17-3** Colorado intrauterine growth charts.
From Lubchenco LO, Hansman C, Boyd E: Intrauterine growth in length and head circumference as estimated from live births at gestational ages from 26 to 42 weeks. *Pediatrics* 1966; 37(3):403. Reproduced by permission of *Pediatrics*, vol. 37, page 403, copyright 1966.

following facial measurements were obtained: outer canthal distance (OC) = 6 cm, inner canthal distance (IC) = 2.25 cm, and interpupillary distance (IP) = 4 cm.

## EXERCISE 3

Given a gestational age of 39 weeks, was this infant's size appropriate for gestational age?

### ■ Discussion:

Growth charts are available for plotting an infant's growth parameters at a given gestational age. This patient's growth parameters can be compared to values obtained from a large group of normal infants. Plot the growth parameters of JK on the charts in Figure 17-3 using a gestational age of 39 weeks.

The length of 46 cm plots at the 20th percentile, the weight of 2,400 g (50th percentile for 35 weeks) falls below the 10th percentile, and the head circumference of 31 cm (50th percentile for 33 weeks) also falls below the 10th percentile. *Therefore, JK is both small for gestational age (SGA) and microcephalic. The head circumference, however, is the smallest measurement.*

## EXERCISE 4

What additional physical parameters would help you to discern whether this child is dysmorphic?

### ■ Discussion:

In 1974, Feingold and Bossert published a landmark study in which they looked at a total of 2,043 children to define normal values for a number of physical features. They hoped physicians would use these standards as screening tools to identify infants or children with possible genetic disorders. These features included head circumference (Fig. 17-3), ear length (Fig. 17-4), ear placement (Fig. 17-5), inner and outer canthal distances (Fig. 17-6), interpupillary distance (Fig. 17-6), nasolabial distance, chest circumference (Fig. 17-7), internipple

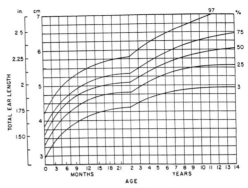

**Figure 17-4**  Maximum ear length.
From Feingold M, & Bossert WH: "Normal values for selected physical parameters: An aid to syndrome delineation." New York: The National Foundation—March of Dimes, BD:OAS X(13):1–16, 1974, with permission of the copyright holder.

distance (Fig. 17-7), and hand, palm, and finger lengths (Fig. 17-8).

*In the case of JK, the tops of his ears fell below an imaginary line extending from the inner canthus of the eye. Therefore, his ears would be considered low set. His interpupillary distance of 4 cm is at the 50th percentile. Therefore, his eye placement is within normal limits.*

Dermal ridge patterns are formed on the palms and soles in early embryonic life. The distal phalanges have a variety of dermal ridge patterns that can be classified into three major pattern groups: arches (A), whorls (W), and loops (L) (Fig. 17-9). In the arch pattern, ridges enter from one side and flow to the other. It is unusual to find eight or more arches in a normal individual (0.9% of healthy controls); however, it is a frequent feature in the Trisomy 18 and XXXXY syndromes. Similarly, loops that open to the radial side of the hand are unusual on the fourth and fifth fingers. Radial loop patterns on these fingers are more common in Down's syndrome children. The frequencies of the different patterns varies from finger to finger. Table 17-3 lists the percentage frequencies of digital pattern types on prints from 500 normal individuals (mainly Caucasian).

Triradii or deltas form at the juncture of three sets of converging ridges, usually where the hypothenar, thenar, and distal palmar patterns converge. Loop patterns have at least one triradius and whorl patterns have at least two.

**Table 17-3**   Percentage Frequencies of Digital Pattern Types on Different Digits

|  | LEFT | | | | | RIGHT | | | | |
|---|---|---|---|---|---|---|---|---|---|---|
|  | 5 | 4 | 3 | 2 | 1 | 1 | 2 | 3 | 4 | 5 |
| Whorl | 12 | 37 | 17 | 33 | 31 | 39 | 36 | 18 | 47 | 15 |
| Ulnar loop | 85 | 60 | 71 | 36 | 63 | 57 | 31 | 71 | 52 | 84 |
| Radial loop | <1 | <1 | 3 | 19 | <1 | <1 | 20 | 3 | <1 | <1 |
| Arch | 3 | 3 | 9 | 11 | 6 | 3 | 13 | 6 | 1 | 1 |

*Source:* From Thompson JS, Thompson MW: *Genetics in Medicine,* 4th ed. Philadelphia, WB Saunders Co, 1986, p. 284. Reprinted with permission of W.B. Saunders Company.

There are usually no triradii between the base of the palm and the interdigital areas of the upper palm. When patterning is present in the hypothenar area, a distal axial triradius often arises (Fig. 17-10). This pattern is found in only 4% of Caucasians, but in 85% of the patients with trisomy 21. A single transverse palma crease (simian crease) (Fig. 17-10) is present in approximately 4% of control subjects and 50% to 55% of newborn infants with Trisomy 21. This crease is also observed in other varieties of trisomies.

The sole of the foot also has a dermal ridge pattern. Usually a loop or whorl pattern is present. A relative lack of complexity in patterning is called an open field or simple arch pattern of the hallucal region (Fig. 17-11). Less than 1% of control subjects have this pattern, while 50% of patients with Trisomy 21 display this pattern.

*In the case of JK, there were bilateral simian creases. His dermal ridge patterns revealed that 9 out of 10 fingers had whorls and 1 of 10 fingers had a loop. (Note that only 3% of normal individuals have 9 or more whorls.)*

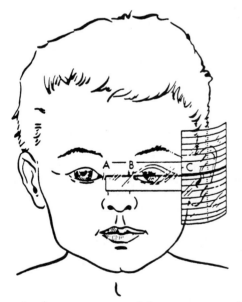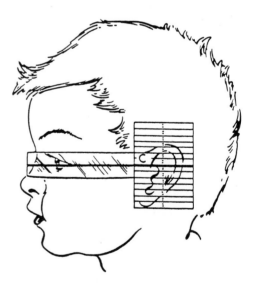

**Figure 17-5**   Depiction of the instrument used for the study of ear positioning. The medial canthi are used as landmarks instead of the outer canthi, since a slant to the palpebral fissures could provide incorrect landmarks.
From Feingold M, & Bossert WH: "Normal values for selected physical parameters: An aid to syndrome delineation." New York: The National Foundation—March of Dimes, BD:OAS X(13):1–16, 1974, with permission of the copyright holder.

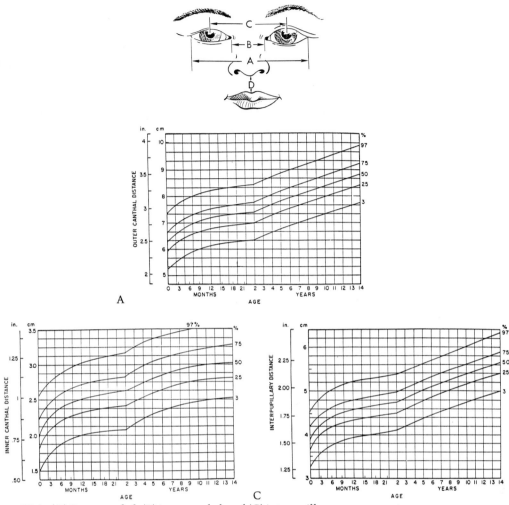

**Figure 17-6** (A) Outer canthal, (B) inner canthal, and (C) interpupillary measurements.
From Feingold M, & Bossert WH: "Normal values for selected physical parameters: An aid to syndrome delineation." New York: The National Foundation—March of Dimes, BD:OAS X(13):1–16, 1974, with permission of the copyright holder.

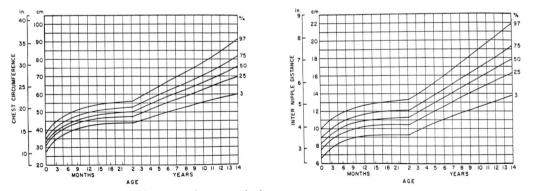

**Figure 17-7** Chest circumference and internipple distance.
From Feingold M, & Bossert WH: "Normal values for selected physical parameters: An aid to syndrome delineation." New York: The National Foundation—March of Dimes, BD:OAS X(13):1–16, 1974, with permission of the copyright holder.

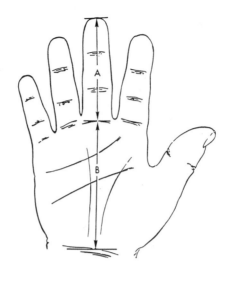

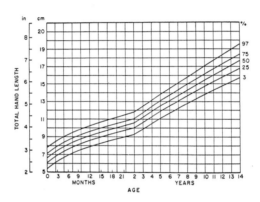

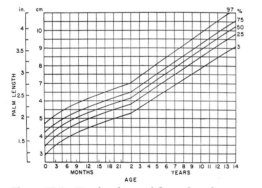

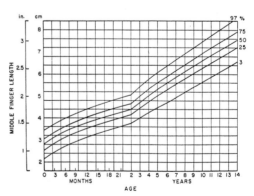

**Figure 17-8** Hand, palm, and finger lengths.
From Feingold M, & Bossert WH: "Normal values for selected physical parameters: An aid to syndrome delineation." New York: The National Foundation—March of Dimes, BD:OAS X(13):1–16, 1974, with permission of the copyright holder.

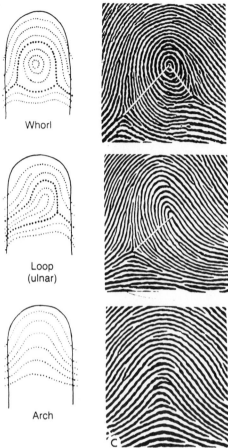

**Figure 17-9**   The three dermal ridge patterns: whorl, loop, and arch.
From Holt SB: Quantitative genetics of finger-print patterns. *Br Med Bull* 1961; 17(3):247. Reproduced with the permission of the British Council from *British Medical Bulletin* (1961) 17:247–250.

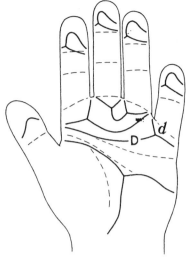

**Figure 17-10**   Distal palmar axial triradius. S = simian crease, T = triradius.
From SB Holt, *The Genetics of Dermal Ridges, 1968.* Courtesy of Charles C Thomas, Publisher, Springfield, Illinois.

*examination was normal. A renal ultrasound examination was performed because of a known association between ear anomalies and renal anomalies. This test demonstrated a single kidney.*

*Chromosomal studies were indicated in this case because of JK's dysmorphic features and multiple anomalies. Such studies can usually be run on peripheral blood samples.*

## EXERCISE 5

What additional consultants or studies would be helpful in this case?

■ **Discussion:**
When a baby has multiple obvious anomalies, it is necessary to look for other less obvious, often internal, anomalies. *In the case of JK, the ophthalmological examination revealed bilateral cataracts, which were not evident on the initial physical examination. A head ultrasound examination was performed because of the small head and hypotonia. This*

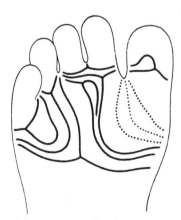

**Figure 17-11**   Hallucal area: Simple arch pattern (open fields).
From SB Holt, *The Genetics of Dermal Ridges, 1968.* Courtesy of Charles C Thomas, Publisher, Springfield, Illinois.

However, if this infant had a life-threatening malformation, a bone marrow aspiration could provide a much quicker result if an abnormality of chromosome number was present. Bone marrow samples are not generally suitable for more sophisticated chromosomal analyses. *The maternal history of two prior miscarriages suggests that one of the parents may be carrying a balanced translocation.* Given the mother's advanced maternal age and history of prior miscarriages, you should compare JK's physical findings with those noted in the three common trisomy syndromes (Trisomy 13, 18, and 21) (Table 17-4).

In summary, JK is a microcephalic, SGA newborn male with bilateral cataracts, low-set ears, cleft palate, micrognathia, postaxial polydactyly, syndactyly of toes two and three, excess whorls, simian creases, a single kidney, cryptorchidism, hypospadias, and hypotonia.

*The clinicians caring for JK felt that his findings were not consistent with any of the common trisomy syndromes. Routine chromosome analysis was performed. The analysis came back normal, 46 XY.*

The absence of a chromosomal abnormality does not mean that a genetic disorder is not present. It simply means that a structural defect was not evident, given the present level of sophistication of genetic analysis. At this stage in the evaluation, you need to consult one or more of the standard reference texts that cross index malformations and list associated syndromes:

1. Bergsma D: *Birth Defects Compendium*, 2nd ed. New York, Alan R Liss, 1979.

2. Gorlin RJ, Cohen, MM, Jr, Levin, SL: *Syndromes of the Head and Neck*, 3rd ed. New York, Oxford University Press, 1990.

**Table 17-4**  Features of Common Autosomal Trisomies

| FEATURE | TRISOMY 21 | TRISOMY 18 | TRISOMY 13 |
|---|---|---|---|
| Eponym | Down's syndrome | Edward's syndrome | Patau's syndrome |
| Liveborn incidence | 1/800 | 1/800 | 1/19,000 |
| Mean birth weight | 3,000 g | 2,340 g | 2,480 g |
| Tone | Hypotonia | Hypertonia | Hypo- or hypertonia |
| Cranium/brain | Mild microcephaly flat occiput, 3 fontanelles | Microcephaly, prominent occiput | Microcephaly, sloping forehead, occipital scalp defects, holoprosencephaly |
| Eyes | Upslanting, epicanthal folds, speckled iris (Brushfield, spots) | Small palpebral fissures, corneal opacity | Micro-ophthalmia, hypotelorism, iris coloboma, retinal dysplasia |
| Ears | Small, low-set, over-folded upper helix | Low-set, malformed | Low-set, malformed |
| Facial features | Protruding tongue, large cheeks, low flat nasal bridge | Small mouth, micrognathia | Cleft lip and palate |
| Skeletal | Clinodactyly 5th digit, gap between toes 1 and 2, excess nuchal skin, short stature | Clenched hand, absent 5th finger distal crease, hypoplastic nails, short stature, thin ribs | Postaxial polydactyly hyperconvex fingernails, clenched hand |
| Cardiac defect | 40% | 60% | 80% |
| Survival | Long term, excluding those with cardiac defects, of whom many die in infancy | 90% die within the first year | 82% die within the first year |
| Other features | Leukemia, Alzheimer's | Rocker bottom feet, polycystic kidneys, dermatoglyphic arch pattern | Genital anomalies, polycystic kidneys, increased nuclear projections in neutrophils |

*Source:* From Donnenfeld AE, Zackai EH: Genetics. In Polin RA, Ditmar MF, eds: *Pediatric Secrets.* Philadelphia, Hanley and Belfus, 1989, p. 121. Reprinted with permission of Hanley and Belfus.

3. Jones KL, ed: *Smith's Recognizable Patterns of Human Malformation*, 4th ed. Philadelphia, WB Saunders Co, 1988.

4. McKusick VA: *Medelian Inheritance in Man Catalogs of Autosomal Dominant, Autosomal Recessive, and X-Linked Phenotypes*. Baltimore, The Johns Hopkins University Press, 1992.

5. Warkany JF: *Congenital Malformations: Notes and Comments*. Chicago, Year Book Medical Publisher, 1971.

## EXERCISE 6

List the malformations identified in JK in the order that you think will be most helpful for cross referencing.

### ■ Discussion:

Aase has written, "The best clues are the rarest. The physical features that will be most helpful on differential diagnosis are those which are infrequently seen either in isolation or as a part of syndromes. Quite often, these are not the most obvious anomalies nor even the ones that have the greatest significance for the patient's health."

Cross referencing, by using the previously listed sources, will help determine what diagnosis these clinical features have in common. When trying to narrow down diagnostic possibilities, it is helpful to cross reference those findings that are less frequently encountered.

A list of the malformations observed in JK from the rarest to most common was constructed from appendix listings in reference text 3 listed in the previous discussion section.

| | |
|---|---|
| *Syndactyly of toes two and three (Caution must be exercised in determining the specificity of this particular finding, since toe syndactyly can be seen as a separate autosomal dominant trait.)* | *2 entries* |
| *Whorls on fingertips* | *4 entries* |

| | |
|---|---|
| *Polydactyly* | *31 entries* |
| *Single palmer creases* | *32 entries* |
| *Cataracts* | *43 entries* |
| *Hypospadias* | *44 entries* |
| *Hypotonia* | *47 entries* |
| *Microcephaly* | *60 entries* |
| *Cleft palate (without cleft lip)* | *69 entries* |
| *Cryptorchidism* | *74 entries* |

## EXERCISE 7

Upon identifying the rarest malformations, use the following lists from reference text 3, and determine the diagnosis in this patient. What additional clues from the history are helpful in supporting your diagnosis?

### *Syndactyly (frequently in)*
Apert syndrome
Carpenter syndrome
de Lange syndrome (syndactyly of second and third toes)
Early amnion rupture sequence
EEC syndrome
Escobar syndrome
FG syndrome
Fraser syndrome
Goltz syndrome
Greig cephalopolysyndactyly syndrome
Holt-Oram syndrome
Jarcho-Levin syndrome
Lenz-Majewski hyperostosis syndrome
Miller syndrome
Neu-Laxova syndrome
Oculodentodigital syndrome (syndactyly of fourth and fifth fingers, and fourth and fifth toes)
Oral-facial-digital syndrome
Oto-palatal-digital syndrome
Pallister-Hall syndrome
Partial Trisomy 10q syndrome
Pfeiffer syndrome
Poland anomaly
Popliteal Pterygium syndrome
Roberts-SC phocomelia
Saethre-Chotzen syndrome
Scerosteosis
Short-rib-polydactyly, Majewski type
Short-rib-polydactyly, non-Majewski type
Smith-Lemli-Opitz syndrome (second and third toe)
Triploidy syndrome (third and fourth fingers)

### *Whorl Dermal Ridge (majority of fingertips)*

Smith-Lemli-Opitz syndrome

9p-syndrome

18q-syndrome

X0 syndrome

### ■ Discussion:

*In the case of JK, his decreased fetal movements, IUGR, microcephaly, cataracts, low-set ears, micrognathia, cleft palate, simian crease, increased incidence of whorls, postaxial polydactyly, syndactyly of toes two and three, hypospadias, cryptorchidism, and kidney anomaly are all consistent with the diagnosis of Smith-Lemli-Opitz syndrome.*

Smith-Lemli-Opitz syndrome is an autosomal recessive disorder characterized by smallness at birth (with subsequent failure to thrive), microcephaly (with a narrow frontal area), ptosis of the eyelids, broad nasal tip with anteverted nostrils, low-set ears, micrognathia, simian crease, high frequency of whorls, syndactyly of second and third toes, and, in males, hypospadias and cryptorchidism. Feeding difficulties and vomiting are frequent problems in early infancy. During the first year of life, 20% of the patients die, usually as a result of pneumonias. Muscle tone, which may be decreased in early infancy, tends to become increased with time. The degree of mental disability is generally moderate to severe. The history of consanguinity in this case is compatible with the autosomal recessive pattern of inheritance found in this syndrome. Therefore, the recurrence risk for future pregnancies is 25%.

---

### Summary of Diagnostic Approach

Pattern recognition of genetic entities involves the comparison of the proband with personal experience, known cases, and literature searching. What if a particular syndrome/diagnosis does not jump out at you? If a patient does have one or more congenital anomalies, you must decide on the underlying nature of the abnormalities. The concepts of malformation, disruption, deformation, and dysplasia are often used (Table 17-5). Multiple anomalies in a given patient may be causally or pathogenically related, may occur together in a statistically associated basis, or may present in the patient simply by chance. This

**Table 17-5**   Alterations of Form or Structure

*Malformation:* A morphological defect of an organ, part of an organ, or a larger region of the body resulting from an intrinsically abnormal developmental process.

*Disruption:* A morphological defect of an organ, part of an organ, or a larger region of the body resulting from the extrinsic breakdown of, or an interference with, an originally normal developmental process.

*Deformation:* An abnormal form, shape, or position of a part of the body caused by mechanical forces.

*Dysplasia:* An abnormal organization of cells into tissue(s) and its morphological result(s).

*Source:* Data from Spranger J, Benirschke K, Hall JG, et al: Errors of morphogenesis: Concepts and terms. *J Pediatr* 1982; 100(1):160–165.

---

relationship can be described by the terms field defect, sequence, syndrome, or association (Table 17-6).

When discussing how to perform a diagnostic evaluation on a malformed infant, we always want to emphasize the importance of arriving at the correct diagnosis. Unfortunately, even under the best of circumstances, this may not be possible. As Aase has written, "Don't panic! The absence of a diagnosis may be distressing to the diagnostician and the family, but it is much less dangerous than the possibility of assigning the wrong diagnosis, with the risk of erroneous genetic and prognostic counseling and possibly hazardous treatment." Except in real emergencies, in which life-threatening anomalies demand immediate therapeutic intervention, there is al-

**Table 17-6**   Patterns of Morphological Defects

*Field defect:* A pattern of anomalies derived from the disturbance of a developmental field.

*Sequence:* A pattern of multiple anomalies derived from a single known or presumed prior anomaly or mechanical factor.

*Syndrome:* A pattern of multiple anomalies thought to be pathogenetically related and not known to represent a single sequence or a field defect.

*Association:* A nonrandom occurrence in two or more individuals of multiple anomalies not known to be a field defect, sequence, or syndrome.

*Source:* Data from Spranger J, Benirschke K, Hall JG, et al: Errors of morphogenesis: Concepts and terms. *J Pediatr* 1982; 100(1):160–165.

ways time to see the patient again, to pursue the pertinent literature, and to follow the clinical course. On the other hand, it is equally important not to defer judgment to the point that important aspects of counseling are neglected. It is equally important not to create a false sense of security in the parents when no definitive diagnosis can be reached. When told that their child "does not have a recognizable diagnosis," the family may conclude that there is nothing really wrong and thus neglect a child's very real needs. The golden rule is: Be sure the family understands everything you know (and don't know) about their child's condition.

## GENETIC COUNSELING

We have discussed a systematic approach to the malformed infant using a specific case in point. In the following section the topic of genetic counseling will be presented in broader terms.

## EXERCISE 8

Identify which of the following individuals and/or families are at increased risk for a genetic condition and therefore deserve genetic counseling.

1. An Afro-American couple who are both healthy

2. A man who has a retarded sibling

3. A couple who are both healthy but who have had three previous pregnancy losses in the first trimester

4. A man who has a sister with Down's syndrome

5. A Jewish couple who are both healthy

6. A woman who has a retarded uncle and a retarded brother

7. A couple who have nuclear family members originating from the Mediterranean area

8. A woman who is 39 years old and is interested in becoming pregnant

9. A couple who have a child with myelomeningocele who are interested in having another child

## ■ Discussion:

*From the preceding sections, it is evident that each of the individuals presented above deserves genetic counseling.* Unfortunately, most of these individuals (and their families) would not be aware of their increased risk for genetic disease, and therefore not seek counseling. They are not alone in that regard, however, for the majority of health care workers would also be unaware of the need for counseling in most such instances. Furthermore, we all tend to forget that in every pregnancy there is an appreciable (baseline) risk for an unfavorable outcome (Table 17-7). Thus, recurrence risks for specific genetic defects that have already appeared in a family represent additive risks to these baseline figures.

Every physician should incorporate the family history into the initial visit of every reproductively active patient. Issues such as ethnicity and consanguinity are important for family planning. In addition, a carefully obtained pedigree can sometimes discover a family member with a birth defect(s) that may warrant further investigation and subsequent genetic counseling.

A major challenge for the treating physician is the identification of heterozygote carriers of autosomal recessive conditions. In autosomal recessive conditions (where neither parent is affected) heterozygote screening is

**Table 17-7** Baseline Risks of Abnormalities in the General Population

| | |
|---|---|
| Risk of a child being born with some birth defect | 1 in 30 |
| Risk of a child being born with some serious physical or mental handicap | 1 in 50 |
| Risk of a child of first-cousin parents being born with some serious physical or mental handicap | 1 in 20 |
| Risk of any pregnancy ending in a spontaneous abortion | 1 in 8 |
| Risk of stillbirth (North America) | 1 in 125 |
| Risk of perinatal death (North America) | 1 in 150 |
| Risk of death in first year of life after first week (North America) | 1 in 200 |
| Risk that couple will be infertile | 1 in 10 |

*Source:* From Thompson JS, Thompson MW: *Genetics in Medicine*, 4th ed. Philadelphia, WB Saunders Co, 1986, p. 284. Reprinted with permission of W.B. Saunders Company.

feasible when the following three criteria are met:

1. The disorder occurs chiefly in a specific population group.

2. A test suitable for mass screening is available.

3. The possibility of prenatal diagnosis exists.

Three disorders that fulfill these criteria (and which are important to cases 1, 5, and 7 in Exercise 8 described above) are sickle-cell disease, Tay-Sachs disease, and β-thalassemia. Sickle-cell disease occurs almost exclusively in the black population with a carrier frequency as high as 45% in parts of Africa and about 8% in the United States. This would mean that an American black couple would have a 1/256 chance ($1/8 \times 1/8 \times 1/4$) of having a child with sickle-cell disease. Tay-Sachs disease has a high incidence in the Ashkenazi (Eastern European) Jewish population. The carrier frequency in this population is 33%. Similarly, β-thalassemia occurs with an increased frequency in people of Italian and Greek ethnic background.

Cytogenetic studies can detect a variety of chromosomal anomalies including aneuploidies (deviations from an exact multiple of the haploid number of chromosomes), translocations, fragile X chromosomes, and mosaicisms (the presence in an individual of two or more cell lines that are karyotypically distinct). Indications for such studies include familial translocations, a history of spontaneous first-trimester pregnancy losses, the prior birth of a trisomic infant, and advanced maternal age, which are exemplified by cases 2, 3, 4, 6, and 8 from Exercise 8. If a family member has mental retardation or Down's syndrome, chromosomal analysis can determine if the basis for that disorder is a structural chromosomal anomaly, such as an unbalanced translocation. Additional chromosomal analysis can then be performed on other family members to see if they are carrying a balanced form of the chromosomal rearrangement. Such an individual will be unaffected, but will carry a risk of passing on an unbalanced form to any of their offspring (see Exercise 2). The fragile X syndrome is a common form of X-linked mental retardation. The cytogenetic appearance of the "fragile X" chromosome (a constriction near the distal end of the long arm of the X chromosome), can be demonstrated only in cells cultured in a special medium that has relatively low concentrations of folic acid and thymidine. Fortunately, the molecular defect in fragile X syndrome has recently been identified. Thus, molecular testing is now available for carrier screening and diagnosis. Sex determination for other X-linked disorders is possible when other more specific tools are unavailable.

As previously mentioned, mothers over the age of 35 have an increased risk for having children with chromosomal abnormalities secondary to nondisjunction (e.g., Down's syndrome). Until recently however, the only ways to suspect that a mother was carrying a Down's syndrome fetus were based on advanced maternal age or a history of delivering a previously affected infant. However, in 1984, Merkatz et al. and Cuckle, Wald, and Lindenbaum reported that maternal serum alpha fetoprotein concentrations were diminished in Down's syndrome pregnancies. These results stimulated research to determine whether other biochemical markers of fetoplacental origin could be used to identify affected pregnancies. Measurements of maternal serum unconjugated estriol and placental human chorionic gonadotropin concentrations also proved to be lower than normal in Down's syndrome pregnancies. Therefore, in 1988 Wald et al. proposed that a new screening method be initiated that would factor in these four variables–maternal age, maternal serum alpha fetoprotein concentration, maternal free estriol concentration, and placental human chorionic gonadotropin concentration. Not surprisingly, this screening panel proved capable of detecting more than 60% of pregnancies with Down's syndrome fetuses. This testing is commonly referred to as AFP Plus or the Triple Screen. The ability of this new screening procedure to provide prenatal screening for chromosomal defects other than Down's syndrome has not been demonstrated. However, maternal serum alpha fetoprotein alone is routinely offered to screen for neural tube defects, such as anencephaly or meningomyelocele (important information for case 9 of Exercise 8), where high serum concentrations are measured. Furthermore, it has recently been reported that folic acid supplementation started before and continued during pregnancy can prevent neural tube abnormalities.

Reproductive options available to couples at risk can be discussed as part of the genetic counseling session. These alternatives include willingness to take the risk, limiting family size, prenatal diagnosis, artificial insemination, *in vitro* fertilization with donor egg, and adoption. A genetic counseling session should ultimately help the family make the best possible adjustment to the disorder in the affected family member and to understand the risk of recurrence of that disorder in future pregnancies. It is critically important to make sure that follow-up sessions are incorporated into long-range planning, because families frequently need to have the same information reinforced on multiple occasions for an extended period of time.

## EXERCISE 9

Name five tests available for prenatal diagnosis.

1.

2.

3.

4.

5.

## ■ Discussion

*The list of tests available for prenatal diagnosis includes ultrasonagraphy, fetal echocardiography, maternal serum testing, amniocentesis, biochemical testing, and molecular testing.* Diagnostic ultrasonography evaluation in skilled hands can identify major structural defects, such as anomalies of the gastrointestinal and urinary tracts, and some of the severe skeletal dysplasias and dwarfing syndromes. Diagnosis of multiple pregnancy and assessment of fetal growth can also be accom-

plished. Fetal echocardiography in the second trimester is a practical way to identify major structural defects of the heart.

Amniocentesis is usually carried out at a gestational age of 16 to 17 weeks. It is regarded as safe and accurate when performed by an individual experienced in the technique and carries an overall risk of 1/200 (0.5%) for fetal demise. Specimens can be used for DNA analysis, chromosomal analysis, biochemical analysis, and measurement of alpha fetoprotein or intestinal enzymes. Chorionic villus sampling had been thought of as an alternative to amniocentesis. However, recent studies reported by Firth et al. suggest an association between this technique and limb-reduction defects. As a result, they and others have raised concerns about the safety of chorionic villus sampling early in pregnancy.

Many biochemical genetic disorders can be detected by assays of specific enzyme activities in cultured fetal cells from amniotic fluid. Most of these biochemical disorders are extremely rare, and the knowledge that a given pregnancy is at risk for a specific biochemical defect requires knowledge of both the ethnic background of the parents (which may predispose them to certain disorders, such as Tay-Sachs disease) or of the family history of a previous affected child.

Physicians should be aware of the availability of DNA testing for carrier detection and prenatal diagnosis. DNA can be obtained from amniocytes and used for direct detection of mutations and linkage analysis. The ability to identify genetic diseases by direct or indirect detection provides valuable information to determine whether the fetus in a given pregnancy is affected and can also identify individuals who are asymptomatic carriers of recessive conditions. When the gene responsible for a condition has been characterized and the mutations identified, direct mutation analysis can be performed. When the gene is unknown, closely linked DNA markers or indirect analysis must be used. Table 17-8 is a list of some of the disorders now being detected by DNA analysis. A full text computer data base of Victor McKusick's reference book *OMIM (Online Medelian Inheritance in Man)* is now available with daily updates. This list continues to grow with each new discovery in molecular genetics.

**Table 17-8**  Genetic Diseases Detected by DNA Analysis

| | |
|---|---|
| Adenomatous polyposis | Ichthyosis due to steroid sulfatase deficiency |
| Adenosine deaminase deficiency | Lesch-Nyhan syndrome |
| Adrenal hyperplasia | Leukocyte adhesion deficiency |
| Alpha-1-antitrypsin deficiency | Lipoprotein lipase deficiency |
| Alport syndrome | Lowe oculocerebrorenal syndrome |
| Antithrombin III deficit | Maple syrup urine disease |
| Carbamoyl phosphate synthetase I deficiency | Marfan syndrome |
| Choroideremia | Menke syndrome |
| Chronic granulomatous disease | Muscular dystrophy (Becker-type and Duchenne-type) |
| Color blindness | |
| Cystic fibrosis | Myotonic dystrophy |
| Ehlers-Danlos syndrome | Neurofibromatosis |
| Elliptocytosis, hereditary | Norrie disease |
| Friedreich ataxia | Ocular albinism |
| Fucosidosis | Ornithine transcarbamylase deficiency |
| G6PD deficiency | Osteogenesis imperfecta |
| Gangliosidosis-GM2 | Pelizaeus-Merzbacher disease |
| Gaucher disease | Phenylketonuria |
| Gyrate atrophy | Polycystic kidney disease |
| Hypoxanthine guanine phosphoribosyl transferase deficiency | Porphyria |
| | Prealbumin amyloidosis |
| Haemochromatosis | Sandhoff disease (type II) |
| Hemophilia A | Sickle-cell anemia |
| Hemophilia B | Skeletal dysplasia X-linked |
| Hereditary persistence of fetal hemoglobin | Stickler syndrome |
| Hunter syndrome | Tay-Sachs disease |
| Huntington disease | Testicular feminization syndrome |
| Hypercholesterolemia, familial | Thalassemias |
| Hypophosphatemia | von Hippel-Lindau syndrome |
| Hypophosphatemia, lethal | von Willebrand disease |
| Hypothyroidism | |

*Source:* From Cutting GR, Antonnarakis SE: Prenatal diagnosis and carrier detection by DNA analysis. *Pediatr Rev* 1992; 13(4):139. Reproduced by permission of *Pediatrics*, vol. 13, page 139, copyright 1992.

## ACKNOWLEDGMENT

We would like to acknowledge Dr. Patrice Trauffer for her review of the case.

## BIBLIOGRAPHY

1. Aase JM: *Diagnostic Dysmorphology.* New York, Plenum Medical Book Co, 1990.
2. Briggs GG, Freeman RK, Yaffe SJ: *Drugs in Pregnancy and Lactation,* 2nd ed. Baltimore, Williams and Wilkins, 1986.
3. Castle D, Bernstein R: Cytogenetic analysis of 688 couples experiencing multiple spontaneous abortions. *Am J Med Genet* 1988; 29:549–556.
4. Cuckle HS, Wald NJ, Lindenbaum RH: Maternal serum alpha-fetoprotein measurement: A screening test for Down syndrome. *Lancet* 1984; 1:926–929.
5. Cutting GR, Antonnarakis SE: Prenatal diagnosis and carrier detection by DNA analysis. *Pediatr Rev* 1992; 13(4):138–143.
6. Donnenfeld AE, Zackai EH: Genetics. In Polin RA, Ditmar MF, eds: *Pediatric Secrets.* Philadelphia, Hanley and Belfus, 1989.
7. Feingold M, Bossert WH: Normal values for selected physical parameters: An aid to syndrome

delineation. In Bergsma D, ed: *The National Foundation–March of Dimes Birth Defects Series: Original Article Series* 1974; 10(suppl 13):1–16.

8. Firth HV, Boyd PA, Chamberlain P, et al: Limb abnormalities and chorion villus sampling. *Lancet* 1991; 338(8758):51.

9. Friedman JM: Genetic disease in the offspring of older fathers. *Obstet Gynecol* 1981; 57(6):745–749.

10. Hall JG, Powers EK, McIlvaine RT, et al: The frequency and financial burden of genetic disease in a pediatric hospital. *Am J Med Genet* 1978; 1:417–436.

11. Hilson D: Malformation of ears as sign of malformation of genitourinary tract. *Br Med J* 1957; 2(pt 2):785–789.

12. Holt SB: Quantitative genetics of fingerprint patterns. *Br Med Bull* 1961; 17:247–250.

13. Holt SB: *The Genetics of Dermal Ridges.* Springfield, IL, Charles C Thomas, 1968.

14. Jones KL, ed: *Smith's Recognizable Patterns of Human Malformation,* 4th ed. Philadelphia, WB Saunders Co, 1988.

15. Karp LE: Older fathers and genetic mutations. *Am J Med Genet* 1980; 7:405–406.

16. Langlois S: Genetic diagnosis based on molecular diagnosis. *Pediatr Clin North Am* 1992; 39(1):91–105.

17. Lubchenco LO, Hansman C, Boyd E: Intrauterine growth in length and head circumference as estimated from live births at gestational ages from 26 to 42 weeks. *Pediatrics* 1966; 37(3):403–408.

18. McLeod PM, Dill F, Hardwick DF: Chromosomes, syndromes, and perinatal deaths: The genetic counseling value of making a diagnosis in a malformed abortus, stillborn and deceased newborn. *Birth Defect* 1979; 15(5A):105–111.

19. Merkatz IR, Nitowsky HM, Macri JN, et al: An association between low maternal serum alphafetoprotein and fetal chromosomal abnormalities. *Am J Obstet Gynecol* 1984; 48:886–894.

20. MRC Vitamin Study Research Group: Prevention of neural tube defects: Results of the Medical Research Council Vitamin Study. *Lancet* 1991; 338(8760):131–137.

21. Scriver CR, Neal JL, Saginur R, et al: The frequency of genetic disease and congenital malformation among patients in a pediatric hospital. *Can Med Assoc J* 1973; 108:111–115.

22. Shepard TH: *Catalog of Teratogenic Agents,* 5th ed. Baltimore, The Johns Hopkins University Press, 1986.

23. Sider D, Wilson WG, Sudduth K, et al: Cytogenetic studies in couples with recurrent pregnancy loss. *South Med J* 1988; 81(12):1521–1524.

24. Smith DW: *Recognizable Patterns of Human Malformation, Genetic Embryologic and Clinical Aspect.* Vol VII in series *Major Problems in Clinical Pediatrics.* Philadelphia, WB Saunders Co, 1970.

25. Smith DW: The fetal alcohol syndrome. *Hosp Prac* 1979; 14(10):121–128.

26. Spranger J, Benirschke K, Hall JG, et al: Errors of morphogenesis: Concepts and terms. *J Pediatr* 1982; 100(1):160–165.

27. Thompson JS, Thompson MW: *Genetics in Medicine,* 4th ed. Philadelphia, WB Saunders Co, 1986.

28. Wald NJ, Cuckle HS, Densem JW, et al: Maternal serum screening for Down's syndrome in early pregnancy. *Br Med J* 1988; 297:883–887.

29. Walker NF: The use of dermal configuration in the diagnosis of mongolism. *Pediatr Clin North Am* 1958; 5:531–543.

# Chapter 18

# SURGICAL EMERGENCIES IN THE NEWBORN

*Frederick J. Rescorla, M.D.*

Surgically amenable conditions of the newborn include a spectrum of defects that necessitate interaction between the neonatologist and pediatric surgeon. These congenital abnormalities consist primarily of abdominal wall defects, obstructive lesions of the gastrointestinal tract, and anatomic pulmonary defects that lead to respiratory insufficiency. Although some defects require immediate surgical intervention (gastroschisis, malrotation with midgut volvulus, tracheoesophageal fistula with respiratory distress), the majority of abnormalities may be systematically evaluated prior to surgical intervention. Some of these defects (meconium ileus, meconium plug, small left colon syndrome) may not require operative intervention and others (congenital diaphragmatic hernia, omphalocele) may benefit from a delayed operative approach. This chapter presents a general overview of the clinical presentation, initial patient management, preferred diagnostic tests, and a discussion of the mode and timing of definitive therapy of several newborn surgical conditions. Case presentations precede formal discussions of several of the more common defects.

## ABDOMINAL WALL DEFECTS

### CASE STUDY 1

A 2,450-g male is delivered by spontaneous vaginal delivery to a 24-year-old, primigravida woman at 36 weeks' gestation. Apgar scores are 7 at 1 minute and 9 at 5 minutes. An abdominal wall defect is noted with "exposed intestinal contents." The umbilical cord appears uninvolved and inserts at the normal location with the defect in the abdominal wall to the right of the umbilicus (Fig. 18-1). The neonatal transport team is summoned to transport the child to the neonatal intensive care unit (NICU). The transporting nurse has placed an intravenous line in an upper extremity.

### EXERCISE 1

#### ■ Questions:

1. What type of defect does this child have?

2. What instructions should be given to the referral facility regarding care of the intestinal contents and general care of the child prior to and during transport?

Answers to these and all other questions are provided in the discussion sections that immediately follow each set of questions.

#### ■ Discussion:

The child in this case has a gastroschisis because the umbilical cord inserts into the abdominal wall. The other condition with this general appearance is a ruptured omphalocele;

**409**

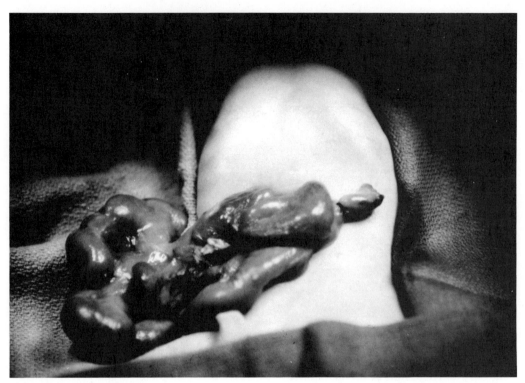

**Figure 18-1** Case Study 1.

however, in this condition the umbilical cord inserts on the most ventral portion of the ruptured sac. The essential points in the initial management of this neonate are to maintain body temperature, administer adequate intravenous fluids, and minimize ongoing fluid losses. The exposed bowel will significantly increase the evaporative fluid losses of the baby and should be covered in some fashion. In addition, the bowel should be briefly inspected to make certain there is no vascular compromise. This can be somewhat difficult because the bowel is frequently edematous and somewhat discolored. The defect can be viewed by gently lifting the bowel and noting that the opening is not tightly constricting the bowel. If the defect is too tight, which is very rare, immediate surgical consultation should be obtained to enlarge the defect. The bowel should be handled in a sterile fashion and covered with warm moist gauze sponges. The lower two-thirds of the infant should then be placed in a sterile bag. A "bowel bag," which is available in most operating rooms, is very useful for this purpose. The drawstrings of the bag can be drawn together loosely above the defect

(Fig. 18-2). The bag reduces heat losses and increases the relative humidity around the baby, thus reducing evaporative fluid losses. A radiant warmer can be used as an additional means to keep the infant warm.

Intravenous fluid requirements in these neonates are increased due to evaporative losses from the abdominal cavity and sequestration of fluid by the exposed bowel. Several options for initial fluid resuscitation are available. A solution containing 10% dextrose and 0.45% saline administered at a rate of 150 to 200 cc/kg/day usually results in adequate hydration. In some instances an initial bolus of 10 to 20 cc/kg of 5% plasmanate, plasma, or saline may be needed for fluid resuscitation. The main concern is to assess the efficacy of therapy continually by observing the infant's skin perfusion and heart rate. Urine output should also be monitored, but may be difficult to assess because of the presence of peritoneal fluid within the bowel bag. Additional aspects of care include placement of an orogastric tube to decompress the stomach. The administration of antibiotics is recommended; most physicians prescribe intravenous ampicillin (100

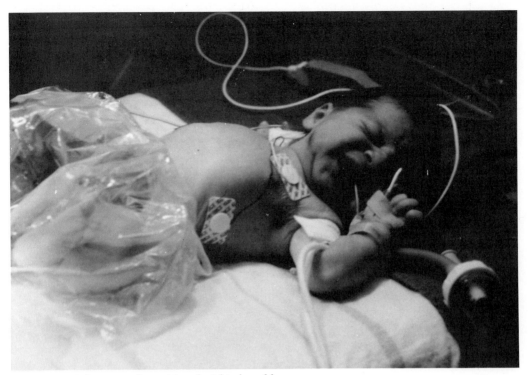

**Figure 18-2** Infant properly positioned within bowel bag.

to 200 mg/kg/day) and gentamicin (5 mg/kg/day) in divided doses.

**CASE STUDY 1 continued**
On arrival at the NICU the child is hemodynamically stable and has voided once. The child is taken to surgery where primary closure of the defect is performed by manually stretching the abdominal wall and replacing the intestinal contents into the abdominal cavity (Fig. 18-3). In addition a central line is inserted for administration of total parenteral nutrition (TPN). After surgery the child's axillary temperature is 35.4°C, the heart rate is 190 beats per minute (BPM) and blood pressure is 55/32. Ventilation is required for several days postoperatively; however, the infant is eventually weaned to room air.

**EXERCISE 2**

■ **Questions:**

1. What kind of intravenous fluids would be

appropriate for this infant and at what rate should they be administered?

2. How would you counsel the family as to expected length of hospital stay?

3. What associated defects can be seen in these children?

■ **Discussion:**
This neonate will continue to require greater than maintenance fluid intake in the postoperative period due to ongoing sequestration of fluid into the abdominal cavity. Daily fluid and electrolyte requirements can be met in one of two general ways. However, no matter what regimen is selected the infant will need to receive 4 to 8 mg/kg/min of dextrose to

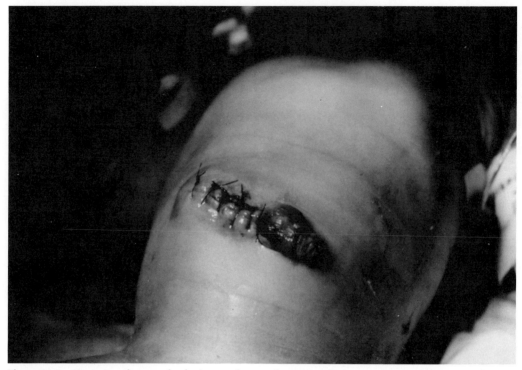

**Figure 18-3** Operative photograph of primary closure of a gastroschisis.

maintain normoglycemia. Glucose requirements can be met with a 10% dextrose solution administered at a rate of 4 cc/kg/hr (100
cc/kg/day). If this fluid plan is chosen, supplemental fluids will need to be administered in
the form of a lactated Ringers solution or plasmanate. Alternatively, 5% dextrose with electrolytes can be administered at a rate of 6 to 8
cc/kg/hr (150 to 200 cc/kg/day). With either
regimen, losses from the orogastric tube will
also need replacement. Most neonates require
175 to 200 cc/kg/day during the first 24 hours
after repair to maintain a urine output of 1 to 2
cc/kg/hr. Continual assessment of the child's
perfusion, urine output, and acid base status is
essential, because an occasional child may require as much as 300 cc/kg/day during the first
24 hours. As urine output increases (usually
24 to 48 hours after surgery), the rate of fluid
administration should be decreased to the
usual level of maintenance requirements.
TPN is generally started 24 to 48 hours after
surgery.

Neonates with gastroschisis typically have
a prolonged adynamic ileus and may require
orogastric decompression of the stomach and
TPN support for 3 to 4 weeks. The child's oral
intake may begin and be advanced as the volume of bilious return from the orogastric tube
ceases and bowel function returns. The family
should be advised to expect at least a 3- to 4-
week hospitalization. Associated anatomic defects are rare and consist primarily of intestinal atresia (10% to 12%) and malrotation.
Atresia may occur as sequelae to an intrauterine volvulus or from vascular compromise of a
segment of bowel by a tight defect.

## Gastroschisis

Gastroschisis is characterized by a defect in
the abdominal wall to the right of the umbilical cord with the intestinal contents herniated
through this defect, unprotected by a sac. The
etiology of gastroschisis is debated. Shaw, in a
careful evaluation of embryos from the 7-mm
to 12-cm size, theorized that with involution
of the right umbilical vein, a weakened area
remained to the right of the remaining umbilical vein. He felt that gastroschisis was a result
of an intrauterine rupture of this amniotic
membrane at the base of a hernia of the umbilical cord. DeVries, in a more recent review,

determined that gastroschisis results from a rupture of the paraumbilical somatopleure and does not represent a rupture omphalacele. The fact that associated defects are much less common with gastroschisis than omphalocele would tend to support different etiologies for the two defects. The eviscerated contents in gastroschisis usually include primarily small bowel with a portion of stomach and proximal colon. The bowel is thickened and foreshortened with adherent loops, which are often covered with an inflammatory exudate. Since the bowel herniates before normal rotation and fixation have occurred, nonrotation (malrotation) is present.

Gastroschisis may be identified by prenatal ultrasound screening. The management of a fetus with gastroschisis diagnosed by ultrasound is controversial. Although cesarean section is advocated by several authors, there is no evidence that this improves outcome. The author's preference is to allow vaginal delivery of these children. Intestinal atresias and malrotation are the most common associated defects.

The preoperative management of a child with gastroschisis is summarized in the case presentation. The goal of operative therapy is primary closure. An orogastric tube is used to decompress the proximal bowel. The rectum and colon can be irrigated with saline just prior to closure in order to decrease the size of the intestine and allow easier closure. At the time of surgery, the abdominal wall is manually stretched to enlarge the abdominal cavity. Several means of assessing the ability to reduce the intestines are available. In some children the contents simply will not fit within the abdominal cavity. If with replacement of the intestinal contents the peak inspiratory ventilator pressure rises above 35 cm of water, a silastic silo is usually constructed to avoid respiratory embarrassment from a tight abdominal closure. In addition, the elevated abdominal pressure can have an adverse effect on renal and intestinal perfusion. Yaster et al. described the use of intragastric pressure and central venous pressure (CVP) measurements to aid as a guide to closure. In this study, a central venous pressure line was placed prior to gastroschisis closure. If the infant maintained an intragastric pressure of less than 20 mm Hg or an increase in CVP of less than 4 mm Hg occurred after the bowel was replaced, primary closure was performed. If the mea-

surements were greater than this, a temporary silastic silo was used. If a silo is required, the defect is enlarged and a temporary housing of Dacron-reinforced silastic is sutured to the skin and constructed as noted in Figure 18-4. A central venous line is placed at the time of the initial procedure for administration of TPN. If intestinal atresia is noted initially, the options include creation of an ostomy or reconstruction with a primary anastomosis. Most pediatric surgeons proceed with an ostomy, planning a secondary procedure to restore bowel continuity. In some infants, an atresia can be suspected but not determined with certainty because of the thickened edematous and matted bowel. In these cases, the bowel is simply replaced into the abdomen and the child observed after surgery. If the usually observed adynamic ileus fails to resolve (3 to 4 weeks) and atresia is suspected, a contrast examination should be obtained to evaluate the bowel when necessary, a secondary procedure can then be performed for relief of the atresia.

Occasionally a child with gastroschisis and atresia may have a prolonged hospital course due to dilatation and ineffective peristalsis in the proximal dilated bowel. These children may require several operative procedures and this can present a difficult psychosocial situation for the family, particularly if they live far from the NICU. Many institutions provide low-cost or free housing for the families to allow them to interact with the child during this prolonged hospitalization. Anticipatory guidance provided by trained surgical nurse specialists and social workers can assist in supporting the family through the long hospitalization.

## Omphalocele

An omphalocele is a defect of the umbilical ring and the medial segments of the lateral abdominal wall folds. This malformation can be primarily epigastric in position related to an embryonic cephalic fold defect, centrally located related to a lateral fold defect, or reside in the hypogastric area related to a caudal fold defect. Since a membranous sac is present, the bowel is well protected and these children do not have the initial evaporative fluid losses associated with gastroschisis (Fig. 18-5). Unfortunately, associated anatomic defects are very common in 30% to 60% of these children.

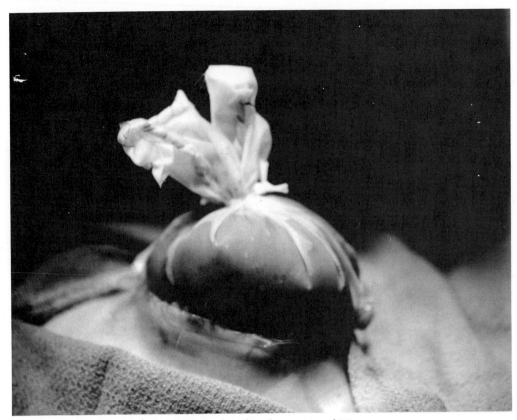

**Figure 18-4**  Photograph of silastic silo in place for a large gastroschisis.

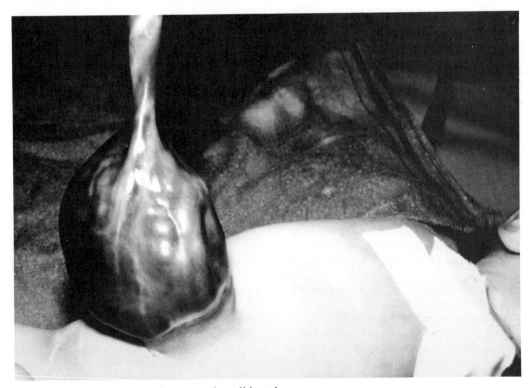

**Figure 18-5**  Omphalocele with contained small bowel.

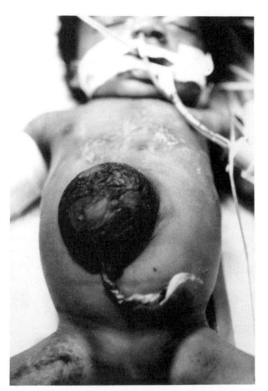

**Figure 18-6** Nonoperative therapy of an omphalocele defect with topical silver nitrate solution in a neonate with complex cyanotic congenital heart disease resulting in a protective eschar.

Cardiac anomalies, primarily tetralogy of Fallot and atrial septal defect, occur in 19% to 25% of children with omphalocele and are associated with increased mortality. Cardiac defects are most commonly seen with the higher (epigastric) omphaloceles and rarely seen with the caudal defects. Other associated malformations include genitourinary anomalies, the pentalogy of Cantrell (omphalocele, anterior diaphragmatic hernia, sternal cleft, pericardial defect, and intracardiac defect), lower midline syndromes such as cloacal exstrophy (omphalocele, bladder exstrophy with vesicointestinal fissure and imperforate anus), Beckwith-Wiedemann syndrome, and various trisomy syndromes.

The initial management of neonates with omphalocele is similar to the approach to patients with gastroschisis. Since evaporative fluid losses are not present to the same degree as with gastroschisis, the membranous sac need only be covered with a sterile dressing. Intravenous fluids (maintenance rate) and antibiotics are routinely administered.

Operative management is similar to that of gastroschisis with the exception that the procedure need not be done on an emergent basis. Other more serious anatomic defects (primarily cardiac) can be dealt with prior to repair of the omphalocele. If delayed repair is desired, topical therapy is useful as a temporizing measure. Silver nitrate solution (0.5%) can be applied on a twice daily basis to allow the sac to thicken as demonstrated in Figure 18-6.

The overall mortality of 30% to 40% is much higher for infants with omphalocele than those with gastroschisis due to the higher incidence of serious associated malformations.

## OBSTRUCTIVE LESIONS OF THE GASTROINTESTINAL TRACT

### Intestinal Obstruction of the Newborn

Neonatal intestinal obstruction is frequently noted in association with several findings including polyhydramnios, bilious vomiting, abdominal distention, and failure to pass meconium within the first 24 to 48 hours of life. Intestinal obstructions in the newborn infant can generally be classified as proximal or distal obstructions (Table 18-1). Proximal ob-

**Table 18-1** Intestinal Obstruction of the Newborn

*Proximal*
Esophageal atresia
Pyloric web/atresia
Duodenal atresia
Malrotation with midgut volvulus
Proximal jejunal atresia

*Distal*
Jejunoileal atresia
Meconium ileus
Neonatal Hirschsprung's disease
Colon atresia
Meconium plug syndrome
Small left colon syndrome
Neuronal intestinal dysplasia
Imperforate anus
Intestinal duplication
Intestinal pseudo-obstruction

structions are more often characterized by the occurrence of polyhydramnios and lack of abdominal distention, except in cases of tracheoesophageal fistula, where a large volume of air may shunt through the fistula into the stomach and bowel. Bilious vomiting occurs in any patient with a lesion obstructing the bowel distal to the ampulla of Vater. Abdominal distention is more characteristic of distal obstructive lesions. Failure to pass meconium within the first 24 to 48 hours of life can occur with any process that interrupts the normal passage of meconium into the distal colon or evacuation of meconium from the rectum.

Polyhydramnios is defined as a volume of amniotic fluid greater than 2,000 cc or an amniotic fluid index of greater than 20.0 cm on ultrasound. In approximately 50% of the pregnancies where polyhydramnios is recognized, there are no identifiable maternal or fetal abnormalities. However, the presence of polyhydramnios should raise the possibility that there may be an impairment in the ability of the fetus to swallow amniotic fluid or an obstruction in the gastrointestinal tract. The prevalence of fetal malformations in a woman with polyhydramnios is 18% to 20%. The most common fetal abnormalities include central nervous system (CNS) lesions (leading to decreased fetal swallowing) followed by digestive system (primarily proximal bowel obstruction) and neuromuscular defects (decreased swallowing).

The presence of bilious vomiting in a newborn infant is frequently indicative of a pathological process. Bile present in the stomach at birth is unusual and any infant presenting with this finding should be investigated for a possible intestinal obstruction. Approximately one-third of the neonates that present with bilious emesis have an identifiable intestinal obstruction. Of interest, more than half of these neonates may require radiographic contrast exams to identify the etiology of the obstruction because initial abdominal radiographs are normal or nonspecifically abnormal.

Abdominal distention is usually a sign of a distal small bowel or colonic obstruction. The loops of intestine are often visualized through the thin neonatal abdominal wall. Failure to pass meconium within the first 24 to 48 hours of life is also a sign of a possible neonatal intestinal obstruction and is commonly seen with a distal obstructive lesion. Other nonsurgical causes of abdominal distention and fail-

ure to pass meconium include an adynamic ileus in a neonate with sepsis, neonatal hypothyroidism, and untoward side effects of maternal medications or drug ingestions (narcotics).

The management of a neonate with a suspected intestinal obstruction should initially include a complete history and physical examination. As soon as abdominal distention is recognized, passage of an orogastric tube to aspirate the gastric material and decompress the proximal bowel is recommended. Blood should be drawn for culture and the child started on antibiotics (ampicillin and gentamicin). Radiographic views of the chest and abdomen are always indicated. A decubitus radiograph of the abdomen may help determine the presence of air fluid levels indicative of an obstructive process.

Proximal obstructive processes (esophageal atresia, duodenal atresia) can frequently be diagnosed accurately on plain radiographs and require no further diagnostic tests. If a distal obstructive process is suspected, the next recommended diagnostic test is usually a barium enema. This procedure must be carefully performed by a radiologist familiar with the technique. The presence of an unused colon or microcolon usually indicates the presence of an obstructive process proximal to the colon (which prevented *in utero* filling of the colon). The following sections discuss several of the more common proximal and distal intestinal malformations with selected case presentations.

### CASE STUDY 2

A 2,500-g full-term female newborn infant is born by spontaneous vaginal delivery. The infant did well for several hours; however, nursery personnel noted that she appeared to salivate excessively. Choking and coughing commenced with the first oral feeding. An NICU was contacted by the nursery staff for advice concerning management and possible transfer of this patient with presumed esophageal atresia.

### EXERCISE 3

■ **Questions:**

1. How can the diagnosis be confirmed in this infant?

2. How should this infant be managed?

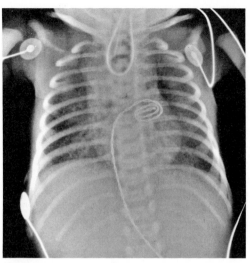

**Figure 18-8**  Case Study 2.

### ■ Discussion:

The quickest and easiest initial diagnostic procedure is to attempt passage of an orogastric tube. In the child presented in the case history, an obstruction was encountered after the catheter was advanced 10 cm, which is indicative of probable esophageal atresia. This catheter should then be placed to suction to prevent aspiration of saliva and a radiograph obtained of the chest and abdomen (Fig. 18-7). The child should be kept in a head-up position in the event that there may be a distal fistula, which would allow aspiration of gastric contents directly into the lungs. Antibiotics are commonly administered to these infants and appropriate intravenous fluid therapy must be provided.

### EXERCISE 4

### ■ Questions:

1. Based on the radiograph in Figure 18-7, what is the child's diagnosis?

2. What other associated anomalies could be present in this child?

3. What type of defect would be present if the radiograph in Figure 18-8 were obtained?

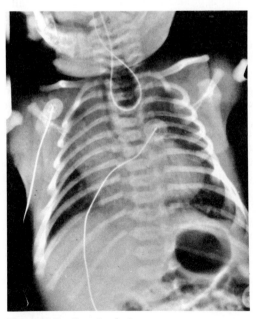

**Figure 18-7**  Case Study 2.

### ■ Discussion:

The child in the present case has esophageal atresia with a distal tracheoesophageal fistula (type C). The catheter placed orally has reached an obstruction in the upper esophagus and air has entered the gastrointestinal tract indicating the presence of a distal fistula. Lack of abdominal gas as in Figure 18-8 generally indicates esophageal atresia without a distal fistula (type A); however, a small percentage of these neonates will have a distal fistula that has not allowed air to pass into the stomach. Children with tracheoesophageal defects have a number of other associated malformations. Cardiac anomalies remain the most common associated defect (29%) followed by imperforate anus (13%) and duodenal atresia (4%). In addition, some children will have the complete VATER (V–vertebral, A–anal, TE–tracheoesophageal, R–renal and radial limb anomalies) association.

---

### CASE STUDY 2 continued

The child has been transferred to the NICU. She is hemodynamically stable and has an oxygen saturation of 94% on room air. She has no other discernable associated malformations. An echocardiogram is normal except for a small patent ductus arteriosus.

### EXERCISE 5

---

#### ■ Question:

What is the appropriate surgical management of this child?

#### ■ Discussion:

This child is physiologically in very stable condition and at most pediatric surgery centers would be a candidate for primary repair through an extrapleural thoracotomy. At the time of surgery the distal tracheoesophageal fistula was divided and an end-to-end esophagoesophagostomy constructed. Seven days after the procedure, an esophagram was obtained demonstrating adequate esophageal continuity. Feedings were advanced and the child released at 9 days of age.

---

### Esophageal Atresia and Tracheoesophageal Fistula

Esophageal atresia and tracheoesophageal fistula (TEF) are thought to arise from an interruption in development occurring around the fourth fetal week. An abnormality occurs in the partitioning of the esophagus and trachea, which results in a persistent fistula and incomplete development of the esophagus. Identification of these defects is usually based on

the Gross classification (Fig. 18-9). Approximately 87% of TEF represent type C defects, followed by 8% for type A and 4% for type E or the "H" type defect. TEF types B and D are quite unusual, representing approximately 1% of defects in most series.

The clinical symptoms of a newborn infant with a TEF vary according to the type of anatomic defect. Types A through D all give rise to excessive salivation. Types B and D may allow direct aspiration of saliva into the trachea from the proximal esophagus and types C and D allow reflux of gastric contents into the trachea through the distal fistula. In addition, neonates with type C or D defects can have significant amounts of tracheal air shunt into their gastrointestinal tracts. This may be particularly pronounced if a child requires endotracheal intubation and mechanical ventilation. Neonates with type A or B defects generally have a scaphoid abdomen, whereas those with type C and D defects may have a fuller, even distended, abdomen. Neonates with type E or the "H" defect are often asymptomatic, presenting later in infancy and childhood with symptoms due to aspiration.

The diagnosis of TEF types A through D can be confirmed by the inability to pass an orogastric tube into the stomach. A radiograph will demonstrate the tip of the tube in the cervical or upper thoracic esophagus. If gas is present in the gastrointestinal tract, a type C defect is probable, although very rarely a type D defect may lead to a similar x-ray appearance. If there is no gas in the abdomen, it is usually a type A or occasionally a type B defect. In addition, as noted previously, an occasional child with a distal fistula will not shunt any air through the fistula due to plugging or obliteration of the fistula.

The optimal operative management of these children is somewhat controversial and recommendations have undergone significant changes over the past two decades. Surgical options include primary repair (as in the case presentation), delayed primary repair with the use of an initial gastrostomy, or a staged repair. The delayed primary repair with use of an initial gastrostomy allows stabilization of the infant while still serving to decompress the stomach and prevent abdominal distention and aspiration through the distal fistula. In the staged repair, the fistula is generally ligated and a gastrostomy placed for feedings. Esophageal continuity is restored through a delayed

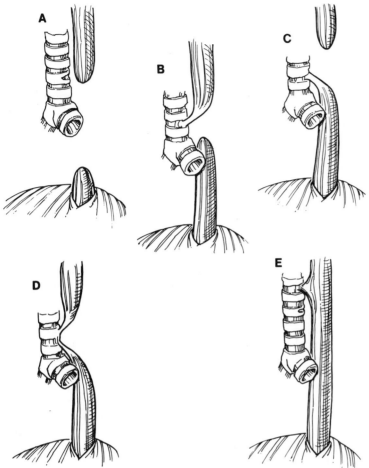

**Figure 18-9** Gross classification of esophageal atresia and tracheoesophageal fistula.

thoracic approach. For many years, a delayed primary repair approach was advocated for infants under 5.5 lb or for those children with higher birth weights but with an associated congenital anomaly or moderate pneumonia. A staged repair was generally advocated for infants with birth weights under 4 lb (1,800 g) or infants with higher birth weights but with concomitant severe pneumonia or severe congenital anomalies.

Recently, a more flexible approach has been advocated where surgical management is individualized for each patient based on clinical and physiological data. In this approach, any infant who is clinically stable is taken for immediate primary repair through a retropleural thoracotomy. No gastrostomy is required for these infants. Those neonates who are physiologically unstable (poor cardiovascular or re-

spiratory function) are taken to the operating room for gastrostomy placement and subsequently undergo delayed TEF repair.

Some newborn infants with a TEF also present with respiratory distress syndrome. This presents a management problem, because in the intubated patient, the amount of air passing through the TEF may compromise the child's tenuous respiratory status by not allowing adequate ventilatory volumes to be delivered. Furthermore, the amount of air passing through the fistula can cause massive gastric distention and gastric perforation and additionally compromise ventilation by elevating the diaphragm. Obliteration of the fistula may become emergently indicated in these patients. Fortunately, several options for management of these patients are available.

A gastrostomy tube can be placed to decompress the stomach, but it should be placed to underwater seal to maintain a determined intragastric pressure. This prevents excessive loss of ventilatory pressure through the tracheoesophageal fistula, while still allowing decompression of the stomach. Alternatively, the endotracheal tube can be manipulated by passing a fiber optic bronchoscope through the endotracheal tube and positioning it so as to occlude the fistula, but not occlude the trachea at the level of the carina. This can be very difficult and requires constant cardiorespiratory monitoring. In addition, in some children the fistula may come off distal to the carina, which makes endotracheal occlusion of the fistula impossible. Another therapeutic maneuver used to occlude the fistula is the insertion of a Fogarty balloon catheter. The catheter can be passed through the gastrostomy into the distal esophagus, or it can be placed from above with the use of a bronchoscope. Manipulating the catheter through the stomach into the distal esophagus may be rather difficult. The balloon should not be overinflated because pressure necrosis of the esophagus can result. Similarly, if placed from above, care should be taken to prevent dislodgement because this may lead to total tracheal occlusion. High-frequency jet ventilation has been useful in providing optimal ventilation in some children with TEF. If Fogarty balloon occlusion and high-frequency ventilation are unsuccessful, the next best option is to ligate the fistula. Although this is very stressful for the child, it is the most efficacious way to occlude the fistula and may also allow primary repair. This can be performed quickly through a retropleural thoracotomy. Other surgical techniques have been described (but are not currently used at most centers), including gastric division with placement of the proximal stomach to water seal, transabdominal closure of the tracheoesophageal fistula with a Nissen fundoplication, and temporary banding of the gastroesophageal junction.

The operative repair for a type C tracheoesophageal fistula is usually rather straightforward. The fourth intercostal space is divided and a retropleural approach used to enter the posterior mediastinum. The distal fistula is identified and divided with closure of the trachea. The proximal esophagus is identified and an end-to-end anastomosis is generally constructed. Occasionally if the gap is significant, a circular myotomy may be required to lengthen the proximal esophagus. Some authors recommend perioperative bronchoscopy to search not only for the distal fistula, but also to identify the rarer upper esophageal fistula (~3%).

The management of a child without a distal fistula is a much more challenging problem for the pediatric surgeon. As noted in Figure 18-9, the distance between the proximal and distal ends of the esophagus is often quite significant in these children. The general approach in most centers is to place a gastrostomy and initiate alimentary feedings. Bronchoscopy can be performed to rule out the presence of a proximal or distal fistula that would put the child at risk for aspiration and also alter the surgical therapy. Numerous options are available for the replacement of the esophagus. Unfortunately, there is no ideal substitute for the esophagus and thus there is tremendous debate among pediatric surgeons as to the optimal conduit. The colon can be placed between the proximal esophagus and the stomach in a retrosternal or retrohilar position. The stomach can also be used in either a gastric pull-up fashion, in which the entire stomach is pulled up into the upper thorax, or as a gastric tube. The gastric tube is fashioned from the greater curvature of the stomach and is then brought up through an opening in the diaphragm into the neck where it is connected to the esophagus. In addition, the small bowel has been used to bridge the gap between the esophagus and the stomach. Another option, which is the current preference at many institutions, is to administer bolus feedings through the gastrostomy and dilate the proximal esophagus on a twice daily basis. A delayed thoracotomy is then performed at 2 to 3 months of age. This usually allows the two ends of the esophagus to come rather close together and in the last several patients at the author's institution, it has allowed an end-to-end anastomosis to be performed. These infants frequently require a circular myotomy of the proximal esophagus to gain adequate length. Postoperative complications are common regardless of the method of restoring continuity. With the use of the native esophagus the occurrence of gastroesophageal reflux is extremely common and these infants frequently require a Nissen fundoplication.

Current survival with esophageal atresia and tracheoesophageal fistula is between 83% and 100%. Most deaths in the current era are due to severe associated malformations (primarily cardiovascular defects) or the occasional child with severe respiratory distress who is unable to be adequately supported because of shunting of inspired gas through a distal tracheoesophageal fistula.

## Pyloric Web

Congenital gastric outlet obstruction is a relatively rare cause of intestinal obstruction in the newborn. It is thought to arise from either an *in utero* vascular accident or from a defect in recanalization. Polyhydramnios is noted in approximately 50% of cases. This type of obstruction can vary from a membranous web blocking the outlet of the stomach to a complete separation between the stomach and duodenum. On rare occasions, pyloric atresia can be associated with epidermolysis bullosa as an autosomal recessive syndrome. The diagnosis of gastric outlet obstruction is usually made by demonstrating gastric distention without any distal gas in a newborn infant with nonbilious emesis. Treatment consists of appropri-

ate fluid resuscitation in association with orogastric tube decompression of the stomach. The surgical management can include excision of the web with a pyloroplasty or, if there is a complete atresia, a gastroduodenostomy. Pyloric obstruction in the newborn has also been reported secondary to aberrant pancreatic tissue and in association with a pyloric duplication, although these are somewhat unusual occurrences.

## CASE STUDY 3

A 2,200-g female infant is delivered by spontaneous vaginal delivery at 36 weeks' gestation. At the time of the first attempted feeding, the child vomits 15 cc of green fluid. The child is taken back to the nursery where further evaluation demonstrates an active child without abdominal distention or tenderness. An orogastric tube is placed with aspiration of an additional 15 cc of bilious material. The abdominal radiograph in Figure 18-10 is obtained.

## EXERCISE 6

### ■ Questions:

1. What is the diagnosis in this child?

2. What other anomalies are associated with this condition?

3. How would the clinical management of this child be altered if her gestational age was 32 weeks and she had developed respiratory distress syndrome?

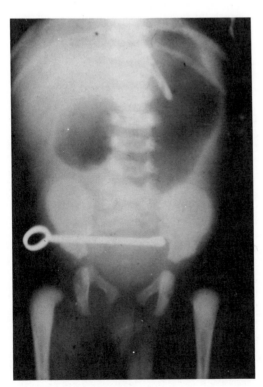

**Figure 18-10** Case Study 3.

### ■ Discussion:

The child in this case has duodenal atresia demonstrated by the classic radiographic appearance of the "double bubble." The plain radiograph is adequate for definitive diagnosis in this case and the child requires no other diagnostic evaluation prior to operative repair. Associated conditions and anomalies can include prematurity (30% to 45%), Down's syndrome (30%), congenital heart disease (30%), esophageal atresia (8%), and imperforate anus (6%). Since operative repair is not emergent, surgery should be delayed in the premature infant with respiratory problems.

### Duodenal Atresia

Duodenal atresia is a relatively common cause of intestinal obstruction in the neonate. The etiology of this defect is probably related to a failure of recanalization of the lumen of the duodenum from the solid cord stage. The vacuolization of the solid cord stage usually begins at 8 to 10 weeks of gestation and normally results in a patent duodenal lumen. Failure of recanalization can result in complete atresia or simply a stenosis. This usually occurs near the ampulla of Vater. This defect is frequently associated with annular pancreas because the ventral pancreas incompletely or partially rotates around the duodenum. Additional intraabdominal abnormalities can occur including preduodenal portal vein and intestinal malrotation.

Increased use of prenatal ultrasound has resulted in the diagnosis of duodenal atresia in a number of children prior to birth. When it is encountered prenatally, families should be counseled regarding the occurrence of Down's syndrome in approximately one-third of these children and the need for appropriate prenatal diagnostic testing. The presence of a proximal obstruction can be suspected by the occurrence of polyhydramnios, which is noted in approximately one-third of these pregnancies. In addition, the examination of the fetus may reveal a dilated, fluid-filled stomach and duodenum. In these neonates the diagnosis can be confirmed by plain radiographs after birth.

Neonates born with an unsuspected duodenal atresia generally present within the first few hours of life with emesis or difficulty with initial feedings. Since the level of obstruction in most children is distal to the ampulla of Vater, the vomiting and orogastric return is usually bilious. Abdominal distention is unusual because the obstruction is very proximal. The initial management of the child includes passage of an orogastric tube and appropriate fluid resuscitation. A careful physical examination is necessary to rule out the

possibility of Down syndrome and congenital heart disease. Abdominal radiographs usually demonstrate an air-filled stomach and first portion of the duodenum, resulting in the classical "double bubble" appearance on x-ray. If no distal air is noted, the diagnosis can be assumed to be duodenal atresia and the child can be prepared for operative management. If air is noted distally, an upper gastrointestinal series may be useful to identify duodenal stenosis or some other defect such as malrotation with volvulus. The operative repair is not emergent and the child can be stabilized, particularly if there are associated anomalies or the presence of respiratory distress.

The operative management of these children consists of construction of a duodenoduodenostomy. The duodenum is opened proximal to the atresia and an attempt is made to identify flow of bile into the duodenum. The duodenum is then opened distal to the obstruction and a duodenoduodenostomy constructed to bypass the obstruction. Occasionally a web is noted, which may be amenable to simple excision. If intestinal malrotation is noted, it is corrected with a Ladd procedure. Postoperatively, these children generally require orogastric tube decompression of their stomach for several days. The survival of neonates with duodenal atresia has improved significantly with most series currently reporting a 90% to 94% survival rate. Mortality is usually due to associated conditions, particularly congenital heart disease.

### CASE STUDY 4

A 2,800-g male is born at 38 weeks' gestation to a 29-year-old, primigravida woman by spontaneous vaginal delivery. The child tolerates feedings for the first 48 hours of life; however, just prior to discharge he has one episode of bilious emesis. A barium enema is performed and interpreted as normal, however, the radiologist notes that the cecum is somewhat high riding. The child resumes feedings and on the fourth day of life develops bilious emesis associated with abdominal distention. The child is transferred by ambulance to the NICU. On arrival, the child has a heart rate of 180 BPM, a respiratory rate of 52, and a systolic blood pressure of 48. The chest is clear. The abdomen is moderately distended. An orogastric tube is placed with bilious return. An abdominal radiograph is obtained (Fig. 18-11).

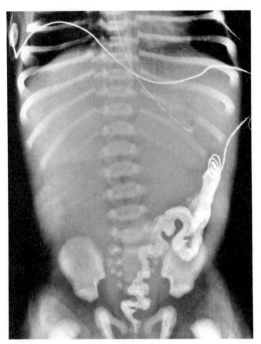

**Figure 18-11**   Case Study 4.

## EXERCISE 7

### ■ Questions:

1. What is the differential diagnosis of this child's condition?

2. What is the appropriate management for this child at this point?

### ■ Discussion:

The most likely diagnosis in this child who has had normal bowel movements and has tolerated feedings intermittently is that of malrotation with midgut volvulus. This is one of the potentially lethal pediatric surgical emergencies. It requires immediate intervention in order to preserve the infant's small bowel. The child should receive an immediate fluid resuscitation with a bolus of 20 cc/kg of saline, plasmanate or lactated Ringers solution. With appropriate surgical consultation, the decision must then be made as to whether to take this child immediately to the operating room for exploration or to proceed with a diagnostic test [repeat barium enema or an upper gastrointestinal (GI) series]. In this particular case, an upper GI series was obtained (Fig. 18-12), which demonstrated a complete cutoff at the level of the duodenum. As noted in the radiograph, the bowel assumed a "bird's beak" appearance as the duodenum entered the neck of the volvulus. The entire midgut consisting of the distal duodenum, entire small bowel, and proximal colon was involved in the volvulus. This child was taken for exploration approximately 90 minutes after arrival at the NICU. A clockwise midgut volvulus was encountered and the bowel was detorsed in a counterclockwise fashion. The entire bowel was viable and the child underwent a Ladd procedure and appendectomy. The infant has subsequently done well.

## Malrotation with Midgut Volvulus

Abnormalities of intestinal rotation and fixation occur between the 4th and 12th weeks of fetal life. Snyder and Chaffin in their classic description of normal rotation noted that at 4 weeks of fetal life the entire bowel is a straight tube with the superior mesenteric artery (SMA) supplying the future small bowel and

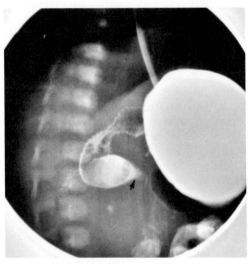

**Figure 18-12**   Radiograph demonstrates complete cutoff of barium in the duodenum (arrow) due to midgut volvulus.

proximal colon (termed the *midgut*). The portion of the bowel proximal to the SMA is the duodenojejunal loop and the portion distal to the SMA is the cecocolic loop. Each of these loops rotates 270 degrees counterclockwise around the SMA as you face the SMA. The duodenojejunal loop starts above the SMA and rotates to the right, then below, and finally to the left of the SMA where it takes its final resting place at the ligament of Treitz. The duodenum therefore forms the usual "C sweep" passing underneath the SMA. The distal cecocolic loop also rotates 270 degrees counterclockwise around the SMA; however, it starts below the SMA, rotates initially to the left, then above, and finally to the right of the SMA, coming to its final resting point in the right lower quadrant.

Interruptions in these events of rotation give rise to various forms of nonrotation or, as it is more commonly referred, malrotation. The term *nonrotation* is the more proper term and refers to events in which the duodenojejunal loop does not rotate around the SMA but remains on the right side of the abdomen. The cecocolic loop remains on the left side of the abdomen. The basic problem, as pointed out by Ladd, is that there is lack of fixation of the small bowel with the entire midgut supported by a narrow pedicle. The entire midgut may therefore undergo a twist (which usually occurs in a clockwise direction), resulting in midgut volvulus.

The clinical presentation of malrotation can include midgut volvulus, which is the most serious problem, or intermittent obstruction of the duodenum due to Ladd's bands, which cross the duodenum. Malrotation with acute midgut volvulus usually occurs in an otherwise healthy child. Presentation within the first month of life is very common and in a recent review 83% of the cases were less than 30 days of age. Presenting features usually include the sudden onset of abdominal pain, bilious emesis, and subsequent abdominal distention. In addition, blood or mucosal tissue can pass per rectum as the process leads to vascular compromise of the intestine. The neonate develops more pain as the ischemic process progresses to involve the serosal surface of the bowel.

Initial treatment for a child with this condition should include prompt fluid resuscitation with simultaneous clinical evaluation and preoperative preparation. An orogastric tube is placed to decompress the stomach and prevent aspiration, and broad spectrum antibiotics are administered.

Radiological examination frequently demonstrates air in the stomach and proximal duodenum in an otherwise gasless abdomen. If the history, physical examination, and plain films are consistent with midgut volvulus, the child is generally taken for immediate operative exploration. If the diagnosis is uncertain, a contrast study can confirm the diagnosis. An upper gastrointestinal study will demonstrate the dilated stomach and duodenum with an abrupt cutoff at the neck of the volvulus. A barium enema will demonstrate an obstruction of the proximal colon as it enters the volvulus.

The midgut volvulus usually occurs in a clockwise fashion and it is therefore detorsed in a counterclockwise direction. After detorsion, toxins may be released from the necrotic or marginally viable bowel into the superior mesenteric vein resulting in a sudden drop in systemic blood pressure. After the bowel is detorsed, it is assessed for viability. If the bowel is clearly viable, a Ladd procedure is performed by dividing the bands arising from the cecum that cross the duodenum and then separating the duodenum and the cecum. This maneuver widens the base of the mesentery and the cecum is then placed in the left lower quadrant. An appendectomy is generally performed since the appendix is not in the usual right lower quadrant position. If a segment of the bowel is necrotic, it is resected with either a primary or delayed anastomosis.

If at the time of initial exploration the entire bowel is necrotic, the surgeon faces few therapeutic options. If the amount of viable small bowel is inadequate to allow survival (estimates range from a minimum of 10 to 15 cm with an intact ileocecal valve), most surgeons recommend closure of the abdomen without a resection and provision of comfort measures to the dying infant. If the family chooses to consider supporting the child with TPN for their lifetime or until small bowel transplantation becomes an achievable alternative, a complete small bowel enterectomy can be performed. This is a difficult decision for the family, surgeon, and neonatologist and must be individualized.

Malrotation with acute midgut volvulus represents one of the most urgent pediatric surgical conditions. Mortality rates within the first 30 days of surgery are currently between 6% and 11%. Any neonate with signs and symptoms consistent with midgut volvulus should undergo immediate evaluation and, if indicated, prompt exploration. Since this condition cannot always be readily differentiated from other obstructive problems, urgent evaluation is necessary for any child in whom acute midgut volvulus remains in the differential diagnosis. Long-term mortality within the first year of presentation and repair ranges from 23% to 28%. These late deaths are due to complications from central line sepsis and liver failure secondary to TPN.

## CASE STUDY 5

A 3,200-g white female infant is delivered by spontaneous vaginal delivery at 38 weeks' gestation. The child does well for the first 18 hours of life and tolerates several feedings. She is then noted to have abdominal distention followed by bilious emesis. The abdominal radiograph in Figure 18-13 (lateral decubitus) is obtained and the child is then referred for evaluation.

## EXERCISE 8

### ■ Questions:

1. How should this child be managed?

2. What is the differential diagnosis of this infant's condition?

3. What is the next most appropriate diagnostic test?

### ■ Discussion:

The child with the symptoms described here, as well as the radiograph demonstrating marked distention of numerous loops of bowel with air fluid levels, most likely has a distal intestinal obstruction. The differential diagnosis would include jejunoileal atresia, colonic atresia, meconium ileus, meconium plug syndrome, small left colon syndrome, and Hirschsprung's disease.

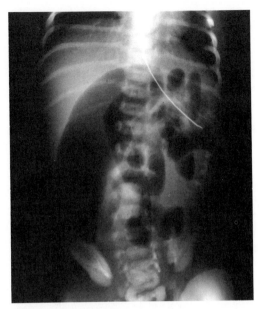

**Figure 18-13**  Case Study 5.

The management of this infant should include placement of an orogastric tube for decompression of the stomach and upper intestine, provision of intravenous fluids, and initiation of antimicrobial therapy. A barium enema would be the next most appropriate diagnostic test. The barium enema illustrated in Figure 18-14 was obtained in this case and the colon was noted to be of very small caliber

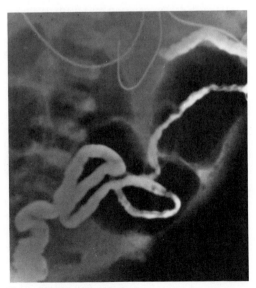

**Figure 18-14**  Case Study 5.

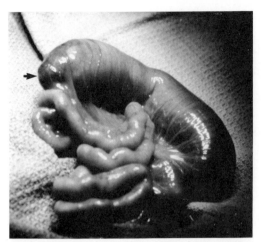

**Figure 18-15** Arrow indicates dilated blind ending proximal bowel in a Type III jejunoileal atresia. The distal bowel is of small caliber.

consistent with a microcolon. As noted in the radiograph, contrast filled the transverse colon and then seemed to meet an intraluminal obstruction. The pediatric radiologists thought this was consistent with material within the colon and that it did not represent a colonic atresia. The child was taken to the operating room where a distal ileal atresia was found (Fig. 18-15). As noted in this operative photograph, the proximal bowel was markedly dilated and the distal bowel was very small. A V-shaped mesenteric anomaly separated the two segments. The child underwent resection of several centimeters of the atonic proximal bowel with reconstruction by a primary end to oblique anastomosis. The child required orogastric tube decompression for 6 days and was then advanced in feedings and released 10 days after surgery.

### Jejunoileal Atresia

Jejunoileal atresia is one of the more common causes of intestinal obstruction in the newborn. The etiology of this type of atresia is presumed to be a mesenteric vascular accident. This type of vascular injury can result from volvulus, intussusception, internal hernia, or strangulation of a segment of the bowel. The vascular supply in a tight gastroschisis may also become compromised and lead to an atresia. The classification of jejunoileal atresia includes a Type I defect in which intact

bowel is separated by a mucosal web (Fig. 18-16), a Type II defect in which the atretic ends are separated by a fibrous cord, and a Type III defect (Case Study 5) in which the atretic ends are separated by a V-shaped mesenteric defect. Type III is the most commonly observed defect. Another type of atresia, sometimes called Type IIIa or Type IV, is the "apple-peel" deformity. This atresia results from a vascular accident involving the superior mesenteric artery, leaving the entire small bowel dependent on a single distal ileal vessel. Figure 18-17 is an operative photograph demonstrating the typical "apple-peel" deformity with the distal bowel encircling the distal ileal vessel.

The clinical presentation of a child with jejunoileal atresia generally includes abdominal distention, bilious vomiting, and failure to pass meconium. If the obstruction occurs very proximal in the jejunum, the child may have associated polyhydramnios. Most infants are full term and do not display any associated malformations. Of interest, 10% to 12% of infants with atresia have cystic fibrosis. Therefore, a sweat chloride test is recommended. The clinical management of an infant with jejunoileal atresia is summarized in the case presentation. The diagnostic procedure of choice is generally a barium enema, which demonstrates a microcolon; a very small ileum may be noted distal to the level of the atresia if reflux of barium occurs through the

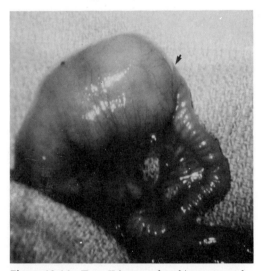

**Figure 18-16** Type II (mucosal web) atresia with dilated proximal bowel (left) and very small distal bowel (right). Arrow indicates location of web.

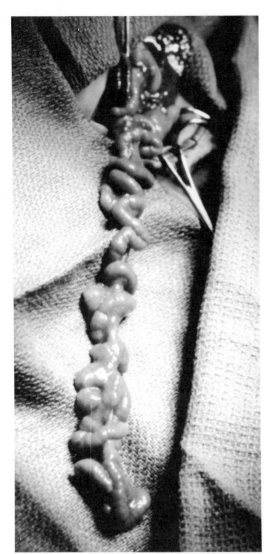

**Figure 18-17** "Apple-peel" atresia with entire small bowel supplied by distal ileal vessel.

13% with deaths occurring in patients whose course is complicated by short gut and the need for prolonged TPN.

### CASE STUDY 6

A 2,750-g male is delivered at 38 weeks' gestation to a primigravida woman by spontaneous vaginal delivery. The child initially does well and is breast fed for the first 24 hours of life. At that point the infant becomes irritable and develops poor feeding. Those signs are followed during the next 12 hours by abdominal distention and bilious emesis. Physical examination reveals a somewhat lethargic child with abdominal distention. No meconium has been passed and the rectal vault is empty. A preliminary evaluation for possible sepsis is unremarkable. An abdominal radiograph (Fig. 18-18) is obtained and the child is then transferred to the NICU for management at 48 hours of age.

### EXERCISE 9

#### ■ Questions:

1. How should this infant be managed?

ileocecal valve. Occasionally with a proximal jejunal atresia (which would have only one or two dilated loops of bowel on a plain radiograph) an upper GI contrast study may demonstrate the defect.

Operative management in children with jejunoileal atresia is usually straightforward. The proximal dilated atretic segment is usually atonic and generally resected. An anastomosis is constructed in a fashion to allow the larger proximal bowel to drain freely into the smaller caliber distal bowel. The distal bowel is irrigated with saline to exclude the presence of a distal atresia. The overall mortality is

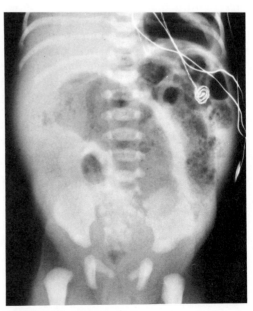

**Figure 18-18** Case Study 6.

2. What is the differential diagnosis based on the history, physical examination, and abdominal radiographs?

3. What is the next appropriate diagnostic or therapeutic procedure?

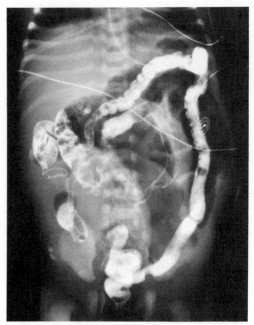

**Figure 18-19** Radiographic appearance of a gastrografin enema in a child with simple meconium ileus.

## ■ Discussion:

Similar to other infants with intestinal obstruction, the initial management of this child should include administration of adequate amounts of intravenous fluids (maintenance plus replacement of preexisting losses from the presumed obstruction). An orogastric tube should be placed to prevent further emesis and to decompress the proximal bowel. Blood cultures should be obtained and the child placed on intravenous antibiotics. In this case the abdominal radiograph demonstrated distention of the bowel as well as air mixed with stool resulting in the so-called "soap bubble" appearance, which is commonly seen in cases of meconium ileus. The differential diagnosis would also include jejunoileal atresia, colonic atresia, and Hirschsprung's disease.

As mentioned previously, the most useful step in the evaluation of a distal neonatal bowel obstruction is generally a barium enema. This would be an appropriate next step in this child. In view of the rather classical appearance of meconium ileus in this present case, however, you could administer a therapeutic gastrografin enema (Fig. 18-19). As noted in the radiograph, the gastrografin filled around the meconium plugs. The hyperosmolar nature of gastrografin draws fluid into the lumen of the bowel and subsequently flushes the meconium pellets into the colon.

A critical aspect of management at the time of the gastrografin enema is the fluid status of the child. Gastrografin is a hyperosmolar agent. This results in fluid shifts from the vascular system into the lumen of the bowel and can result in hypovolemic shock. Additional intravenous fluids are always required and the neonate must be carefully monitored. In the current case, the child passed numerous meconium plugs over the first 6 to 8 hours after the enema and then began passing softer meco-

nium. The abdomen became less distended and the child was advanced to a diet approximately 48 hours later. The diagnosis of cystic fibrosis was confirmed by a subsequent sweat chloride test. The child was placed on appropriate enzyme replacements, the parents were instructed in the pulmonary care of an infant with this disorder, and the child was released from the hospital.

## Meconium Ileus

Cystic fibrosis remains the most common autosomal recessive condition affecting the Caucasian population. Approximately 10% to 20% of neonates with cystic fibrosis develop an intraluminal obstruction of the terminal ileum from viscid meconium. If a simple mechanical obstruction occurs from the meconium plugging the lumen, it is referred to as simple meconium ileus. If the proximal bowel dilates and perforates, twists, or becomes ischemic, the child may develop a complicated meconium ileus, which can include volvulus, perforation, ileal atresia, or giant cystic meconium peritonitis. In most series in the literature, a simple meconium ileus occurs in approximately 50% of cases. The etiology of the abnormal meconium and intraluminal obstruction has been debated for a number of years. The meconium in these neonates has been noted to contain albumin at a concentration 5 to 10 times higher than that of the meconium of unaffected neonates. Protein levels in the meconium have been as high as 85%, whereas normal meconium contains only 7% protein. Recent studies by Brock concerning the concentrations of microvillar enzymes and albumin in affected and unaffected fetuses have determined that the contents of albumin, gamma glutamyltranspeptidase, and 5' nucleotidase within the lumen of the bowel are abnormally concentrated at the duodenal and jejunal level. Other enzymes that are secreted into the meconium at a more distal location are in similar concentration between affected and unaffected fetuses, signifying that the abnormal concentration of meconium constituents occurs at the level of the duodenum and jejunum.

Aggressive therapy for these affected neonates is indicated particularly in view of recent progress in cystic fibrosis research. Researchers have recently located the cystic fibrosis gene in the long arm of chromosome 7 and have also identified the delta F508 mutation, which is responsible for approximately 70% of the abnormal cystic fibrosis genes. Future therapy for cystic fibrosis may include administration of the normal protein to affected children or gene therapy, which could possibly insert the normal gene into defective cells. The long-term survival for cystic fibrosis continues to improve and new therapies for its complications have also been developed including the use of aerosolized amiloride, a medication that alters sodium transport and thins bronchial secretions. In addition, lung transplantation has been successfully used in increased numbers of patients with end-stage pulmonary disease due to cystic fibrosis. Cystic fibrosis does not recur in the transplant because the abnormal gene is not present in the transplanted lung.

The clinical presentation of meconium ileus is generally that of a term neonate who develops abdominal distention and bilious vomiting and who fails to pass meconium. Infants who have simple, uncomplicated meconium ileus or complicated cases with atresia will often tolerate feedings initially and develop signs and symptoms consistent with an obstruction at 24 to 48 hours of age. Children with complicated cases consisting of perforation or giant cystic meconium peritonitis usually present with distention and bilious gastric aspirate or emesis shortly after birth. The initial care of a newborn infant with a bowel obstruction is summarized in the case discussion. Radiographic examination in children with uncomplicated meconium ileus frequently demonstrates several loops of dilated bowel without air fluid levels. The viscid meconium does not permit an air/fluid interface, which results in air mixing with meconium and a radiograph appearance that resembles "soap bubbles" in the right lower quadrant. Cases complicated by atresia or volvulus generally have more impressive bowel dilatation with air fluid levels (see Fig. 18-13). In neonates with perforation or giant cystic meconium peritonitis, calcifications are frequently seen within the peritoneal cavity (Fig. 18-20). As noted previously, the initial diagnostic test in most children with lower intestinal obstruction is a barium enema (occasionally a therapeutic enema may be the procedure of choice if plain films strongly suggest uncomplicated meconium ileus). The barium enema in meconium ileus generally demonstrates a small, unused colon (microcolon). In cases of simple meconium ileus, some of the meconium pellets may be seen within the terminal

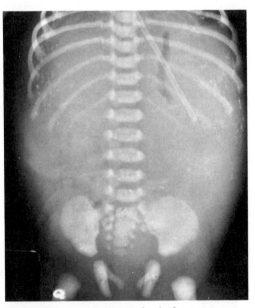

**Figure 18-20** Intraperitoneal calcification in a child with giant cystic meconium peritonitis.

ileum. The barium enema will also exclude several other disease states in the differential diagnosis including meconium plug syndrome, small left colon syndrome, and colonic atresia. Total colonic Hirschsprung's disease can exhibit a similar appearance to an uncomplicated case of meconium ileus and neonates with jejunoileal atresia can also demonstrate a microcolon. Neonates who after initial evaluation are felt to have complicated meconium ileus are taken to the operating room for laparotomy. Infants with uncomplicated meconium ileus are candidates for a nonoperative therapeutic enema.

Noblett in 1969 reported the use of full-strength gastrografin (diatrizoate meglumine) enemas with an added wetting agent, 0.1% polysorbate 80 (Tween 80), to treat four neonates with meconium ileus. In her original description, she emphasized the need for adequate intravenous fluid replacement as well as the requirement that there be no evidence of a volvulus, perforation, or atresia. Although Noblett used full-strength gastrografin, most radiologists currently dilute it approximately 4 to 1 with water to decrease the osmolarity, which is approximately 1,900 mOsm/L. As mentioned above, the major factor responsible for clearing the bowel in these cases is thought to be the hyperosmolar nature of the gastrografin solution, which draws fluid into the bowel lumen and results in a flushing of the meconium out of the intestinal lumen. Numerous complications including perforation, necrotizing enterocolitis, shock, and death have been reported. Other solutions have also been effective including Tween 80, N-acetylcysteine with or without gastrografin, diatrizoate sodium (Hypaque), and iothalamate meglumine (Conray). Some radiologists do not recommend gastrografin due to the risks noted above and instead use dilute Hypaque or Conray mixed with N-acetylcysteine. The current preference at the author's institution is to use dilute gastrografin.

Neonates should receive at least 1.5 times maintenance fluid requirements during and after the procedure. Urine output, urine specific gravity or osmolarity, and serum values of urea nitrogen, creatinine, and osmolarity should be closely followed. Broad-spectrum antibiotics should be continued and the child's clinical picture (the degree of abdominal distention, tenderness) and stool output carefully monitored. In general, rapid passage of the meconium pellets and then semiliquid meconium occurs during the first 24 hours after the enema. If the obstruction does not resolve and the child is stable, a second enema may be attempted. In addition, 5% to 10% N-acetylcysteine can be given through the orogastric tube at a volume of approximately 5 to 10 cc every 6 hours to aid in clearing the thick meconium. As the obstruction resolves, feedings are resumed.

Prior to Noblett's introduction of the gastrografin enema, surgical therapy for simple meconium ileus was associated with a very high mortality. Numerous procedures were devised in an attempt to perform a simple procedure; however, most of these included an ostomy in order to irrigate the bowel postoperatively. This subsequently required a second procedure in a group of children who represented a very high risk population in terms of anesthetic administration. The use of simple enterotomy with irrigation and then enterotomy closure was originally described by Hiatt and Wilson in 1948; however, that procedure was not widely utilized until the 1970s and 1980s. It is currently the procedure of choice for children with simple meconium ileus who fail nonoperative enema treatment. Saline or dilute gastrografin can be used to irrigate the bowel intraoperatively and remove the meconium pellets and thick meconium.

Neonates with complicated meconium ileus, as mentioned above, are treated operatively. Cases complicated with atresia or volvulus are generally treated with resection and primary anastomosis. In cases of perforation or giant cystic meconium peritonitis, a temporary ostomy is usually required. With advances over the past two decades in neonatal intensive care management and pediatric anesthesia, the mortality for neonates with meconium ileus has markedly decreased. In a recent review, the 1-year survival was 92% in neonates with uncomplicated meconium ileus and 89% in those with complicated meconium ileus.

### Colonic Atresia

Colonic atresia is a relatively uncommon cause of distal bowel obstruction in the neonate. The most widely held theory is that it is the result of an *in utero* vascular accident. The type of atresia can be a simple intraluminal diaphragm (Type I), a fibrous cord with intact mesentery between the two segments of bowel (Type II), or a complete gap in the mesentery with the two segments separated (Type III). The Type III defect is the most common. Although most of the children reported are otherwise normal, it has been observed with increased frequency in association with gastroschisis and jejunoileal atresia.

The clinical presentation is usually that of a classic distal intestinal obstruction. The child may feed well for a variable period of time; however, abdominal distention and bilious emesis eventually develop. In addition, failure to pass meconium is noted. The plain abdominal radiograph demonstrates multiple loops of dilated small bowel with air fluid levels indicative of a complete distal obstruction. The diagnostic procedure of choice is a barium enema, which reveals a microcolon up to the level of the atresia. The child in Figure 18-21 presented at approximately 36 hours of age with abdominal distention and bilious vomiting. At exploration, a Type III defect was noted at the splenic flexure with an extremely dilated proximal bowel. The proximal colon was converted to a colostomy and 1 month later the child was taken back to surgery for reversal of the colostomy and performance of an end-to-end anastomosis. Management of these children is identical to that described above for other infants with intestinal obstruction.

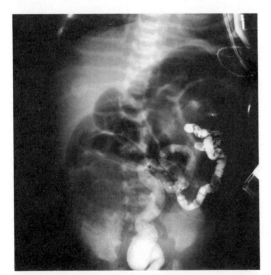

**Figure 18-21** Barium enema in a child with a low intestinal obstruction demonstrates a microcolon with complete obstruction near the splenic flexure.

Surgical alternatives include either colostomy with delayed anastomosis or resection of the dilated segment with a primary anastomosis. Both of these are acceptable alternatives and a decision is generally made in the operating room. Several authors prefer to use a colostomy for those neonates with atresia distal to the splenic flecture and primary anastomosis for those lesions proximal to the splenic flexure.

### Small Left Colon Syndrome

The small left colon syndrome was originally described in 1974 in a group of 20 neonates presenting with colonic obstruction. Of interest, 8 of these patients were infants of diabetic mothers and this strong association was subsequently described by other authors. These children frequently present with a classic colonic obstruction with proximal distention and bilious emesis. A barium enema frequently reveals a transition zone in the left colon (Fig. 18-22). Although the exact etiology of this disorder is unknown, it has been suggested that the syndrome results from a transient dysmotility state rather than from an actual mechanical obstruction due to the meconium. The diagnosis is confirmed by barium enema. The usual course for these children is that the obstruction resolves with provision of supportive care. Reports have been made of rare intestinal perforations in association with the small left colon syndrome. The child in Figure 18-22 presented with bilious emesis and abdominal distention and had the barium enema performed. A full thickness rectal biopsy was obtained, which demonstrated the presence of ganglion cells (Hirschsprung's disease was initially suspected). After several days with orogastric decompression of the stomach and proximal bowel, the obstruction resolved. The child has since been asymptomatic.

### Meconium Plug Syndrome

The meconium plug syndrome was originally described by Clatworthy, Howard, and Lloyd in 1956, in a brief report of nine infants with colonic obstructions. Seven of the infants resolved with enemas or rectal examinations and passed large plugs of thick meconium per rectum. Two of the infants had enterostomies for presumed Hirschsprung's disease. The eti-

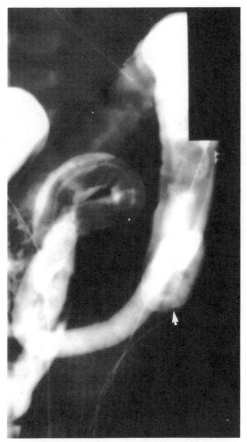

**Figure 18-22** Barium enema in a child with small left colon syndrome. Arrow indicates transition from narrow distal to dilated proximal colon.

ology of this obstructive process is thought to be meconium inspissating within the rectosigmoid area, leading to a complete obstruction. These children may present with emesis at 24 to 48 hours of age after initially tolerating feedings. Management of these children is similar to that of any infant with intestinal obstruction. Meconium plug syndrome usually cannot be differentiated from the small left colon syndrome, neonatal Hirschsprung's disease, colonic atresia, or even perhaps ileal atresia until a barium enema is performed. The barium enema is usually both diagnostic and therapeutic because the large meconium plug within the rectosigmoid portion of the colon commonly passes during the procedure. This is followed by the rapid passage of the meconium that was just proximal to the plug. The child's symptoms usually resolve within 24 hours, following which an oral diet can be resumed.

## CASE STUDY 7

A 790-g white female is delivered at 26 weeks' gestation to a 27-year-old, primigravida woman. The infant passes meconium on the third day of life and drip feedings begun at 1 week of life are well tolerated. At 14 days of age, she develops abdominal distention with increased gastric residuals, which subsequently turned bilious. Abdominal radiographic examinations are thought to demonstrate small bowel distention (Fig. 18-23). A laboratory evaluation including platelet count, white blood cell count, and arterial blood gas is completely normal.

## EXERCISE 10

### ■ Questions:

1. What is the differential diagnosis of this infant's condition?

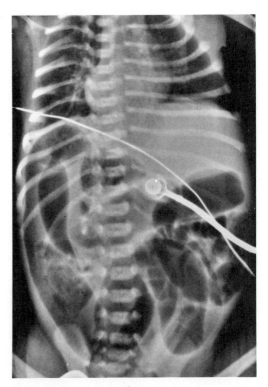

**Figure 18-23** Case Study 7.

2. How should this child be managed?

## ■ Discussion:

This child is at high risk for developing necrotizing enterocolitis (NEC) and in view of the distention and bilious return she would undergo a septic workup and be placed on appropriate antibiotics. In addition, orogastric tube decompression of the stomach would be instituted. Serial physical examinations, laboratory tests, and radiographs would be obtained to follow this child for the development of NEC.

The child in the current case did not develop a picture consistent with NEC and simply appeared to have a persistent complete mechanical bowel obstruction. A contrast enema (Fig. 18-24) demonstrated normal caliber colon with intraluminal material within the right transverse and right colon. A dilute gastrografin enema was used in an attempt to remove this material. This was successful in removing only a portion of the meconium and the child

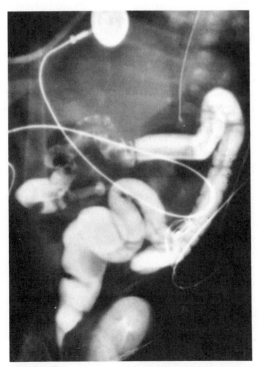

**Figure 18-24** Contrast enema demonstrates meconium pellets within the right colon.

remained completely obstructed. The child was subsequently taken to the operating room where inspissated meconium and material consistent with a lactobezoar were found obstructing the small bowel. This material was irrigated free and an enterostomy constructed.

## Meconium Disease in Premature Infants

This entity was originally described by Rickham and Boeckman in 1965 in a study of neonatal meconium obstruction without cystic fibrosis. In this disorder, the meconium is noted to be inspissated in the terminal ileum and proximal colon. This disorder, although somewhat different in etiology, is similar to the "milk curd" syndrome secondary to thick meconium or milk in preterm and term infants. The typical patient develops obstructive symptoms at several days of age after passing meconium within the first few days of life. This process, although rare, appears to be more common in preterm infants. The clinical presentation is usually similar to the case presentation. Plain films as in the current case demonstrate bowel distention. Most infants respond positively to a dilute gastrografin enema. If the child fails to respond, a repeat enema may be necessary. Vinograd et al., in a report of seven preterm children with this disorder, had a 100% success rate with enema clearance; four of the children required more than one enema. Several preterm infants at the author's institution have been treated with this disorder and some who have failed enema treatment have required operative intervention to clear the obstructing meconium.

## Hirschsprung's Disease

Hirschsprung's disease or aganglionic megacolon is defined as an absence of ganglion cells in the myenteric (Auerbach's) and submucosal (Meissner's) plexuses. This disorder is thought to arise from incomplete migration of neuroblasts. If these ganglion stem cells fail to reach the rectum, the child has Hirschsprung's disease. In approximately 80% of children, the ganglion cell migration stops in the rectosigmoid area leaving the child with relatively short segment disease. In another 10%, the cells stop their migration somewhat more proximally in the colon, and in the remaining 10%, the cells do not reach the colon, leaving the child with total colonic aganglionosis. Of interest, Hirschsprung's disease is also associated with Down syndrome in approximately 5% of cases. In addition, the risk of recurrence to the "normal" population in a second child after an initial index case is approximately 6%.

The clinical presentation of a child with Hirschsprung's disease is related to the failure of relaxation of the aganglionic internal anal sphincter and any other aganglionic portion of bowel. Infants can present at birth with complete obstruction and associated bilious vomiting, distention, and failure to pass meconium. Alternatively, children may present later in life with chronic constipation. In newborn infants diagnosed with Hirschsprung's disease, 95% will fail to pass meconium within 48 hours of birth. A common presentation in infancy is a neonate who fails to pass meconium within the first 24 to 48 hours of life and then passes meconium but remains chronically constipated.

Unfortunately, a small percentage of neonates with Hirschsprung's disease will develop enterocolitis. This is usually characterized by a sudden onset of abdominal distention, explosive diarrhea, and fever. It is often accompanied by subsequent hypovolemic shock. Enterocolitis carries a significant morbidity and mortality and is more common in cases that have been delayed in diagnosis and in children with Down syndrome.

In the neonate with Hirschsprung's disease, useful information can be obtained from plain films, barium enema, anorectal manometry, suction rectal biopsy, and full thickness rectal biopsy. Plain films may occasionally demonstrate distention of the colon to the level of the transition zone between the proximal ganglionic bowel and the distal aganglionic bowel. The barium enema is frequently normal in neonates with Hirschsprung's disease. If a child presents with obstructive symptoms in the newborn period, a barium enema is frequently required to exclude other causes of low intestinal obstruction including meconium plug syndrome, colonic atresia, distal ileal atresia, and meconium ileus. Although a transition zone is commonly observed between the unaffected and affected segments of the bowel in older infants, it is rarely seen in the newborn infant (Fig. 18-25). Occasionally, neonates with total colonic Hirschsprung's will present with a microcolon due to persis-

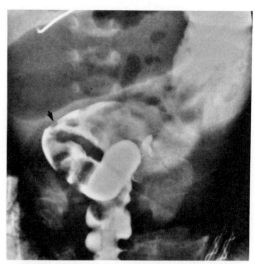

**Figure 18-25** Barium enema demonstrates a transition zone (arrow) between the dilated proximal bowel and the small caliber distal bowel.

tent contraction of the entire colon. These neonates are generally taken for operative exploration where the transition zone is readily recognizable. The barium enema can be a useful diagnostic test in infants with Hirschsprung's disease in that they commonly retain the barium for 24 to 48 hours rather than empty the material in less than 24 hours.

The suction rectal biopsy is performed with a device that can be used at the bedside to obtain a biopsy of the bowel mucosa and submucosa. This will determine the presence or absence of ganglion cells in Meissner's plexus. If ganglion cells are present, it excludes the diagnosis of Hirschsprung's disease. If ganglion cells are absent and the specimen is completely consistent with Hirschsprung's disease, the child should undergo operative exploration of the abdomen and colostomy. If there is any question about the validity of the results from the suction rectal biopsy, a full thickness rectal biopsy should be performed in the operating room before exploring the abdomen. Acetylcholinesterase levels can also be determined on suction rectal biopsy material and increased activity has been described in Hirschsprung's disease specimens. The full thickness rectal biopsy is the most definitive means to confirm or exclude Hirschsprung's disease. It does, however, require a general anesthetic and carries some associated risks. If Hirschsprung's disease is confirmed, the therapeutic choice at most centers is operative exploration with placement of a decompressing ostomy just proximal to the transition zone. A frozen section at the time of operation should confirm the presence of ganglion cells at the site of the ostomy. Although some centers are reporting successful pull-through procedures in the neonatal and early infancy periods (<3 months), most pediatric surgeons delay this procedure to approximately 6 months to 1 year of age.

### Imperforate Anus

Imperforate anus is one of the more common causes of distal intestinal obstruction in the neonate. It can generally be identified by a careful examination of the child's perineum shortly after delivery; however, if the defect is not initially noted, the child will usually develop signs consistent with a distal colonic obstruction. Abdominal distention usually occurs within 24 to 48 hours of life followed by bilious emesis. The perineum must be inspected closely, looking for a bulge in the area of the normal anal canal or an opening on the skin anterior to the normal location. This may be located at the base of the scrotum in a little boy or at the vulvar or vestibular areas in a little girl.

If no fistula is present, most pediatric surgeons generally wait approximately 24 hours to allow meconium to push its way down into the lowest portion of the bowel. Additional evaluation during this time can include sacral radiographs to assess for possible associated anomalies, ultrasound of the pelvis to determine the level of the pouch, and an invertogram to determine the level of the air-filled rectal pouch in relation to the pubococcygeal line. In some children, meconium may be seen bulging from the area of the external sphincter area within 24 hours. These children may simply have anal atresia with a thin membrane covering the normal anal canal. This malformation can be treated by simply opening the skin and dilating the opening.

Imperforate anus is generally classified as low, intermediate, or high based on whether the rectum has descended below the levator ani muscles, is at the level of the muscles, or remains above this level. Males with low defects and a fistula usually have an opening just anterior to the normal anal opening or near the base of the scrotum. This defect is usually treated with a cutback anoplasty in the newborn period. Females with low defects and an opening on the skin just anterior to the normal location are also treated with a cutback anoplasty. Infant females with a rectovestibular fistula are usually treated with a transplant anoplasty due to the proximity to the vagina. This can be performed in the newborn period or at approximately 3 months of age. If the anoplasty is delayed, the fistula can be dilated in the neonatal period to allow adequate evacuation of stool.

Intermediate lesions are those where the rectum has descended into but not through the levator muscles. In females the fistula usually enters the back of the vagina and in males there is usually a rectobulbar urethral fistula. High lesions are those defects in which the rectum has not descended to the level of the levator muscles. In males these children usually have a fistula to the prostatic urethra. In females, the high defects may either have no fistula or else a fistula that joins with the upper portion of the vagina. High and intermediate lesions in males and females are treated with an initial colostomy. These malformations are then corrected at approximately 9 to 12 months of age with division of the fistula and a posterior sagittal anorectoplasty. This procedure brings the rectum through the levator muscle and external sphincter muscles in an attempt to restore continence. The colostomy serves to protect the pull-through procedure by diverting the fecal stream and is usually taken down approximately 3 months after the pull-through procedure. Procedures for imperforate anus are quite difficult and should be performed with the goal to return the child to normal continence. This is usually possible in all children with low defects because they normally have a very good external sphincter muscle mechanism. The higher the defect, the more likely the child may have problems with continence later in life.

## OTHER ABDOMINAL CONDITIONS

### Necrotizing Enterocolitis

See Chapter 19.

### CASE STUDY 8

A 45-day-old, white male, the product of a 28-week gestation, has required ventilatory assistance since birth. The child has been known to

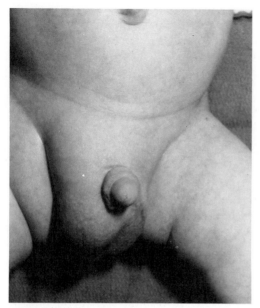

**Figure 18-26** Case Study 8.

have a right inguinal hernia for the past 2 weeks. Six hours ago, a firm mass in the inguinal-scrotal region (Fig. 18-26) was noted. The child currently has abdominal distention and exhibited a large gastric residual 3 hours after his most recent feeding. On physical examination, the child's abdomen is distended but soft. The inguinal-scrotal mass is tender and does not transilluminate. The right testicle cannot be identified with certainty. An abdominal radiograph demonstrates small bowel distention.

### EXERCISE 11

■ **Questions:**

1. What is the most probable diagnosis?

2. How should this infant be managed?

3. Is emergency care required or can surgical consultation be deferred?

■ **Discussion:**

A neonate presenting with the history, physical examination, and the signs and symptoms described here most likely has an incarcerated inguinal hernia, perhaps with strangulation of the contained intestinal contents. This is a surgical emergency that requires prompt intervention to prevent loss of the entrapped bowel. The initial management of this child would generally consist of an attempt at nonoperative reduction of the bowel into the abdominal cavity. This is performed by applying gentle downward pressure over the area of the external inguinal ring (to prevent reduction superficial to the ring) and then manually attempting to push the bowel contents into the abdominal cavity (Fig. 18-27). If this is unsuccessful, the child is sedated for a second attempt at reduction. This can be accomplished with the careful use of intramuscular or intravenous morphine (0.1 to 0.2 mg/kg) or meperidine hydrochloride (Demerol) (1 mg/kg) and

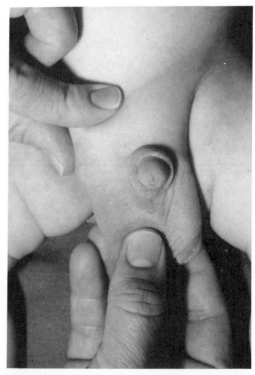

**Figure 18-27** Manual reduction of an incarcerated inguinal hernia. The thumb and index finger of one hand form an inverted "V" at the level of the external inguinal ring. Gentle pressure is applied to the hernia and contained bowel with the opposite hand.

secobarbital sodium (Seconal) (1 mg/kg). In addition, elevation of the foot of the bed may be a useful maneuver to aid reduction. After the child is quiet and well relaxed, gentle pressure is again applied in an attempt to reduce the hernia manually. If this attempt is unsuccessful, the child is taken to the operating room for operative reduction. If the attempt is successful, the hernia can be repaired electively.

---

## Incarcerated Inguinal Hernia

Inguinal hernias in infancy and childhood are one of the more common conditions requiring surgical intervention. Nearly all of these hernias are indirect inguinal hernias, which result from persistent patency of the embryologic processus vaginalis. This structure appears normally during the third fetal month as an outpouching in the peritoneum at the internal ring level. The processus vaginalis then accompanies the testicle during its descent through the internal ring during the seventh through ninth months of gestation. The proximal portion of the processus vaginalis is patent in approximately 80% of neonates at birth. The processus generally proceeds to close through infancy and childhood; however, patency does persist into adulthood in approximately 10% to 20% of patients. This congenital hernia remains the most common type of hernia, even in adults. The opening at the level of the internal ring can allow abdominal contents to move into the processus vaginalis and down into the scrotum. If the opening at the internal ring level is very small, occasionally only fluid will be found in the scrotal sac and this would be termed a *communicating hydrocele.*

A hernia is usually noted as a bulge in the inguinal or scrotal region. It is observed more frequently when the child strains and may disappear when the child relaxes or is sleeping. Hernias are noted with increased frequency in infants with increased intra-abdominal pressure such as infants with bronchopulmonary dysplasia (Case Study 8), ventriculoperitoneal shunts, abdominal wall defects, ambiguous genitalia, extrophy of the bladder, cloacal extrophy, or liver disease with ascites. In addition, hernias are more common in premature infants, particularly in association with cryptorchid testes.

The contained structures consist of the small bowel, colon, or, in female patients, an ovary or fallopian tube. The major clinical problem with inguinal hernias is incarceration or entrapment of abdominal contents as noted in the present case. The frequency of occurrence of incarceration of an inguinal hernia in the general pediatric population ranges from 6% to 20% with the highest incidence occurring during infancy. Presenting symptoms with incarceration include the presence of an irreducible inguinal or scrotal mass and varying degrees of irritability, pain, abdominal distention, and vomiting. The mass does not transilluminate, thus distinguishing it from a hydrocele.

Occasionally, a neonate may be rather asymptomatic from an incarcerated inguinal hernia. This can occur if the internal ring is large enough to allow normal bowel function to continue through the entrapped intestine and the vascular supply is not compromised. In addition, female neonates with an irreducible ovary presenting as a labial or inguinal mass frequently have a rather asymptomatic incarceration.

If the intestinal contents become compromised from a vascular standpoint, strangulation may develop. Venous occlusion develops initially and as further distention occurs arterial compromise will produce bowel necrosis. A complete mechanical bowel obstruction can ultimately ensue and lead to further abdominal distention and bilious emesis. In addition, injury to the gonad can occur from strangulation of an ovary in a female infant or from vascular compromise of the testes in a male infant. Plain films, in this situation, may demonstrate a mechanical bowel obstruction. The differential diagnosis in a male infant includes an acute hydrocele and testicular torsion. A hydrocele will usually transilluminate and is usually unassociated with gastrointestinal symptoms. An acute hydrocele occurs when the processus vaginalis fills with fluid leading to an enlarged scrotal or inguinal-scrotal region. If the proximal opening to the abdominal cavity is small, the lesion may remain tense and distended. The infant usually displays little or no discomfort related to this fluid collection. Torsion commonly produces a swollen, extremely tender testes.

The management of an incarcerated inguinal hernia usually includes an attempt at reduction with the assistance of sedation and elevation. Most pediatric surgeons attempt nonoperative reduction even if there is radiological evidence of a bowel obstruction. If peritoneal irritation is present, the child will need urgent operative exploration. As noted in the discussion of the previous case study, if nonoperative reduction is successful, the hernia can be repaired electively. If the hernia is irreducible, the child should be taken to surgery for immediate operative reduction and repair of the inguinal hernia. In the operating room the hernia occasionally reduces with the induction of anesthesia. These infants then undergo a standard exploration with high ligation of the processus vaginalis at the level of the internal ring. If the bowel remains within the hernia sac, the operative approach is similar; however, the hernia sac is opened and the bowel is carefully inspected. If the bowel is viable, it is reduced into the abdominal cavity followed by a standard hernia repair. If the bowel is not viable, a resection can usually be performed through the inguinal incision. On occasion, the internal inguinal ring may require enlargement or a separate abdominal incision may be necessary to complete the procedure.

In general, an inguinal hernia can be repaired in a neonate with little morbidity. The timing of hernia repair may vary between institutions; however, most centers repair an inguinal hernia in a premature neonate prior to discharge due to the risk of incarceration. If the operative situation is not emergent, most pediatric surgeons explore the opposite side due to the high incidence of bilateral hernias in this age group. The morbidity associated with hernia repair increases significantly in instances of incarceration and strangulation. Rowe and Clatworthy, in a series of 68 irreducible incarcerations, noted that 5 required intestinal resection. In addition, the incidence of testicular infarction with incarceration varies between 2.2% and 14%. The incidence of recurrent hernias is also higher in cases of incarcerated hernias than in uncomplicated inguinal hernias. The rate of recurrence in uncomplicated hernias is generally between 0.3% and 1.0%, whereas the rate with incarcerated hernias varies between 3% and 6%.

## SURGICALLY CORRECTABLE NEONATAL RESPIRATORY PROBLEMS

### CASE STUDY 9

A 3,940-g white male infant is born to a 24-year-old woman at 40 weeks' gestation by spontaneous vaginal delivery. Apgar scores were 8 at 1 minute and 8 at 5 minutes. The child did well initially; however, shortly after birth he developed respiratory distress and 15 minutes later required intubation. The following ventilator settings were needed to maintain adequate oxygenation: $FiO_2 = 1.0$, rate = 60, inspiratory pressure = 30 cm $H_2O$, PEEP = 6 cm $H_2O$, and mean airway pressure (MAP) = 13.8 cm $H_2O$. The chest x-ray depicted in Figure 18-28 was obtained. An umbilical arterial line was placed and the following blood gas determinations were performed during the next two hours:

| $PaO_2$ | $PaCO_2$ | pH |
|---------|----------|------|
| 54 | 39 | 7.40 |
| 166 | 23 | 7.57 |
| 435 | 17 | 7.63 |

## EXERCISE 12

### ■ Questions:

1. What is this infant's diagnosis?

2. What are the important steps in the initial management of this child?

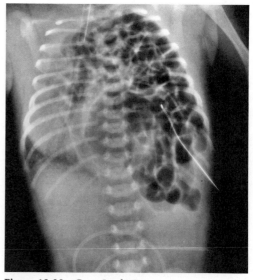

**Figure 18-28**   Case Study 9.

■ **Discussion:**

This child has a left-sided diaphragmatic hernia with distention of the bowel and mediastinal shift to the right. Newborn infants with this malformation are generally intubated shortly after birth because of severe respiratory distress. In addition, an orogastric tube should be placed to decompress the stomach and prevent further distention of the bowel contents within the hemithorax. The child's blood gas determinations demonstrate the presence of well-developed lung parenchyma as evidenced by a $PaO_2$ as high as 435 mm Hg and relative ease of $CO_2$ elimination with moderate ventilatory assistance.

The child obviously will require repair of his diaphragmatic hernia; however, the timing of this repair is controversial and will be discussed in the next section. The plan for this particular child was to proceed with observation for a few days before undertaking repair of the diaphragmatic defect. Unfortunately, between 36 and 48 hours of age, the child proceeded to deteriorate and was unresponsive to maximal medical management. The best arterial blood gas determination during a 4-hour period was $PaO_2$, 45 mm Hg; $PaCO_2$, 34 mm Hg; and pH, 7.54. ($FiO_2$, 1.0; ventilatory rate, 80; inspiratory pressure/PEEP pressure, 38/4 cm $H_2O$; and mean airway pressure, 19.4 cm $H_2O$.)

■ **Question:**

What is the appropriate management of the child at this point?

■ **Discussion:**

Although perhaps controversial, the decision for this child was to proceed with extracorporeal membrane oxygenation (ECMO). This was instituted and the child stabilized with the assistance of cardiopulmonary bypass. Forty-eight hours later the child underwent uneventful repair of the diaphragmatic hernia on ECMO. The radiograph shown in Figure 18-29 demonstrates the final repair of the diaphragm, which was closed primarily. A small left lung was noted at the time of surgery. The child tolerated a gentle wean from ECMO support and was taken off bypass after 132 hours. Ventilatory assistance was required for an additional 6 days following which he was extu-

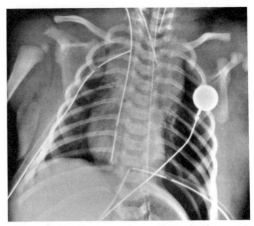

**Figure 18-29** Postoperative radiograph after repair of a congenital diaphragmatic hernia. ECMO cannulas in place.

bated and weaned to room air within 24 hours. The child has subsequently done well.

**General Overview**

Numerous congenital abnormalities of the oral cavity, neck, larynx, and upper airway can cause severe airway compromise in the newborn. In addition, abnormalities of the trachea and bronchi including agenesis, stenosis, and anomalous bronchi can cause severe respiratory problems. Anomalous vessels such as a pulmonary artery sling or aortic arch anomaly can lead to extraluminal obstruction of the airway. Parenchymal problems noted at birth include intrinsic processes such as lung cysts and congenital cystic adenomatoid malformations or extrinsic lesions such as congenital diaphragmatic hernia that cause displacement of the developing lung. This section is limited to a discussion of cystic malformations and congenital diaphragmatic hernia.

**Congenital Diaphragmatic Hernia**

Congenital diaphragmatic hernia results from a defect in the pleuroperitoneal membrane of the developing diaphragm. The anomaly is located on the left side in 88% of patients, usually at the area of the posterolateral foramen of Bochdalek. The opening in the diaphragm allows the viscera to enter the chest between the 8th and 12th week of fetal life. The herniated intestine, spleen, and occasionally stomach and liver act as a mass effect in the thoracic cavity preventing normal lung development. This defect is often diagnosed by prenatal ultrasound, and the presence of polyhydramnios on ultrasound in association with diaphragmatic hernia is a very poor prognostic sign. If the diaphragmatic hernia is diagnosed antenatally, the child should be delivered at a facility with a neonatal intensive care unit.

Neonates delivered with an unsuspected diaphragmatic hernia usually develop respiratory distress in the delivery room or shortly thereafter, depending on the degree of pulmonary hypoplasia and the occurrence of pulmonary hypertension. Air passing into the intestinal tract can lead to an increase in the volume of the herniated viscera producing further mediastinal shift, which interferes with ventilation of the contralateral lung. On physical examination, bowel sounds may be noted on the left side of the chest. Breath sounds on that side of the chest are almost always decreased compared to the contralateral hemithorax. The diagnosis can usually be confirmed by the chest radiograph. The presence of the stomach or liver in the left hemithorax correlates with a poorer prognosis.

The treatment of congenital diaphragmatic hernia is currently controversial. Several factors, however, are not controversial and those include the stabilization and preoperative preparation, which would include endotracheal intubation and control of ventilation. An orogastric tube is placed to decompress the stomach and decrease passage of air through the gastrointestinal tract. The child is monitored with an umbilical arterial line as well as a right radial arterial line if possible, allowing measurement of $PaO_2$, pH, and $PaCO_2$. Fluid management must be carefully monitored to avoid hypovolemia or fluid overload because a significant number of these neonates may demonstrate inappropriate antidiuretic hormone release after surgery.

Controversy centers on the type of ventilation, timing of operative repair of the diaphragmatic hernia, and use of ECMO should the child fail conventional management. The ventilatory management of a child with diaphragmatic hernia includes attempts to minimize or reverse any element of pulmonary hypertension. This is beyond the scope of this section and is discussed in Chapter 13 on pulmonary hypertension. The controversy over the use of ECMO centers around the actual criteria at which to institute ECMO. Despite

the controversy, numerous studies have demonstrated ECMO improves survival of patients with congenital diaphragmatic hernia.

Numerous parameters have been established to characterize the severity of the child's respiratory status including the alveolar-arterial gradient ($AaDO_2$), oxygenation index (OI) and ventilatory index (VI):

$$AaDO_2 = FiO_2 \ (P_B - P_{H_2O}) - PaCO_2/0.8 - PaO_2, \ [P_B = \text{barometric pressure (760 mm Hg)}, \ P_{H_2O} = \text{water vapor pressure (47 mm Hg)}]$$

$$OI = \text{mean airway pressure (MAP)} \times FiO_2 \times 100/PaO_2$$

$$VI = \text{ventilatory rate} \times MAP.$$

Based on the initial blood gas values in the case presentation, the following calculations were made: $AaDO_2 = 610$, OI = 25, and VI = 828. Although the $AaDO_2$ is quite high, the other values are not as elevated. Furthermore, with subsequent blood gas determinations, the $AaDO_2$ and OI fell dramatically. As the $PaO_2$ and $PaCO_2$ improved, the ventilatory pressure was dropped and the MAP subsequently decreased. At the time of deterioration, the MAP was 19.4 cm $H_2O$. The following calculations were made at that point: $AaDO_2 = 626$, OI = 43, and VI = 1,552. According to criteria established for our patient population, all of the values indicate an unfavorable prognosis, and the patient was placed on ECMO with parental consent.

Although the field of extracorporeal support is in considerable flux, the current preference at the author's institution is to use ECMO to support those patients that fail standard ventilatory management including the use of high-frequency ventilation. Definitive criteria for ECMO include an OI greater than 40 for 2 hours or an $AaDO_2$ greater than 630 for 4 hours. If a neonate is in the process of deteriorating and has an OI greater than 35 for 2 to 4 hours or an $AaDO_2$ greater than 600 for 2 to 4 hours, consideration would be given to instituting ECMO.

In the current case, an excellent $PaO_2$ was documented early in the patient's course, indicating that the deterioration was in large part a result of reactive pulmonary hypertension and not severe pulmonary hypoplasia (in which case a high PaO$_2$ would never be achievable). Neonates who have a diaphragmatic hernia who never achieve a PaO$_2$ > 100 torr or a PaCO$_2$ < 40 torr while receiving assisted ventilation exhibit a much lower survival rate than those who do. Note, however, that when high-risk criteria are applied to a large group of infants with diaphragmatic hernias, some infants will survive with the help of ECMO who would have been predicted to die based on blood gas criteria or other unfavorable prognostic indices. These high-risk neonates with diaphragmatic hernia can present a difficult ethical and psychosocial issue for the neonatologist. The data on the child must be carefully reviewed in an attempt to estimate the degree of overall pulmonary hypoplasia. If ECMO is considered to be a supportive option, the family must be carefully counseled as to the nature of the therapy (risks and benefits) and must be aware that if the pulmonary hypoplasia is severe, ECMO will likely be of no benefit.

The timing of repair of congenital diaphragmatic hernia has changed over the past decade. Bohn's group noted decreased compliance of the chest after repair and suggested that the role of urgent surgery should be reevaluated. In view of these data, most centers throughout the country currently tend to delay operative repair of the diaphragmatic hernia in an attempt to allow stabilization of the child. A recent report with operative delay and preoperative ECMO did not demonstrate any improvement in survival but did note fewer late deaths and fewer pulmonary sequelae when compared to immediate surgery with postoperative ECMO.

The current preference at the author's institution is to use an approach of delayed surgical management. The child is stabilized with ventilatory support in an attempt to keep the PaCO$_2$ below 40 (preferably 35) and pH ≥ 7.45. If the child stabilizes with an adequate PaO$_2$ (>100 torr), the child is taken for diaphragmatic hernia repair at 48 to 72 hours. If the child deteriorates pre- or postoperatively and meets criteria for ECMO (as stated above), we would proceed with the use of ECMO. If the child has never achieved an acceptable PaO$_2$ or PaCO$_2$, the use of ECMO must be carefully considered because the infant may have severely hypoplastic lungs.

In a child who requires ECMO preoperatively, the diaphragmatic hernia can be repaired while on ECMO, usually 48 to 72 hours after going on bypass. This is a difficult procedure in the face of systemic heparinization; however, with the use of meticulous hemostasis, the procedure can usually be safely accomplished. The operative repair of diaphragmatic hernia is a relatively straightforward procedure. A standard posterolateral defect in the diaphragm can usually be repaired primarily. In cases compounded by herniation of the stomach and/or liver, there is frequently an absent diaphragm, which may require replacement with a prosthetic patch.

Intrauterine repair of congenital diaphragmatic hernias has been reported by Harrison and colleagues. This approach may offer a therapy to interrupt the pathophysiological process that, undeterred, results in pulmonary hypoplasia. This early success of this repair on a small number of patients is encouraging, but needs further evaluation before it can be applied to the general population of patients diagnosed *in utero* with diaphragmatic hernia.

### Congenital Cystic Lung Disease

Congenital cystic adenomatoid malformation (CCAM) is a result of overgrowth of terminal bronchiolar structures with a lack of mature alveoli. These lesions can be primarily cystic or solid. Approximately one-third of affected fetuses are hydropic and stillborn. Those infants discovered to have CCAM after birth usually present immediately with pulmonary compromise secondary to pulmonary hypoplasia or they soon exhibit respiratory compromise as the cyst fills with air. CCAM can also present in an older child with a primary cystic lesion. Figure 18-30 demonstrates a rather typical appearance for an infant with CCAM. This child did well with excision of the left upper lobe and lingula. Management of these children is primarily aimed at controlling the airway and optimizing the respiratory status prior to surgical excision. ECMO has occasionally been utilized to salvage some of these infants who have developed severe pulmonary hypertension around the time of surgical excision. The fetus diagnosed with a solid CCAM and fetal hydrops rarely survives and may be a candidate for open fetal surgery. This procedure has been performed successfully by Harrison and colleagues.

Simple congenital lung cysts can also present in the newborn due to mass displace-

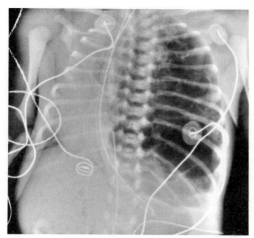

**Figure 18-30** Radiograph of a primarily cystic CCAM.

ment of the hemithorax. The patient in Figure 18-31 presented shortly after birth with severe respiratory distress and was noted to have an air- and fluid-filled cyst occupying the entire left hemithorax. The child needed an emergent left lower lobectomy for removal of the cystic malformation and then, because of severe pulmonary hypertension, required ECMO support. The child subsequently did well.

Congenital lobar emphysema or hyperinflation of a single lobe can present with tachy-

pnea, retractions, and wheezing. Approximately one-half of these infants present shortly after birth, with the remainder presenting within the first few months of life. These lesions are characterized by hyperexpansion of the involved lobe with mediastinal shift to the contralateral side. The left upper lobe is the most commonly involved lobe followed by the right middle lobe. Congenital heart disease can be associated in 13% of the affected infants and an echocardiogram should be performed preoperatively in these children. A pulmonary artery sling can lead to right-sided congenital emphysema and should be treated with transposition of the vessel rather than lobectomy. Therapy for a symptomatic infant or child with congenital lobar emphysema is generally lobectomy. Children with lobar emphysema but few or no symptoms require no treatment and many have normal pulmonary function.

## BIBLIOGRAPHY

### Abdominal Wall Defects

1. Mollitt DL, Ballantine TVN, Grosfeld JL, et al: A critical assessment of fluid requirements in gastroschisis. *J Pediatr Surg* 1978; 13:217.
2. Philippart AI, Canty TG, Filler RM: Acute fluid requirements in infants with anterior abdominal wall defects. *J Pediatr Surg* 1972; 7:353.
3. Grosfeld JL, Dawes L, Weber TR: Congenital abdominal wall defects: Current management and survival. *Surg Clin N Am* 1981; 61:1037.
4. Grosfeld JL, Weber TR: Congenital abdominal wall defects: Gastroschisis and omphalocele. In Ravitch MM, ed: *Current Problems in Surgery*. Chicago, Year Book Medical Publishers, 1982, p. 159.
5. Shaw A: The myth of gastroschisis. *J Pediatr Surg* 1975; 10:235.
6. deVries PA: The pathogenesis of gastroschisis and omphalocele. *J Pediatr Surg* 1980; 15:245.
7. Lenke RR, Hatch EI Jr: Fetal gastroschisis: A preliminary report advocating the use of cesarean section. *Obstet Gynecol* 1986; 67:395.
8. Schipul AH, Roberts EF, Hunter VP, et al: Diagnosis and management of fetal gastroschisis. *Perinatol Neonatol* 1987; (Nov/Dec): 19.
9. Sipes SL, Weiner CP, Sipes DR II: Gastroschisis and omphalocele: Does either antenatal diagnosis or route of delivery make a difference in perinatal outcome? *Obstet Gynecol* 1990; 76:195.
10. Bethel CA, Seashore JH, Touloukian RJ: Cesarean section does not improve outcome in gastroschisis. *J Pediatr Surg* 1989; 24:1.
11. Yaster M, Scherer LR, Stone MM, et al: Prediction of successful primary closure of congeni-

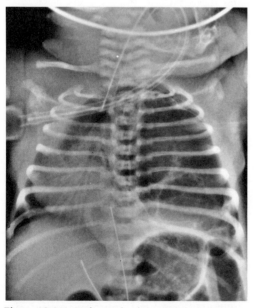

**Figure 18-31** Radiograph of a congenital cyst of the left lower lobe.

tal abdominal wall defects using intraoperative measurements. *J Pediatr Surg* 1989; 24:1217.

12. Amoury RA, Ashcraft KW, Holder TM: Gastroschisis complicated by intestinal atresia. *Surgery* 1977; 82:373.

13. Muraji T, Tsugawa C, Nishijima E, et al: Gastroschisis: A 17-year experience. *J Pediatr Surg* 1989; 24:343.

14. Hrabovsky EE, Boyd JB, Savrin RA, et al: Advances in the management of gastroschisis. *Ann Surg* 1980; 192:244.

15. Caniano DA, Brokaw B, Ginn-Pease ME: An individualized approach to the management of gastroschisis. *J Pediatr Surg* 1990; 25:297.

16. Greenwood RD, Rosenthal A, Nadas AS: Cardiovascular malformations associated with omphaloceles. *J Pediatr* 1974; 85:818.

17. Allen RG: Omphalocele and gastroschisis. In Holder TM, Ashcraft KW, eds: *Pediatric Surgery*. Philadelphia, WB Saunders Co, 1980, p. 572.

18. Cantrell JR, Haller JA, Ravitch MM: A syndrome of congenital defects involving the anterior abdominal wall, sternum, diaphragm, pericardium and heart. *Surg Gynecol Obstet* 1958; 107:602.

## Obstructive Lesions of the Gastrointestinal Tract

19. Phelan JP, Ahn MO, Smith CV, et al: Amniotic fluid index measurements during pregnancy. *J Reprod Med* 1987; 32:601.

20. Phelan JP, Martin GI: Polyhydramnios: Fetal and neonatal implications. *Clin Perinatol* 1989; 16:987.

21. Desmedt EJ, Henry OA, Beischer NA: Polyhydramnios and associated maternal and fetal complications in singleton pregnancies. *Br J Obstet Gynaecol* 1990; 97:1115.

22. Phelan JP, Park YW, Ahn MO, et al: Polyhydramnios and perinatal outcome. *J Perinatol* 1990; 10:347.

23. Lilien D, Srinivasan G, Pyati SP, et al: Green vomiting in the first 72 hours in normal infants. *AJDC* 1986; 140:662.

24. Berdon WE, Baker DH, Santulli TV, et al: Microcolon in newborn infants with intestinal obstruction. Its correlation with the level and time of onset of obstruction. *Radiology* 1968; 90:878.

25. Gutman FM, Braun P, Bensoussan AL, et al: The pathogenesis of intestinal atresia. *Surg Gynecol Obstet* 1975; 141:203.

26. Leonidas JC: Microcolon in the absence of small bowel obstruction in the newborn. *J Pediatr Surg* 1989; 24:180.

## Esophageal Atresia and Tracheoesophageal Fistula

27. Ein SH, Shandling B, Wesson D, et al: Esophageal atresia with distal tracheoesophageal fistula: Associated anomalies and prognosis in the 1980's. *J Pediatr Surg* 1989; 24:1055.

28. Gross RE: *Surgery of Infancy and Childhood*. Philadelphia, WB Saunders Co, 1953, p. 75.

29. Holder RM, Cloud DT, Lewis JE Jr, et al: Esophageal atresia and tracheoesophageal fistula. A survey of its members by the Surgical Section of the American Academy of Pediatrics. *Pediatrics* 1961; 34:542.

30. Randolph JG: Esophageal atresia and congenital stenosis. In Welch KJ, Randolph JG, Ravitch MM, et al, eds: *Pediatric Surgery*. Chicago, Year Book Medical Publishers, 1986, p. 682.

31. Goh DW, Brereton RJ, Spitz L: Esophageal atresia with obstructed tracheoesophageal fistula and gasless abdomen. *J Pediatr Surg* 1991; 26:160.

32. Grosfeld JL, Ballantine TVN: Esophageal atresia and tracheoesophageal fistula: Effect of delayed thoracotomy on survival. *Surgery* 1978; 84:394.

33. Waterston BJ, Bonham-Carter RE, Aberdeen E: Oesophageal atresia: Tracheoesophageal fistula. A study of survival in 218 infants. *Lancet* 1962; 1:819.

34. Randolph JG, Altman RP, Anderson KD: Selective surgical management based upon clinical status in infants with esophageal atresia. *J Thoracic Cardiovasc Surg* 1977; 74:335.

35. Randolph JG, Newman KD, Anderson KD: Current results in repair of esophageal atresia with tracheoesophageal fistula using physiologic status as a guide to therapy. *Ann Surg* 1989; 209:526.

36. Pohlson EC, Schaller RT, Tapper D: Improved survival with primary anastomosis in the low birth weight neonate with esophageal atresia and tracheoesophageal fistula. *J Pediatr Surg* 1988; 23:418.

37. Fann JI, Hartman GE, Shochat SJ: "Waterseal" gastrostomy in the management of premature infants with tracheoesophageal fistula and pulmonary insufficiency. *J Pediatr Surg* 1988; 23:29.

38. Richenbacher WE, Ballantine TVN: Esophageal atresia, distal tracheoesophageal fistula, and an air shunt that compromised mechanical ventilation. *J Pediatr Surg* 1990; 25:1216.

39. Filston HC, Chitwood WR, Schkolne B, et al: The Fogarty balloon catheter as an aid to management of the infant with esophageal atresia and tracheoesophageal fistula complicated by severe RDS or pneumonia. *J Pediatr Surg* 1982; 17:149.

40. Donn SM, Zak LK, Bozynski MA, et al: Use of high-frequency jet ventilation in the management of congenital tracheoesophageal fistula associated with respiratory distress syndrome. *J Pediatr Surg* 1990; 25:1219.

41. Templeton JM, Templeton JJ, Schnaufer L, et al: Management of esophageal atresia and tracheoesophageal fistula in the neonate with severe respiratory distress syndrome. *J Pediatr Surg* 1985; 20:394.

42. Randolph JG, Tunell WP, Lilly JR: Gastric division in the critically ill infant with esophageal atresia and tracheoesophageal fistula. *Surgery* 1968; 63:496.

43. Ogita S, Tokiwa K, Takahashi T: Transabdominal closure of tracheoesophageal fistula: A new procedure for the management of poor-

risk esophageal atresia with tracheoesophageal fistula. *J Pediatr Surg* 1986; 21:812.

44. Fagelman KM, Boyarsky A: Temporary banding of the gastroesophageal junction in the critically ill neonate with esophageal atresia and tracheoesophageal fistula. *Surgery* 1985; 98:594.

45. Kosloske AM, Jewell PF, Cartwright KC: Crucial bronchoscopic findings in esophageal atresia and tracheoesophageal fistula. *J Pediatr Surg* 1988; 23:466.

46. Anderson KD: Replacement of the esophagus. In Welch KJ, Randolph JG, Ravitch MM, et al, eds: *Pediatric Surgery.* Chicago, Year Book Medical Publishers, 1986, p. 704.

47. Campbell JR, Webber BR, Harrison MW: Esophageal replacement in infants and children by colon interposition. *Am J Surg* 1982; 144:31.

48. Anderson KD, Randolph JG: The gastric tube for esophageal replacement in children. *J Thoracic Cardiovasc Surg* 1973; 66:333.

49. Saeki M, Tsuchida Y, Ogata T, et al: Long-term results of jejunal replacement of the esophagus. *J Pediatr Surg* 1988; 23:483.

50. Lindahl H, Rintala R, Louhimo I: Failure of the Nissen fundoplication to control gastroesophageal reflux in esophageal atresia patients. *J Pediatr Surg* 1989; 24:985.

**Pyloric Web/Atresia**

51. Lloyd JR, Clatworthy HW Jr: Hydramnios as an aid to the early diagnosis of congenital obstruction of the alimentary tract: A study of the maternal and fetal factors. *Pediatrics* 1958; 21:903.

52. Bar-Maor JA, Nissan S, Nevo S: Pyloric atresia: A hereditary anomaly with autosomal-recessive transmission. *J Med Gen* 1972; 9:70.

53. Bull MJ: Epidermolysis bullosa-pyloric atresia. An autosomal-recessive syndrome. *Am J Dis Child* 1983; 137:449.

54. Muller M, Morger R, Engert J: Pyloric atresia: Report of four cases and review of the literature. *Pediatr Surg Int* 1990; 5:276.

55. Ishihara M, Yamazaki T, Ariwa R, et al: Aberrant pancreatic tissue causing pyloric obstruction. *Pediatr Surg Int* 1990; 5:140.

56. Mogilner JG, Vinograd I, Presman A, et al: Pyloric duplication in children. *Pediatr Surg Int* 1990; 5:61.

**Duodenal Atresia**

57. Grosfeld JL, Rescorla FJ: Duodenal atresia and stenosis: Reassessment of treatment and outcome based on antenatal diagnosis, pathologic variance and long-term follow-up. *Surgery* 1993; in press.

58. Tandler J: Entwicklungsgeschichte des menschlichen Duodenum. *Morhol Jahrb* 1902; 29:187.

59. Hancock BJ, Wiseman NE: Congenital duodenal obstruction: The impact of an antenatal diagnosis: *J Pediatr Surg* 1989; 24:1027.

60. Rescorla FJ, Grosfeld JL: Duodenal atresia in infancy and childhood: Improved survival and longterm followup. *Contemp Surg* 1988; 33:22.

61. Kullendorf CM: Atresia of the small bowel. *Ann Chir Gynecol* 1983; 72:192.

**Malrotation and Midgut Volvulus**

62. Snyder WH, Chaffin L: Embryology and pathology of the intestinal tract: Presentation of 48 cases of malrotation. *Ann Surg* 1954; 140:368.

63. Ladd WE: Congenital obstruction of the duodenum in children. *N Engl J Med* 1932; 206:277.

64. Ladd WE: Surgical diseases of the alimentary tract in infants. *N Engl J Med* 1936; 215:705.

65. Rescorla FJ, Shedd FJ, Grosfeld JL, et al: Anomalies of intestinal rotation in childhood: Analysis of 447 cases. *Surgery* 1990; 108:710.

66. Powell DM, Othersen HB, Smith CD: Malrotation of the intestines in children. The effect of age on presentation and therapy. *J Pediatr Surg* 1989; 24:777.

67. Filston HC, Kirks DR: Malrotation—the ubiquitous anomaly. *J Pediatr Surg* 1981; 16:614.

**Jejunoileal Atresia**

68. Louw JH: Investigations into the etiology of congenital atresia of the colon. *Dis Colon Rectum* 1964; 7:471.

69. Santulli TV, Blanc WA: Congenital atresia of the intestine: Pathogenesis and treatment. *Ann Surg* 1961; 154:939.

70. Abrams JS: Experimental intestinal atresia. *Surgery* 1968; 64:185.

71. Koga Y, Hayashida Y, Ikeda K, et al: Intestinal atresia in fetal dogs produced by localized ligation of mesenteric vessels. *J Pediatr Surg* 1975; 10:949.

72. Louw JH, Barnard CN: Congenital intestinal atresia: Observations on its origin. *Lancet* 1955; 2:1065.

73. Grosfeld JL, Ballantine TVN, Shoemaker R: Operative management of intestinal atresia and stenosis based on pathologic findings. *J Pediatr Surg* 1979; 14:368.

74. Rescorla FJ, Grosfeld JL: Intestinal atresia and stenosis: Analysis of survival in 120 cases. *Surgery* 1985; 98:668.

**Meconium Ileus**

75. Donnison AB, Shwachman H, Gross RE: Review of 164 children with meconium ileus seen at the Children's Hospital Medical Center. *Boston Pediatr* 1966; 37:833.

76. Rescorla FJ, Grosfeld JL, West KW, et al: Changing patterns of treatment and survival in neonates with meconium ileus. *Arch Surg* 1989; 124:837.

77. Brock D: A comparative study of microvillar enzyme activities in the prenatal diagnosis of cystic fibrosis. *Prenat Diag* 1985; 5:129.

78. Riordan J, Rommens JM, Kerem BS, et al: Identification of the cystic fibrosis gene: Cloning and characterization of complimentary DNA. *Science* 1989; 245:1066.

79. Rommens JM, Iannuzzi MC, Kerem BS, et al: Identification of the cystic fibrosis gene. Chro-

mosome walking and jumping. *Science* 1989; 245:1059.

80. Kerem BS, Rommens JM, Buchanan JA, et al: Identification of the cystic fibrosis gene: Genetic analysis. *Science* 1989; 245:1073.

81. Collins FS, Riordan J, Tsui LL: The cystic fibrosis gene: Isolation and significance. *Hosp Practice* 1990; 25:47.

82. Trulock EP, Cooper JD, Kaiser LR, et al: The Washington University Barnes Hospital experience with lung transplantation. *JAMA* 1991; 266:1943.

83. Fleischer AC, Davis RJ, Campbell L: Sonographic detection of a meconium-containing mass in a fetus: A case report. *JCU* 1983; 11:103.

84. Noblett HR: Treatment of uncomplicated meconium ileus by Gastrografin enema: A preliminary report. *J Pediatr Surg* 1969; 4:190.

85. Stringer DA: Congenital and developmental anomalies of the small bowel. In Stringer DA, ed: *Pediatric Gastrointestinal Imaging*. Philadelphia, BC Decker, 1989, p. 259.

86. Hiatt RB, Wilson PE: Celiac syndrome: Therapy of meconium ileus: Report of eight cases with a review of the literature. *Surg Gynecol Obstet* 1948; 87:317.

87. Rescorla FJ, Grosfeld JL: Comtemporary management of meconium ileus. *Surgery* 1993; in press.

**Colonic Atresia**

88. Schiller M, Aviad I, Freund H: Congenital colonic atresia and stenosis: *Am J Surg* 1979; 138:721.

89. Boles ET, Vassy LE, Ralston M: Atresia of the colon. *J Pediatr Surg* 1976; 11:69.

90. Coran AG, Eraklis AJ: Atresia of the colon. *Surgery* 1969; 65:828.

91. Powell RW, Raffensperger JG: Congenital colonic atresia. *J Pediatr Surg* 1982; 17:166.

**Meconium Plug Syndrome/Small Left Colon Syndrome**

92. Davis WS, Allen RP, Favara BE, et al: The neonatal small left colon syndrome. *Am J Roentgenol Radium Ther Nucl Med* 1974; 120:322.

93. Davis WS, Campbell JB: Neonatal small left colon syndrome. *Am J Dis Child* 1975; 129:1024.

94. Philippart AI, Reed JO, Georgeson KE: Neonatal small left colon syndrome: Intramural not intraluminal obstruction. *J Pediatr Surg* 1975; 10:733.

95. Philippart AI: Atresia, stenosis, and other obstructions of the colon. In Welch KJ, Randolph JG, Ravitch MM, et al, eds: *Pediatric Surgery*. Chicago, Year Book Medical Publishers, 1986, p. 984.

96. Nixon GW, Condon VR, Stewart DR: Intestinal perforation as a complication of the neonatal small left colon syndrome. *Am J Roentgenol* 1975; 125:75.

97. Clatworthy HW Jr, Howard WH, Lloyd J: The

98. Eillis DG, Clatworthy HW Jr: The meconium plug syndrome revisited. *J Pediatr Surg* 1966; 1:54.

**Meconium Disease of Preterm Infants**

99. Rickham PP, Boeckman CR: Neonatal meconium obstruction in the absence of mucoviscidosis. *Am J Surg* 1965; 106:173.

100. Shigemoto H, Isomoto T, Horiga Y, et al: Inspissated meconium syndrome: Neonatal meconium obstruction in the ileum without mucoviscidosis. *Kaws Med J* 1978; 4:293.

101. Cremin BJ, Smagthe PM, Cywes S: The radiological appearance of the "inspissated milk syndrome": A cause of intestinal obstruction in infants. *Br J Radiol* 1970; 43:856.

102. Konvolinka CW, Frederick J: Milk curd syndrome in neonates. *J Pediatr Surg* 1989; 24:497.

103. Vinograd I, Mogle P, Peleg O, et al: Meconium disease in premature infants with very low birth weight. *J Pediatr* 1983; 103:963.

**Hirschsprung's Disease**

104. Rescorla FJ, Morrison AM, Engles D, et al: Hirschsprung's disease: Evaluation of mortality and long term function in 260 cases. *Arch Surg* 1992; 127:934–942.

105. Smith GHH, Cass D: Infantile Hirschsprung's disease—Is a barium enema useful? *Pediatr Surg Int* 1991; 6:318.

106. Taxman TL, Barry SY, Rothstein FC: How useful is the barium enema in the diagnosis of infantile Hirschsprung's disease? *Am J DC* 1986; 140:881.

107. Carcassonne M, Guys JM, Morisson-Lacombe G: Management of Hirschsprung's disease: Curative surgery before 3 months of age. *J Pediatr Surg* 1989; 24:1032.

**Imperforate Anus**

108. Donaldson JS, Black CT, Reynolds M, et al: Ultrasound of the distal pouch in infants with imperforate anus. *J Pediatr Surg* 1989; 24:465.

109. Smith ED: The bath water needs changing, but don't throw out the baby: An overview of anorectal anomalies. *J Pediatr Surg* 1987; 22:335.

110. deVries PA, Pena A: Posterior sagittal anorectoplasty. *J Pediatr Surg* 1982; 17:638.

**Other Abdominal Conditions**

**Incarcerated Inguinal Hernia**

111. Shrock P: The processus vaginalis and gubernaculum. *Surg Clin North Am* 1971; 51:1263.

112. Rowe MI, Clatworthy HW: Incarcerated and strangulated hernias in children. *Arch Surg* 1970; 101:136.

113. Rowe MI, Marchildon MD: Inguinal hernia and hydrocele in infants and children. *Surg Clin North Am* 1981; 61:1137.

114. Farrow GA, Thompson S: Incarcerated inguinal hernia in infants and children: A five year

review at the Hospital for Sick Children, Toronto, 1955 to 1959 inclusive. *Can J Surg* 1963; 6:63.

115. Puri P, Guiney EJ, O'Donnel B: Inguinal hernia in infants: The fate of the testis following incarceration. *J Pediatr Surg* 1984; 19:44.

116. Rescorla FJ, Grosfeld JL: Inguinal hernia repair in the perinatal period and early infancy: Clinical considerations. *J Pediatr Surg* 1984; 19:832.

117. Slowman JG, Mylius RE: Testicular infarction in infancy: Its association with irreducible inguinal hernia. *Med J Aust* 1958; 1:242.

118. Grosfeld JL, Minnick K, Shedd F, et al: Inguinal hernia in children: Factors affecting recurrence in 62 cases. *J Pediatr Surg* 1991; 26:283.

119. Clatworthy HW, Thompson AG: Incarcerated and strangulated inguinal hernia in infants: A preventable risk. *JAMA* 1954; 154:123.

## Thoracic Problems

120. Luck SR, Reynolds M, Raffensperger JG: Congenital bronchopulmonary malformations. In Ravitch MM, ed: *Current Problems in Surgery.* Chicago, Year Book Medical Publishers, 1986, p. 251.

## Surgically Correctable Neonatal Respiratory Problems

### Congenital Diaphragmatic Hernia

121. Adzick NS, Vacanti JP, Lillehei CW, et al: Fetal diaphragmatic hernia: Ultrasound diagnosis and clinical outcome in 38 cases. *J Pediatr Surg* 1989; 24:654.

122. Adzick NS, Harrison MR, Glick PL, et al: Diaphragmatic hernia in the fetus: Prenatal diagnosis and outcome in 94 cases. *J Pediatr Surg* 1985; 20:357.

123. Burge DM, Atwell JD, Freeman NV: Could the stomach site help predict outcome in babies with left sided congenital diaphragmatic hernia diagnosed antenatally? *J Pediatr Surg* 1989; 24:567.

124. Touloukian RJ, Markowitz RI: A preoperative x-ray scoring system for risk assessment of newborns with congenital diaphragmatic hernia. *J Pediatr Surg* 1984; 19:252.

125. Rowe MI, Smith SD, Cheu H: Inappropriate fluid response in congenital diaphragmatic hernia: First report of a frequent occurrence. *J Pediatr Surg* 1988; 23:1147.

126. Bohn DJ, James RM, Filler SH, et al: The relationship between $PaCO_2$ and ventilation parameters in predicting survival in congenital diaphragmatic hernia. *J Pediatr Surg* 1984; 19:666.

127. Beck R, Anderson KD, Pearson GD, et al: Criteria for extracorporeal membrane oxygenation in a population of infants with persistent pulmonary hypertension of the newborn. *J Pediatr Surg* 1986; 21:297.

128. Johnston PW, Bashner B, Liverman R, et al: Clinical use of extracorporeal membrane oxygenation in the treatment of persistent pulmonary hypertension following surgical repair of congenital diaphragmatic hernia. *J Pediatr Surg* 1988; 23:908.

129. Heiss K, Manning P, Oldham KT, et al: Reversal of mortality for congenital diaphragmatic hernia with ECMO. *Ann Surg* 1988; 209:225.

130. Bartlett RH, Toomasian J, Roloff D, et al: Extracorporeal membrane oxygenation (ECMO) in neonatal respiratory failure. *Ann Surg* 1986; 204:236.

131. O'Rourke PP, Lillehei CW, Crone RK, et al: The effect of extracorporeal membrane oxygenation on the survival of neonates with high-risk congenital diaphragmatic hernia: 45 cases from a single institution. *J Pediatr Surg* 1991; 26:147.

132. Bohn D, Tamura M, Perrin D, et al: Ventilatory predictors of pulmonary hypoplasia in congenital diaphragmatic hernia, confirmed by morphologic assessment. *J Pediatr* 1984; 19:666.

133. Karl SR, Ballantine TV, Snider MT, et al: High-frequency ventilation at rates of 375 to 1800 cycles per minute in four neonates with congenital diaphragmatic hernia. *J Pediatr Surg* 1983; 18:822.

134. Newman KD, Anderson KD, Meurs KV, et al: Extracorporeal membrane oxygenation and congenital diaphragmatic hernia: Should any infant be excluded? *J Pediatr Surg* 1990; 25:1048.

135. Sakai H, Tamura M, Hosokawa Y, et al: Effect of surgical repair on respiratory mechanics in congenital diaphragmatic hernia. *J Pediatr Surg* 1987; 111:432.

136. Langer JC, Filler RM, Bohn DJ, et al: Timing of surgery for congenital diaphragmatic hernia: Is emergency operation necessary? *J Pediatr Surg* 1988; 23:731.

137. Breaux CW, Rouse TM, Caine WS, et al: Improvement in survival of patients with congenital diaphragmatic hernia utilizing a strategy of delayed repair after medical and/or extracorporeal membrane oxygenation stabilization. *J Pediatr Surg* 1991; 26:333.

138. Wilson JM, Lund DP, Lillehei CW, et al: Delayed surgery and preoperative ECMO does not improve survival in high risk congenital diaphragmatic hernia. Presented at 7th Annual Children's National Medical Center ECMO Symposium, Breckenridge, Colorado, February 24–28, 1991.

139. Connors RH, Tracy T, Bailey PV, et al: Congenital diaphragmatic hernia repair on ECMO. *J Pediatr Surg* 1990; 25:1043.

140. Harrison MR, Adzick NS, Longaker MT, et al: Successful repair in utero of a fetal diaphragmatic hernia after removal of herniated viscera from the left thorax. *N Engl J Med* 1990; 322:1582.

141. Harrison MR, Langer JC, Adzick NS, et al: Correction of congenital diaphragmatic hernia in utero. V. Initial clinical experience. *J Pediatr Surg* 1990; 25:47.

### Congenital Cystic Lung Disease

142. Adzick NS, Harrison MR, Glick PL, et al: Fetal cystic adenomatoid malformation: Prenatal di-

agnosis and natural history. *J Pediatr Surg* 1985; 20:483.

143. Rescorla FJ, West KW, Vane DW, et al: Pulmonary hypertension in neonatal cystic lung disease: Survival following lobectomy and ECMO in two cases. *J Pediatr Surg* 1990; 25:1054.

144. Longaker MT, Golbus MS, Filly RA, et al: Maternal outcome after open fetal surgery. *JAMA* 1991; 265:737.

145. Eigen H, Lemen RJ, Waring WW: Congenital lobar emphysema: Long-term evaluation of surgically and conservatively treated children. *Am Rev Resp Dis* 1976; 113:823.

# Chapter 19

# NECROTIZING ENTEROCOLITIS: DIFFERENTIAL DIAGNOSIS AND MANAGEMENT

☐ ☐ ☐ ☐ ☐ ☐

## *Robert M. Kliegman,* M.D.

Necrotizing enterocolitis (NEC) is the most common, acquired serious gastrointestinal illness among neonates. Manifestations of NEC cover a broad spectrum from mild abdominal distention with hematochezia to a fulminant septic shock-like picture with transmural necrosis of the entire gastrointestinal tract. Because of its wide range of clinical manifestations, NEC may be confused with other common benign or serious primary gastrointestinal diseases affecting the infant. Furthermore, many systemic illnesses that affect the infant (e.g., sepsis) often produce secondary gastrointestinal disturbances such as ileus and hemorrhage that many mimic NEC. A careful and detailed assessment of the history, the physical examination, specific laboratory tests and radiological studies (including, on occasion, contrast roentgenograms and abdominal ultrasonography) will usually help differentiate NEC from these other disorders. A rapid and accurate diagnosis is essential because most patients with NEC may be managed with medical therapy alone, while other acute neonatal gastrointestinal emergencies not only require immediate medical management for stabilization but may need prompt surgical intervention.

This chapter provides the reader with the knowledge to differentiate NEC from other gastrointestinal and nongastrointestinal disturbances. The management of each disorder will be discussed as if the reader had direct patient care responsibilities for that patient. Therefore, the reader is asked to make diagnostic and management decisions each step of the way. Choices will be made along a "decision tree" and the consequences of each decision discussed prior to proceeding to the next step in determining a diagnosis or planning therapy. Answers are given in italics in the Discussion/Answer section after each exercise.

### EPIDEMIOLOGY

NEC is a disease that occurs predominantly in Level II (15% of cases) and Level III (85% of cases) neonatal intensive care units (NICUs) and primarily affects preterm infants (85% to 90% preterm) who are recovering from common neonatal cardiopulmonary diseases such as respiratory distress syndrome. Thus NEC is often a disease noted among convalescing "gainers and growers" whose mean gestational age at birth is 30 to 32 weeks. The onset of NEC is unusual on the first day of life and exceedingly uncommon among patients who have not received enteral nutrition. Indeed, more than 95% of patients have received some enteral formula or human milk feeding prior to the onset of signs or symptoms. NEC may occur sporadically but often affected patients are clustered in place and time. Although an infectious agent(s) has been thought to cause NEC, no consistent bacteria or virus has been isolated from all reported epidemics. Purported responsible agents include *E. coli*, Klebsiella, *Staphylococcus epidermidis*, rotavirus, and coronavirus.

The day of onset of NEC is usually between the third and tenth day of life with a wide range depending on when enteral feedings are begun and the degree of immaturity of the infant: The more immature the infant, the longer the period of susceptibility and the later the onset of disease. NEC has rarely occurred on the 90th day of life among very low birth weight infants.

Since the early 1960s a variety of risk factors for NEC have been suggested. While many of these are clearly just associations, several have been proposed as etiologic factors involved in the pathogenesis of this disease. Unfortunately, most of these purported risk factors are common to all premature infants and are not necessarily associated with the pathogenesis of NEC. Thus, when investigated in carefully controlled studies, risk factors such as respiratory distress syndrome, birth asphyxia, umbilical catheters, patent ductus arteriosus, hypotension, and anemia have not been demonstrated to be more common among patients who developed NEC than among unaffected age-matched controls. Indeed, the most dominant risk factor for NEC is the degree of immaturity as determined by gestational age.

## STAGING OF NEC BASED ON CLINICAL AND ROENTGENOLOGICAL MANIFESTATIONS

Infants developing NEC demonstrate a wide range of clinical signs that vary in severity (Table 19-1). Many patients will not progress from the presenting level of clinical illness to the next level of severity; however, fulminant cases of NEC may progress from minimal signs and symptoms to intestinal transmural necrosis, intestinal perforation, peritonitis, and death within 12 hours.

Stage I NEC may, in fact, actually be subclinical or mild NEC. More often, however, it represents a variety of other benign neonatal gastrointestinal disturbances that have clinical manifestations similar to NEC. These other mild diseases include milk protein allergy, feeding intolerance, and intestinal infections by agents such as rotavirus.

Infants with stage II NEC demonstrate the pathognomonic roentgenographic signs of NEC, pneumatosis intestinalis, and hepatic portal venous gas (Fig. 19-1). Pneumatosis intestinalis represents gas-filled cysts in the submucosal or subserosal layers and is universally associated with gaseous distention of the bowel lumen (Fig. 19-2). Stage II is definitive, moderately severe disease and is not usually associated with severe extraintestinal disturbances (Table 19-1).

Stage III is advanced, documented NEC and affected infants demonstrate signs of cardiovascular and/or pulmonary insufficiency, peritonitis, and gastrointestinal perforation (Table 19-1).

Remember that for all three stages, sepsis (or sepsis syndrome) should be high on the list of differential diagnoses.

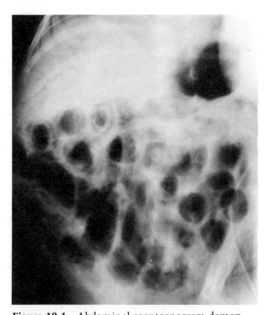

**Figure 19-1** Abdominal roentgenogram demonstrating pneumatosis intestinalis in right lower quadrant and hepatic portal venous gas over the liver in the right upper quadrant.
Roentgenogram courtesy of Dr. Stuart Morrison, Department of Pediatric Radiology, Case Western Reserve University School of Medicine, Rainbow Babies and Children's Hospital, Cleveland, Ohio.

**Table 19-1** Modified Bell's Staging Criteria for Neonatal Necrotizing Enterocolitis

| STAGE | SYSTEMIC SIGNS | INTESTINAL SIGNS | RADIOLOGICAL SIGNS | TREATMENT |
|---|---|---|---|---|
| IA—Suspected NEC | Temperature instability apnea, bradycardia, lethargy | Elevated pregavage residuals, mild abdominal distention, emesis, guaiac positive stool | Normal or intestinal dilation; mild ileus | NPO, antibiotics for 3 days pending cultures, gastric decompression |
| IB—Suspected NEC | Same as IA | Bright red blood from rectum | Same as IA | Same as IA |
| IIA—Definite NEC, mildly ill | Same as IA | Same as IA-IB plus diminished or absent bowel sound ± abdominal tenderness | Intestinal dilation, ileus, pneumatosis intestinalis | Same as IA plus NPO, antibiotics for 7 to 10 days if examination is normal in 24 to 48 hours |
| IIB—Definite NEC, moderately ill | Same as IIA, plus mild metabolic acidosis and mild thrombocytopenia | IIA plus definite abdominal tenderness, ± abdominal cellulitis, or right lower quadrant mass, absent bowel sounds | Same as IIA, ± portal vein gas, ± ascites | Same as IIA plus NPO, antibiotics for 14 days, NaHCO$_3$ for acidosis, volume replacement |
| IIIA—Advanced NEC, severely ill, bowel intact | Same as IIB, plus hypotension, bradycardia, severe apnea, combined respiratory and metabolic acidosis, DIC, neutropenia, anuria | IIB plus signs of generalized peritonitis, marked tenderness, distention, and abdominal wall erythema | Same as IIB; definite ascites | Same as IIB plus as much as 200 mL/kg fluids, fresh frozen plasma, inotropic agents, intubation, ventilator therapy, paracentesis; surgical intervention if patient fails to improve with medical management within 24 to 48 hours |
| IIIB—Advanced NEC, severely ill bowel perforated | Same as IIIA; sudden deterioration | Same as IIIA; sudden increased distention | Same as IIB, plus pneumoperitoneum | Same as IIIA plus surgical intervention |

*Source:* Adapted from Bell MJ, Ternberg JL, Feigin RD, et al: Neonatal necrotizing enterocolitis: Therapeutic decisions based upon clinical staging. *Ann Surg* 1978; 187:1–7; and Kliegman RM, Walsh MC: Neonatal necrotizing enterocolitis: Pathogenesis, classification and spectrum of disease. *Curr Prob Pediatr* 1987; 17:213–288. Adapted with permission of J.B. Lippincott Company, Mosby-Year Book, Inc., and M.J. Bell.

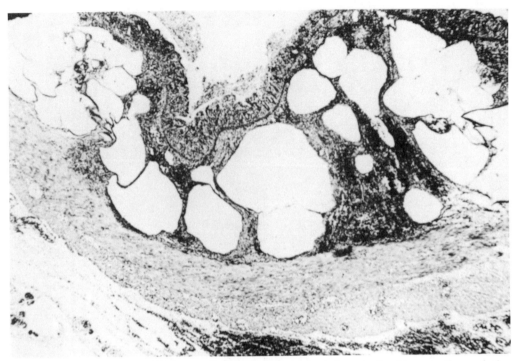

**Figure 19-2** Submucosal gas-filled cysts diagnostic of pneumatosis intestinalis. Also note the marked hemorrhage and inflammatory response. (Hematoxylin and eosin; 56×).
Photograph courtesy of Dr. Beverly Dahms, Chief, Department of Pediatric Pathology, Case Western Reserve University School of Medicine, Rainbow Babies and Children's Hospital, Cleveland, Ohio.

## DIFFERENTIAL DIAGNOSIS

### CASE STUDY 1

A 3,100-g male infant was born following an uncomplicated term pregnancy. Labor and delivery were normal as were the immediate 48 hours after birth. The child was discharged home on regular cow's milk protein-based formula. He did well at home during the first week of life except for occasional nonbilious emesis after feedings and fussiness between formula feedings. The pediatrician believed this was due to gastroesophageal reflux and colic and reassured the mother that the child was all right. The child passed meconium normally after birth and routinely had three to four normally formed and colored stools each day.

On the 10th day of life the emesis increased in frequency and became bilious. On physical examination the pulse rate was 175/minute, respiratory rate was 70/minute, and the mean blood pressure was 30 mm Hg. The abdominal examination revealed distention, tenderness, and diminished bowel sounds. A rectal examination demonstrated black stool that was he-matest positive; no masses were palpated and the sphincter tone was normal. An arterial blood gas had a $pH = 7.12$, $PCO_2 = 25$ mm Hg, $PaO_2 = 100$ mm Hg, and a bicarbonate of 10 mEq/L. Additional laboratory studies demonstrated an indirect bilirubin of 15.5 mg/dL and a hemoglobin of 8 gm/dL.

### EXERCISE 1:

#### ■ Question:

Which of the following steps would you undertake now?

1. Obtain a blood culture, place the patient NPO (nothing by mouth), and administer broad spectrum antibiotics.

2. Administer 20 cc/kg of normal saline intravenously and insert a nasogastric tube. Send blood to the laboratory for a type and cross match and order a plain film of the abdomen.

3. Obtain a stool culture and examination for fecal leukocytes.

4. Initiate antireflux precautions and begin thickened feedings. Administer Reglan (to improve gastric emptying) if the emesis continues.

## ■ Discussion/Answer:

1. Given the signs of shock, *antibiotics are indicated in this case. However, it is important to realize that this child's presentation is an unusual presentation for NEC (and even sepsis).* NEC is less likely in this patient because the child is 1.5 weeks old and was born following a full-term gestation. Even if the patient demonstrates pneumatosis intestinalis on an abdominal roentgenograph, other acute gastrointestinal diseases must be considered (Table 19-2). The prior history of recurrent emesis (which progressed to bile-stained emesis) and colic is also not typically noted in patients with NEC. However, any infant with these signs should be placed NPO.

2. The patient has manifestations of shock, gastrointestinal blood loss, anemia, and intestinal obstruction. *The initial resuscitative effort with normal saline is appropriate and is needed to improve tissue perfusion.* If the anemia worsens with the intravascular resuscitation, blood products can then be administered.

   *The placement of a nasogastric tube is appropriate in this case (and ultimately revealed 30 cc of bile-stained gastric fluid).* There was no evidence of free intraperitoneal gas or pneumatosis intestinalis on the abdominal radiograph. However, there was a paucity of gas in the right lower quadrant and marked gastric and duodenal distention.

**Table 19-2** Differential Diagnosis of Neonatal Pneumatosis Intestinalis

Necrotizing enterocolitis*
Midgut volvulus
Acute-chronic diarrhea
Postoperative gastrointestinal surgery
Hirschsprung disease
Short bowel syndrome
Neutropenia
Idiopathic
Mesenteric thrombosis
Imperforate anus
Congenital malignancy
Congenital heart disease postcatheterization

* Common etiology.

**Table 19-3** Differential Diagnosis of Gastrointestinal Hemorrhage in Neonates

*Upper Gastrointestinal*

Swallowed maternal blood at delivery*
Ingested maternal blood during breast feeding*
Gastritis*
Esophagitis
Peptic ulceration (primary or secondary)
Hemorrhagic disease of newborn
Other coagulopathy
Vascular malformation
Necrotizing enterocolitis
Iatrogenic trauma
Tumor (polyps, leiomyoma)

*Lower Gastrointestinal*

Anal fissure*
Upper tract bleeding*
Swallowed blood*
Milk protein allergy*
Infectious colitis*
Midgut volvulus*
Necrotizing enterocolitis*
Idiopathic
Coagulopathies*
Intussusception
Stricture from NEC
Vascular malformations
Hirschsprung enterocolitis
Meckel's diverticulum
Iatrogenic
Munchausen
Tumor
Asphyxial intestinal necrosis
Pseudomembranous colitis
Eosinophilic gastroenteritis
Lymphonodular hyperplasia

* Common etiology.

3. Although emesis may be the sole initial manifestation of gastroenteritis, this patient never had diarrhea (enteritis). *Therefore, a stool culture and examination for fecal leucocytes are not indicated.* Furthermore, the melanotic stool is not characteristic of dysentery and should not lead one to suspect infection but rather gastrointestinal hemorrhage (Table 19-3). The absence of blood in the gastric fluid suggests that the bleeding has originated from the lower gastrointestinal tract. Although lower gastrointestinal bleeding often manifests as bright red blood per rectum, a darker melanotic stool does not rule that condition out.

4. *Antireflux precautions are not indicated.* Although this child may have had reflux earlier in life, the emesis was most likely

due to a more distal intermittent or partial gastrointestinal obstruction. Furthermore, idiopathic colic is an unusual problem in the first week of life. Both symptoms are suggestive of an intermittent or partial intestinal obstruction.

### ■ Question:

After fluid resuscitation and transfusion, the child's vital signs stabilize. The patient demonstrates distention and moderate abdominal tenderness; however, the surgical consultant does not think peritonitis exists. Which of the following steps would you undertake now?

1. Obtain an immediate contrast enema.

2. Screen the mother for diabetes mellitus.

3. Perform a suction biopsy of the rectal mucosa.

4. Obtain an upper gastrointestinal contrast study.

### ■ Discussion/Answer:

1. A contrast enema is an appropriate way to diagnose *certain, but not all,* gastrointestinal obstructions. In the early neonatal period (day 1 to 2 of life) a patient presenting with obstipation, bile-stained emesis, and abdominal distention (without tenderness) probably has a lower intestinal obstruction. A contrast enema in these infants will help identify the "microcolon" (unused colon), which follows the atretic jejunal or ileal segment. *A contrast enema is of little use in identifying infants with malrotation and is not indicated in this case.* In infants with malrotation and midgut volvulus, a barium enema will demonstrate obstruction of the proximal colon as it enters the volvulus. Furthermore, the cecum will not be present in the right lower quadrant. Note, however, that the absence of the cecum in the right lower quadrant is not pathognomonic for malrotation, since it can also be observed when the cecum is excessively mobile. Remember that a contrast study is only indicated in those instances where the diagnosis is uncertain. If the history, physical examination, and abdominal radiographs are consistent with the diagnosis of malrotation and midgut volvulus, the child should be taken directly to the operating room after an appropriate resuscitation.

2. Gestational diabetes mellitus in the mother may adversely effect neonatal gastrointestinal function. The small left colon syndrome, observed in some infants of diabetic mothers, presents in the first 48 hours of life with obstipation and abdominal distention. This is an unlikely diagnosis in an infant with this patient's symptoms who is 10 days old. Furthermore, the maternal glucose tolerance test reverts to normal soon after delivery and would not identify a gestational diabetic on the 10th postpartum day. *This mother does not need to be screened for diabetes mellitus.*

3. Hirschsprung disease is more common in males and presents after birth with obstipation, constipation, and rarely with severe toxic megacolon (shock, enterocolitis, *Clostridium difficile* infection). This patient's predominant findings include bilious vomiting, hemorrhage, and abdominal distention, a disease pattern atypical for Hirschsprung disease. *A suction biopsy is not indicated and may be dangerous in this case.*

4. *This is a correct answer.* An upper intestinal contrast study is considered by many to be the method of choice to visualize disorders of rotation. In this case the contrast study demonstrated that the duodenum had not crossed to the left side of the vertebral column to assume its normal location next to the ligament of Treitz. Normally during fetal development (~12 weeks' gestation) the intestinal tract enters the abdominal cavity as the duodeno-jejunal and cecocolic loops rotate 270 degrees counterclockwise behind the superior mesenteric artery. This 270-degree counterclockwise rotation places the colon anterior to the superior mesenteric artery and the cecum in the right lower quadrant (Fig. 19-3). Obstruction in malrotation can be due to fibrous bands crossing the duodenum or due to wrapping of the freely mobile bowel around the superior mesenteric artery (midgut volvulus). The latter may produce ischemic necrosis of the bowel receiving blood from the superior mesenteric circulation.

   This patient was diagnosed as having intestinal malrotation and midgut volvulus. While the differential diagnosis of intestinal disorders presenting in a similar fashion

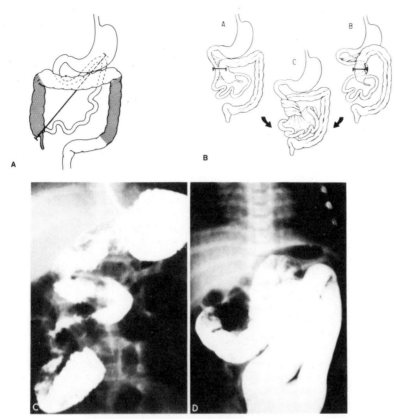

**Figure 19-3** (A) Normal intestinal rotation with broad attachment of the mesentery from the ligament of Treitz in the left upper quadrant high behind the stomach to the ileocecal region low in the right lower quadrant. (B) Malrotation (A, B) of various types can lead to midgut volvulus (C) and bowel ischemia due to narrowing of the attachment of the small bowel mesentery and accompanying superior mesenteric artery. (C) Classic upper gastrointestinal contrast study in malrotation showing failure of the C-loop of the duodenum to return to the left upper quadrant behind the stomach. (D) Barium enema in malrotation showing the cecum in the right upper quandrant.
Modified with permission from Bill, AH: Malrotation of the intestine. *In* Ravitch, MM, et al. (eds): Pediatric Surgery, 3rd ed., Chicago: Yearbook Medical Publishers, Inc., 1979.

is extensive (Table 19-4), midgut volvulus can be most difficult to distinguish from NEC. Careful analysis of the clinical signs, symptoms, and diagnostic test results enables the clinician to differentiate NEC from midgut volvulus (Table 19-5).

## CASE STUDY 2

An 1,800-g female infant was born by spontaneous vaginal delivery at 33 weeks' gestation, following a pregnancy complicated by oligohydramnios secondary to chronic leakage of amniotic fluid since 28 weeks' gestation. Apgar scores were 8 and 9 at 1 and 5 minutes of life, respectively. The child developed significant

cyanosis, grunting, flaring, and retractions immediately after birth, and required endotracheal intubation, 100% inspired oxygen ($FiO_2$), and mechanical ventilation with a pressure cycled infant ventilator. Blood cultures were obtained and ampicillin and gentamicin were administered by intravenous route.

At 18 hours of age the patient developed a right-sided pneumothorax, which was successfully treated with tube thoracostomy drainage. A chest roentgenogram taken after chest tube placement demonstrated that the tube was in an appropriate position; both lungs were expanded and there was bilateral pulmonary interstitial emphysema. At 24 hours of age the infant developed marked abdominal disten-

**Table 19-4** Differential Diagnosis of Gastrointestinal Obstruction in the Neonate, Which May Stimulate NEC

*Intestinal Atresia (Stenosis) (Webs-Membranes)*..........................

Duodenum*

Jejuneum*

Ileum*

Pyloric

Multiple

Colon

*Anal-Rectal*_____

Imperforate anus

Hirschsprung disease

*Malrotation*_____

Volvulus*

Ladds bands

*Functional*_____

Adynamic ileus*

Drugs (morphine, magnesium sulfate)*

Pseudo-obstruction

*Other*_____

Meconium plug*

Meconium ileus*

Small left colon syndrome (infant of diabetic mother)

Lactobezoar (inspissated milk)

Duplication

Annular pancreas

Gastric volvulus

Incarcerated hernia

* Common etiology.

**Table 19-5** Distinguishing Features of NEC and Volvulus

|  | NEC | VOLVULUS |
|---|---|---|
| Preterm (%) | 85–90 | 30–35 |
| Onset by day of life 14 (%) | 85–90 | 50–60 |
| Male : female | 1 : 1 | 2 : 1 |
| Associated anomalies (%) | Rare | 25–40 |
| Bilious emesis (%) | Unusual | 75 |
| Grossly bloody stools | Common | Less common |
| Pneumatosis intestinalis (%) | 80–90 | 1–2 |
| Marked proximal duodenal obstruction (x-ray) | Rare | Common |
| Thrombocytopenia without DIC | Common | Rare |

tion, and a tympanitic abdomen with a blue discoloration over the anterior abdominal wall. The child's vital signs remained stable.

## EXERCISE 2

### ■ Question:

The initial diagnostic evaluation of this patient should include which of the following studies?

1. Complete blood count, platelet count, and coagulation studies (prothrombin time, partial thromboplastin time, fibrinogen, D-dimers)

2. Chest and abdominal radiographs

3. Blood culture

4. Contrast enema

### ■ Discussion/Answer:

1. The blue discoloration of the anterior abdominal wall accompanied by abdominal distention could be due either to gastrointestinal perforation, an hepatic, adrenal, or splenic hematoma, or hemorrhage from a punctured umbilical artery. Disseminated intravascular coagulation and hemorrhagic shock with subsequent anemia could also be present, especially in such a sick infant. *Therefore, it is important to monitor hemoglobin values and to obtain baseline coagulation studies.*

2. *Radiographs of the abdomen and chest are clearly indicated in this case.* Not surprisingly, the abdominal roentgenograms demonstrate a pneumoperitoneum. The chest x-ray, however, demonstrates the unexpected finding of a left-sided pneumothorax, which you treat appropriately with a new chest tube. The differential diagnosis of pneumoperitoneum in the neonate is listed in Table 19-6 and the relative frequencies of the most common conditions are shown in Figure 19-4. Figure 19-5 illus-

**Table 19-6** Differential Diagnosis of Pneumoperitoneum in the Neonate

| *Gastrointestinal Obstruction* | *Traumatic* |
|---|---|
| Meconium ileus* | Ventilatory associated* |
| Atresia* | Nasogastric tube* |
| Stenosis | Suction catheter |
| Midgut volvulus (malrotation) | Thermometer |
| Hirschsprung disease | Enema |
| Gastroschisis | Ventriculoperitoneal shunt |
| Duplication | Gastric perforation with TEF† during ventilator therapy |
| Incarcerated hernia | |
| Imperforate anus | |
| Small left colon syndrome | |
| Intussusception | |
| Meconium plug | |
| *Other* | |
| Necrotizing enterocolitis* | |
| Spontaneous gastric perforation* | |
| Catheter-associated intestinal infarction | |
| Peptic ulceration (duodenum) | |
| Meckel's diverticulum | |
| Appendicitis | |
| Drugs (indomethacin, dexamethasone) | |
| Gastric lactobezoar | |

* Common etiology.
† TEF = tracheoesophageal fistula.

## ETIOLOGY OF PNEUMOPERITONEUM IN THE NEONATE

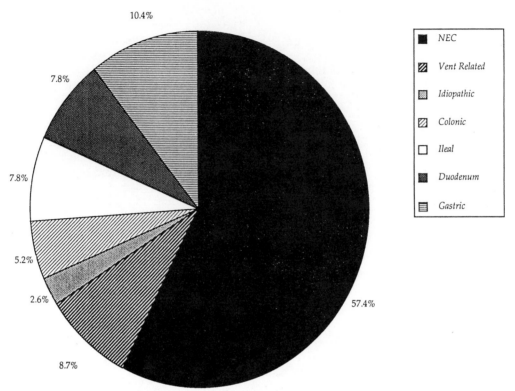

**Figure 19-4** Etiology of pneumoperitoneum in the neonate.

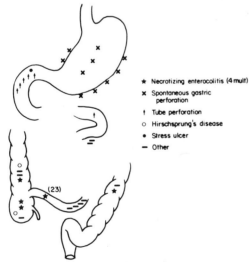

**Figure 19-5** Sites of intestinal perforation among 60 neonates.
From Bell M: *Pediatr Clin North Am* 1985; 32:1181.
Reprinted with permission of W.B. Saunders Company.

trates the sites of intestinal perforation for several of these conditions.

3. *A blood culture is appropriate in any child in whom an intestinal perforation is suspected.*

4. *A contrast enema is contraindicated whenever an intestinal perforation is highly suspected.*

### ■ Question:

Considering the differential diagnosis of pneumoperitoneum in this infant, the most likely diagnosis is which?

1. NEC

2. Spontaneous gastric perforation

3. Feeding tube related trauma

4. Dissection of extra-alveolar gas to the peritoneum

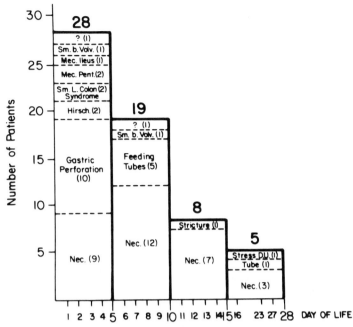

**Figure 19-6** Time of intestinal perforation in 60 neonates.
From Bell M: *Pediatr Clin North Am* 1985; 32:1181. Reprinted with permission of W.B. Saunders Company.

■ **Discussion/Answer:**

1. *It is unlikely that this patient has NEC.* This patient is relatively young for the onset of NEC (i.e., the first day of life, Fig. 19-6) and she has never been fed. Furthermore, it is very unusual to develop NEC during the acute phase of respiratory distress syndrome.

2. *A gastric perforation is unlikely in this case.* Spontaneous gastric perforation is a sudden, often catastrophic, event affecting both premature and full-term infants. Asphyxia and a requirement for resuscitation in the delivery room are common preceding events. The onset is usually during the first 5 days of life and the greater curvature of the stomach is involved in 65% to 86% of patients. Pneumoperitoneum is often extensive, while peritonitis is uncommon. This patient did not have spontaneous gastric perforation.

3. *This answer is incorrect.* The child was never fed, and did not have a feeding tube in place.

4. Extra-alveolar gas from a pneumothorax, pneumomediastinum, pulmonary interstitial emphysema, or intravascular pulmonary venous air embolism, can dissect below the diaphragm to produce pneumoperitoneum. *This patient had a component of pulmonary hypoplasia (secondary to the prolonged oligohydramnios) necessitating the use of high peak inspiratory pressures. These high pressures ultimately resulted in the alveolar air leaks.* The evaluation of this patient should be entirely noninvasive and should not include a diagnostic exploratory laparotomy (see Fig. 19-7). Once gastrointestinal perforation is excluded, expectant management is all that is needed.

## ACUTE NECROTIZING ENTEROCOLITIS

### CASE STUDY 3

A 25-day-old, 1,050-g, male infant suddenly developed temperature instability, an increased frequency of apnea and bradycardia, hematest-positive stools, and abdominal distention. Born in mid-January, he initially had respiratory distress syndrome and required intubation, mechanical ventilation, and exogenous surfactant therapy. He developed a patent ductus arteriosus on the third day of life, which required three doses of intravenous indomethacin. By

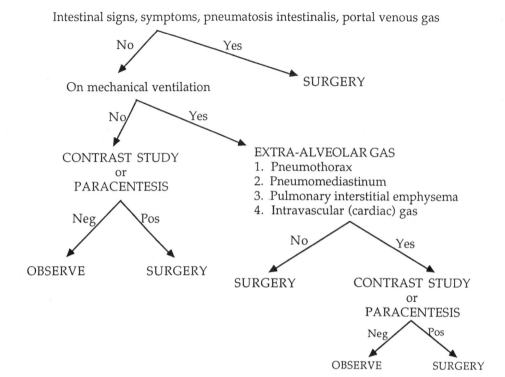

Intestinal signs, symptoms, pneumatosis intestinalis, portal venous gas

**Figure 19-7** Algorithm for approach to neonatal pneumoperitoneum.
Adapted from Stevens M, Ricketts RR: Pneumoperitoneum in the newborn infant. *Ann Surg* 1987; 53:226.

day 7 of life, he was extubated and 2 days later he was weaned to room air (when his umbilical arterial catheter was removed). A head ultrasound study was normal at that time. Enteral feedings with a high caloric density premature infant formula were begun on the 10th day of life and "full" enteral feedings were accomplished by the 13th day of life. Because of poor weight gain, the formula was supplemented with medium-chain triglycerides on the 16th day of life. The charge nurse informs you that two neonates from that same room in the nursery developed NEC last week.

## EXERCISE 3

### ■ Question:

List three findings in this infant that might be indicative of serious systemic and gastrointestinal disease?

1.

2.

3.

### ■ Discussion/Answer:

1. *Temperature instability* in the premature neonate more commonly manifests itself as hypothermia rather than hyperthermia. An increasing or sustained incubator or radiant warmer heater output (ambient temperature) may also indicate a temperature regulation problem. Temperature instability may be due to infection, metabolic disturbances (hyper- or hypothyroidism, hypoglycemia), central nervous system disease, NEC, a faulty isolette, etc.

2. *An increasing frequency of apnea and bradycardia*, especially when the onset is in the third week of life (when prior episodes were self-limited and not significant enough to mention), is an ominous sign and deserves immediate attention. The differential diagnoses include infection, NEC, metabolic disturbances, airway obstruc-

tion, intracranial hemorrhage, seizures, heart failure, etc.

3. *The sudden occurrence of hematest-positive stools and the abdominal distention* should focus attention on the possibility of an intra-abdominal process, especially since both signs occurred together and were not present prior to the 25th day of life. Nonetheless, systemic illnesses (sepsis) may produce an adynamic (functional) ileus, while gastrointestinal bleeding may be due to an acquired (disseminated intravascular coagulation, heparin overdose, thrombocytopenia) or congenital coagulopathy. Indomethacin therapy has been associated with gastrointestinal bleeding while the drug was being administered. It would be unusual to have such symptoms 3 weeks later.

■ **Question:**

List four risk factors for the development of serious gastrointestinal disease in this infant.

1.

2.

3.

4.

■ **Discussion/Answer:**

1. *The achievement of "full" enteral feedings in a 1,050-g neonate, 3 days after beginning them, is too rapid.* This places the patient at risk for feeding intolerance and NEC. Indeed, the risk of NEC is greatest among very low birth weight infants who are enterally fed with formula increments that exceed 20 to 30 cc/kg/day. To achieve "full feeds" (120 cc/kg/day) within 72 hours, this patient would have had formula increments of 40 cc/kg/day! Often house staff and nurses are tempted to increase the rate of formula increments at times (e.g., the middle of the night) when an intravenous line infiltrates and a new vein is difficult to cannulate. Avoid this temptation if the increment of formula advancement is greater than 20 to 30 cc/kg/day.

2. *Supplementation of high caloric premature formula with medium-chain triglycerides has been reported to produce gastrointesti-*

nal disturbances. One such problem is the gastric lactobezoar, which can present with abdominal distention, gastrointestinal bleeding, emesis due to gastric outlet obstruction, and, rarely, intestinal perforation. There may also be a palpable mass in the left upper quadrant, which may be visible with plain roentgenography or abdominal ultrasound.

3. *The occurrence of NEC in two neonates from the same nursery suggests that an epidemic of NEC may be brewing.* It is also noteworthy that mid-January often coincides with epidemics of rotavirus among inpatients and among families and personnel outside of the hospital. Indeed, rotavirus has been associated with epidemics of NEC (in patients without antecedent diarrhea). Furthermore, during these epidemics of documented NEC, there are additional patients (stage I, Table 19-1) who do not fulfill criteria for documented NEC, but who have manifestations similar to that of the patient. Nursery personnel may also become symptomatic during these epidemics of NEC.

4. *This patient's prematurity is clearly a significant risk factor for NEC and sepsis.* The presence of respiratory distress syndrome, a patent ductus arteriosus, and an umbilical artery catheter have *not* been consistent risk factors for NEC.

■ **Question:**

The immediate clinical approach to this patient should include which of the following?

1. Assess vital signs and respiratory status.

2. Obtain a blood and stool culture and no other cultures at this time. (Antibiotics are not necessary at this time.)

3. Place the patient NPO, insert a nasogastric tube, and obtain an abdominal radiograph.

4. Obtain a head ultrasound examination.

■ **Discussion/Answer:**

1. A preterm neonate presenting with temperature instability and frequent episodes of apnea and bradycardia may have impending circulatory or respiratory failure requiring immediate therapy. *Therefore, an initial assessment of vital signs, perfusion (capillary refill time and urine specific gravity*

and output) oxygenation, ventilation, and acid-base balance is urgently needed to determine the severity of cardiopulmonary impairment. Such assessment must be performed concomitantly with more specific diagnostic procedures. The arterial blood gas is particularly useful because it can detect hypoxia, the presence of a respiratory acidosis (due to central hypoventilation, pneumonia, or compromise of diaphragmatic excursion due to abdominal distention), or the presence of a metabolic acidosis (due to hypoxia or poor peripheral tissue perfusion from shock).

This patient's vital signs included a heart rate of 135/minute, a respiratory rate of 42/minute, and a mean blood pressure of 39 mm Hg. The arterial blood gas had a pH = 7.36, $PCO_2$ = 37 mm Hg, and $PaO_2$ = 78 mm Hg. Perfusion appeared to be adequate.

2. *It would be inappropriate in this case to obtain* only *stool and blood cultures.* Prior to establishing the diagnosis of NEC, blood, urine, and cerebrospinal fluid cultures should be obtained. Indeed 1% to 2% of patients with NEC actually have meningitis. Antibiotics should always be initiated if sepsis or NEC is suspected. The specific antimicrobial agents chosen should be based on a knowledge of the prevailing microorganisms responsible for sepsis or NEC in a given NICU and additional risk assessments (e.g., the presence of a central venous catheter or the suspicion of bowel perforation).

In addition to these microbiological tests, a test for rotavirus should be performed. This is particularly helpful in light of the season (January) and the presence of other cases of NEC in the nursery.

3. *Immediately after determining that the patient is not in shock or respiratory failure, you should insert a nasogastric tube and obtain an abdominal roentgenogram.* The x-ray will help to identify portal venous gas over the liver, pneumatosis intestinalis, pneumoperitoneum, or an isolated dilated loop of bowel. The plain film of the abdomen in this patient demonstrated minimally distended loops of bowel, which were distributed throughout the abdomen. The bowel wall was not thickened; there was no evidence of ascites and pneumatosis intestinalis was not evident.

4. *A head ultrasound study would only be indicated in this case if posthemorrhagic hydrocephalus was suspected.* It is very unusual to develop an intraventricular hemorrhage at 3 months of age. Because this patient did not have an intraventricular hemorrhage on routine head ultrasound on the seventh day of life, the head ultrasound is not indicated now.

■ **Question:**

During the initial assessment, the patient has a bowel movement that contains blood mixed with stool and mucus. The vital signs remain stable, perfusion appears normal, and with the nasogastric tube in place the abdominal distention resolves. You should now do which of the following?

1. Check the stool for *Clostridium difficile* toxin.

2. Administer vitamin K.

3. Check the hematocrit, platelet count, prothrombin time, and partial thromboplastin times.

4. Perform an abdominal Doppler ultrasound scan to detect an aortic thrombus.

■ **Discussion/Answer:**

1. *C. difficile* (more specifically *C. difficile* toxin) is responsible for pseudomembranous colitis in older children and adults. Premature infants, however, may be colonized with *C. difficile* (and its toxins), and not become symptomatic. *Therefore, this test is not indicated for this patient.*

2. Assuming this patient received vitamin K prophylaxis at birth, and has not been receiving human milk, hemorrhagic disease of the newborn is an unlikely diagnosis. *Additional vitamin K is not required.*

3. The gastrointestinal bleeding may, with time, result in anemia, hypovolemic shock, or both. *Therefore, a baseline hematocrit is clearly indicated. It is also important to assess this infant's coagulation status,* especially when sepsis or NEC is suspected. Isolated thrombocytopenia or disseminated intravascular coagulation may be noted in patients with NEC or sepsis. Although gastrointestinal hemorrhage may be one symptom of disseminated intravascular coagulation, you would also expect to see petechiae, ecchymosis, and bleeding from

puncture-wound sites. Nonetheless, the early diagnosis of disseminated intravascular coagulation, prompt correction of the initiating event, and judicious use of platelet and fresh frozen plasma transfusions are all beneficial to the outcome of the patient.

4. Aortic thrombi may be noted in very low birth weight infants who have had an umbilical artery catheter in place. Presenting manifestations of such thrombi often include hematuria and hypertension with subsequent cardiac failure, although thrombi may be present in asymptomatic infants. Most infants with aortic thrombi exhibit symptoms during the time the catheter is in place or within 1 week of catheter removal.

An occasional infant may present 2 to 3 weeks after catheter removal. *The presenting symptoms of this patient are not suggestive of a catheter-related aortic thrombosis,* because hematochezia is an unusual isolated symptom of such thromboembolism. If evidence of hematuria existed, in the absence of a coagulopathy, a Doppler ultrasound study of the abdominal aorta might be indicated. The relationship between such thrombi and NEC is highly controversial but most case-control studies suggest that there is little or no relationship between large vessel thrombi and NEC or between the use of umbilical arterial catheters and NEC.

■ **Question:**

Seventy-two hours after the initial presentation, the infant's symptoms have resolved, the abdominal roentgenograms are normal, and all laboratory tests are normal, except the test for rotavirus, which is positive. The patient continues to have hematest-positive stools without evidence of frank blood or mucus. There are normal bowel sounds and the distention has resolved. You should do which of the following?

1. Administer an oral dose of an intravenous immunoglobulin preparation.

2. Begin human milk feedings.

3. Begin total parenteral alimentation for a total of 21 days.

4. Slowly begin formula feedings to achieve "full feeds" over a 10- to 14-day feeding advance.

■ **Discussion/Answer:**

1. Oral administration of standard intravenous immunoglobulin (IVIG) preparations has been anecdotally reported as a way to treat infants with rotavirus diarrhea and possibly as a way to prevent rotavirus infection. Nonetheless, this is not standard therapy, nor has it been tested in large randomized controlled clinical trials. Furthermore, uncomplicated rotavirus infection in neonates is usually a self-limited infection. *Therefore, IVIG should not be administered.*

Oral administration of a specially prepared IgA-IgG immunoglobulin preparation has been demonstrated to reduce the incidence of NEC in a single clinical trial. Nonetheless, it has not been demonstrated to be of benefit in infant's who are symptomatic.

2. Human milk feedings have been demonstrated to reduce the incidence of infectious diarrhea and in one randomized clinical study to reduce the incidence of NEC. *Although human milk may be of benefit to this patient, it is not the standard of care to refeed such patients with human milk.* Furthermore, it would be difficult to reestablish maternal milk production 3 weeks after the delivery of a premature infant when the mother had not been breast feeding during this time. In addition, pooled human milk may be inappropriate, because the antibody spectrum from unrelated mothers may not contain activity against rotavirus and the nutritional composition of mature human milk may not be optimal for the growth of the premature infant.

3. There are few indications for total parenteral alimentation in the neonatal period. These include severe NEC, short bowel syndrome, intestinal pseudo-obstruction, and possibly intractable diarrhea of infancy. Total parenteral alimentation among preterm infants is associated with significant risks such as "line" sepsis, osteopenia of prematurity (rickets), cholestatic jaundice, which may progress to cirrhosis, and the induction of gastrointestinal mucosal atrophy (see Chapter 6). *This particular patient does not need total parenteral alimentation because bowel function has returned to normal and NEC has not been documented.*

4. In stage I NEC enteral feedings can be reintroduced after more serious gastrointestinal diseases are ruled out and bowel function has returned to normal. Furthermore, rotavirus gastroenteritis can be managed successfully with careful attention to the state of hydration and regular formula feeding. *Refeeding the patient after a 72-hour period of observation is quite appropriate.*

## CASE STUDY 4

A 1,500-g, appropriate for gestational age, male twin A was born by spontaneous vaginal delivery. The Apgar scores were 8 and 9 at 1 and 5 minutes, respectively. The serum glucose concentration was 75 mg/dL and the hematocrit was 48% at 1 hour of life. The infant developed mild retractions and was administered supplemental oxygen (maximum $FiO_2$ = 40%) via an oxyhood. He was weaned to room air on the second day of life. Enteral feedings (given every 2 hours) were initiated on the third day of life with a standard 20 cal/oz. premature infant formula. The infant tolerated feedings well for 48 hours. On the fifth day of life the evening nurse noticed that the child was lethargic and had 7 cc of undigested food in his stomach immediately before the next scheduled feeding. Two stools passed in the late afternoon tested hematest positive (all previous stools were hematest negative).

The physical examination reveals a heart rate of 180/minute, a respiratory rate of 75/minute, and mean blood pressure of 29 mm Hg. In addition, the infant is hypotonic, has decreased activity, and lies motionless. Abdominal distension and abdominal tenderness are present, and bowel sounds are absent. During your examination the infant becomes apneic.

## EXERCISE 4

### ■ Questions:

Which of the following should be accomplished immediately? Identify the choice with the highest priority:

1. Initiate enteric precautions.

2. Obtain a surgical consultation.

3. Insert a nasogastric tube, place the infant NPO, and obtain a plain film of the abdomen.

4. Insert an endotracheal tube and administer 20 cc/kg of normal saline.

### ■ Discussion/Answer:

1. *Enteric isolation is important for all patients with suspected or proven NEC.* Indeed, the use of gown and glove precautions with cohorting of patients and nurses and meticulous hand washing have been shown to abate epidemics of NEC. *However, while enteric isolation may be important in this case (depending on your level of suspicion for NEC), it is not the first thing to do for this patient.*

2. A surgical consultation is indicated for any patient with a suspected intra-abdominal process including NEC. *Therefore, it is appropriate to ask the surgeons to evaluate this infant, but it is not your highest priority.*

3. *Insertion of a nasogastric tube to decompress the abdomen and cessation of feedings are important therapeutic approaches for all patients with suspected NEC. Furthermore, a plain film of the abdomen should be high on your list of essential diagnostic procedures. Nonetheless, this is not your highest priority.* Half credit is given if you placed a nasogastric tube to evacuate the distended stomach prior to intubation.

4. *This infant requires immediate endotracheal intubation and fluid resuscitation.* The ABCs of resuscitation—Airway, Breathing, & Circulation—are applicable in this case. This patient is apneic (due to increased abdominal pressure, sepsis, shock) and has poor circulatory function (hypotension due to septic shock, third space fluid losses). Therefore, endotracheal intubation and fluid resuscitation are urgently indicated.

### ■ Question:

After endotracheal intubation and fluid administration, the infant's skin perfusion improves and the mean blood pressure increases to 40 mm Hg. The plain film of the abdomen reveals generalized areas of distended bowel but no evidence of pneumatosis intestinalis, pneumoperitoneum, or portal venous gas over the liver.

You obtain appropriate cultures, initiate broad spectrum antibiotics, place the patient

NPO, and continue mechanical ventilation. The postintubation arterial blood gas demonstrates a pH = 7.31, $PCO_2$ = 35 mm Hg, and $PaO_2$ = 75 mm Hg. The CBC reveals a hematocrit of 45%, 85,000 platelets/$mm^3$, and a total white blood cell count of 5,100/$mm^3$ with 10% neutrophils and 5% band forms. Four hours later the abdominal girth increases from 22 to 25 cm and faint erythema is now present over the anterior abdominal wall. Which of the following should be done now?

1. Administer a monoclonal IgM antibody against endotoxin.

2. Administer a granulocyte transfusion.

3. Check for disseminated intravascular coagulation.

4. Repeat the plain film of the abdomen.

### ■ Discussion/Answer:

1. Monoclonal IgM antibodies directed against endotoxin have proven effective in the treatment of gram-negative sepsis in one study among adult patients. There is little experience with this preparation in neonates and it is currently not licensed for that age group. However, NEC is associated with bacteremia in 30% of documented cases. *E. coli*, Klebsiella, and *Staphylococcus epidermidis* are the most common bacterial isolates. Fortunately, in this particular patient, vital signs and perfusion normalized after the fluid resuscitation. *Therefore, monoclonal antibodies against endotoxin are not indicated.*

2. This patient has neutropenia (an absolute neutrophil count less than 1,000/$mm^3$), which is most likely due to sepsis or necrotizing enterocolitis. Neutropenia associated with sepsis is due either to excessive neutrophil margination or neutrophil bone marrow storage pool depletion, while in NEC the former mechanism appears to dominate. Patients with bone marrow storage pool depletion have a poorer prognosis than those with sufficient marrow neutrophil stores.

   The use of granulocyte transfusions for neonatal sepsis is an unresolved controversy. Nonetheless, there is little evidence that such therapy is beneficial in patients with NEC. *Therefore, granulocytes should not be administered to this infant.*

3. The presence of thrombocytopenia with or without disseminated intravascular coagulation is common in patients with NEC. Given this infant's decrease in platelet number, it would be appropriate to determine the prothrombin time, partial thromboplastin time, D-dimers, and fibrinogen levels so that disseminated intravascular coagulation can be ruled out. *The thrombocytopenia in this patient does not require therapy unless it declines significantly (<50,000) or is associated with hemorrhage.*

4. *A repeat abdominal radiograph should be your highest priority.* Although the initial abdominal plain film did not reveal pneumatosis intestinalis, pneumoperitoneum, or hepatic portal venous gas, NEC is a disease that can progress quite rapidly. We recommend that abdominal roentgenograms be repeated every 6 hours during the acute, unstable period of the disease (first 72 hrs) and whenever clinical deterioration occurs. The repeat abdominal film now reveals pneumatosis intestinalis and portal venous gas over the liver (see Fig. 19-1).

### ■ Question:

Twenty-four hours later the patient develops additional signs of generalized peritonitis, has bright red blood per rectum, hypotension, oliguria, and a metabolic acidosis. The prothrombin time and partial thromboplastin time are prolonged and the fibrinogen level is 45 mg/dL. You initially administer normal saline and, when the coagulopathy is diagnosed, you infuse fresh frozen plasma until the blood pressure and urine output improve. Because perfusion and blood pressure remain unstable you begin a dopamine infusion, titrating the rate of infusion against blood pressure.

A surgical consultant concurs with the diagnosis of NEC and agrees to continue medical management for another 24 hours. Thirty-six hours after the onset of the illness the patient develops a sudden increase in abdominal size and peripheral cyanosis. The infant's mean blood pressure is 28 mm Hg. You should immediately do which of the following?

1. Obtain an arterial blood gas.

2. Administer sodium nitroprusside.

3. Obtain a repeat abdominal plain film.

4. Obtain a cross table lateral abdominal roentgenogram.

■ **Discussion/Answer:**

1. Peripheral cyanosis may be due to hypoxia or poor peripheral perfusion. The blood gas (pH = 7.12, $PCO_2$ = 51 mm Hg, and $PaO_2$ = 70 mm Hg ($FiO_2$ = 80%) demonstrates a mixed respiratory and metabolic acidosis and a significant alveolar-arterial oxygen gradient. This latter problem suggests the development of adult respiratory distress syndrome, which often accompanies sepsis or peritonitis. *This is a correct response.*

2. Afterload reduction using nitroprusside or other vasodilators may help improve peripheral perfusion in patients with septic shock. *However, vasodilators are not indicated at this time because the infant's blood pressure is unstable.*

3. This infant's plain abdominal radiograph is shown in Figure 19-8. On superficial examination it demonstrates only pneumatosis intestinalis in the right lower quadrant and dilated loops of bowel. However, on careful inspection a lucent appearance is visible over the liver and a linear density is apparent in the midliver region representing the umbilical vein. These signs signify the

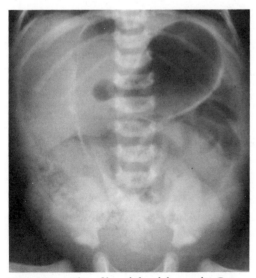

**Figure 19-8** Plain film of the abdomen for Case Study 4.
Roentgenogram courtesy of Dr. Stuart Morrison, Department of Pediatric Radiology, Case Western Reserve University School of Medicine, Rainbow Babies and Children's Hospital, Cleveland, Ohio.

presence of pneumoperitoneum due to gastrointestinal perforation from NEC. *The plain abdominal radiograph is an appropriate test, but is not the best way to identify a pneumoperitoneum.*

4. *The cross table lateral radiograph is the correct way to detect pneumoperitoneum* (Fig. 19-9). The presence of the radiolucent (black gas bubble) beneath the anterior abdominal wall is diagnostic of free intraperitoneal gas from an intestinal perforation. (For other causes of pneumoperitoneum, review Table 19-6.)

## CHRONIC SEQUELAE

■ **Question:**

The surgeon returns to the NICU and together you stabilize the patient in preparation for surgery. At exploratory laparotomy, generalized peritonitis is found with brown-green peritoneal fluid present. In addition, the bowel looks dusky-blue but appears to be viable except for 10 cm surrounding the site of perforation near the terminal ileum (see Fig. 19-5 for common sites of perforation in NEC). An ileostomy is performed after the bowel resection, a Broviac catheter is inserted, and the patient is returned to the NICU in excellent condition. Subsequently, the patient does well, tolerates central hyperalimentation, and is extubated on the third postoperative day.

This patient is at risk for development of which of the following conditions?

1. Short bowel syndrome

2. Pernicious anemia

3. Severe episodes of gastroenteritis

4. Cholestatis jaundice

5. "Line" sepsis

■ **Discussion/Answer:**

1. NEC is the second most common cause of short bowel syndrome in infancy (after multiple small bowel atresias). Other causes of this syndrome include midgut volvulus, gastroschisis, and aganglionosis. Complications of short bowel include failure to thrive secondary to malabsorption, "line" sepsis, cholelithiasis, cholecystitis, cholestatic jaundice leading to cirrhosis and hepatic failure, nephrolithiasis, os-

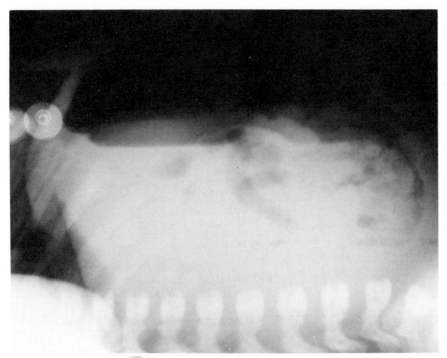

**Figure 19-9**  Cross table lateral film for Case Study 4.
Roentgenogram courtesy of Dr. Stuart Morrison, Department of Pediatric Radiology, Case Western Reserve University School of Medicine, Rainbow Babies and Children's Hospital, Cleveland, Ohio.

teopenic bone disease, pancreatitis, and gastrointestinal obstruction secondary to peritoneal adhesions. The minimal amount of viable bowel required for survival with enteral nutrition ranges from 8 to 15 cm if the ileocecal valve is present to 29 to 40 cm if the ileocecal valve has been resected. The shorter the bowel length, the longer the time needed for intestinal adaptation (e.g., 27 months for less than 40 cm of remaining bowel or 14 months if 40 to 80 cm of bowel remains). Rehabilitation requires a fine balance between minimizing the risks of total parenteral alimentation with the enteral tolerance of an elemental formula. *A minimal amount of bowel was resected in this patient. Therefore, short bowel syndrome would be highly unlikely.*

2. Low vitamin $B_{12}$ levels and even megaloblastic anemia have occurred in childhood among patients who had resection of the terminal ileum during the neonatal period. Anemia often takes 5 to 15 years to develop and is a very late manifestation of such surgery. *Therefore, this patient is at risk for pernicious anemia.*

3. Patients who have an ileostomy after NEC often develop protracted episodes of watery diarrhea due to common gastrointestinal viral pathogens. This results in severe dehydration, electrolyte abnormalities, and failure to thrive. Because of this risk, it is recommended that all patients undergo a bowel reanastamosis before being discharged from the hospital. *Our patient was at risk for this complication prior to having his bowel reanastamosed at 2 months of age.*

4. *Cholestatic jaundice is a common problem among patients who cannot tolerate enteral feedings and who require prolonged central intravenous hyperalimentation* (see Chapter 6). All patients recovering from NEC should begin enteral alimentation as soon as possible. Enteral nutrients can reduce the toxicity of intravenous alimentation fluid through stimulation of bile salt secretion and normal hepatic function (by local paracrine or direct nutrient mechanisms). Hepatic failure is now an unfortunately common cause of death among patients receiving prolonged intravenous

hyperalimentation due to short bowel syndrome. Fortunately, this infant required central intravenous alimentation for only 1 month and exhibited only mildly abnormal liver function studies, which rapidly reverted to normal after enteral feedings were restarted.

5. "Line" sepsis is another significant problem for infants receiving prolonged central hyperalimentation (see Chapter 6). Signs and symptoms are often nonspecific. Common pathogens include *Staphylococcus epidermidis*, *Staphylococcus aureus*, and *Candida albicans*. Patients with short bowel syndrome are at particular risk to develop line sepsis due to gram-negative bacteria.

## CASE STUDY 5

A 35-day-old, formula fed, former 1,500-g, appropriate for gestational age infant develops marked abdominal distention and bile-stained emesis. The nurse informs you that he has not stooled for 7 days. Past history reveals that he had transient tachypnea and was weaned to room air by the fifth day of life. Enteral feeding were successfully initiated on the third day of life and full feedings were achieved by day 12. On day 14 of life, he developed abdominal distention and had two hematest-positive stools. The workup did not reveal a cause for this previous episode and he was slowly refed after being kept NPO for 7 days because of possible NEC.

## EXERCISE 5

### ■ Question:

Which of the following disorders should be included in the differential diagnosis?

1. Pyloric stenosis

2. Milk protein allergy

3. Recurrent NEC

4. Post-NEC colonic stricture

### ■ Discussion/Answer:

1. *Pyloric stenosis is unlikely.* Patients with pyloric stenosis often have a scaffoid abdomen and recurrent projectile nonbilious emesis over several days. Furthermore, the early phase of the disease is not preceded by obstipation.

2. Infants with milk protein allergy may present with emesis, but more often exhibit hematest-positive stools with or without diarrhea. Obstipation and bile-stained emesis are not usually present. *Therefore, milk protein allergy is an unlikely diagnosis.*

3. Recurrent NEC occurs in approximately 5% of patients. The recurrences usually manifest with typical features of NEC, within 1 to 4 weeks after the initial episode. *This patient does not have symptoms compatible with recurrent NEC.*

4. *This infant most probably has a post-NEC intestinal stricture.* Obstipation, bile-stained emesis, and abdominal distention are classic signs of intestinal obstruction. While this patient could have a congenital cause of intermittent intestinal obstruction (such as malrotation with midgut volvulus), the previous episode of abdominal distention (on the 14th day of life) most likely was NEC. Indeed, not all patients with NEC demonstrate pneumatosis intestinalis at the time the roentgenogram is obtained. Furthermore, some roentgenographic signs of NEC may be subtle and interpreted as normal by experienced pediatric radiologists and neonatologists.

Intestinal stricture formation is a common late sequela of NEC occurring 2 to 8 weeks after the acute episode. Strictures may develop in medically and surgically treated patients. Because most patients with NEC respond to medical management alone, stricture formation probably occurs at the site where inflammation is most severe. During the recovery phase, stricture formation results from continued acute and chronic inflammation and reparative processes. Strictures often develop in the colon or terminal ileum; rarely is there more than one stricture.

The incidence of strictures following NEC varies from 5% to 25%. The higher incidence is reported from centers that routinely order contrast enemas in all patients who have had NEC. Other centers obtain a routine screening upper gastrointestinal contrast study followed by a contrast enema in those patients demonstrating abnormalities on the small bowel follow-through study. It is important to remember, however, that many areas of narrowing detected on contrast studies do not represent sites of complete obstruction. Therefore some centers simply refeed infants who have recovered from NEC, and only study those infants who display signs of feeding intolerance.

If undetected, strictures following NEC may lead to intestinal obstruction. However, more serious complications of strictures include an increased predisposition for the development of bacterial sepsis, intestinal perforation, and dehiscence of the anastamosis site following intestinal re-anastamosis. Resection of the stricture is indicated for these complications, but not necessarily for mild gastrointestinal bleeding (or anemia) from a nonobstructive healing stricture.

If a contrast roentgenographic study is not performed prior to refeeding an infant who has been medically managed, you must pay close attention to the clinical course of the patient. Strictures should be suspected in patients recovering from NEC who develop signs and symptoms of gastrointestinal obstruction. Contrast enemas are usually performed on all surgically managed patients before enteral feedings are initiated. The risk of distal obstruction and anastamotic perforation is considered by many too high a risk to take.

## BIBLIOGRAPHY

### Epidemiology

1. Kosloske AM: A unifying hypothesis for pathogenesis and prevention of necrotizing enterocolitis. *J Pediatr* 1990; 117:S68–S74.
2. Holman RC, Stehr-Green JK, Zelasky MT: Necrotizing enterocolitis mortality in the United States, 1979–85. *Am J Publ Health* 1989; 79:987–989.
3. Palmer SR, Biffin A, Gamsu HR: Outcome of neonatal necrotizing enterocolitis: Results of the BAPM/CDSC surveillance study, 1981–1984. *Arch Dis Child* 1989; 64:388–394.
4. Jason JM: Infectious disease-related deaths of low birth weight infants, United States, 1968 to 1982. *Pediatrics* 1989; 84:296–303.
5. Kliegman RM: Neonatal necrotizing enterocolitis: Bridging the basic science with the clinical disease. *J Pediatr* 1990; 117:833–835.
6. Anderson DM, Kliegman RM: The relationship of neonatal alimentation practices to the occurrence of endemic necrotizing enterocolitis. *Am J Perinatol* 1991; 18:62–67.
7. Ballance WA, Dahms BB, Shenker N, et al: Pathology of neonatal necrotizing enterocolitis: A ten year experience. *J Pediatr* 1990; 117:S6–S13.
8. Coombs RC, Morgan MEI, Durbin GM, et al: Gut blood flow velocities in the newborn: Effects of patent ductus arteriosus and parenteral indomethacin. *Arch Dis Child* 1990; 65:1067–1071.
9. Downing GJ, Horner SR, Kilbride HW: Characteristics of perinatal cocaine-exposed infants with necrotizing enterocolitis. *Am J Dis Child* 1991; 145:26–27.

### Differential Diagnosis

10. Kliegman RM, Walsh MC: Neonatal necrotizing enterocolitis: Pathogenesis, classification and spectrum of disease. *Curr Prob Pediatr* 1987; 17:213–288.
11. Bell MJ: Perforation of the gastrointestinal tract and peritonitis in the neonate. *Surg Gyn Obstet* 1985; 160:20–26.
12. Eggli KD, Loyer E, Anderson K: Neonatal pneumatosis cystoides intestinalis caused by volvulus of the mid intestine. *Arch Dis Child* 1989; 64:1189–1190.
13. Wilde J, Yolken R, Willoughby R et al: Improved detection of rotavirus shedding by polymerase chain reaction. *Lancet* 1991; 337:323–326.
14. Ghory MJ, Sheldon CA: Newborn surgical emergencies of the gastrointestinal tract. *Surg Clin North Am* 1985; 65:1083–1098.
15. Aschner JL, Deluga KS, Metlay LA et al: Spontaneous focal gastrointestinal perforation in very low birth weight infants. *J Pediatr* 1988; 113:364–367.
16. Stevens M, Ricketts RR: Pneumoperitoneum in the newborn infant. *Am Surg* 1987; 53:226–230.
17. Bell MJ: Perforation of the gastrointestinal tract and peritonitis in the neonate. *Surg Obstet Gyn* 1985; 160:20–26.
18. Shashikumar VL, Bassuk A, Pilling GP, et al: Spontaneous gastric rupture in the newborn: A clinical review of nineteen cases. *Ann Surg* 1973; 182:22–25.
19. Leonidas JC, Magid N, Soberman N, et al: Midgut volvulus in infants: Diagnosis with US. Work in progress. *Pediatr Radiol* 1991; 179:491–493.
20. Rescorla FJ, Shedd FJ, Grosfeld JL, et al: Anomalies of intestinal rotation in childhood: Analysis of 447 cases. *Surgery* 1990; 108:710–716.
21. Boulton JE, Ein SH, Reilly BJ, et al: Necrotizing enterocolitis and volvulus in the premature neonate. *J Pediatr Surg* 1989; 24:901–905.
22. Powell DM, Othersen HB, Smith CD: Malrotation of the intestines in children: The effect of age on presentation and therapy. *J Pediatr Surg* 1989; 24:777–780.
23. Sherman NJ, Clatworthy HW Jr: Gastrointestinal bleeding in neonates: A study of 94 cases. *Surgery* 1967; 62:614–619.
24. Yoss BS: Human milk K lactobezoars. *J Pediatr* 1984; 105:819–822.
25. Erenberg A: Lactobezoar. In Sunshine P, ed: *Feeding the Neonate Weighing Less Than 1500 Grams: Nutrition and Beyond.* Proceedings of

the Seventy-ninth Ross Conference on Pediatric Research, Columbus, Ohio, 1980, Ross Laboratories, pp. 190–202.

26. Caniano DA, Beaver BL: Meconium ileus: A fifteen-year experience with forty-two neonates. *Surgery* 1987; 102:699–703.

27. Kwong MS, Dinner M: Neonatal appendicitis masquerading as necrotizing enterocolitis. *J Pediatr* 1980; 96:917–918.

28. Smith VS, Giacoia GP: Intussusception associated with necrotizing enterocolitis. *Clin Pediatr* 1984; 23:43–45.

29. Stine MJ, Harris H: Intussusception in a premature infant simulating neonatal necrotizing enterocolitis. *Am J Dis Child* 1982; 136:76–77.

30. Berkowitz GP, Buntain WL, Cassady G: Milk curd obstruction mimicking necrotizing enterocolitis. *Am J Dis Child* 1980; 134:989–990.

31. Lilien LD, Srinivasan G, Pyati SP, et al: Green vomiting in the first 72 hours in normal infants. *Am J Dis Child* 1986; 140:662–664.

32. O'Niel EA, Chwals WJ, O'Shea MD, et al: Dexamethasone treatment during ventilator dependency: Possible life threatening gastrointestinal complications. *Arch Dis Child* 1992; 67:10–11.

## Acute NEC

33. Ricketts RR, Jerles ML: Neonatal necrotizing enterocolitis: Experience with 100 consecutive surgical patients. *World J Surg* 1990; 14:600–605.

34. Caplan MS, Hsueh W: Necrotizing enterocolitis: Role of platelet activating factor, endotoxin, and tumor necrosis factor. *J Pediatr* 1990; 117:S47–S51.

35. Rotbart HA, Johnson ZT, Reller LB: Analysis of enteric coagulase-negative staphylococci from neonates with necrotizing enterocolitis. *Pediatr Infect Dis J* 1989; 8:140–142.

36. Buras R, Guzzetta P, Avery G, et al: Acidosis and hepatic portal venous gas: Indications for surgery in necrotizing enterocolitis. *Pediatrics* 1986; 78:273–277.

37. Brill PW, Olson SR, Winchester P: Neonatal necrotizing enterocolitis: Air in Morison pouch. *Radiology* 1990; 174:469–471.

38. Weinberg B, Peralta VE, Diakoumakis EE, et al: Sonographic findings in necrotizing enterocolitis with paucity of abdominal gas as the initial symptom. *Mt. Sinai J Pediatr* 1989; 56:330–333.

39. Cullen DJ, Coyle JP, Teplick R, et al: Cardiovascular, pulmonary, and renal effects of massively increased intra-abdominal pressure in critically ill patients. *Crit Care Med* 1989; 17:118–121.

40. Scheifele DW, Ginter GL, Olsen E, et al: Comparison of two antibiotic regimens for neonatal necrotizing enterocolitis. *J Antimicrobial Chemotherapy* 1987; 20:421–429.

## Chronic Sequelae

41. Radhakrishnan J, Blechman G, Shrader C, et al: Colonic strictures following successful management of necrotizing enterocolitis: A prospective study evaluating early gastrointestinal contrast studies. *J Pediatr Surg* 1991; 26:1043–1046.

42. Hancock BJ, Wiseman NE: Lethal short-bowel syndrome. *J Pediatr Surg* 1990; 25:1131–1134.

43. Weber TR, Tracy T Jr, Connors RH: Short-bowel syndrome in children: Quality of life in an era of improved survival. *Arch Surg* 1991; 126:841–846.

44. Goulet OJ, Revillon Y, Jan D, et al: Neonatal short-bowel syndrome. *J Pediatr* 1991; 119:18–23.

45. Hartman GE, Drugas GT, Shochat SJ: Post-necrotizing enterocolitis strictures present with sepsis or perforation: Risk of clinical observation. *J Pediatr Surg* 1988; 23:562–566.

# INDEX